Radiology Noninterpretive Skills

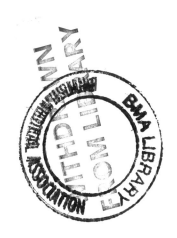

SERIES EDITOR

James H. Thrall, MD
Radiologist-in-Chief Emeritus
Massachusetts General Hospital
Distinguished Juan M. Taveras Professor of Radiology
Harvard Medical School
Boston, Massachusetts

OTHER VOLUMES IN THE REQUISITES RADIOLOGY SERIES

Breast Imaging
Cardiac Imaging
Emergency Imaging
Gastrointestinal Imaging
Genitourinary Imaging
Musculoskeletal Imaging
Neuroradiology Imaging
Nuclear Medicine
Pediatric Imaging
Radiology Noninterpretive Skills
Thoracic Imaging
Ultrasound
Vascular and Interventional Imaging

Radiology Noninterpretive Skills

Hani H. Abujudeh, MD, MBA, FSIR, FACR
Chairman of Radiology
Cooper University Hospital
Cooper Medical School of Rowan University
Camden, New Jersey

Michael A. Bruno, MS, MD, FACR
Professor of Radiology and Medicine
Vice Chair for Quality and Patient Safety
Chief, Division of Emergency Radiology
Penn State Milton S. Hershey Medical Center and Penn State College of Medicine
Hershey, Pennsylvania

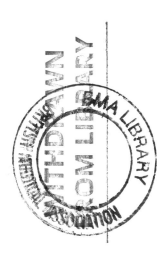

ELSEVIER

ELSEVIER

1600 John F. Kennedy Blvd.
Ste 1800
Philadelphia, PA 19103-2899

RADIOLOGY NONINTERPRETIVE SKILLS: THE REQUISITES   ISBN: 978-0-323-46297-6

Library of Congress Cataloging-in-Publication Data

Names: Abujudeh, Hani H., editor. | Bruno, Michael A., editor.
Title: Radiology noninterpretive skills / [edited by] Hani H. Abujudeh,
    Michael A. Bruno.
Other titles: Requisites series. | Requisites in radiology.
Description: Philadelphia, PA : Elsevier, [2018] | Series: Requisites |
    Series: Requisites in radiology series | Includes bibliographical
    references and index.
Identifiers: LCCN 2017012727 | ISBN 9780323462976 (hardcover : alk. paper)
Subjects: | MESH: Radiologists–standards | Radiography–standards | Quality
    Improvement–standards | Clinical Competence | Quality Assurance, Health
    Care–methods | Patient Safety
Classification: LCC RC78.15 | NLM WN 21 | DDC 616.07/572076–dc23 LC record available at
https://lccn.loc.gov/2017012727

Executive Content Strategist: Robin Carter
Senior Content Development Specialist: Margaret Nelson
Publishing Services Manager: Patricia Tannian
Senior Project Manager: Carrie Stetz
Design Direction: Amy Buxton

Printed in the United States of America

Last digit is the print number: 9 8 7 6 5 4 3 2 1

Working together
to grow libraries in
developing countries

www.elsevier.com • www.bookaid.org

Contributors

Hani H. Abujudeh, MD, MBA, FSIR, FACR
Chairman of Radiology
Cooper University Hospital
Cooper Medical School of Rowan University
Camden, New Jersey

Cory Angelini, BA, MBA
Adjunct Assistant Professor of Lean Six Sigma
Cooper Medical School of Rowan University;
Lean Six Sigma Champion/Senior Director of Operational
    Excellence
Cooper University Health System
Camden, New Jersey

Lindsey Berkowitz, PhD
Imaging Physicist
Department of Radiology
Maine Medical Center
Portland, Maine;
Assistant Professor
Tufts University School of Medicine
Boston, Massachusetts

Bruce Berlanstein, MD, MBA
Vice Chair for Safety and Quality
Radiology
Johns Hopkins Hospital
Baltimore, Maryland

Leonard Berlin, MD, FACR
Radiology Department
Skokie Hospital
Skokie, Illinois;
Professor of Radiology
Rush University and University of Illinois
Chicago, Illinois

Puneet Bhargava, MD, FSAR
Associate Professor
Department of Radiology
University of Washington
Seattle, Washington

Chandni Bhimani, DO
Resident Physician
Department of Radiology
Cooper University Hospital
Cooper Medical School of Rowan University
Camden, New Jersey

C. Craig Blackmore, MD, MPH
Director
Center for Health Care Improvement Science
Virginia Mason Medical Center
Seattle, Washington

Einat Blumfield, MD
Associate Professor
Department of Radiology
Jacobi Medical Center
Albert Einstein College of Medicine
New York, New York

Michael A. Bruno, MD, FACR
Professor of Radiology and Medicine
Vice Chair for Quality and Patient Safety
Chief, Division of Emergency Radiology
Penn State Milton S. Hershey Medical Center and Penn State
    College of Medicine
Hershey, Pennsylvania

Joseph James Cavallo, MD
Chief Resident
Department of Radiology and Biomedical Imaging
Yale School of Medicine
New Haven, Connecticut

Paul Chang, MD
Professor and Vice Chair
Department of Radiology
University of Chicago
Chicago, Illinois

Linda E. Chen, MD
Radiology Resident
Department of Radiology
University of Washington School of Medicine
Seattle, Washington

Paul Cronin, MD, MS
Associate Professor
Department of Radiology
University of Michigan
Ann Arbor, Michigan

Adam Danielson, MD, MPH
Radiology Fellow
Chief Resident of Quality and Safety
Department of Radiology
University of California, San Diego
San Diego, California

Manjiri Dighe, MD
Professor
Department of Radiology
University of Washington
Seattle, Washington

James R. Duncan, MD, PhD
Professor of Radiology
Vice Chair for Quality and Safety
Mallinckrodt Institute of Radiology, Interventional
    Radiology Section
Washington University in St. Louis School of Medicine
St. Louis, Missouri

Jeffrey J. Farrell, MD
Chief Diagnostic and Interventional Radiology Resident
Department of Radiology
University Hospitals
Cleveland, Ohio

Irina S. Filatova, MD
Resident Physician
Department of Radiology
Penn State Milton S. Hershey Medical Center
Hershey, Pennsylvania

Howard Paul Forman, MD, MBA
Professor
Department of Radiology and Biomedical Imaging
Yale School of Medicine
New Haven, Connecticut

Joseph Fotos, MD
Assistant Professor
Department of Radiology
Penn State Milton S. Hershey Medical Center
Hershey, Pennsylvania

Ron Gefen, MD
Assistant Professor
Department of Radiology
Cooper University Hospital
Cooper Medical School of Rowan University
Camden, New Jersey

Andrew J. Gunn, MD
Assistant Professor of Radiology
Department of Radiology
Division of Vascular and Interventional Radiology
University of Alabama at Birmingham
Birmingham, Alabama

Matthew T. Heller, MD, FSAR
Associate Professor of Radiology
Abdominal Imaging
Director, Radiology Residency Program
University of Pittsburgh School of Medicine and Medical Center
Pittsburgh, Pennsylvania

Christopher S. Hollenbeak, PhD
Professor
Departments of Surgery and Public Health Sciences
Penn State College of Medicine
Hershey, Pennsylvania

Jason N. Itri, MD, PhD
Assistant Professor
Department of Radiology
University of Virginia
Charlottesville, Virginia

Ramesh S. Iyer, MD
Associate Professor
Department of Radiology
Seattle Children's Hospital
Seattle, Washington

Saurabh Jha, MD
Associate Professor of Radiology
Hospital of the University of Pennsylvania
Philadelphia, Pennsylvania

Nadja Kadom, MD
Associate Professor
Department of Radiology and Imaging Sciences
Emory University School of Medicine
Atlanta, Georgia

Mannudeep K. Kalra, MD
Radiologist
Division of Thoracic and Cardiac Imaging
Massachusetts General Hospital;
Associate Professor
Harvard Medical School
Boston, Massachusetts

Aine M. Kelly, MD, MS, MA
Professor
Department of Radiology
University of Michigan
Ann Arbor, Michigan

Christos Kosmas, MD
Assistant Professor
Department of Radiology
University Hospitals/Case Western Reserve University
Cleveland, Ohio

James E. Kovacs, DO
Head, Division of Body Imaging
Department of Radiology
Cooper University Hospital
Cooper Medical School of Rowan University
Camden, New Jersey

Jonathan Larson, MD
Clinical Instructor
Department of Radiology
Tufts Medical Center
Tufts University School of Medicine
Boston, Massachusetts

Frank J. Lexa, MD, MBA
Adjunct Professor of Marketing
Project Faculty
Spain and East Asia Regional Manager
Global Consulting Practicum
The Wharton School
University of Pennsylvania
Philadelphia, Pennsylvania;
Chief Medical Officer
The Radiology Leadership Institute;
Chair, Commission on Leadership and Practice
    Development
American College of Radiology

Behrang Litkouhi, MD
Attending Radiologist
Radiology and Outpatient Diagnostic Testing
Cooper University Hospital
Cooper Medical School of Rowan University
Camden, New Jersey

Neel Madan, MD, BSc
Assistant Professor of Radiology and Pediatrics
Department of Radiology
Tufts Medical Center
Tufts University School of Medicine
Boston, Massachusetts

Mohammad Mansouri, MD, MPH
Postdoctoral Research Fellow
Radiology
Massachusetts General Hospital
Boston, Massachusetts

Zachary Masi, MD
Resident, Diagnostic Radiology
Cooper University Hospital
Camden, New Jersey

Anika L. McGrath, MD
Resident Physician
Department of Radiology
University of Washington School of Medicine
Seattle, Washington

Jared Meshekow, MD, MPH
Chief Radiology Resident
Department of Radiology
Cooper University Hospital
MD Anderson at Cooper
Camden, New Jersey

David C. Mihal, MD
Resident and Clinical Instructor
University of Cincinnati Medical Center
Cincinnati, Ohio

Jeff M. Moirano, MS, DABR
Medical Physicist
Department of Radiology
University of Washington
Seattle, Washington

Michael M. Moore, MD
Associate Professor of Radiology and Pediatrics
Department of Radiology
Penn State Health–Children's Hospital
Hershey, Pennsylvania

Elena Motuzko, MD
Clinical Instructor
Cooper Medical School of Rowan University;
Chief Resident
Department of Diagnostic Radiology
Cooper University Hospital
Camden, New Jersey

John P. Nazarian, MD
Neuroradiology Fellow
Mallinckrodt Institute of Radiology
Washington University in St. Louis School of Medicine
St. Louis, Missouri

Ryan B. O'Malley, MD
Assistant Professor
Department of Radiology
University of Washington Medical Center
Seattle, Washington

Alexi Otrakji, MD
Department of Radiology
Massachusetts General Hospital
Boston, Massachusetts

Atul M. Padole, MD
Research Fellow
Department of Radiology
Massachusetts General Hospital
Harvard Medical School
Boston, Massachusetts

Tarun Pandey, MD, FRCR
Associate Professor of Radiology
University of Arkansas for Medical Sciences
Little Rock, Arkansas

David M. Paushter, MD
Professor and Chair
Department of Radiology
University of Chicago
Chicago, Illinois

Prabhakar Rajiah, MD
Associate Professor of Radiology, Cardiothoracic Imaging
Associate Director of Cardiac CT and MRI
Department of Radiology
University of Texas Southwestern Medical Center
Dallas, Texas

Dushyant Sahani, MD
Associate Professor of Radiology
Department of Radiology
Massachusetts General Hospital
Boston, Massachusetts

Khalid W. Shaqdan, MD
Postdoctoral Research Fellow
Department of Radiology
Massachusetts General Hospital
Boston, Massachusetts

Steven Tandberg, MD
Assistant Professor of Radiology
Department of Radiology
University of New Mexico
Albuquerque, New Mexico

Eric A. Walker, MD, MHA, FACR
Associate Professor
Department of Radiology
Penn State Milton S. Hershey Medical Center
Hershey, Pennsylvania;
Uniformed Services University of the Health Sciences
Bethesda, Maryland

Michael R. Williamson, MD
Professor of Radiology
Department of Radiology
University of New Mexico
Albuquerque, New Mexico

Franz J. Wippold II, MD
Mallinckrodt Institute of Radiology
Washington University in St. Louis School of Medicine
St. Louis, Missouri

Foreword

Radiology Noninterpretive Skills is a new and unique addition to *THE REQUISITES* series. The motivation behind adding this book is straightforward—in the era of health care reform, the circumstances surrounding the practice of medicine and radiology have become steadily more complex. There are higher expectations on the part of all stakeholders with respect to the patient experience; provider compliance with innumerable new rules, regulations, and laws; and objective demonstration of improved quality and safety. Moreover, new payment systems for physicians now include the need to meet quality and service metrics and the need to comply with other new measures that are often tangential to the delivery of medical care. *Radiology Noninterpretive Skills: THE REQUISITES* brings together a discussion of these diverse topics that will increasingly affect the success and professional satisfaction of physicians in the future and that are crucial to achieving patient satisfaction.

Physicians engaged in every medical specialty face the similar need to acquire an array of noninterpretive skills and learn how to use them efficiently to meet new compliance requirements and other expectations of health reform. This new addition to the series, edited by Drs. Hani Abujudeh and Michael Bruno, brings together a stellar group of contributors with extraordinary experience and expertise. They discuss key topics related to quality and safety, interactions with patients, practice management, and practice improvement among many other topics that face radiologists in training and active radiology practitioners every day. No other book brings these topics together in a single place for the radiologist.

Radiology Noninterpretive Skills will serve as both an educational tool and reference resource. The first section, entitled "Quality, Safety, and Process Improvement," introduces these topics. In Section III, these topics are again addressed in more detail relative to the special issues that arise in subspecialty areas of radiology and with the different imaging modalities. For example, no topic in the quality and safety arena has had more publicity than radiation exposure in computed tomography. Every radiologist would be well served to know more about this issue—how to discuss it and put it into perspective for patients, how to optimize radiation doses, and how to maintain appropriate records. There is an entire chapter devoted to this topic.

For the resident in radiology, Section II is especially important. This section provides several chapters with the basic information necessary to meet Accreditation Council on Graduate Medical Education (ACGME) educational requirements. Beyond acquiring the necessary medical knowledge, the ACGME specifically requires training in Practice-Based Learning, Professionalism, Interpersonal and Communications Skills, and Systems-Based Practice. These topics are all covered and placed into the context of what radiologists encounter in the real world along with additional topics required to run a successful practice.

Section IV provides chapters on several topics that are outside the ACGME curriculum for radiology trainees. These topics—malpractice, leadership, social media, and ACR Guidelines and Criteria—are of great interest and are discussed in a radiology-specific context.

As with other books in *THE REQUISITES* series, this text is designed to be efficient for the reader. It is manageable in length, and topics are discussed in practical terms without unnecessary material that is too often included in textbooks for the sake of "completeness."

Having a strong working knowledge about the noninterpretive aspects of radiology and, more broadly, about the practice of medicine in general, is a fundamental necessity to meet current educational and compliance requirements and stakeholder expectations. Furthermore, being conversant with these skills will become an increasingly important key to career success and to establishing a successful practice. Drs. Abujudeh and Bruno are to be congratulated for carefully choosing the content of their book and for bringing together an outstanding group of contributors who have the expertise and experience necessary to address the issues effectively. I am confident that readers of *Radiology Noninterpretive Skills: THE REQUISITES* will find substantial value in this book.

James H. Thrall, MD
Radiologist-in-Chief Emeritus
Department of Radiology
Massachusetts General Hospital
Distinguished Taveras Professor of Radiology
Harvard Medical School
Boston, Massachusetts

Preface

We are very pleased to present this new volume, *Radiology Noninterpretive Skills: THE REQUISITES*, an entirely new radiology textbook designed to provide a comprehensive tutorial and reference for the unusually broad and diverse range of topics that comprise the American Board of Radiology's Noninterpretive Skills Domain. This volume contains 30 chapters written by leading experts and thought leaders that summarize the current state of knowledge in their areas of expertise. These chapters also include some forward-looking special topics, such as change management and leadership, malpractice litigation, and the evolving world of social media and internet applications in radiology. We believe these topics are particularly relevant to the rapidly changing healthcare environment in which we now practice.

The many topics in the Noninterpretive Skills Domain are indeed diverse, and their number and range continue to grow and evolve. They include quality and safety in all of its many aspects, professionalism and ethics, informatics, organizational leadership, payment models, guidelines for evidence-based utilization of imaging, imaging appropriateness and clinical decision support, the use of social media and internet applications, coding/billing and accounting, medicolegal issues, and statistical methods for quantitative reasoning, among others. Because of the wide range of topics covered, we have organized this material into four major sections: Quality, Safety, and Process Improvement (9 chapters); Core Concepts in Radiology Noninterpretive Skills (9 chapters); Practice-Specific and Subspecialty Topics (8 chapters); and Special Topics (4 chapters).

Although this new textbook is designed to be particularly useful for candidates preparing for the American Board of Radiology's core, certification, and MOC examinations, we also hope to provide all readers with a solid base on these topics from which to grow their own personal knowledge and expertise as this area continues to evolve across many disciplines, not just radiology. In fact, much of the included material has been drawn from other disciplines, including manufacturing, aviation, mathematics, finance, and law. For those preparing for the ABR examinations, we also recommend the companion volume *Noninterpretive Skills for Radiology: Case Review Series,* published by Elsevier in 2016, edited by Dr. David M. Yousem and coauthored by the many trainees of the Johns Hopkins Department of Radiology. This separate title includes more than 600 practice questions for exam review and supplements this textbook.

This is the second radiology textbook we have had the privilege of writing and editing together; we have once again been extremely fortunate to have received the help of a truly outstanding group of volunteer chapter contributors. Our friends and distinguish colleagues have generously given their time, energy, perspectives, expertise, and outstanding depth of knowledge to this yearlong project. We are also grateful for the unflagging support of series editor Dr. James H. Thrall and our expert team at Elsevier. We welcome the feedback of our readers.

Hani H. Abujudeh, MD, MBA, FSIR, FACR
Michael A. Bruno, MS, MD, FACR

About the Authors

Hani H. Abujudeh, MD, MBA, FSIR, FACR

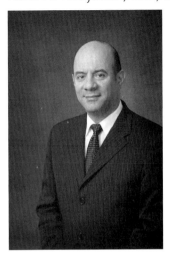

Dr. Abujudeh is Professor and Chairman of the Department of Radiology at the Cooper University Hospital of Rowan University in Camden, New Jersey. He previously served as Associate Professor of Radiology and Director for Quality and Safety at the Massachusetts General Hospital and Harvard Medical School. He was elected to Phi Beta Kappa at Rutgers University and is a 1995 graduate of the New Jersey Medical School UMDNJ. He completed his residency in Diagnostic Radiology in 2001 also at the New Jersey Medical School UMDNJ, as well as a residency in Nuclear Medicine at New York Medical College/St. Vincent's Hospital in 1997 and a fellowship in Interventional Radiology at the Weil Cornell Sloan Kettering Cancer Center in New York in 2002. He earned his MBA from the Columbia University Business School in 2004, prior to joining the Harvard faculty in that same year. He became a fellow of the Society of Interventional Radiology in 2013 and was elected to fellowship of the American College of Radiology in 2015. He has received numerous accolades and awards for his research and teaching.

Dr. Abujudeh is the author of three prior textbooks: *Cases in Radiology: Emergency Radiology Cases,* published in 2014; *Emergency Radiology (Rotations in Radiology),* published in 2016; and *Quality and Safety in Radiology*, published in 2012 and coauthored with Dr. Bruno. He served as an editor for the *Journal of Emergency Radiology.* He chairs the ACR RadPeer Committee and the RSNA Policy and Practice Committee, along with the International Relations Committee of the American Society of Emergency Radiology (ASER), and currently serves as the MOC Committee Chair of the American Society of Emergency Radiology. He previously served on the ABR Core Exam Quality and Safety Committee.

Dr. Abujudeh has authored or coauthored more than 100 articles in peer-reviewed medical journals as well as more than 160 book chapters, case reports, clinical guidelines and practice parameters, commentaries, and reviews. He is a frequent speaker on radiology quality and safety and emergency radiology imaging topics throughout the United States and internationally.

Dr. Abujudeh and Dr. Bruno have also together presented numerous formal continuing medical education courses on radiology quality and safety, practice management, process improvement, and other noninterpretive skills topics at national radiology meetings, including the ARRS Annual Meeting, the ACR Annual Meeting, and the Association of University Radiologists (AUR) Annual Meeting.

Michael A. Bruno, MS, MD, FACR

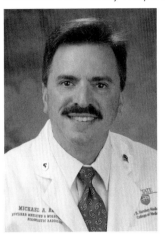

Dr. Bruno is Professor of Radiology and Medicine, Vice Chair for Quality and Patient Safety, and Chief of the Division of Emergency Radiology for the Department of Radiology at the Penn State Milton S. Hershey Medical Center in Hershey, Pennsylvania. He is a 1982 graduate of The Johns Hopkins University and the University of California, Irvine School of Medicine, where he earned his medical degree, along with a Master of Science in Biophysics, in 1987. He completed his residency in Diagnostic Radiology at UC Irvine in 1992 and a Fellowship in Nuclear Radiology at Vanderbilt University in 1996. Dr. Bruno is certified in Diagnostic Radiology (1992) with Special Competence in Nuclear Radiology (1997). He became a Fellow of the American College of Radiology in 2012.

Dr. Bruno is the coauthor of two prior textbooks: *Quality and Safety In Radiology*, published in 2012 and coauthored with Dr. Abujudeh, and *Arthritis In Color*, published in 2009. He chairs the ACR Emergency Radiology Committee and currently serves on the ACR Commission for the Patient and Family Experience as well as the ACR Commission for General, Emergency, and Small/Rural Practice, the ACR RadPeer Committee, the e-learning committee of the American Roentgen Ray Society, and the Research Committee of the Society to Improve Diagnosis in Medicine. He formerly chaired the ABR Core Exam Committee for Quality & Safety and served as a member of the Distinguished Roster of Scientific Advisors for the RSNA Research & Education Foundation, the Committee on Policy & Practice of the RSNA, and the ACR Expert Panel on Musculoskeletal Imaging as well as the Editorial Advisory Panel for the *American Journal of Roentgenology.*

He has authored or coauthored more than 40 articles in peer-reviewed medical journals as well as numerous clinical guidelines and practice parameters, book chapters, commentaries, and reviews and is a frequent speaker on radiology quality and safety and musculoskeletal imaging topics throughout the United States and internationally. Dr. Bruno has been recognized with numerous awards for teaching, clinical service, and academic excellence over the span of his career. His work has been featured in the *ACR Bulletin*, the ARRS *In Practice* magazine, *Diagnostic Imaging* magazine, *Inside Medical Liability,* and *The Wall Street Journal.* Dr. Bruno and Dr. Abujudeh have also together presented several formal continuing medical education courses for practicing radiologists on radiology quality and safety, practice improvement, and other noninterpretive skills topics in recent years at national radiology meetings, including the ARRS, the ACR, and the Association of University Radiologists (AUR).

Contents

SECTION I

Quality, Safety, and Process Improvement

Chapter 1

History and Current Status of Quality Improvement in Radiology

Joseph James Cavallo and Howard Paul Forman

TO ERR IS HUMAN

When the Institute of Medicine (IOM, now the Academy of Medicine) first released its report, *To Err Is Human*, in 1999, headlines were made throughout the world. The notion that our healthcare delivery system was not only *not* achieving the positive exceptionalism that one might expect from the most expensive system in the world, but also guilty of contributing to the demise of nearly 100,000 people each year, was more than unsettling. The report was widely credited for blowing the whistle on an immense problem with our healthcare system. Many knew of these errors few had an idea of the scope, but all wanted to reduce them. Improvement would never come about if the collective knowledge of medical errors was sequestered to the confines of morbidity and mortality talks, hospital board rooms, and isolated court cases. The report better defined the magnitude of the issue and ultimately helped to bring about a change in attitude; this was a monumental problem, and a difficult one, that required candid discussion, accurate quantification, effective collaboration, and measureable solutions.

After the whistle was blown, 2 years later the IOM released a second report, *Crossing the Quality Chasm*. With this, the IOM threw down the gauntlet, challenging the leadership of US healthcare delivery to make good on its promises. The report issued six aims for improvement:

1. Healthcare must be safe.
2. Healthcare must be effective.
3. Healthcare must be patient centered.
4. Healthcare must be timely.
5. Healthcare must be efficient.
6. Healthcare must be equitable.

Realizing the magnitude of the systemic dysfunction and the enormity of the task that healthcare faced, the IOM rightfully made no attempt to specify a plan for improvement. Rather, they set forth 10 rules for redesign, looking to establish a framework within which individuals and entities would be free to innovate their own solutions. Although all 10 of these rules are important, we feel there are a few that should be stressed as paramount principles considered when undertaking quality improvement initiatives:

- It must be patient centered.
- Free exchange of patient information and knowledge (including errors) is a necessity.
- Safety should focus on systems rather than individuals.
- Transparency must exist for patients (and clinicians).
- Waste should be continually decreased.

Together, the IOM reports successfully kick-started a culture of patient safety. It is a culture that has begun to permeate the halls of all healthcare institutions, public and private, as the field seeks to achieve these aims. Quality improvement initiatives have been undertaken and published with increasing frequency. *To Err Is Human* has served as the de facto benchmark against which progress can be measured. How is the healthcare sector doing? Results are mixed to say the least. There are published accounts of meaningful progress but often at a brutally slow pace. Some suggest that problems are worsening. Others, such as the Consumers Union Safe Patient Project 10-year review of the industry response to the IOM reports are not shy in giving the healthcare response a failing grade.

How can this be? Although some problems appear to be worsening, it is logical to conclude that some of this can be attributed to better recognition, measurement, and reporting of the issues at hand, something that should be taken as a positive and worthy step on the road to better healthcare. The number of and use of incident report systems have grown, in large part secondary to the Joint Commission requiring their use by hospitals. Despite this, (1) accurate and well-defined measurement,

(2) standardization of data, and (3) proper implementation of this data-driven improvement continue to be an issue for a multitude of reasons. These include underreporting, lack of accepted standards, fragmentation of systems, and the inherent variability among different patient populations and care settings. There is increasing need to identify data that actually affect patient outcomes, and, of course, balance quality data with the cost and time required to collect it. In the continued efforts for improvement, healthcare has begun to embrace the practice of high-reliability organizations (HROs), learning from multiple other industries. The application of this concept to healthcare has been summarized based on three main tenets: (1) strong and committed leadership at all levels, (2) an institution-wide culture of safety, and (3) a methodical identification of root problems allowing for robust process improvement.

Better quantification of errors and their prevention in the delivery of care are only part of the problem. Some patients are directly or indirectly harmed before any attempt at treatment is even made. The need for improvements in patient diagnosis, of particular interest to the field of radiology, was recently examined in a 2015 IOM publication, *Improving Diagnosis in Health Care*. It is currently estimated that on a yearly basis, 5% of adults seeking outpatient care are improperly diagnosed. This harms the patient and adds cost to the system in the form of wasted resources. Much like *To Err Is Human*, perhaps this will serve as another much-needed benchmark for improvement.

RADIOLOGY'S PREEMPTIVE WORK IN QUALITY IMPROVEMENT

To Err Is Human was a major wakeup call to medicine. It was a necessary call to attention to the fact that physicians and other care providers, no matter how skilled or competent, do not operate in a bubble. Despite their best intentions, care providers were still at risk of causing substantial harm, even if it was mainly secondary to systemic problems. Healthcare workers needed to be aware of the care settings, systems, and governing policies that were a part of their daily clinical duties and how each of these impacts the quality of care they were delivering. As such, many of the principles written about in *To Err Is Human* and *Crossing the Quality Chasm* could and would parallel the extradiagnostic aspects of radiology that are important today. That being said, the field of radiology was not oblivious to the issues at hand in 1999.

Just prior to the publication of *To Err Is Human*, through the leadership of Philip Alderson, noninterpretive skills for radiologists—in particular residents—was getting attention. He rightfully questioned the growing gap between a radiologist's adequate interpretation skills and a lack of understanding of one's place within the general healthcare delivery system. This was recognized in 1997 by the Association of Program Directors in Radiology (APDR), which later collaborated with the American College of Radiology (ACR) to produce a curriculum of noninterpretive skills that was further publicized by the *American Journal of Radiology* (AJR).

Much of this series focused on aspects of radiology care delivery that correlated with the IOM's call for a more effective and patient-centered approach to healthcare. In particular, there was an in-depth look at the ACR's efforts to create practice standards, accreditation of subspecialty programs, and the appropriateness criteria for imaging that had already been instituted. These published standards provided radiologists and other care providers with practice guidelines that, if followed, would increase the quality of care provided by radiologists. Accreditation programs, the first being the program in radiation oncology in 1966, ensured that techniques or practices underwent an evidence-based formal review process to ensure that specific quality standards were met. The widely recognized success of the mammography accreditation program, established in 1985 in response to disparities in mammography quality, led to measurable improvements in the quality of mammography throughout the United States and was eventually adopted by the US Food and Drug Administration (FDA). The ACR Appropriateness Criteria, introduced in 1993 and continually refined, defined evidence-based best use standards for selection of imaging exams or therapeutic processes for specific clinical conditions. This not only allowed radiologists and medical clinicians to deliver the most appropriate and effective care to each patient, but also preempted yet-to-be implemented future developments in healthcare that would require valid justification for and evidence supporting tests ordered prior to payment.

Around the same time that the IOM was releasing these pivotal reports, the American Board of Radiology (ABR) also recognized the importance of noninterpretive skills in the education and competence of our workforce. Today, the Diagnostic Radiology Boards include examination in noninterpretive skills, as does the Maintenance of Certification (MOC) Program. Recently, the number of ways to fulfill this requirement has greatly expanded, giving radiologists more flexibility and allowing for more creativity in fulfilling the required competencies in practice quality improvements. The ABR has maintained a syllabus, the Noninterpretive Skills Domain Specification and Resource Guide, which is available online and continually updated. The syllabus directly addresses the IOM aims for quality care and embraces the 10 guidelines for healthcare redesign. It provides valuable information for today's radiologist and serves as a framework within which to examine efforts made by the field over the past 2 decades in addressing the IOM aims. The syllabus is divided into six sections, each of which receives a brief overview in the following pages and helps introduce some of the concepts that will be evaluated in this text. Despite the value and wealth of information provided by the syllabus, it is by no means a comprehensive work; it is the intention of this book to fill in the gaps and further develop these important aspects of radiology.

Part I: General Quality Improvement

The complexity of healthcare demands a continuous effort of all involved parties to achieve meaningful quality *improvement*. The unremitting nature of improvement can be contrasted with the more traditional, and much more static notion of quality assurance, in which the goal is merely compliance with predefined standards. There are multiple approaches to quality improvement. One of the most recognized is the Plan-Do-Study-Act (PDSA) cycle, which by its very name implies continuous improvement efforts. It embraces the isolation of and quantification of a specific problem, targeted interventions, and measurable outcomes. "Lean" process improvement focuses on elimination of waste and an institution-wide culture of mutual trust and continual improvement. Failure mode and effect analysis can be used to proactively assess complex processes for possible errors. Innumerable other methodologies exist and can be used to complement one another. Specific quality improvement tools that can be applied to any of these methods include establishing key performance indicators, value stream maps, cause-and-effect diagrams, time series plots, Pareto charts, prioritization matrices, and simulation walk-throughs.

Regardless of the methods and tools used, there are key components in all successful quality improvement projects. A specific opportunity for improvement should be identified. A qualified and inclusive team should be assembled. A clear aim statement should define specific goals of the project. Appropriate measures and benchmarks should be selected. Objective data sources should be identified and appropriately collected, including baseline values. Thorough process analysis should be performed to obtain a complete understanding of specific problems that are obstacles to improvement. A project plan should be constructed, implemented, and continuously evaluated. Initially, when doing quality improvement projects, things may appear to get worse before they get better. This situation is probably due to the Hawthorne effect, which is the initial part of the *Abujudeh curve* and results from an increase in awareness and observations (Fig. 1.1). When appropriate, the project should be closed, at which time there is documentation of what was learned, proposals for other areas in which this change could be applicable, and ideas for future exploration.

Part II: Patient Safety

There are a multitude of errors that can result in harm to a patient and they can be grouped into a few categories. Diagnostic errors encompass incorrect or missed diagnoses, failure to select appropriate tests, and outdated studies and therapy. Treatment errors include technical mistakes, administration errors, incorrect dosing, unnecessary delay, and nonindicated care. Preventive errors include lack of indicated prophylactic treatment and inadequate screening or follow-up. Systemic errors include, but are not limited to, breakdowns in the chain of communication, equipment malfunction, and process failure. Recent progress in the field of radiology related to safety will be explored later.

Part III: Professionalism and Ethics

A seminal publication on modern professionalism, titled *Medical Professionalism in the New Millennium: A Physician Charter*, was published in 2002 and was a joint project of multiple medical societies. This charter has been adopted by many medical societies including, in 2005, the Radiological Society of North America (RSNA) Professional Committee. Professional responsibilities in today's complex healthcare climate are too numerous to adequately detail here. However, they are best summarized as the basis of medicine's contract with society. This contract is composed of three fundamental principles: primacy of patient welfare, patient autonomy, and social justice.

More recently, Halpern and Spandorfer sought to better frame professionalism within the context of the radiologist. They expanded on some of the more opaque concepts not fully described, such as the learning, teaching, and evaluation of professionalism. Even more importantly, they brought attention to some of the challenges to professionalism faced by current physicians. Managing conflict of interest has become increasingly significant because healthcare is, without a doubt, big business. The dangers of self-referral are still present, especially for those practicing in independent groups. Teleradiology has furthered the loss of contact between radiologists and clinicians and often driven contracts to the lowest price rather than the highest quality. Efforts to incentivize clinical productivity, without caveat, will apply negative pressure to the important but non–revenue-generating aspects of radiology such as resident education and clinician consultation.

Diagnostic errors occur in radiology that are often not discovered until subsequent examinations. There are currently no guidelines for error disclosure by the major radiologic societies. The idea of personally communicating errors to patients, who almost certainly have never met the radiologist and may even be unaware of his or her role, creates complex situations, not to mention potentially litigious challenges. However, simply ignoring that these errors occurred directly refutes the Physician Charter, potentially eroding patient and societal trust. At least one large-scale case study at the University of Michigan, although not specific to radiology, demonstrated that medical error disclosure programs can be implemented without increasing total claims and liability costs. Equitable allocation of limited resources is yet another ethical challenge for radiology as a profession. As a supplemental source to the information provided in this book, the ACR offers a set of online ethics and professionalism courses for its members, most recently revised in January 2015.

Part IV: Compliance, Regulatory, and Legal Issues

Compliance, regulatory, and legal issues are topics typically neglected by many medical schools and residencies. However, that does not diminish their importance and makes self-education all the more crucial. It is nearly impossible to eliminate diagnostic errors in radiology and the resulting litigation that may arise from them, but there are ways to minimize their occurrence as well as their effects on patients and practices. Not surprisingly, diagnostic errors, the genres of which were discussed previously, are the most common cause of malpractice suits against radiologists. An additional pitfall are lapses in communication with providers and patients. Departments or hospitals should have systems in place to prevent this from occurring. It is important to keep accurate documentation of communication efforts, even so-called curbside consultations. Radiologists often engage in activities that involve direct patient care, and, whenever possible, authorized chaperones should be used during these encounters.

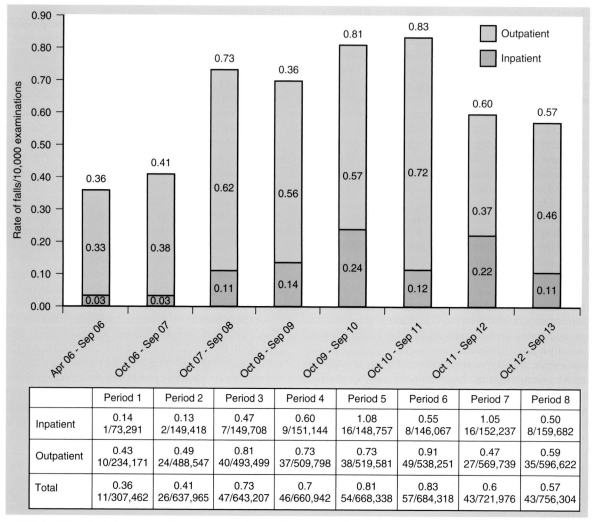

	Period 1	Period 2	Period 3	Period 4	Period 5	Period 6	Period 7	Period 8
Inpatient	0.14 1/73,291	0.13 2/149,418	0.47 7/149,708	0.60 9/151,144	1.08 16/148,757	0.55 8/146,067	1.05 16/152,237	0.50 8/159,682
Outpatient	0.43 10/234,171	0.49 24/488,547	0.81 40/493,499	0.73 37/509,798	0.73 38/519,581	0.91 49/538,251	0.47 27/569,739	0.59 35/596,622
Total	0.36 11/307,462	0.41 26/637,965	0.73 47/643,207	0.7 46/660,942	0.81 54/668,338	0.83 57/684,318	0.6 43/721,976	0.57 43/756,304

FIG. 1.1 The Abujudeh curve refers to a curve observed in some quality improvement projects. A program designed and implemented to decrease the incidence of falls in a radiology department observed the opposite effect, a statistically significant *increase*, rather than decrease, in the reported incidents of falls in radiology. A plateau and then a decrease followed this increase. The initial increase is attributed to the Hawthorne effect. (From Abujudeh HH, Aran S, Daftari Besheli L, Miguel K, Halpern E, Thrall JH. Outpatient falls prevention program outcome: an increase, a plateau, and a decrease in incident reports. *Am J Roentgenol.* 2014;203[3]:620–626.)

While the appropriateness criteria are aimed at improving compliance with best use practices of imaging, there are a multitude of extradiagnostic clinical duties that also warrant standardized conduct. The ACR publishes General Practice Parameters and Technical Standards to provide goals for competency in these areas. The practice parameters offer guidelines on topics including, but not limited to, communication of findings, properly obtaining informed consent, imaging of pregnant patients, patient sedation, and even more unique circumstances such as proper conduct and responsibilities of expert witnesses. The Technical Standards are provided to set necessary levels of performance, mainly regarding equipment specifications. This includes requirements for imaging acquisition equipment as well as diagnostic workstations.

Part V: Research and Screening

Evidence-based medicine, formulated from the reported outcomes of quality research, is the foundation for the proper practice of medicine. With this in mind, it is important for all physicians to understand how appropriate research is conducted and how to properly evaluate new research findings that could impact changes to their practice. The noninterpretive skills domain provides radiologists with a primer on the essentials of research terminology and practice. At a minimum, radiologists should understand the strength of various types of research ranging from cross-sectional studies to randomized controlled trials. Additionally, familiarity with statistical basics such as *P* values, confidence intervals, sensitivity, specificity, odds ratios, and relative risks will allow one to evaluate the presented data beyond what is described in the discussion or conclusion.

Part VI: Imaging Informatics

A 2003 national survey attempted to gauge physician involvement in quality improvement. It concluded that the majority of physicians do not routinely use data to assess their performance and are reluctant to share available data. In many industries, especially those in the technology sector, the concept of quarterly and yearly performance reviews is quickly falling out of favor; medicine should take notice and be a part of this trend. The amount of real-time data at our fingertips is growing exponentially. Electronic medical record (EMR) integration is allowing radiologists to access vast amounts of patient data; arguably, the format, ease of access, and usability of this data are varied, but that is outside the scope of this discussion. Picture archiving and communication systems (PACS) and workflow managers are increasingly robust, offering tools for tracking personal performance, seamless follow-up of interesting or indeterminate cases, and alerts for pathology/surgical reports of previously viewed studies. Peer-review systems can tap into the knowledge and expertise of our colleagues. Radiologists must make it a priority to use all tools at their disposal in an effort to measure and improve personal performance. In the spirit of transparency, practice-wide data, anonymized or not, should also be made available.

As we attempt to harness this data to drive improvement, informatics systems and the information technology personnel who build and manage these systems, will become increasingly important. Making sense of this data will not only drive quality improvement, it can also demonstrate the value and effectiveness of care, an increasingly important metric as payment models continue to evolve. Informatics systems can be harnessed by radiologists to track exam appropriateness, patient wait times, timely result communication, and patient safety to name just a few such metrics. It can also be used to evaluate the ordering patterns of clinicians. By identifying trends pertaining to inappropriately ordered exams or nonindicated imaging studies, the radiologist can help better direct hospital initiatives on clinician imaging education, providing value to patients and their referring caregivers, while having the added benefit of saving money.

RADIOLOGY CROSSES THE QUALITY CHASM

Patient Safety

Patient safety is of paramount importance and is likely the reason it topped the IOM's list of aims for improvement. Radiology is somewhat unique in the practice of medicine, considering that many of our tools may add some degree of risk for patient harm. Adverse radiation effects were first reported within a year of the discovery of x-rays and the concept of "as low as reasonably achievable" (ALARA) can be traced back to 1977. Radiology has made great strides over the past decades in making diagnostic imaging and therapeutic procedures safer for the patient. In 2006, the Society for Pediatric Radiology formed a committee that ultimately led to the Alliance for Radiation Safety in Pediatric Imaging. At its inception, this alliance focused on decreasing computed tomography (CT) utilization and dose reduction. Coinciding nicely with the efforts of the Alliance, the rate of CT use in the pediatric population, which had increased two- to threefold from 1996 to 2005, stabilized from 2006 to 2007 and began to decline thereafter. As the campaign matured, it extended its efforts to other areas of radiology. The dedicated Pause and Pulse campaign in fluoroscopy and the Step Lightly campaign in interventional radiology followed soon thereafter.

Not wanting to limit these efforts to children, in 2009 the ACR and the RSNA established the Joint Task Force on Adult Radiation Protection; this ultimately created the Image Wisely campaign for adult radiation protection. In addition to eliminating unnecessary exams, future goals of this campaign aim to create a stronger link between optimization of radiation dose and accreditation, increase participation in a national dose registry, and allow providers to compare radiation doses with national benchmarks.

Many tools are provided to educate radiologists on dose reduction techniques, which are unfortunately often left for medical physicists and technologists to manage. The *Journal of the American College of Radiology* maintains a dose optimization website that serves as an educational repository for radiologists at all levels. Institution-specific dose reduction workshops comprised of multidisciplinary teams have been demonstrated to be effective tools for evaluation and improvement of imaging protocols and increasing the staff's dose reduction knowledge. Additionally, the comprehensive clinical knowledge of radiologists, when combined with specific provider questions, provides a unique opportunity to add further value by customizing protocols to reduce dosage on a patient-by-patient basis.

Advances in ultrasound have improved image quality and expanded its indications for use, including some that are now commonly independent of the radiologist. Drawbacks remain, especially its operator-dependent nature. However, as a nonionizing imaging modality, it should be further embraced moving forward. There has been a strong push toward first-line ultrasound imaging in many aspects of pediatric radiology, especially in the case of the Safe and Sound campaign concerning appendicitis. Focused assessment with sonography in trauma (FAST) examinations, when properly implemented, have been shown to decrease the use of abdominal CTs in the trauma setting. Factor in the cost savings and portability of ultrasound, and it is not hard to imagine an increasingly important role for this imaging modality in the future.

Obstacles to patient safety in radiology go beyond radiation risk. The use of contrast media in radiology, while often a necessary part of diagnosis, introduces risks to patient health ranging from potentially fatal allergic-like reactions to kidney damage. In an effort to standardize contrast practices and provide the safest care possible, the ACR publishes the *ACR Manual on Contrast Media*, most recently released in 2016 (Version 10.2). This manual provides evidence-based guidelines for the appropriate use of contrast, prevention and management of adverse events secondary to contrast administration, and management of allergic-like contrast reactions. Additionally, some institutions have demonstrated that high-fidelity simulation training is an effective tool to educate radiologists on the proper management of these rare, but sometimes life-threatening, circumstances.

Although safety is centered on the patient, it should not and cannot be blind to the staff and environment responsible for delivering care. Magnetic resonance imaging (MRI) suites, in particular, introduce risk to staff and patients that must be appropriately managed. With the increased use of MRI, and perhaps coupled with an unevenly weighted focus on CT radiation safety, the FDA reported MRI adverse events increased steadily in the 2000s. Proper education of MRI personnel and appropriate planning of an MRI facility layout remain important. Increased awareness and future progress in reducing the number of these events are certainly areas of future need in radiology, especially as the use of, and indications for, MRI increase. Recent efforts by the ACR Magnetic Resonance Safety Subcommittee have established standardized terminology for the magnetic resonance (MR) industry to help decrease confusion surrounding safety tests.

Effectiveness and Efficiency

Effective care is quality care. Many tools are available to aid radiologists in their pursuit of maximal effectiveness. This starts with selecting the appropriate exam. The ACR appropriateness criteria, although not comprehensive, is an excellent source for clinicians and radiologists alike to select the most effective exam for the clinical question. Even once clinician selection of imaging studies is optimized, there is considerable variation in the performance of such studies (use of oral and/or intravenous contrast, sequences, presentation of images for interpretation, etc.). It would be impossible to imagine complete standardization across our nation now, but there is a great opportunity to validate best practices and promote their wide diffusion.

Contemporaneous interpretation of urgent and emergent studies has been an active area of investigation. Some of the largest research efforts on this topic have focused on academic (training program) practices. They have demonstrated that resident interpretation error rates are low and have minimal adverse effects on patient care. Expectedly, resident performance increases with experience. Full attending coverage allows for more inexperienced (postgraduate years 2 and 3) residents to actively participate in and benefit from the educational experiences of the call pool. Literature review supports the ability of residents, especially more senior residents, to provide accurate reports with discrepancy rates equal to that of attending radiologists. However, from a statistical standpoint, it is difficult to accurately represent the small subset of difficult cases within these large cohorts where having an attending or subspecialized read *could* make a difference in management. If, as a field, we are indeed striving for the highest possible quality of patient care, we must closely evaluate the currently time-dependent availability of attending-level and subspecialty interpretations.

Standardization is another important aspect of effective and efficient care. The acceptance of PACS and Digital Imaging and Communications in Medicine (DICOM) standards, coupled with their widespread adoption, allowed for the seamless exchange and evaluation of images from which we benefit today, something that is conspicuously absent from the current status of fragmented and isolated general EMRs. Throughout healthcare, the adoption and use of published standards for diagnostic interpretation have become commonplace, helping patients and consulting clinicians by diminishing the impact of variability among radiologists. This situation is a result of various ACR Reporting and Data Systems (RADS) developed by the radiology community and accepted as reliable diagnostic tools for oncology of breast, liver, lung, and prostate. Additional systems are in development, including some systems outside of oncology, such as head imaging in traumatic brain

injuries. There has been a justifiable push to reduce the huge variation in reporting through standardization and templates. In addition to simplification for clinicians, potential advantages include easier data mining for research, quality improvement, and other analyses. Structured reports could support compliance with accepted guidelines. The RSNA radiology reporting initiative maintains a library of suggested reporting templates for those looking to institute structured reporting in their practice.

Patient Centeredness

So much of what we do in radiology, and medicine in general, is done with the physician rather than the patient in mind. Measured outcomes are centered too often around the hospital or physician, when more focus is needed on the patient. Outcomes based on the overall patient experience with care, including how their care, or lack thereof, has impacted their quality of life or ability to deal with a chronic condition, need to be given proper weight. As healthcare becomes increasingly data driven, it is important to establish and incorporate outcome measures that prioritize the patient. To address this, the Patient Protection and Affordable Care Act (PPACA) included a provision to establish the Patient-Centered Outcomes Research Institute (PCORI). This organization's goal is to develop and fund research that places the patient's voice at the center of healthcare assessment. Radiologists need to be active in this movement because the outcomes determined as a result of this research will undoubtedly have implications for future standards and reimbursement. The PCORI, which will have funding totaling $3.5 billion by 2019, is currently funding only a small amount of research that centers on imaging. Given the central role that imaging plays in modern healthcare, this presents a huge opportunity for the radiology community to participate in and direct research shaping future patient care. Potential foci of research are limited only by the innovation within our field. For those seeking inspiration, Zygmont et al. offer a thorough review of opportunities currently unexplored.

Research aside, it is easy to think of instances in the everyday practice of radiology where the patient experience can be improved. Oral contrast is an easy example, given its unsettling taste and the added wait time it introduces; it should be used only when necessary. Abundant evidence suggests that we, collectively, could use it much less. The timing of inpatient exams can be disruptive to the patient schedule. Hospitals often fit these studies in where possible, regardless of patient interruption, often in the middle of the night.

Patients now have access to their radiology reports, sometimes even before their clinician has reviewed it. There is enormous variability in the transmission medium of reports, time interval to access, and the party responsible for disclosing information. Additionally, these reports are still predominantly written to address only the clinician. Perhaps radiologists can add value with patient-directed reports or even, when appropriate, an additional section following the traditional impression. This could be tailored to patients with simple, rather than technical, language that helps them understand the significance of their imaging results. Patients have also expressed strong preferences for being able to view their actual images upon receiving their report. Perhaps key images can be attached to reports for further explanation, satisfying patient curiosity with ease and succinctness.

Finally, personal encounters with patients, even if for just a few minutes, have been reported to increase patient understanding of the radiologist's role in care and improve the overall patient care experience. These practices, and others yet to be explored, should be increasingly incorporated to our practices to improve patient experience and alleviate the anxiety that can often be associated with medical imaging.

Timeliness

Achieving temporal balance within a radiology department can be a challenging task as the time requirements of different studies can vary widely from emergent traumas to outpatient studies. Despite this, meeting appropriately selected turnaround times is important to our patients, our colleagues ordering exams, and even the department when one considers reimbursement implications. At academic institutions, turnaround times can create barriers to education. Time requirements, although beneficial for patient care, have been suggested to have negative effects on resident caseload and the amount and quality of faculty teaching provided.

With regard to the Emergency Department (ED) setting, in house ED-dedicated staff radiologists have been shown to decrease turnaround time. The ED can be a stressful environment and may require creative solutions to keep things moving smoothly. Nonphysician providers, including radiology assistants (RAs), can be employed to increase efficiency, quality, and timeliness within a radiology department. Unlike their nurse practitioner and physician assistant counterparts, RAs are not yet recognized as billable providers. However, they can still perform basic procedures and release trainees from repetitive tasks with little educational value. Additionally, more innovative uses for RAs should be explored, and their utility and value will ultimately be limited only by the creativity of the radiology administrators employing them.

Turnaround time is generally less of an issue in the outpatient setting. However, multiple instances exist where more rapid report generation is necessary, and departments should have systems in place to identify these appropriately. For example, in an effort to save patients from multiple care visits, patients may get their imaging performed the same day they have clinician visits. Although in theory this offers convenience, it can be less efficient if the patient gets to the clinician visit and a radiologist has yet to look at the study. Clear communication between ordering clinicians, schedulers, and reporting radiologists is needed to avert scenarios like this. It is also important to ensure adequate staffing so that efforts to improve turnaround time do not adversely affect report accuracy or quality.

Quality improvement can prove a helpful tool in the on-time performance of a radiology department. This can result in improved patient satisfaction due to decreased waiting time and can improve a department's bottom line through increased overall imaging utilization and throughput. An excellent example of this was recently published by Pianykh and Rosenthal. As expected, data and data collection are of paramount importance. They used a total of 25 wait time–related parameters to develop models that ultimately allowed them to display real-time wait estimates for patients. The collected data simultaneously identifies congestion and excessive downtime that can help schedulers be more efficient. Scheduling an exam, especially advanced imaging, begins long before a patient is appointed a time slot. Any number of steps can introduce inefficiency and delay including, but not limited to, protocol completion, prior authorization, patient screening, and scanner availability. As an institution-specific example, Wessman and colleagues used the Lean Method and PDSA cycles to decrease the scheduling time of outpatient MRI exams from 117 to 33 hours.

Equity

Healthcare equity in this country was boosted significantly by the passage of the PPACA. As these changes are relatively recent, the data pertaining to the magnitude of its effect are limited. Some implications, such as the state-optioned expansion of Medicaid, only implemented in January 2014, are in their infancy. Early results demonstrate improved access to care and affordability for states using Medicaid expansion as well as those using the private option (the use of Medicaid funds to purchase private insurance). The refusal of some states to accept the expansion of Medicaid has allowed for built-in comparative cohorts. Not surprisingly, low-income adults in states that refused expansion were worse off than their counterparts in numerous markers of health and healthcare including access to a usual source of care and utilization of appropriate preventative services. Although these issues may be beyond the efforts of individual radiologists, it is important to be aware of them.

CONCLUSION

The Requisites Series, since its inception, has been keen to strike the right balance between consummate coverage and the necessary fundamental requirements of practice. The authors of the following chapters have stayed true to this mission in covering some of the most important themes in radiology today, many of which are all too often not given appropriate weight during training. Adherence to these themes can help drive radiology toward more patient-centric care and ultimately enable the current and next generation of radiologists to be more accessible, marketable, indispensable, and central to a dynamic and increasingly complex healthcare system.

SUGGESTED READINGS

American Board of Radiology. Noninterpretive Skills Resource Guide. Available at: https://www.theabr.org/sites/all/themes/abr-media/pdf/Noninterpretive_Skills_Domain_Specification_and_Resource_Guide.pdf.

American College of Radiology. ACR Appropriateness Criteria. Available at: https://www.acr.org/Quality-Safety/Appropriateness-Criteria.

American College of Radiology. *ACR Manual on Contrast Media*. Version 10.2, 2015. Available at: https://www.acr.org/~/media/ACR/Documents/PDF/QualitySafety/Resources/Contrast-Manual/2016_Contrast_Media.pdf?la=en.

American College of Radiology. Practice Parameters and Technical Standards. Available at: https://www.acr.org/Quality-Safety/Standards-Guidelines.

Alderson PO. Noninterpretive skills for radiology residents. Introduction to series. *Am J Roentgenol*. 1999;173(6):1451.

Amis ES. American College of Radiology Standards, Accreditation Programs, and Appropriateness Criteria. *Am J Roentgenol*. 2000;174(2):307–310.

Audet AM, Doty MM, Shamasdin J, Schoenbaum SC. Measure, learn, and improve: physicians' involvement in quality improvement. *Health Aff (Millwood)*. 2005;24(3):843–853.

Balogh EP, Miller BT, Ball JR. *Improving Diagnosis in Health Care.* Washington, DC: National Academies Press; 2015.

Brennan T. Medical professionalism in the new millennium: a physician charter. *Ann Intern Med.* 2002;136(3):243-246.

Cabarrus M, Naeger DM, Rybkin A, Qayyum A. Patients prefer results from the ordering provider and access to their radiology reports. *J Am Coll Radiol.* 2015;12(6):556-562.

Chassin MR, Loeb JM. The ongoing quality improvement journey: next stop, high reliability. *Health Aff (Millwood).* 2011;30(4):559-568.

Clarke R, Valentin J. A history of the international commission on radiological protection. *Health Phys.* 2005;88(6):717-732.

Cooper VF, Goodhartz LA, Nemcek AA Jr, Ryu RK. Radiology resident interpretations of on-call imaging studies: the incidence of major discrepancies. *Acad Radiol.* 2008;15(9):1198-1204.

Cunningham L, McGregor J. *Why Big Business Is Falling Out of Love With the Annual Performance Review.* Washington Post; 2015.

Dentzer S. Still crossing the quality chasm—or suspended over it? *Health Aff (Millwood).* 2011;30(4):554-555.

Donnelly LF, Mathews VP, Laszakovits DJ, Jackson VP, Guiberteau MJ. Recent changes to ABR maintenance of certification part 4 (PQI): acknowledgment of radiologists' activities to improve quality and safety. *J Am Coll Radiol.* 2016;13(2):184-187.

Ellenbogen PH. The radiologist assistant: best new thing since sliced bread or Trojan horse? *Radiology.* 2008;248(1):4-7.

England E, Collins J, White RD, Seagull FJ, Deledda J. Radiology report turnaround time: effect on resident education. *Acad Radiol.* 2015;22(5):662-667.

Gilk T, Kanal E. Planning an MR suite: what can be done to enhance safety? *J Magn Reson Imaging.* 2015;42(3):566-571.

Guillerman RP. From "Image Gently" to image intelligently: a personalized perspective on diagnostic radiation risk. *Pediatr Radiol.* 2014;44(suppl 3):444-449.

Halpern EJ, Spandorfer JM. Professionalism in radiology: ideals and challenges. *Am J Roentgenol.* 2014;202(2):352-357.

Han X, Nguyen BT, Drope J, Jemal A. Health-related outcomes among the poor: Medicaid expansion vs. non-expansion states. *PLoS One.* 2015;10(12):e0144429.

Hawkins CM, Bowen MA, Gilliland CA, Walls DG, Duszak Jr R. The impact of nonphysician providers on diagnostic and interventional radiology practices: regulatory, billing, and compliance perspectives. *J Am Coll Radiol.* 2015;12(8):776-781.

Hernanz-Schulman M, Goske MJ, Bercha IH, Strauss KJ. Pause and pulse: ten steps that help manage radiation dose during pediatric fluoroscopy. *Am J Roentgenol.* 2011;197(2):475-481.

Institute of Medicine. *Crossing the Quality Chasm: A New Health System for the 21st Century.* Washington, DC: The National Academies Press; 2001.

Kachalia A, Kaufman SR, Boothman R, et al. Liability claims and costs before and after implementation of a medical error disclosure program. *Ann Intern Med.* 2010;153(4):213-221.

Kahn CE Jr, Heilbrun ME, Applegate KE. From guidelines to practice: how reporting templates promote the use of radiology practice guidelines. *J Am Coll Radiol.* 2013;10(4):268-273.

Kanal E, Froelich J, Barkovich AJ, et al. Standardized MR terminology and reporting of implants and devices as recommended by the American College of Radiology Subcommittee on MR safety. *Radiology.* 2015;274(3):866-870.

Kohn LT, Corrigan JM, Donaldson MS. To err is human: building a safer health system. In: Kohn LT, Corrigan JM, Donaldson MS, eds. *To Err Is Human: Building a Safer Health System.* Washington DC: National Academy of Sciences; 2000.

Kotagal M, Richards MK, Chapman T, et al. Improving ultrasound quality to reduce computed tomography use in pediatric appendicitis: the Safe and Sound campaign. *Am J Surg.* 2015;209(5):896-900. discussion 900.

Lamb L, Kashani P, Ryan J, et al. Impact of an in-house emergency radiologist on report turnaround time. *CJEM.* 2015;17(1):21-26.

Mahesh M, Haines GR. JACR radiation dose optimization in CT: an online resource center for radiologists. *J Am Coll Radiol.* 2013;10(6):477.

Miglioretti DL, Johnson E, Williams A, et al. The use of computed tomography in pediatrics and the associated radiation exposure and estimated cancer risk. *JAMA Pediatr.* 2013;167(8):700-707.

Miller P, Gunderman R, Lightburn J, Miller D. Enhancing patients' experiences in radiology: through patient-radiologist interaction. *Acad Radiol.* 2013;20(6):778-781.

Nachiappan AC, Valentin LI, Metwalli ZA, et al. CT dose reduction workshop: an active educational experience. *J Am Coll Radiol.* 2015;12(6):610-616. e1.

Pfeifer K, Staib L, Arango J, et al. High-fidelity contrast reaction simulation training: performance comparison of faculty, fellows, and residents. *J Am Coll Radiol.* 2016;13(1):81-87.

Pham JC, Girard T, Pronovost PJ. What to do with healthcare incident reporting systems. *J Public Health Res.* 2013;2(3):e27.

Pianykh OS, Rosenthal DI. Can we predict patient wait time? *J Am Coll Radiol.* 2015;12(10):1058-1066.

RSNA. Radiology Reporting Templates. *RadReport.org;* 2016.

Rubin DL. Informatics in radiology: measuring and improving quality in radiology: meeting the challenge with informatics. *Radiographics.* 2011;31(6):1511-1527.

SafePatientProject. To Err Is Human—To Delay Is Deadly: 10 Year Follow Up. *Consumers Union.* 2009.

Selby JV, Beal AC, Frank L. The Patient-Centered Outcomes Research Institute (PCORI) national priorities for research and initial research agenda. *J Am Med Assoc.* 2012;307(15):1583-1584.

Shartzer A, Long SK, Anderson N. Access to care and affordability have improved following Affordable Care Act implementation; problems remain. *Health Aff (Millwood).* 2016;35(1):161-168.

Sheng AY, Dalziel P, Liteplo AS, Fagenholz P, Noble VE. Focused assessment with sonography in trauma and abdominal computed tomography utilization in adult trauma patients: trends over the last decade. *Emerg Med Int.* 2013;2013:678380.

Sidhu M. Radiation safety in pediatric interventional radiology: step lightly. *Pediatr Radiol.* 2010;40(4):511-513.

Sommers BD, Blendon RJ, Orav EJ. Both the 'private option' and traditional Medicaid expansions improved access to care for low-income adults. *Health Aff (Millwood).* 2016;35(1):96-105.

Tamm EP, Szklaruk J, Puthooran L, Stone D, Stevens BL, Modaro C. Quality initiatives: planning, setting up, and carrying out radiology process improvement projects. *Radiographics.* 2012;32(5):1529-1542.

Teplick SK. Medical professionalism in the new millennium: a physicians' charter. *Radiology.* 2006;238(2):383-386.

Thornton E, Brook OR, Mendiratta-Lala M, Hallett DT, Kruskal JB. Application of failure mode and effect analysis in a radiology department. *Radiographics.* 2011;31(1):281-293.

Wang Y, Eldridge N, Metersky ML, et al. National trends in patient safety for four common conditions, 2005-2011. *N Engl J Med.* 2014;370(4):341-351.

Weinberg BD, Richter MD, Champine JG, Morriss MC, Browning T. Radiology resident preliminary reporting in an independent call environment: multiyear assessment of volume, timeliness, and accuracy. *J Am Coll Radiol.* 2015;12(1):95-100.

Wessman BV, Moriarity AK, Ametlli V, Kastan DJ. Reducing barriers to timely MR imaging scheduling. *Radiographics.* 2014;34(7):2064-2070.

Zygmont ME, Lam DL, Nowitzki KM, et al. Opportunities for patient-centered outcomes research in radiology. *Acad Radiol.* 2016;23(1):8-17.

Chapter 2
Key Concepts in Quality Improvement

Nadja Kadom

CONCEPTS FOR QUALITY IMPROVEMENT

Quality improvement (QI) methods are not new; they are just relatively new to the healthcare industry and the field of radiology. As a result, there is currently a gap between the high desire and need to apply QI methods in daily practice and a lack of radiologists who are sufficiently trained in the proper use of these methods. In response to this gap, many medical schools and radiology residency programs have now started to teach QI methods to medical students and residents, and the American Board of Radiology (ABR) has incorporated QI into the certification exam curriculum.

Before delving into the study and application of QI methods, several key concepts in QI need to be understood. For example, to solicit and motivate a local QI team, one needs to understand and communicate the reasons why we embark on QI initiatives. A basic understanding of the major domains of QI is necessary when identifying QI projects that support the greater mission for improvement in healthcare. To execute QI methods successfully, several basic philosophical principles need to be applied and are described here.

DRIVERS OF QUALITY IMPROVEMENT

What drives us to do QI in radiology? How can we persuade the skeptics to join our efforts? The rationale for doing QI encompasses ethics, the economy, science, and gripping patient narratives (Fig. 2.1).

Physicians practice according to high *ethical standards and principles*, such as those attributed to Hippocrates in the *Hippocratic Oath*. The statement *Primum non nocere (First, do no harm)* is frequently quoted when promoting QI in healthcare. Just how do we harm patients in healthcare today? According to the 1999 Institute of Medicine (IOM) report *To Err Is Human*, preventable causes of patient deaths are the result of erroneous or delayed diagnoses, treatment errors such as a wrong operation and medication errors, failure to give prophylaxis, inadequate monitoring/follow-up, and communication and equipment failures. The IOM reported in 1999 that between 44,000 and 98,000 people died in hospitals each year as a result of preventable medical errors. An analysis published in 2013 estimated that there are more than 400,000 premature deaths associated with preventable harm to patients per year. How can we simply go on about our business in light of such shocking numbers? What happened to *Primum non nocere*? I do not know

about you, but I have a sense of urgency to start improving patient care!

There is also an *economic argument* supporting QI in healthcare. As of the first quarter of 2014 the total US net worth was estimated to be $269.6 trillion, the national debt was $145.8 trillion, and the annual gross domestic product (GDP) was $123.8 trillion. Very plainly, we are in debt because we spend more than we produce, and healthcare is one of the areas where we spend a lot (Kaiser Family Foundation [KFF]). In 2009, health spending per capita in the United States was $7598, which was 48% higher than in the next highest spending country, Switzerland (KFF). Despite this high investment in healthcare, the United States does not appear to achieve substantially better health outcomes. For example, in 2015 the Central Intelligence Institute (CIA) ranked US life expectancy No. 43, while Switzerland ranked No. 9 (CIA). The discrepancy between high spending and suboptimal outcomes is explained by a multitude of factors. About half of the spending growth in healthcare is being attributed to the availability of new medical technology. The development and use of healthcare technology are thriving because health insurance bears a substantial share of the incurred cost to patients (KFF). Another factor contributing to rising healthcare costs is the aging of the US baby boomer population. Baby boomers are expected to have more health problems and require more care between 2012 and 2022. In addition, about 20% or more of total healthcare expenditures are being attributed to various forms of waste (overutilization, failed care coordination or failed care delivery, and administrative waste, fraud, and abuse) (KFF). According to a Kaiser Health Tracking Poll, rising healthcare costs have caused many American families to cut back on medical care by using home remedies rather than medical professionals, cutting back on dental care, or postponing the care they need. Many of these issues need to be addressed at a political level, through legislation and modifications to our insurance payer system. However, eliminating waste from the system can be done locally, by anyone, right now.

Another big driver for QI in healthcare is to provide more *effective care*, meaning care that is proven to achieve its purpose. There is currently a wide temporal gap between publication of scientific knowledge and its application to patient care. It is said, for example, that it takes 17 years for research evidence to reach clinical practice, due to the time required and the complexities of performing basic research, translating lab results into human trials, using experiences in humans for clinical

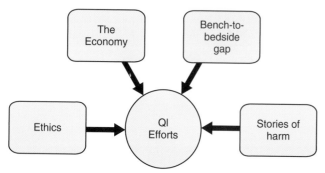

FIG. 2.1 Drivers of QI efforts in healthcare. *QI,* Quality improvement.

trials, becoming a practice guideline, and becoming an established practice. There are time-consuming matters of getting access to facilities and funding, addressing human subject protection, federal regulations for drug and device development, and efforts invested in manuscript writing that have to be surmounted prior to publication. In addition, all practitioners harbor a wealth of cognitive biases against new treatments and processes and it has been shown that these cognitive biases can cause underuse of effective new strategies in favor of old suboptimal therapies. Closing the gap between research and clinical practice can be as simple as review and implementation of one of the many clinical guidelines or American College of Radiology (ACR) appropriateness criteria, which are built on current scientific knowledge.

When logic and science fail to persuade others of the importance of QI in radiology, there is still a possibility that a *narrative of harm* can do so. The *story of harm* is very similar to an account given in mortality and morbidity (M&M) meetings. In contrast to M&M accounts, the story of harm may be told by the person who experienced the harm (usually the patient or a relative) or by the caregiver involved in events that caused harm and is always told in a setting that is supportive of the narrator and with an emphasis on learning from mistakes. A story of harm appeals at an emotional level and can be a strong motivator for joining or initiating QI efforts.

Twenty-eight-year-old Angela Myers was awaiting an outpatient angiogram for an arteriovenous malformation on her leg. She was very anxious about the impending procedure. The patient spoke English and appeared to be of average intelligence. David, a 45-year-old interventional radiology (IR) technologist: "I went to the waiting room to meet my next patient. I picked up the chart that was next to this patient. The chart had the correct name for my next patient. I verbally stated the patient's name and this woman confirmed her name. She also confirmed other information, including the type of procedure. I walked the patient to the IR suite and had her positioned on the IR table. The certified nurse anesthetist checked the patient's wristband and alerted me that this was not the correct patient for the uterine fibroid embolization procedure. I was shocked. I apologized. I explained she was in the wrong room. I had to take the patient off the IR table and return her to the waiting room." *Upon reflection David realized:* "This patient was so anxious she was not actually hearing much of anything I said to her. She continued to agree and confirm whatever I said to her. The error on my part was that I stated her name, and did not

check her wristband." *Luckily, the error was caught and the patient was not harmed. As David recalled,* "I learned a serious lesson, which I certainly had been taught by my supervisor, which is to always check the wristband. I don't know just how far this mistake would have gone, because the patient is frequently asleep when the surgeon enters the suite. I now reinforce the importance of always checking the wristband whenever I have an opportunity to with my colleagues."

Modified from the Patient Safety Network (PSN)

DOMAINS OF QUALITY IMPROVEMENT

Once we start looking for QI projects, the number of possibilities may result in a need to prioritize projects. Frequently we are drawn into projects that address a problem, but solving the problem does not result in improved patient care. There are established patient care domains that can help in selecting improvement projects that are relevant to patient care.

The *Donabedian model* divides the aspects of patient care into structure, process, and outcomes (Fig. 2.2). The *structure* category pertains to the facilities, equipment, and manpower involved in the patient care process. It is assumed that the optimal healthcare delivery structure is conducive to providing good care. Under this category, quality improvement metrics would reflect the type and amount of resources used in a particular structure to deliver good care, such as the number of staff, beds, supplies, buildings, and cost to run the facility. In radiology, these metrics could be the number and age of computed tomography (CT) scanners, magnetic resonance imaging (MRI), and radiographic equipment; the number of radiologists with subspecialty training; the number of certified technologists; compliance with facility policies and equipment maintenance; and compliance with continuing medical education (CME) requirements. The *process* category pertains to the quality of the delivered care itself. Under this category, quality improvement metrics would reflect the activities and tasks during every patient encounter. In radiology, these metrics could be the appropriateness of the exams performed, patient wait times, radiation dose, and rates of critical results reporting. The *outcome* category pertains to the end result of care. The outcome is a state of health that is the result of the process delivered within the structure. Outcomes may be classified by the 5 D's: death, disease, disability, discomfort, and dissatisfaction. Examples of outcome metrics in radiology include adherence to diagnostic imaging-reporting and data systems such as the Breast Imaging Reporting and Data System (BI-RADS), wrong patient/wrong exam, patient falls, outcomes of contrast extravasations and reactions, patient satisfaction scores, and critical result reporting.

More granular domains for patient care are the *six IOM aims* proposed in the 2001 IOM report *Crossing the Quality Chasm.* These six aims can be remembered by the acronym STEEEP: safe care, timely care, efficient care, effective care, equitable care, and patient-centered care. The definition of *safe* care is "avoiding injuries to patients from the care that is intended to help them." In radiology, the major hazards include adverse outcomes in interventional radiology, MRI safety incidents,

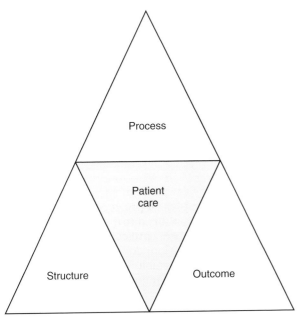

FIG. 2.2 Donabedian model.

contrast reactions and extravasations, imaging the wrong patient or choosing the wrong exam, and radiation exposure.

The definition of *timely* care is "reducing waits and sometimes harmful delays for both those who receive and those who give care." In radiology, timeliness can apply to report turnaround times, critical result reporting, patient access to radiology results, timely response to patient calls for scheduling or inquiries regarding their exams, patient wait times in radiology, and the ability to get a walk-in radiology exam.

The definition of *efficient* care is "reducing waits and sometimes harmful delays for both those who receive and those who give care." The most effective method of quality improvement targeting waste is the lean approach. There are five major categories of waste: transport, waiting, production, inventory, and processing. Some radiology examples of reducing waste are decreasing repeat imaging studies, decreasing patient wait times, decreasing equipment/staff idle times, limiting overutilization of imaging studies, optimizing storage of interventional radiology supplies, and decreasing reporting times through structured templates.

The definition of *effective* care is "providing services based on scientific knowledge to all who could benefit, and refraining from providing services to those not likely to benefit." Examples of metrics in this domain could be adherence to medical subspecialty guidelines in the diagnosis and treatment of certain diseases, and use of the ACR Appropriateness Criteria.

The definition of *equitable* care is "providing care that does not vary in quality because of personal characteristics such as gender, ethnicity, geographic location, and socioeconomic status." In radiology, this could mean bringing advanced imaging technology to remote locations or making imaging more affordable.

The definition of *patient-centered* care is "providing care that is respectful of and responsive to individual patient preferences, needs, and values, and ensuring that patient values guide all clinical decisions." In radiology, this

may include procedure consents in patient-appropriate language, respecting religious and ethnic preferences that patients may have, providing translation services for foreign languages, or providing convenient access to the imaging facility.

CONCEPTS FOR QUALITY IMPROVEMENT

QI efforts thrive best in an environment that is supportive of these efforts. Successful QI efforts depend on commitment by the organization to improvement of patient care, the people who drive the improvements, and a culture that enables these improvements.

One of the key ideas in QI is that organizations desire to become *high-reliability organizations* (HROs) (Chassin). Becoming an HRO means that the organization has succeeded in avoiding catastrophes in an environment with many risk factors and high levels of complexity, where adverse outcomes would be expected to happen all the time. The most frequently cited examples of successful HROs in the United States are nuclear power plants, air traffic control systems, and aircraft carriers. Healthcare has much catching up to do to become an HRO industry! Becoming an HRO involves five major features: (1) HROs are preoccupied with failure, meaning that they are always fixing any issues that occur and are alert and on the lookout for the next possible adverse event, and eager to prevent it. (2) HROs always get to the root of a problem, no matter how complex, never dismissing anything with simple explanations. (3) HROs take the pulse of frontline workers who are generally the first to discover problems as they run their daily operations. (4) HROs are resilient, meaning they recover quickly from issues, and they adapt and develop innovative solutions on the fly. (5) HROs use on-the-ground subject matter experts to address problems, not just the next authority in line.

In his work, W. Edwards Deming, one of the most influential pioneers of scientific quality control, outlined a system of profound knowledge (SoPK). He emphasized the following four areas of knowledge: appreciation for a system, knowledge of variation, theory of knowledge, and psychology. In radiology, we are embedded within the healthcare system, raising the levels of *system* complexity tremendously. Deming thought that in complex systems, individual parts work together for the benefit of the whole, and not at the expense of any of the other parts. He used the analogy of an orchestra, which is judged by the listeners, not by the players, and the need to work together to achieve a favorable outcome. The conductor, similar to a manager, fosters cooperation among the players, where every player supports the others. This framework encourages us to look beyond the confines of our QI goals and initiatives and have greater goals in mind. It also fosters collaboration with other professional disciplines and medical subspecialties to reach these goals. For example, to achieve the greater goals of limiting radiation exposure, we should not just change the technique on our CT scanners by working with our technologists and physicists but educate clinicians and their practice staff on the proper use of appropriateness criteria and other scientific evidence to use CT more appropriately.

Another area in which we need profound knowledge is *variation*. Any activity we perform or any item we produce is of varying quality. Variation is an expected outcome, but we have a chance to use QI methods to decrease the degree of variation. Studying variation by plotting data in control charts can help differentiate common-cause from special-cause variation. Common-cause variation can be likened to the noise in the system, something that is always active, whereas special-cause variation can be likened to a signal, a special event, often worth studying further. For example, when baking bread, the oven's thermostat will allow the oven temperature to drift up and down slightly throughout the baking process, a common-cause variation. If we open the oven door or turn the temperature switch, we introduce a special cause variation into the baking process. Deming stated that managers often think they *know* because they have information, opinions, theories, hypotheses, hunches, or beliefs. Deming postulated that profound *knowledge* requires profound experience, which can be gained through a cycle of forming a hypothesis, making a prediction based on past experience, testing the theory, and checking the results. Hypotheses are proven with data. The caveat is that if you base your decisions on data, the data must be of high quality. This involves precise definitions of data, reliable data collection and data documentation systems, and consistent data interpretation. For example, if you tell your data collector to document the report turnaround times, the data collector must clearly understand what you mean by *time*. Is it the time from study completion to signed report, or is it the time from patient arrival to preliminary report? How reliable are the time points? Are they being documented manually or are these times reliably documented electronically? Finally, Deming emphasized human *psychology*. Organizations need to understand what motivates people to do a good job. Deming had the two key beliefs that people are different and that they are mostly motivated intrinsically. Based on these beliefs, Deming opposed the top-to-bottom management style. Based on his philosophy, QI initiatives are almost always team driven and recognize the tremendous value of frontline workers in the process of improvement.

In 1990, Reason developed a model for the dynamics of accident causation that is frequently referred to as the *Swiss cheese* model. This model postulates that errors occur as a result of fatefully aligned latent system failures, human factors, event triggers, and failure of the system's defenses. This model helps us understand error, not as the fault of an individual, but as a complex issue that requires complex analysis and solutions. In the past, many individuals involved in errors lost their jobs as a result, which was not always fair.

To mitigate the effects of blame and scapegoating, we now use the system of *just culture*. In just culture, human behavior is analyzed. If an error was an honest mistake, the individual should be consoled because they likely suffer from having committed an error, especially if a patient was harmed. For example, if the wrong imaging study was performed because the operator clicked the wrong choice on a drop-down menu on the computer, the person would feel bad about that *slip* and should be consoled in order to move on and practice better in the future. If a mistake is made as a result of at-risk behavior, the individual should receive corrective action and coaching. For example, if you always do the imaging protocols in 10 minutes, whereas your colleagues take 60 minutes, because you do not follow the policy of looking up patient information and prior studies, you are taking shortcuts on diligence. You would benefit from coaching on the importance of reviewing the patient history and prior exams before selecting an imaging protocol, on the importance of following departmental rules and guidelines, and perhaps someone would monitor you for a time to make sure that you spend as much time on the task as your more diligent colleagues do. If the behavior causing errors is reckless, punishment is appropriate. If you protocol every brain MRI as a routine brain with contrast because it fits the clinical question most of the time, without reviewing the actual order or the patient's history, you may be subject to disciplinary action; termination may even be the appropriate outcome. Employing the just culture system creates an environment where employees feel safe about reporting their own mistakes, because they know that their managers understand an unintended *slip* and are willing to forgive and coach *at-risk behavior*, as long as the employee is willing and able to improve.

Reason also recognized that there are *active and latent errors*. Active errors are obvious, whereas latent errors are hidden in the system. In the example of selecting an imaging protocol, the radiologist clicking the wrong study from the drop-down menu made an active error, but the computer system that allowed the mouse to slip by a line and did not provide a double-check option makes this latent error possible, which is a situation that is just waiting to create more problems.

There are many other concepts of quality improvement in healthcare to consider. A great resource for further reading is the *Journal of the American College of Radiology (JACR)* and, of course, this book!

SUGGESTED READINGS

American Public Health Association (APHA). Gun Violence Prevention. <https://www.apha.org/~/media/files/pdf/factsheets/gun_violence_prevention.ashx>.

Centers for Disease Control and Prevention (CDC). Impaired Driving: Get the Facts. <http://www.cdc.gov/motorvehiclesafety/impaired_driving/impaired-drv_factsheet.html>.

Central Intelligence Agency. The World Factbook: Country Comparison: Life Expectancy at Birth. <https://www.cia.gov/library/publications/the-world-factbook/rankorder/2102rank.html>.

Donabedian A. Quality of care: problems of measurement. II. Some issues in evaluating the quality of nursing care. *Am J Public Health Nations Health.* 1969;59(10):1833–1836.

Eaglstein WH. Evidence-based medicine, the research-practice gap, and biases in medical and surgical decision making in dermatology. *Arch Dermatol.* 2010;146(10):1161–1164.

Greenhalgh T, Russell J, Swinglehurst D. Narrative methods in quality improvement research. *Qual Saf Health Care.* 2005;14(6):443–449.

Harvey HB, Hassanzadeh E, Aran S, Rosenthal DI, Thrall JH, Abujudeh HH. Key performance indicators in radiology: you can't manage what you can't measure. *Curr Probl Diagn Radiol.* 2016;45(2):115–121.

Institute of Medicine (IOM). *Crossing the Quality Chasm: A New Health System for the 21st Century.* Washington, DC: National Academy Press; 2001.

Institute of Medicine. *To Err Is Human: Building a Safer Health Care System.* Washington, DC: National Academy Press; 1999.

James JT. A new, evidence-based estimate of patient harms associated with hospital care. *J Patient Saf.* 2013;9(3):122–128.

Kadom N, Watson H, Nagy P. Making quality improvement projects relevant to the 6 Institute of Medicine aims. *J Am Coll Radiol.* 2015;12(4):415–416.

Kruskal JB, Reedy A, Pascal L, Rosen MP, Boiselle PM. Quality initiatives: lean approach to improving performance and efficiency in a radiology department. *Radiographics.* 2012;32(2):573–587.

Mainz J. Defining and classifying clinical indicators for quality improvement. *Int J Qual Health Care.* 2003;15(6):523–530.

Morris ZS, Wooding S, Grant J. The answer is 17 years, what is the question: understanding time lags in translational research. *J R Soc Med*. 2011;104(12):510–520.

Patient Safety Network. Check the Wristband. <https://psnet.ahrq.gov/webmm/case/22>.

Reason J. *Human Error*. New York, NY: Cambridge University Press; 1990.

The Deming Institute. The Deming System of]profound knowledge. <https://deming.org/theman/theories/profoundknowledge>.

The Henry J. Kaiser Family Foundation. Health Care Costs: A Primer. <http://kff.org/report-section/health-care-costs-a-primer-2012-report>.

The Joint Commission: High Reliability Health Care: Getting There From Here. <http://www.jointcommission.org/assets/1/6/chassin_and_loeb_0913_final.pdf>.

Wikipedia. Financial Position of the United States. <https://en.wikipedia.org/wiki/Financial_position_of_the_United_States>.

Chapter 3
Quality Improvement: Definition and Limitations

Eric A. Walker

CURRENT AND TRADITIONAL DEFINITIONS OF QUALITY IN HEALTHCARE

How do we best define quality in healthcare? The quality literature includes several definitions. The Institute of Medicine (IOM) defines quality of care as the degree to which health services for individuals and populations increase the likelihood of desired health outcomes and are consistent with current professional knowledge. How care is administered should demonstrate appropriate use of the most current knowledge about scientific, clinical, technical, interpersonal, manual, cognitive, and organizational and management elements of healthcare. The Agency for Healthcare Research and Quality (AHRQ) defines quality healthcare as "doing the right thing for the right patient, at the right time, in the right way to achieve the best possible results." The American College of Radiology (ACR) defines the quality of healthcare in radiology as "the degree to which health services for individuals and populations increase the likelihood of desired health outcomes and are consistent with current professional knowledge. Specifically with regard to diagnostic imaging and image-guided treatment, quality is the extent to which the right procedure is done in the right way, at the right time, and the correct interpretation is accurately and quickly communicated to the patient and referring physician. The goals are to maximize the likelihood of desired health outcomes and to satisfy the patient."

The IOM offers six overarching characteristics of high-quality care (Table 3.1), which have been widely adopted by other organizations active in improving the quality of healthcare. These are discussed in greater detail in Chapter 1.

An important component of improving the quality of healthcare involves the reduction of both diagnostic and treatment errors. A significant stimulus to the current quality and safety movement in the United States was the IOM's 1999 landmark monograph, *To Err Is Human*. This report stated that 44,000 to 98,000 deaths each year are a result of medical errors.

Other reports since then have also highlighted the need for quality improvement (QI) in healthcare, including *Crossing the Quality Chasm* and the *National Healthcare Quality Report,* published annually since 2003 by the AHRQ. Diagnostic error in medicine continues to be a major cause of patient harm, with the rate of missed, incorrect, or delayed diagnoses estimated to be as high as 10% to 15%. Two broad error categories in diagnostic radiology include perceptual errors and cognitive (interpretive) errors. Perceptual errors are far more frequent, accounting

for 60% to 80% of radiologists' errors. This topic is further discussed in Chapter 14 of this book.

An important consideration in healthcare quality is the appropriate use of available resources. Inappropriate use of resources can be further classified as underuse, overuse, or misuse. *Underuse* is prevalent, and many evidence-based recommendations are not used as often as recommended. As an example, although biannual screening in women age 50 to 75 years has been proven to be beneficial, less than 75% of women in this age group report obtaining a mammogram in the previous 2 years. *Overuse* occurs when testing and treatments are used to a greater extent than the available clinical evidence supports. Overuse, by this definition, contributes significantly to current healthcare costs. An example of overuse is obtaining a magnetic resonance imaging (MRI) scan of the lumbar spine for acute uncomplicated low back pain or radiculopathy. The *ACR Appropriateness Criteria* rates MRI in this example as "usually not appropriate." *Misuse* involves using the wrong resource. An example of misuse is a physician ordering a radiograph of the skull after an acute closed head injury rather than the clinically indicated head computed tomography exam.

QUALITY CONTROL, QUALITY ASSURANCE, AND QUALITY IMPROVEMENT

Quality control (QC) is defined as "a management process where actual performance is measured against expected performance, and actions are taken on the difference." QC in the industrial or healthcare setting establishes ranges of acceptability for specific measures or data points. Action is taken when a measurement falls outside the acceptable range. QC sets the baseline for a minimal level of quality. Efforts must be made to reduce variation as much as possible. Examples of QC include the regular, intermittent testing of medical equipment, the measurement of radiation dosage, or the evaluation of image quality. The radiologist practicing QC may request a repeat chest radiograph if the lung apices are excluded. QC establishes the range of acceptability including the accuracy, which refers to the proximity of a measurement to the true value; the precision, which refers to the reproducibility of a measurement; and the reliability, which refers to the accuracy and precision of a measurement. QC is a process by which we review the quality of all factors involved in producing an item.

Quality assurance (QA) is a comprehensive quality management program used to ensure healthcare excellence through the systematic collection and evaluation of data. QA involves focusing on specific indicators that are

TABLE 3.1 Institute of Medicine's Six Aims of High-Quality Care

Safe	Avoiding injuries to patients from the care that is intended to help them.
Effective	Providing services based on scientific knowledge to all who can benefit, and refraining from providing services to those not likely to benefit.
Patient centered	Providing care that is respectful of and responsive to the individual patient preferences, needs, and values, and ensuring that patient values guide all clinical decisions.
Timely	Reducing waits and sometimes harmful delays for those who receive and those who give care.
Efficient	Avoiding waste, including waste of equipment, supplies, ideas, and energy.
Equitable	Providing care that does not vary in quality because of personal characteristics such as gender, ethnicity, geographic location, and socioeconomic status.

Modified from Committee on Quality of Health Care in America. *Crossing the Quality Chasm.* Washington, DC: National Academy Press; 2001.

believed to affect the quality of services. Key performance indicators (KPIs) are measures that are used to evaluate the health of an organization and define and quantitatively measure progress toward the organization's goals. In diagnostic imaging, performance indicators may include access to services, utilization appropriateness, timeliness of scheduling, waiting times, patient safety, or image modality and protocol selection. QA includes all activities related to proper operational and strategic planning, preassessment, and self-evaluation. QA involves compliance with specifications, requirements, or standards and implementing methods for conformance. QA has lost its earlier popularity because it may be interpreted as reactive, retrospective, and policing and could result in disciplinary means. QA often involved determining who was at fault after something went wrong. QA is an older term not frequently used today.

Quality improvement (QI), sometimes called continuous quality improvement or total quality management, is defined as an ongoing, organization-wide framework in which employees are committed to and involved in monitoring and evaluating all aspects of an organization's activities including inputs, processes, and outputs to continuously improve them. QI is a holistic approach focusing on the entire system to provide services that meet or exceed the patient's or referring clinician's expectations. A QI program should have a clear idea of patient needs, be familiar with all the individual steps in a system, understand potential sources of variability in the system, encourage teamwork, embrace experimentation, and implement ideas for process improvement. In radiology, QI dictates that all activities in an imaging facility be identified and that clear standards (performance indicators) be set and measured to allow processes to be improved continuously. Process QI activities involve a retrospective and prospective evaluation of the system to identify unacceptable variability or occurrence of defects and encourage experimenting with methods to minimize the variability and eliminate defects. The steps in a process may be mapped with a simple flow chart and the Plan-Do-Study-Act (PDSA) cycle can be used for the QI process.

A few valuable QI tools include the "5 Whys," the histogram, the flowchart, cause-and-effect diagrams (fishbone or Ishikawa diagrams), Pareto charts, run charts, control charts (Shewhart charts), and the PDSA cycle (Shewhart cycle, Deming cycle). These topics are discussed in greater detail in Chapter 4.

Practice quality improvement (PQI) is a QI project or activity undertaken at least once per 3-year period to satisfy the American Board of Radiology (ABR) Maintenance of Certification (MOC) Part 4 requirements. A PQI activity involves the continuous engagement of healthcare professionals in efforts expected to lead to better health outcomes for patients and better system performance with the desired outcome of improved patient care and/or enhanced professional development. PQI projects use any standard QI methodology, such as the PDSA cycle approach. An individual radiologist, a group practice, a department at a healthcare or academic institution, a healthcare system, or a society at the local, regional, or national level may develop a PQI project.

QUALITY IMPROVEMENT AND VALUE

Value in healthcare has been defined as the health outcomes achieved per dollar spent. By this definition, both quality and cost play a major role in determining value. Although reducing costs can sometimes increase value, the term *value* is not synonymous with cost cutting. Cost reduction without consideration of outcomes is dangerous and self-defeating. Because value is defined as outcomes relative to costs, it encompasses efficiency. Increasing value involves an efficient (lowest cost) use of resources that produces the desired level of quality. To measure value, we must first be able to measure quality, and then compare the costs to accepted benchmarks. Value-based payment systems offer incentives to increase quality and transparency, while offering disincentives, such as decreased payment, for overtreatment and opacity. The goal of the value-based payment system is to shift from volume-based (fee-for-service) to value-based reimbursement.

LIMITATIONS OF TRADITIONAL QUALITY IMPROVEMENT TECHNIQUES

In an attempt to provide healthcare of optimal quality, healthcare providers traditionally assess or measure performance and then ensure that it conforms to standards. In cases where performance fails to conform, providers attempt to modify or improve physician behavior. According to an article by Laffel et al., traditional approaches to healthcare quality have several limitations. First, the classic definition of quality of care is too narrow to meet the needs of modern healthcare providers. Second, traditional medical QA features a static approach to quality with a goal of conforming to standards and assuming that some rate of poor outcomes is acceptable. Instead, QI in healthcare should be a dynamic and continuous process. A third limitation of traditional techniques is that they tend to focus on physician performance and to underemphasize the contributions of nonphysicians and organizational systems in general. A fourth limitation is that QA tends to emphasize certain aspects of physician performance, such as technical expertise and interpersonal relations, rather than the physician's ability to mobilize an organization's resources to meet the needs of individual patients and reach the organization's goals.

As stated earlier, traditional QA may be interpreted as reactive, retrospective, policing, and possibly resulting in disciplinary or punitive actions. QA often involves identifying an individual or individuals at fault rather than identifying why the current system allowed the error to occur. When there is fear of blame or punishment (such as disciplinary action or litigation), a provider who makes a medical error will most likely not come forward and report his or her own participation in the undesirable event. But when errors are not discovered, the system cannot be adapted to prevent similar errors in the future. Establishment of a *just culture*, that is, an organizational culture that is a compromise between a *blame-free culture* and a *highly punitive culture*, is widely viewed as imperative in an organization's ability to identify and mitigate risk.

QUALITY IMPROVEMENT METRICS

Choosing the wrong quality metric may result in undesirable system adaptations. In the traditional fee-for-service pay model, an obvious institutional metric is the volume of care delivered, often measured in relative value units. The value of the service provided is not considered in this measurement. This is the classic *volume over value* problem. In medical imaging, tracking a volume metric will incent radiologists to finalize the maximum number of reports. Many undesirable shortcuts may be taken to achieve this goal. Images may be interpreted without proper clinical history or comparison to prior studies, the radiologist may avoid valuable clinical consultations with referring clinicians because they are time consuming and unrecognized by the volume metric. Individuals may be tempted to cherry-pick the easiest studies from the work list and may not make the proper effort to communicate critical results to referring physicians in person or by phone and may choose a faster and less reliable communication tool such as email or fax.

APPLICATION OF INDUSTRIAL QUALITY MANAGEMENT SCIENCE TO HEALTHCARE

The healthcare quality movement has incorporated many valuable quality management principles from industry. A few of the more notable examples of quality thought leaders and their QI systems and theories are presented along with industrial QI processes and approaches in the following paragraphs. Many of these concepts are explored in more detail in later chapters.

The Hawthorne effect (or the *observer effect*) was first reported following an investigation examining methods of increasing productivity in the Western Electric Hawthorne Works plant in Chicago during the 1920s and 1930s. The interesting finding is that no matter what change was introduced in working conditions, the result was increased worker productivity. For example, improving the lighting in the plant resulted in increased worker productivity, but reducing the lighting in production areas produced a similar productivity increase. The Hawthorne effect has been defined as an "increase in worker productivity produced by the psychological stimulus of being singled out and made to feel important." For example, a PQI project on imaging radiation measurements may result in shortening fluoroscopic times unrelated to an intervention, simply because the process is under observation. Subsequently, the Hawthorne effect definition has been broadened and may also be used to describe treatment responses in addition to productivity.

Walter A. Shewhart (1891–1967), a PhD physicist, used his understanding of statistical methods to design tools to respond to variation. After his arrival at Western Electric in 1924, he prepared a short memorandum of about a page in length, one-third of which was devoted to a simple diagram that would be recognized today as a control chart (Fig. 3.1). In his manuscript "Economic Control of Quality Manufactured Product," he introduced the concept of statistical process control.

W. Edwards Deming (1900–1993) is often referred to as the father of quality. He began as a statistics professor and physicist and was greatly influenced by the works of Shewhart. Deming was an advisor to Japanese auto industry leaders in the 1950s and provided advice on design, product quality, testing, and sales. He emphasized

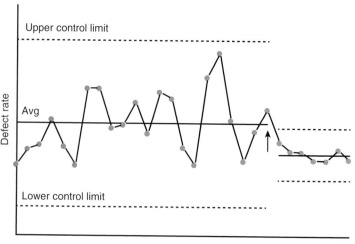

FIG. 3.1 The control chart (Shewhart chart) is a graphical quality tool used to study how a process changes over time with data plotted in time order. The control chart has a central line for the average, an upper line for the upper control limit, and a lower line for the lower control limit. Without the upper and lower control lines, it is simply a run chart. The upper and lower control limits are traditionally placed three standard deviations (sigmas) from the average. In a stable process, 99.7% of all data points will fall between the upper and lower control limits. This control chart shows a stable process. The data points do not fall outside the upper and lower control limits. During a quality improvement process, an intervention is performed (arrow). After the intervention, the average defect rate decreases and variability is reduced. Reduction in variability is demonstrated by contraction of the upper and lower control limits.

the importance of practicing continuous QI and thinking of manufacturing as a system. He proposed that around 15% of poor quality was due to workers and the remaining 85% was because of bad management and improper systems and processes. Deming built on the concepts he learned from Shewhart to develop the PDSA cycle and named this synthesis the Shewhart cycle (also called the Plan-Do-Check-Act cycle or the Deming cycle). This tool may be used with multiple cycles in sequence, with the initial PDSA cycle performed to obtain baseline data and subsequent cycles to assess the results of QI initiatives.

Joseph M. Juran (1904–2008) was an American engineer and management consultant who worked for Western Electric's inspection department. In 1941, Juran focused on the previous work of Italian economist Vilfredo Pareto and began to extrapolate on Pareto's finding that 80% of the income in Italy was received by 20% of the Italian population. The Pareto principle as it relates to quality suggests that roughly 80% of the effects come from 20% of the causes. This is also known as "the vital few and the trivial many." Like Deming, Juran also consulted with the Japanese auto industry in the 1950s. He is also noted for the *Juran Trilogy*, which describes three interrelated processes: quality planning, QI, and QC.

Kaoru Ishikawa (1915–1989) was a student of Deming and a member of the Union of Japanese Scientists and Engineers. A noted contribution of Ishikawa to the quality movement is the cause-and-effect diagram (Fishbone diagram, Ishikawa diagram).

The concept of total QC began in a 1951 book titled *Total Quality Management* by Armand Vallin Feigenbaum (1922–2014). He was an American QC expert and businessman. Feigenbaum defines total quality management as an excellence-driven rather than a defect-driven process. It is a system that integrates quality development, QI, and quality maintenance. He introduced the concept of the *hidden plant*, noting that so much extra work is performed in correcting mistakes that there is effectively a hidden plant within any factory.

APPLICATION OF LEAN AND SIX SIGMA TO HEALTHCARE

The Massachusetts Institute of Technology first used the term *lean* in 1987 to describe product development and production methods that produce more products with fewer defects in a shorter time. The Lean Process Improvement System (also known as the Toyota Production System) is an organizational style of continuous improvement workflow management that emerged from postwar Japan with an emphasis on smooth workflow from end to end. Lean describes a set of tools designed to eliminate or reduce waste. Waste is considered to be any element of the workflow that does not add value in the eyes of the end user. Principal forms of waste include transportation, inventory, motion, waiting, overproduction, overprocessing, and defective steps or products. The just-in-time (JIT) principle is an inventory strategy that companies employ to increase efficiency and decrease waste by receiving goods only as they are needed in the production process, thereby reducing inventory costs. Toyota adopted JIT as a means of eliminating waste associated with overproduction, waiting, and excess inventory. Much of the literature

written about JIT is limited to manufacturing, although JIT is equally applicable to all businesses, including hospitals. Pull systems and kanbans (alert systems) control the flow of resources in a production process by replacing only what has been consumed. Pull systems work to emulate one-piece flow where the subsequent step of work on a product or process occurs immediately at the completion of the prior step, the prior step does not create any more than the subsequent step can handle, and the subsequent step is not idly waiting on the prior step. This is achieved by producing a small buffer of inventory and instituting alert systems (kanbans) that signal readiness for additional parts or work.

The Six Sigma model is a set of techniques and tools for process improvement developed by Hewlett-Packard, Motorola, and General Electric in the 1980s and 1990s. Six Sigma seeks to improve quality by identifying and removing the causes of defects (errors) and minimizing variability in manufacturing and business processes. A Six Sigma process is statistically expected to be free of defects (3.4 defective features/million opportunities).

Industrial quality science emphasizes use of statistics to analyze production and service provision processes. It is based on the assumption that employees and top leadership should continuously strive to improve processes and stresses interdepartmental cooperation, training, and experimentation.

AMERICAN COLLEGE OF RADIOLOGY'S IMAGING 3.0

Imaging 3.0 is an initiative developed by the ACR to aid in the transformation of radiologists from being solely image interpreters to also becoming organizational leaders integrated into the new healthcare environment focused on adding value. Imaging 3.0 principles assist radiologists in using their expertise to expertly manage all aspects of imaging care prior to and following image interpretation to improve patient safety and outcomes, and deliver more cost-effective care. Imaging 3.0 positions radiologists as expert consultants to referring clinicians, coordinates service and technology tools to support radiologists as diagnosticians and consultants in new healthcare models, empowers and informs patients and providers to improve efficiency and quality of care, and helps sensibly align payment incentives as medicine shifts from a volume to a value-based payment model.

Radiologists using Imaging 3.0 must go beyond providing accurate image interpretation by making themselves available as expert consultants to referring physicians and healthcare systems and helping providers decide the optimal imaging studies using appropriateness criteria, decision support tools, previous imaging, and medical history. They should discuss imaging results with referring clinicians and provide meaningful, actionable reports by way of electronic medical records and decision support systems. They should use the principles of Image Gently and Image Wisely to optimize imaging radiation dose. Radiologists should acquire a working knowledge of information technology standards as they relate to equipment purchasing and operational decisions that support an infrastructure that enables implementation of Imaging 3.0. Radiologists must become local and national leaders and participate in shaping the future of the healthcare system by participating in discussions with other physician groups, medical facilities, and payers in their communities to work within integrated payment models such as accountable care organizations (ACOs) and capitated care agreements.

Imaging 3.0 offers a toolbox including the ACR appropriateness criteria, ACR Select Clinical Decision Support, ACR facility accreditation, ABR board certification and maintenance of certification, Image Gently and Image Wisely, patient consultations, image exchanges, the ACR Dose Index Registry, and ACR Imaging Centers of Excellence.

According to Dr. Paul Ellenbogen, former chair of the ACR Board of Chancellors, "Imaging 3.0 is a call to action for radiologists, policymakers, payers, referring physicians, and patients to provide optimal imaging care from the moment a clinician considers ordering an imaging study or treatment until that referring physician receives and understands an actionable report with evidence-based recommendations." The ultimate goal is to deliver all the imaging care that is beneficial and necessary to the patient and none that is not.

SUGGESTED READINGS

American Board of Radiology. Maintenance of Certification. Part 4: Practice Quality Improvement. <http://www.theabr.org/moc-dr-comp4/>.

American Board of Radiology. Noninterpretive Skills Resource Guide. <http://theabr.org/sites/all/themes/abr-media/pdf/Noninterpretive_Skills_Domain_Specification_and_Resource_Guide.pdf/>.

Abujudeh HH, Bruno MA. *Quality and Safety in Radiology*. New York, NY: Oxford University Press; 2012.

Abujudeh HH, Kaewlai R, Asfaw BA, Thrall JH. Quality initiatives: key performance indicators for measuring and improving radiology department performance. *Radiographics*. 2010;30(3):571-580.

American College of Radiology. ACR Appropriateness Criteria: Low Back Pain. <https://acsearch.acr.org/docs/69483/Narrative/>.

AHRQ. A quick look at quality. <http://archive.ahrq.gov/consumer/qnt/qntqlook.htm/>.

Allen B, Wald C. Imaging 3.0™. American College of Radiology; 2013:1-11. Available at: http://www.acr.org/~/media/ACR/Documents/PDF/Advocacy/IT%20Reference%20Guide/IT%20Ref%20Guide%20Imaging3.pdf.

Applegate KE. Continuous quality improvement for radiologists. *Acad Radiol*. 2004;11(2):155-161.

Brown JA. *The Healthcare Quality Handbook*. Pasadena, CA: JB Quality Solutions; 2011.

Bruno MA, Walker EA, Abujudeh HH. Understanding and confronting our mistakes: the epidemiology of error in radiology and strategies for error reduction. *Radiographics*. 2015;35(6):1668-1676.

Chapman SN. Adapting just-in-time inventory control to the hospital setting. *Hosp Mater Manage*. 1986;11(10):8-12.

Ellenbogen PH. Imaging 3.0: what is it? *J Am Coll Radiol*. 2013;10(4):229.

Erturk SM, Ondategui-Parra S, Ros PR. Quality management in radiology: historical aspects and basic definitions. *J Am Coll Radiol*. 2005;2(12):985-991.

Hillman BJ, Amis ES, Neiman HL. FORUM Participants. The future quality and safety of medical imaging: proceedings of the third annual ACR FORUM. *J Am Coll Radiol*. 2004;1(1):33-39.

Hynes DM. Quality management. *Can Assoc Radiol J*. 1994;45(5):353-354.

Institute of Medicine Committee to Design a Strategy for Quality Review and Assurance in Medicare. *Medicare: A Strategy for Quality Assurance*. Vol. 1. Washington, DC: National Academies Press; 1990.

Institute of Medicine. *Crossing the Quality Chasm*. Washington, DC: National Academies Press; 2001.

Institute of Medicine. *To Err Is Human: Building a Safer Health System*. Washington, DC: National Academies Press; 2001.

Joshi M, Nash DB, Ransom SB. *The Healthcare Quality Book: Vision, Strategy, and Tools*. 3rd ed. Chicago, IL: Health Administration Press; 2014.

Laffel G, Blumenthal D. The case for using industrial quality management science in healthcare organizations. *J Am Med Assoc*. 1989;262(20):2869-2873.

Margolis NE, Mackey RA, Sarwar A, Fintelmann FJ. 15 Practical ways to add value in daily practice: an imaging 3.0 primer for trainees. *J Am Coll Radiol*. 2015;12(6):638-640.

McCarney R, Warner J, Iliffe S, van Haselen R, Griffin M, Fisher P. The Hawthorne effect: a randomised, controlled trial. *BMC Med Res Methodol*. 2007;7(1):30.

Porter ME. What is value in health care? *N Engl J Med*. 363(26):2477-2481.

Chapter 4
Quality Improvement Tools

Cory Angelini and Elena Motuzko

INTRODUCTION

The challenge of a changing economy and increasing pressure in healthcare for optimal performance while dealing with limited resources and maintaining the high quality levels of medicine is becoming increasingly difficult. There is increasing demand for quality improvement to drive improved outcomes and reduce costs. The primary methodology used to deliver improved quality with lower costs is a process improvement methodology known as Lean Six Sigma. Lean Six Sigma originated in manufacturing and has since migrated to almost all industries, including healthcare. It has proven highly effective in its application to all aspects of care delivery, including patient satisfaction.

In all practices and industries there are processes that generate specific outcomes. The outcomes are measured by the level of quality. The level of quality is measured and defined by the specific customers of the processes. These customers may be internal to the organization or considered external customers. Examples of internal customers are a hospital or radiology group, and an external customer would be a patient or an insurance carrier.

A process is a combination of tasks in a specified order designed to create a specific outcome. An example would be the activities necessary to perform a radiologic study and generate a report. The outcome of this process is a completed radiology report.

The quality measures of this process are the metrics used to measure specific attributes of the process and the outcomes. However, before this can be done, a baseline performance of the metric in question must be established. Typically, a dashboard made up of key performance indicators is used to assess the current state of operations. We can use key performance indicators that represent high-level metrics to assess the performance of the operation. For the indicators that are not performing at the target level, the quality metrics impacting that indicator will be deduced.

It is important to explicitly define how all quality metrics will be measured, and for this reason operational definitions are used. It is extremely important to be as specific as possible in clearly stating operational definitions, because the accuracy of the operational definition will directly impact the accuracy of the metric being used to measure quality. If the measurement system of the process is not clearly defined through operational definitions, it may introduce increased variation in results.

The general approach in many industries emphasizes continuous improvement of processes to maintain and sustain high-quality performance. The foundation of Lean Six Sigma is based upon key quality improvement tools. Quality improvement tools can be applied as standalone tools or as part of an overall improvement effort, such as a process improvement project or activity. Finally, the quality activities should represent a continuous system that strives to improve the process.

CASE STUDY

To illustrate the application of some key quality improvement tools we will use examples of process improvement activities in a radiology department.

Case Description

A radiology department has a problem with a large study queue. The large study queue results in increased lag time to process the requested studies. This has a negative impact on other departments' metrics, such as emergency department wait time and length of hospital stay. Examination of dashboard key performance indicators shows an unexpected decrease in productivity along with a decreased number of generated reports when compared to prior years. The department head has asked his team to look into the process and apply various quality improvement tools to understand the problem and identify the root cause issues; this information will be applied to drive corrective actions. The goal is to improve the number of generated reports without negatively impacting the report quality and patient satisfaction.

Case Workup

The first step is to examine the process and define its outcomes. The number of reports generated will be the outcome metric.

The operational definition of the outcome metric (reports generated) is the following: A report is generated once the report is completed, finalized, submitted to the electronic health record, and the critical findings have been communicated to the ordering physician.

The following steps outline the sequence of further analysis and the quality tools used for that analysis:

1. The first step is to examine the outcome metric of how many reports were produced year over year. This is done by creating a *run chart*.
2. The second step is to define the process or the combination of tasks in a specified order to create the report and identify the responsible parties. This is done by creating a *flow chart* (also known as a *process map*).
3. The third step is to categorize and quantify high-level factors to narrow the focus and provide a general idea of where the main issue is occurring. This is done by generating a *Pareto chart*.
4. The fourth step is to analyze the contributing factors that influence the creation of the report by generating a *cause-and-effect diagram (fishbone diagram)*.

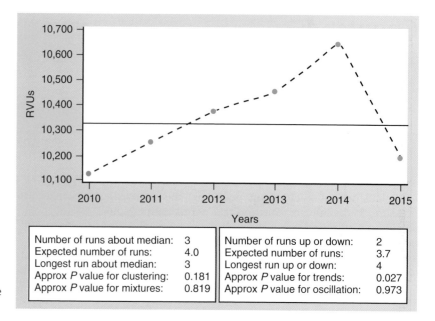

FIG. 4.1 Run chart of number of reports in relative value units.

Once the key specific factors (root causes) have been identified, the appropriate corrective actions can be determined and then taken to improve the established quality metric.

Run Chart

Definition. A run chart, also known as a run-sequence plot, is a graph that displays observed data plotted with respect to time. Often, the data displayed represent some aspect of the performance of a business process. This chart may be used to establish basic trends in relation to specific time periods. However, the interpretation is limited due to the characteristics of the data used. Run charts can be used to examine potential special causes of nonrandom variation in the data, specifically oscillation, clustering, mixtures, and trends. For instance, a cluster pattern may indicate variation due to special events such as a point of introduced change in the process, whereas mixture and oscillating patterns occur when the data fluctuate around a certain point or baseline, which can occur due to several factors affecting the process. The following example represents a sustained drift in the data, which can be interpreted as an upward trend until a turning point, after which the number of relative value units (RVUs) starts to trend down.

Example. The number of study reports produced by the radiology department, normalized by RVUs, will be used to account for the difference in complexity of the studies plotted per year. Fig. 4.1 demonstrates a drastic decrease in RVUs in 2015.

Flow Chart

Definition. Flowcharts are used in designing and documenting processes. Like other types of diagrams, they help visualize what is going on and thereby help users understand a process, and perhaps also find flaws, bottlenecks, and other factors contributing to the detriment of the quality improvement metric. There are many different types of flowcharts, and each type has its own repertoire of boxes and notational conventions. A flowchart is described as *cross-functional* when the page is divided into different swimlanes describing the activities of different organizational units or work performed by specific roles. Each symbol represents a particular category of activity.

Example. A simplified process is outlined that lists the basic steps involved in creating a radiology report in an inpatient setting (Fig. 4.2).

1. The order is placed in the electronic health record by the ordering physician.
2. The technician checks the laboratory results, allergies, and other factors that may represent contraindications for the study. At this decision point, the study proceeds or an alternative action is suggested.
3. The technician calls for patient transport.
4. The transport team picks up the patient from the room and brings the patient to the radiology department.
5. The technician enters the patient information into the system, chooses the appropriate protocol, and generates the accession number.
6. The radiology technician positions the patient in the scanner and performs the study.
7. Images are generated at the console.
8. Images are sent to the picture archiving and communication system.
9. The radiologist opens the study in the queue and evaluates the images.
10. The radiologist generates and finalizes the report.
11. The radiologist calls the ordering physician to review the findings and communicate the critical results.
12. The radiologist confirms that the ordering physician understands and acknowledges the results, upon which the appropriate note is documented in the report.

Practical Tips.
1. The programs that are most commonly used to create process maps or flow charts are:
   - Visio
   - Microsoft Excel
   - Flowgorithm
   - Raptor

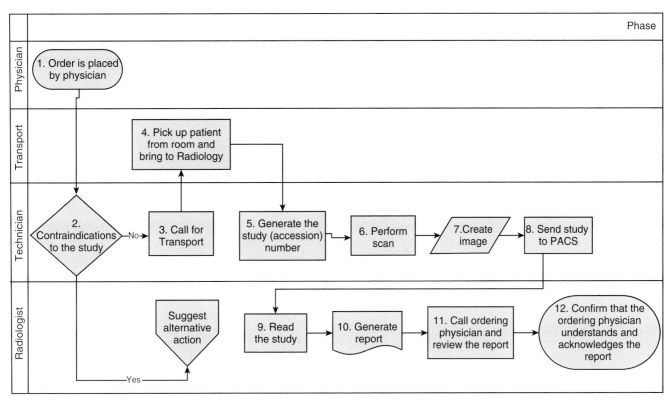

FIG. 4.2 Report creation in radiology for an inpatient study. *PACS,* Picture archiving and communication system.

- LARP
- Visual Logic
- VisiRule
- Logical Scheme Compiler
2. The following are best practices for creating a process map/flow chart:
   - Flowcharts flow from top left to bottom right.
   - Labeled connectors are used in complex or multi-sheet diagrams with arrows. For each label, the *outflow* connector must always be unique, but there may be any number of *inflow* connectors.
   - A concurrency symbol is represented by a double transverse line with any number of entry and exit arrows. These symbols are used whenever two or more control flows must operate simultaneously.
   - Horizontal rows, or *swimlanes*, may represent distribution or a category assignment, in this case these rows represent responsible parties (*Physician, Transport, Technician, Radiologist*).

Table 4.1 shows some of the shapes commonly used in flowcharts.

Pareto Chart

Definition. A Pareto chart, named after Vilfredo Pareto, is a chart that contains both bars and a line graph, where individual values are represented in descending order by bars, and the cumulative total is represented by the line.

The left vertical axis is the frequency of occurrence, but it can alternatively represent another important unit of measure. The right vertical axis is the cumulative percentage of the total number of occurrences or the total of the particular unit of measure. Because the reasons are in decreasing order, the cumulative function is concave.

The purpose of the Pareto chart is to highlight the most important among a (typically large) set of factors. In quality control, it often represents the most common contributing factors with numerical values and their relative percentage.

Example. Continuing the example of the radiology report creation process and factors contributing to lower report production, the contribution of the steps primarily responsible for the decreased number of reports was identified (Fig. 4.3). The largest contributing factor to be analyzed in more detail was circled.

Practical Tips.
- When creating a Pareto chart, focus on the factors contributing to about 80% of the output. The largest contributing factors or reasons for the impact upon output are further investigated to uncover the root causes.
- Wilkinson (2006) devised an algorithm for producing statistically based acceptance limits (similar to confidence intervals) for each bar in the Pareto chart.
- These charts can be generated by simple spreadsheet programs, such as Apache OpenOffice/LibreOffice Calc and Microsoft Excel, visualization tools such as Tableau Software, specialized statistical software tools, and online quality chart generators.

Cause-and-Effect Diagram

Definition. The cause-and-effect diagram, also known as a *fishbone or Ishikawa diagram*, is used to identify variation sources or factors contributing to a specific problem. Traditionally there are two versions of the primary factors used in this brainstorming diagram. The choice to use one version over the other depends on the nature of the business and its specific needs. Typically the *5 M's and an E* (man, machine, materials, measurement, methods,

TABLE 4.1 Shapes Commonly Used in Flowcharts

Shape	Name	Description
→	Flow line	An arrow starting at one symbol and ending at another symbol represents the flow of the process from one step to the next. The line for the arrow can be solid or dashed. The meaning of an arrow with a dashed line may differ from one flowchart to another and can be defined in the legend.
	Annotation	Annotations represent comments or remarks about the flowchart.
	Terminator	Represented as circles, ovals, stadiums, or rounded rectangles. They usually contain the word "Start" or "End," or another phrase signaling the start or end of a process.
	Decision	Represented as a diamond (rhombus) showing where a decision is necessary, commonly a yes/no question or true/false test.
	Input/output	Represented as a parallelogram. Involves receiving data and displaying processed data. Can only move from input to output and not vice versa. Example: If A, then B.
	Predefined process	Represented as rectangles with double-struck vertical edges; these are used to show complex processing steps, which may be detailed in a separate flowchart.
	Process	Represented as rectangles. This shape is used to show that an action occurred. Examples: "scan is performed," "study is read," etc.
	Off-page connector	Represented as a home plate–shaped pentagon. Symbol allows for placing a connector that connects to another page or reference.

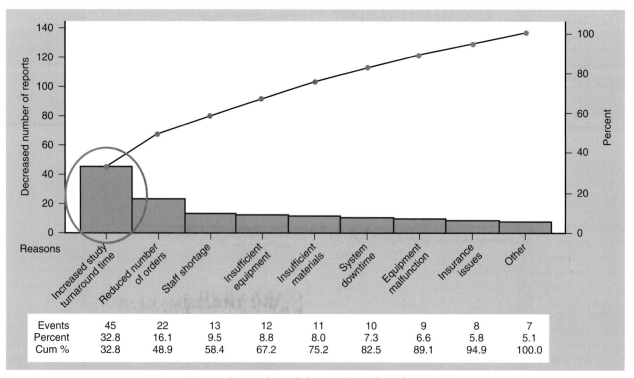

Events	45	22	13	12	11	10	9	8	7
Percent	32.8	16.1	9.5	8.8	8.0	7.3	6.6	5.8	5.1
Cum %	32.8	48.9	58.4	67.2	75.2	82.5	89.1	94.9	100.0

FIG. 4.3 Pareto chart of decreased number of reports.

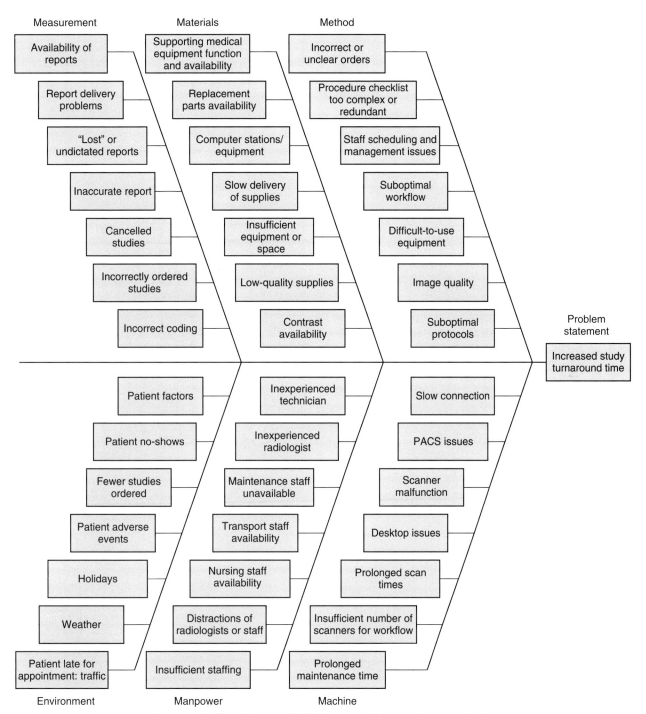

FIG. 4.4 Cause-and-effect diagram. *PACS,* Picture archiving and communication system.

and environment) approach is used for manufacturing and healthcare. The *6 P's* (people, product, price, place, promotion, positioning and environment) is typically used in service-related industries.

Example. Using the example provided in Fig. 4.1, showing the number of produced radiologic reports plotted for each month, it was identified that there were significantly fewer reports in certain months compared with others. To look further into the process, the major contributing factors that may affect the productivity of the radiology department will be outlined (Fig. 4.4).

Practical Tips.

1. On a large sheet of paper, draw a long arrow horizontally across the middle of the page pointing to the right, and label the arrowhead with the issue/problem to be analyzed. This is the backbone of the fish.

2. Draw spurs coming off the backbone at about 45 degrees, one for every category (man, machine, materials, measurement, methods, and environment), and label each at its outer end.
   - Add subspurs to represent potential root causes.
   - Highlight any causes that appear more than once; they may be significant.

3. The group considers each spur/subspur, taking the simplest first, partly for clarity but also because a good simple explanation may make more complex explanations unnecessary.

4. Circle anything that seems to be a key cause, so it can be examined in detail later.
   - Do not use the cause-and-effect diagram as an alternative form of process mapping.
   - Causes on the diagram must be verified with data.
   - Problems (effects) must be focused and specific before using this tool.
   - Broad definitions lead to too many items, are tedious to construct, are time consuming, and are very difficult to verify.

CASE STUDY SUMMARY

This case study used quality tools to illustrate a quality improvement activity for radiology. The example showed an expected decrease in the number of radiology studies for a given year as demonstrated in the run chart. With the flow chart, the workflow was mapped to identify the key players and events. The Pareto chart gave us the percentage and numerical value for the main events that were responsible for the decrease in the number of reports and their relative percentage. The largest contributing factors were analyzed using the cause-and-effect diagram to further dissect the causes of the delayed study turnaround time. This analysis provides a guide for further actions and interventions to consider to improve this process and address the issue of reduced report production.

CONCLUSION

In summary, quality improvement tools can be used effectively to analyze a complex problem and uncover the contributing factors to address the root causes. The previously mentioned quality improvement tools help drive changes in specified metrics and enhance the overall quality of the process output. To maintain a high level of quality in our processes, we need to continuously monitor, measure, and modify processes to yield improved outcomes. This pursuit of quality improvement drives the continuous improvement cycle advocated by the Lean Six Sigma methodology.

SUGGESTED READINGS

Arthur J. *Lean Six Sigma for Hospitals: Simple Steps to Fast, Affordable, and Flawless Health Care*. New York: McGraw-Hill; 2011.

Breyfogle FW. *Implementing Six Sigma: Smarter Solutions Using Statistical Methods*. 2nd ed. New York: John Wiley & Sons; 2013.

DeFeo JA. *Juran's Quality Handbook: The Complete Guide to Performance Excellence*. 7th ed. New York: McGraw-Hill; 2016.

Kiemele MJ. *Basic Statistics: Tools for Continuous Improvement*. 4th ed. Colorado Springs, CO: Air Academy Press; 1997.

Kubiak TM, Benbow DW. *The Certified Six Sigma Black Belt Handbook*. 2nd ed. Milwaukee, WI: ASQ Quality Press; 2009.

Pande PS, Neuman RP, Cavanah RR. *The Six Sigma Way*. New York: McGraw-Hill; 2014.

Chapter 5
Patient Safety

Bruce Berlanstein

Safety in radiology is expected by our patients, colleagues, administrators, providers, national organizations, oversight organizations, and the government. It is no longer enough to provide accurate reports of findings on imaging studies. Radiologists and their coworkers in the radiology department are also expected to provide patient-centered care and safe experiences prior to, during, and after imaging and procedures in radiology. To meet this need, considerable educational and other resources have evolved to guide radiologists and their staffs to carry out meaningful improvements in patient safety and have raised the awareness of existing tools to help assess and improve safety in radiology.

Today, radiologists are expected to be fully engaged in all aspects of radiology and to add value to the patient experience by ensuring that safety is at the forefront of care. Performing the right examination at the right time for the right reasons is now a basic assumption. Providing timely results is expected and communicating critical values in short time frames with appropriate follow-up is a widely expected outcome. Consistently delivering actionable recommendations based upon the best evidence available is on the horizon. Within the whirlwind of all these laudable goals is the patient who is likely to be ill and may be overwhelmed and confused by the medical system. As radiologists and staff working in radiology we must now, more than ever, examine our culture, processes, and experiences to do our best to ensure that the patient is kept as safe as possible, while accepting that no system is perfect and that adverse events are not completely preventable. Our goal is to consistently improve our processes and use adverse events and outcomes as opportunities for learning and making patient safety more robust. We do this realizing that it is the right thing to do and the right way to practice medicine. We accept that often there will not be additional reimbursement for better safety measures and that sometimes our leaders and those in positions of greatest power will talk about safety first but actually be less than devoted to the execution of safety measures when they conflict with financial targets. Still, we must keep our eyes on the patient and pursue our patients' safety as a core duty and basic element of our work in radiology.

SAFETY AND ERROR

A basic aspect of improving safety is understanding error. The study of human error has been important in industries like manufacturing and aviation for several decades. Medicine has more slowly embraced the study of error. Many cite 1996, with the publication of the monograph *To Err Is Human,* as the beginning of the serious study of safety and quality in medicine. At that time, the realization

began that the current state of affairs in medical care with respect to safety was unacceptable and urgent action was necessary to insure safe treatment of patients.

Quality improvement (QI) is a goal as well as a *hot topic* for discussion in many healthcare organizations. QI replaces the concept of quality assurance, which was more often than not reactive, punitive, and focused on assigning blame. QI has the goal of actually making things better. It involves retrospective and prospective reviews and data collection, which should be used to create systems that prevent errors from happening, or at least minimize errors and reduce their impact. It should attempt to avoid attributing blame, but people being people, that goal is not always achievable. Ideally, QI is a continuous process, hence the term *continuous quality improvement* (CQI). In CQI, the challenge is to closely examine a process that is working fairly well and tweak it to make it better still. However, once a process is *improved*, we tend to move on with other work and it is often a poor outcome or adverse event that forces us to go back to the process and look again to find and correct latent defects. Ideally, such discovery and improvement should be prospective, ongoing, and iterative, not episodic, sporadic, and reactive.

Quality control (QC) is often useful or essential as part of a practice quality improvement (PQI) project. PQI projects are the focus of a later chapter. QC is the process by which we review the quality of all elements and factors in producing an item of outcome. QC often involves evaluation of *accuracy*, *precision*, and *reliability*. Accuracy refers to the closeness of a measurement to the true value. Precision refers to the reproducibility of a measurement. Reliability includes both the accuracy and precision of a measurement. Therefore, QC evaluates a process for accuracy, precision, and reliability and provides data to validate the conclusions of a QI project.

QUALITY SCIENCE AND THE SIX AIMS

Quality in healthcare is sometimes referred to as *quality science*. Perhaps it is less rigorous than physics or mathematics, but it has come a long way in the past 20 or so years. Currently, quality efforts often include measurement, data analysis, and assessment for variation. In the past, variation was accepted or ignored; now variation is viewed as a potential concern and mainly something to be avoided. Leadership that supports QI, and the efforts necessary to obtain and analyze data, is essential to strides that have been made in this field, as well as ongoing progress.

Much of the focus on quality in healthcare and radiology derives from goals and publications originating from an organization known as the Institute of Medicine (IOM). Very recently the name changed to the National Academy of

Medicine (NAM), which is a nonprofit, nongovernmental organization that is part of the National Academies of Sciences, Engineering and Medicine. NAM provides advice on issues relating to biomedical science, medicine, and health. The advice should be evidence-based and may be used by policy makers as well as the public at large. The NAM has proposed the Six Aims of High-Quality Care: namely, that healthcare should be (1) safe, (2) timely, (3) effective, (4) efficient, (5) equitable, and (6) patient centered.

An integral part of the quality movement in healthcare is the Maintenance of Certification or MOC. In theory, MOC provides value by promoting lifelong learning that encourages incorporating new information and knowledge into routine clinical practice. The American Board of Radiology looks back at three previous years and determines if each diplomate is meeting MOC requirements. MOC touches on six core competencies: (1) patient care, (2) medical knowledge, (3) interpersonal and communication skills, (4) professionalism, (5) systems-based practice, and (6) practice-based learning and improvement. A central tenet is that patient care should be compassionate, appropriate, and effective and based upon established and evolving knowledge. Communication should be effective with patients, families, and professional associates. Performance of duties should be ethical and sensitive to diverse patient populations. Care givers should be able to work well as part of the team and help to improve the practice of medicine.

QUALITY METRICS AND DASHBOARDS

We all hope to practice quality medicine. However, quality can be an elusive goal, and choosing metrics that truly reflect the quality we seek can be challenging. Dashboards help us to assess quality and avoid unnecessary variation. A dashboard is a visual display of important information, just like in a car. As in driving, the information should be displayed so that it can be monitored at a glance. Benchmarking also helps us make some decisions regarding whether we are practicing quality medicine. It involves comparing a product, policy, program, or outcome with those of a similar organization or a peer. Hopefully we can learn from others how to achieve high performance and they can learn from us.

QUALITY AND VALUE: MEASUREMENT AND GRAPHICAL TOOLS

Just as *quality* can be hard to pin down conceptually, so can *value*. The term *value* brings to mind concepts like quality, cost, and efficiency. It may be useful to think of value as efficient use of resources to produce a desired result. Most analyses of value include a comparison of costs to benchmarks.

Thought leaders working in the field of value in healthcare often refer to key performance indicators (KPIs), which are measures used to define and evaluate the success of an organization. KPIs are specific to an organization's goals and strategies. One can look at progress in KPIs over time to determine whether an organization is making progress toward its goals.

There are a variety of methods that may be useful in the performance of a CQI project. One of the best-known

methods is the plan-do-study-act (PDSA) cycle (Fig. 5.1). This series of steps for gaining knowledge about a process was made well known by Dr. W. Edwards Deming and Walter Shewhart at the highly respected Bell Laboratories. It is meant to be an iterative process that identifies a goal, puts a plan into action, monitors outcomes with data collection, and acts on the information acquired to change and hopefully improve the process of a plan. It is important to have an appropriate measure or measures and to set a target level of performance desired. At the end of the first cycle, one can determine how well the data compares with the desired goal and also consider root causes for failure to meet the goal. After the first cycle, an improvement plan should be created and another PDSA cycle begins until the goal is achieved.

A method commonly used in QI projects involves graphical tools as a picture, which can often be more illuminating than a long discourse. An example of a graphical tool is the flow chart, where the steps in a process are presented as a diagram using commonly accepted symbols to illustrate the process and help clarify stress points as well as opportunities for improvement. A Pareto chart is another graphical tool where risk factors are displayed in order of importance. The fishbone diagram, also known as an Ishikawa diagram, is often used in root cause analysis (RCA) to help identify all causes that contribute to an identified problem in a manner that is visually inclusive and comprehensible (Fig. 5.2). The control chart is another method and is used to determine if a process is stable with variation coming only from sources common to the process. Analysis of a control chart may also help determine the sources of variation. Typically, control charts are used for time series data and therefore variation at a given time of day may be discovered. For further detail on these topics, the reader is directed to the suggested reading list at the end of this chapter.

THE HAWTHORNE EFFECT

In the performance of a QI project it is important to be aware of sources of bias. In particular, it is important to be aware of the *Hawthorne effect*, also known as the observer effect. This effect is exhibited in the fact that individuals modify or improve an aspect of their behavior simply in response to their awareness of being observed. As an example, in a study looking at radiation dose measurement during fluoroscopy, there was an initial decrease in fluoroscopic times when radiologists were monitored, which could be attributed to the Hawthorne effect. Interestingly, there is not universal acceptance of this effect by experts in the field, and some feel that it attenuates over time.

LEAN/SIX SIGMA

Yet another methodology used in the QI sphere is *Lean Six Sigma*. This methodology relies on a collaborative team effort to improve performance by systematically analyzing processes step by step, removing waste from each step, and finding ways to eliminate defects. The interest in this method was inspired by the success of the Toyota Motor Company. It was also central to the strategy of General Electric and Motorola. A core principle of Lean Six Sigma is respect for the relationships among employees, suppliers,

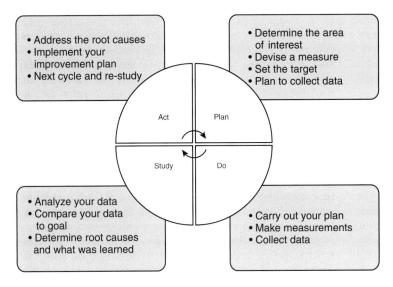

FIG. 5.1 Plan-do-study-act cycle of Deming and Shewhart, the core action in process improvement. (From Scottish Government. A Guide to Service Improvement: Measurement, Analysis, Techniques, and Solutions–Tools and Techniques for the Delivery of Modern Health Care: http://www.gov.scot/Publications/2005/11/04112142/21444. Copyright Institute for Healthcare Improvement.)

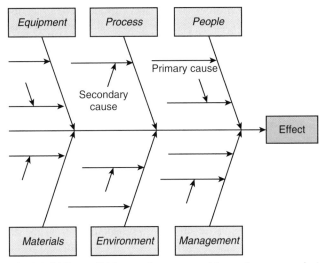

FIG. 5.2 Ishikawa fishbone diagram used in root cause analysis to map the multiple causes for any adverse event. (From Kodyaz Development Resources: http://www.kodyaz.com/pmp/ishikawa-diagram.aspx.)

and customers based upon mutual trust and dedication to improvement. This speaks to a healthy organizational culture, and although the sentiments are admirable, even Toyota seems to have had difficulty bringing this concept to fruition as it deals with large settlements for concealing safety issues with unintended acceleration and defective air bags. A focus on data collection, elimination of waste, and reduction in unnecessary variation suggests why Lean has become popular in healthcare. However, it is also important to accept that not all companies practicing Lean Six Sigma (including Toyota) have had sustained success. Some business leaders caution that "the process triumphs over judgment" (John Boyle, founder of the Vanguard Group).

In addition to the methods described previously, another technique used since the 1950s is brainstorming. It began in the advertising industry as a method for creative problem solving. It relies on a group process where a list of ideas is spontaneously contributed by the members of the group. Brainstorming seeks quantity of ideas, welcomes out-of-the-box thinking, and prohibits initial criticism. After ideas are accumulated, the group may vote on the value of the ideas, and retained ideas are eventually used as the basis of action plans. Brainstorming, along with all of the methods discussed, has its place and value. However, it is important to realize that the value of any of these techniques is open to skepticism, and, in fact, there is little objective evidence to support the inherent value of any given QI method. Still, experience suggests that each tool may have positive applications when combined with insight and wisdom.

THE JOINT COMMISSION

The Joint Commission (TJC) is an independent, not-for-profit organization that accredits and certifies healthcare organizations. Thus organizations seriously consider the goals of TJC and usually embrace its goals as part of the organization's safety priorities. Examples of some of the goals are prevention of falls, patient identification, reducing hospital infections, improving hospital staff communication, and avoiding abbreviations that lead to misinterpretation. These are part of the National Patient Safety Goals (NPSGs). Other goals that often impact radiology departments include reporting of critical results of tests in a timely manner, labeling all medications, maintaining accurate patient medication records, complying with hand hygiene guidelines, preventing central line–associated infections, conducting a preprocedure verification process, marking the proposed procedure site, and performing a time-out before the procedure. Adherence to these priorities and goals is important every day and not just when TJC inspection for accreditation is imminent.

TO ERR IS HUMAN

In 1999, the IOM (now known as the NAM) issued a report entitled *To Err Is Human: Building a Safer Health System.* The report highlighted the significant role of medical errors in patient deaths and ignited serious attention to improvement in the prevention of errors. Medical errors were defined as "the failure of a planned action to be completed as intended or the use of a wrong plan to achieve an aim." Most errors were felt to be due to flawed systems rather than problems related to individuals. The report suggested a strategy to significantly reduce errors and focused on an improved knowledge base regarding errors, learning from errors, motivating leadership to embrace error reduction, and raising expectations for improvements in safety. The end result of the report has been significant. The creation of the Agency for Healthcare Research and Quality (AHRQ), the creation of private enterprises focused on improving safety, and the creation of a list of mandatory reporting of adverse events are all outgrowths of *To Err Is Human*.

To prevent errors, it is useful to understand the type and nature of errors. Diagnostic errors are usually related to an error or delay in diagnosis. They may also involve a failure to employ an indicated test, use of an inappropriate test, or the failure to act on the results of tests. Treatment errors refer to errors in the performance of a procedure or treatment. This may include an error in drug dose, delay in treatment, or inappropriate treatment. Communication errors are failures to communicate information important for patient care. This is increasingly relevant in the practice of radiology. Prevention errors are those due to failure to provide follow-up or prophylactic treatment. There are yet other errors related to equipment and system failures, which are significant in the highly technical nature of radiology.

HIGH-RELIABILITY ORGANIZATION AND THE CULTURE OF SAFETY

An often-stated goal in healthcare is to become a *high-reliability organization*, that is, an organization that despite the stresses and risks involved in caring for patients, somehow manages to function with the fewest number of errors possible. These sorts of organizations tend to be mindful of potential sources of error and are consistently vigilant in reducing error. They also have a focus on the possibility of failure, avoid oversimplification, respect expertise, are sensitive to fine-tuning operations, and are resilient in the face of adversity. A prime example is Navy Aviation.

Ultimately, safety-focused organizations aspire to strive toward a *culture of safety*. It should not be surprising that the *safety culture* concept originated in organizations that valued high reliability. They acknowledged that to be highly reliable, they needed to maintain a commitment to safety from frontline providers to managers and executives. Organizations that embrace this culture of safety acknowledge the high-risk nature of their activities. They try to be as free of blame as possible and thus motivate individuals to report errors and near misses. Collaboration across disciplines and ranks is also viewed as a positive. Resources and money are devoted to help achieve safety goals, and, as such, the commitment is far from trivial. In fact, achieving a *culture of safety* is difficult, time-consuming, and sometimes expensive. In reality, although most organizations profess a culture of safety, it is a challenge to find examples that *walk the walk* on a daily basis. Fear of punishment for errors and lack of resources to prevent errors are unfortunately a reality. Safety teams, safety surveys, and executive walkarounds are likely well-intentioned and possibly effective approaches to achieving a greater safety culture, but they have yet to demonstrate links to lower error rates.

In theory, the concept of *no blame* sounds nice. However, we accept that humans are capable of good and bad behaviors. It is not challenging to consider a scenario where bad behavior or poor judgment contributed to an error or adverse outcome. Consider the healthcare worker who comes to work impaired by drugs or alcohol or is distracted by non-work–related texting. One can imagine poor outcomes related to these behaviors, and the newspapers chronicle real-life examples. Hence, the concept of a *just culture* has been proposed to reconcile the combined need for no blame and appropriate accountability. In the just culture model, there is a focus on correcting system issues that contribute to errors, and driving down and (as much as possible) eliminating reckless behaviors and poor judgment. For example, in a just culture, someone who made a good-faith human error would be consoled or provided with opportunities for remediation or education, whereas failure to observe an established safety norm would still merit significant punishment.

Some actions fall in an in-between space and are considered *at-risk behaviors*. An example might be a work-around of a safety norm to possibly reduce time or cost. At-risk behaviors are dealt with by improving incentives to do things the right way along with counseling, coaching, and monitoring the potentially at-risk behavior.

In achieving a safety culture, it might be useful to have an identified safety coach/champion. This individual fosters the culture of safety in the organization and takes ownership of the processes that support safety. The safety champion may help collect and disseminate safety data and promote solutions to potential safety breaches. The champion might consider a *forcing function* that would prevent a target action from being performed only if another action is performed first. For example, a patient in magnetic resonance imaging (MRI) may not be allowed to move closer to the magnet until a history is obtained indicating that he or she does not have a pacemaker in place that might be impacted by the magnet.

ACTIVE VERSUS LATENT ERRORS, AND THE *SENTINEL EVENT*

Attempts have been made to define error types. One classification considers *active errors* as different from *latent errors*. Active errors occur at a point of contact between a human and a system, such as pushing an incorrect button. Latent errors are the result of failures of design or process. Latent errors are often considered *accidents waiting to happen*. Understaffing a healthcare team is an example of a latent error. Active errors are sometimes referred to as errors on the *sharp end* of a symbolic scalpel, whereas latent errors are errors on the *blunt end*.

In the analyses of healthcare-related errors, a well-known term is the *sentinel event*. TJC describes a sentinel event as "an unexpected occurrence involving death or serious physical or psychological injury, or the risk thereof." An example might be unintentionally exposing a patient to a level of radiation that inflicts physical damage during a common test such as a computed tomography (CT) exam. Sentinel events require prompt investigation and a response or explanation, if possible.

PERCEPTUAL ERRORS OF RADIOLOGISTS

In radiology many errors are thought of as a *miss*. Inspecting a so-called *miss* with more attention reveals that the *miss* is often a failure to perceive a significant finding. Studies suggest that perceptual errors account for 60% to 80% of radiologist errors. It is frustrating and often embarrassing for the radiologist to know that the miss is evident in retrospect but was not noted or appreciated at the time of interpretation. Distractions and fatigue may contribute to perceptual error, yet this seems to be something inherent in visual processing that cannot be eliminated completely. Most radiologists are aware of the phenomenon of *satisfaction of search*, where one abnormality is identified but others are not because the radiologist directs too much attention on the first abnormality seen. This may also produce a perceptual error regarding the second, third, or more abnormalities in the study. Cognitive errors are less common and involve perceiving a finding and then ascribing a wrong significance or association to the finding. An example might be noting a lung nodule on a chest x-ray and wrongly attributing it to a benign process due to a relatively smooth shape and failing to realize that the nodule has been enlarging progressively based upon prior exams. Another cognitive error might arise from a lack of sufficient background knowledge. If a radiologist has never heard of Gardner syndrome for example, the radiologist might fail to look for desmoid tumors in the anterior abdominal wall.

ROOT CAUSE ANALYSIS, FAILURE MODE AND EFFECTS ANALYSIS, AND THE *SWISS CHEESE MODEL*

To some extent, errors are an inherent feature of the extremely complex system in which radiologists operate, yet there are tools for evaluating risk and adverse events that may be useful. Failure mode and effects analysis (FMEA) is a process that can be used to identify error risk. It begins by mapping all the steps in a given process. Next, each step is evaluated to determine how it might go wrong. The probability that an error will be detected and the impact of an error at each step are predicted to produce a criticality index. The criticality index is a rough estimate of the magnitude of hazard associated with each step in a process. In this way, targets for improvement can be identified and ideally a process can be made safer. In practice, assumptions and predictions are to some degree subjective, and the reliability of the technique is not guaranteed.

Unlike FMEA, which is prospective, RCA is a retrospective technique. RCA analysis has the goal of identifying problems that make errors more likely. RCA begins with data collection and reconstruction of the events leading to an adverse outcome. A multidisciplinary team works together to analyze the timeline and look for preventable errors. The focus is on system or latent errors with avoidance of assigning blame. The desired outcome from an RCA is the implementation of system changes that will reduce the likelihood of a future, similar adverse event. During the course of an RCA, it may become apparent that multiple errors intersected allowing the adverse event to impact a patient. This is known as the *Swiss cheese model* because events must pass through holes in the symbolic cheese to ultimately reach the patient. Ideally, an understanding of the model serves as a springboard to prevention of a potential future error.

In error analyses, a vocabulary of acronyms and terms has arisen and it is often assumed that those around the table speak the same language and understand the acronyms and terms. So far we have covered several of the acronyms such as FMEA, RCA, and the like. Two terms sometimes confused or wrongly used interchangeably are *accuracy* and *precision*. Accuracy is used to describe the closeness of a measurement to the true value. Precision is the closeness of agreement among a set of results. Using a target-shooting analogy, an accurate result hits the center bull's eye, or is very close. In target shooting, a precise result clusters all the bullets or arrows closely together even though they may be significantly away from the bull's eye.

PRACTICAL APPLICATIONS IN PATIENT SAFETY: THE UNIVERSAL PROTOCOL

Patient identification is central to safe care. To that end, two patient identifiers, such as name, date of birth, phone number, or medical record number, should be used to confirm patient identification prior to any procedure or treatment. Prior to an interventional image-guided procedure, a patient should be assessed by a focused history and physical exam and appropriate laboratory tests when needed. Informed consent is also necessary prior to an invasive image-guided procedure. Final responsibility for addressing patient concerns prior to a procedure rests with the provider performing or supervising the procedure. Elements of informed consent include a description of the procedure, the benefits of the procedure, and the risks and reasonable alternatives. Some patients may not be capable of giving consent due to illness or impairment, and consent should be obtained from a guardian, healthcare representative, or close family member. Physicians may provide treatment or perform a procedure without consent in situations where the patient might otherwise suffer death, major suffering, or disability.

The *Universal Protocol* was created to prevent wrong person, wrong procedure, and wrong site surgery. The first part is to conduct a preprocedure verification process to verify the correct procedure, the correct patient, and the correct site. If possible, the patient should be involved in the verification process. The next step is to identify the presence of items that must be available for the procedure. The items include the history and physical, signed consent forms, preanesthesia assessment, laboratory reports, imaging studies, equipment, devices, and possible blood products. Then, the procedure site is marked with involvement of the patient if possible. There are some situations and some sites where site marking is not possible or practical, for example, when going through a natural orifice or mucosal surface. The final step in the University Protocol is to perform a time-out to resolve any final concerns or questions. All relevant members of the procedure team communicate during the time-out and confirm the correct patient identity, the correct site, and the procedure to be done. Finally, the time-out is documented and the procedure may commence.

MAGNETIC RESONANCE IMAGING SAFETY

In radiology an area of intense interest and concern relates to safety in the MRI suite and scanner. The magnetic field is always on, and some healthcare personnel may not appreciate the implications of working in the MR environment. A key concept in MR safety is the division of the MR suite into four zones, based on proximity to the magnet and the magnetic field. There is progressive monitoring and restriction of entry into the higher-numbered zones closer to the magnet. Zone 1 is unrestricted but is the portal to the more controlled zones. Zone 2 is the interface zone where patients are greeted and screened. In zone 2, patients are under the supervision of MR personnel. Zone 3 houses the scanner control room and is very restricted. Zone 4 is the scanner room and the highest risk area. Access to zone 4 is under direct supervision of MR personnel. When a medical emergency occurs in the scanner room, the patient should be removed from zone 4 to a safe location while resuscitation is begun. In some instances a patient cannot cooperate for screening for MR safety and decisions must be made based on information from family members and available medical records. Another consideration in MRI safety is a quench event. When there is unexpected heating of magnetic coils, a quench event may occur with displacement of room air by helium gas. Emergency venting systems should activate, and all personnel must evacuate the scanner room.

INTRAVENOUS CONTRAST SAFETY

Contrast is widely used in radiology, particularly in CT, MR, and interventional procedures. Therefore, the safest possible use of contrast is paramount. Fortunately, contrast reactions are not common with less than 1% of patients experiencing reactions, which are usually mild or self-limited. Severe or life-threatening reactions are fortunately rare, with an incidence as low as 0.01% to 0.02% of all IV contrast administrations. When using contrast, it is optimal to consider if contrast is appropriate for a patient, to do what is possible to minimize the likelihood of reactions, and to always be prepared to treat a reaction. Because the greatest risk for a patient is a history of a prior reaction, it is important to take a careful patient history with respect to contrast allergy. Previously, a shellfish allergy was thought to be a significant risk factor, but that is now known not to be the case. However, a history of asthma is felt to increase the risk of contrast allergy.

It is appropriate to premedicate patients at increased risk of an acute allergic-like reaction to contrast. The concept is to limit the release or the effects of histamine and other mediators of allergic reactions by administration of corticosteroids. There are a variety of regimens but most include oral corticosteroids at least 6 hours prior to contrast with an H-1 antihistamine agent. *The ACR Manual on Contrast Media* provides guidance on specific regimens, but one widely suggested regimen is oral prednisone 50 mg at 13 hours, 7 hours, and 1 hour before contrast injection, plus 50 mg diphenhydramine given intravenously, intramuscularly, or by mouth 1 hour before contrast. Another recommendation would be methylprednisolone 32 mg by mouth 12 hours and 2 hours before contrast media injection. An antihistamine (as mentioned above) can also be added to this regimen injection. If the patient is unable to take oral medication, 200 mg of hydrocortisone intravenously may

be substituted for oral prednisone. Premedication regimens have been shown to reduce minor reactions, but there is a lack of evidence to show that severe reactions are prevented with premedication. Therefore, it is important to be prepared to treat a contrast reaction whether mild or severe in all patients, even those patients who have been premedicated. The *ACR Manual on Contrast Media* provides guidance regarding treatment. Diphenhydramine is recommended for hives. Epinephrine is used for moderate or severe reactions involving facial or laryngeal edema, bronchospasm, or hypotension. Vagal reactions (hypotension with bradycardia) may require IV atropine. Pulmonary edema may require IV diuretics, and seizures may need treatment with IV diazepam. In addition to becoming familiar with appropriate therapy, it is helpful to have treatment options posted and available for review when needed. In addition, it is advisable to have practice walk-throughs including how to get help from a rapid response team that is more experienced in treating cardiovascular and respiratory emergencies.

In addition to being aware and capable of treating a contrast reaction, it is important to be knowledgeable regarding contrast-induced nephropathy (CIN). It is a sudden deterioration in renal function following recent intravascular contrast media. There is some latitude in the definition of CIN as well as uncertainty in pathogenesis. Usually there is a rise in serum creatinine within 24 hours of contrast administration with a return to baseline within 7 to 10 days. The dose of contrast given may be a risk factor, but the evidence is not conclusive. Without overwhelming evidence to support the approach to CIN, there is a consensus that preexisting renal insufficiency confers an increased risk. The *ACR Manual on Contrast Media* suggests a serum creatinine of 2.0 gm/dL as a risk factor and other potential risk factors may include diabetes mellitus, dehydration, advanced age, and multiple myeloma.

In light of what is known, the *ACR Manual on Contrast Media* suggests obtaining a serum creatinine measurement in patients older than 60 years and in patients with a history of significant renal disease, diabetes mellitus, and hypertension requiring medical therapy. If the patient is stable, a creatinine value within 30 days of contrast administration is adequate. For patients taking metformin, it is also considered prudent to obtain a creatinine level, because they have an increased risk of lactic acidosis with renal failure. In patients who are considered to be at increased risk for CIN, exams that avoid contrast, such as ultrasound, should be looked at as alternatives. If essential information can only be provided with the use of contrast, then the lowest dose of contrast possible is suggested, even though there is no clear proof of a dose-related risk. Patients should also be well hydrated preexam and postexam using IV 0.9% saline if there is concern for potential CIN. Recent studies question this long-held belief and suggest that "no prophylaxis to be noninferior and cost saving in preventing contrast-induced nephropathy compared with intravenous hydration according to current clinical practice guidelines" (Nijssen et al). Therefore, if the results are reproduced in follow up studies, the practice of precontrast and postcontrast hydration may be no longer recommended. Patients on chronic hemodialysis who receive intravenous contrast do not require immediate postcontrast dialysis.

In general, similar precautions should be followed when using gadolinium-based MR contrast agents as when using iodine-based CT contrast agents. Reactions to gadolinium-based contrast media (GBCM) are less frequent than reactions to iodinated contrast media. Severe reactions to MR contrast agents have been reported but are extremely rare. GBCM is relatively contraindicated in pregnant patients because there may be prolonged presence of the chelate in the amniotic fluid and risk of dissociation of the gadolinium ion to the fetus is a concern, although the actual risk is unknown.

Much has been discussed in the medical literature and in the popular press regarding the use of GBCM and the risk of nephrogenic systemic fibrosis (NSF), a fibrosing disease primarily noted in the skin and subcutaneous tissues but also involving other organs. Affected patients often experience skin thickening and pruritus, but may also have contractures at joints and involvement of the heart, lungs, and gastrointestinal tract that could lead to death. There is much that is uncertain about NSF, however, and there appears to be an association between chronic kidney disease or acute kidney injury, administration of GBCM, and the development of NSF. Some gadolinium agents appear to have a greater risk for the development of NSF than others. Therefore, agents with the highest association with NSF should be avoided in patients with a history of renal disease and the lowest dose possible should be used. The *ACR Manual on Contrast Media* recommends obtaining an estimated glomerular filtration rate (eGFR) within 6 weeks of anticipated GBCM and avoiding contrast in patients with a eGFR <30 mL/minute per 1.73 m^2 or with an acute kidney injury.

Another area of concern regarding the use of intravenous contrast is extravasation when contrast enters the soft tissues rather than a vein. So-called extravasation of contrast is more likely to be significant when a power injector is used because a large volume of contrast is injected over a shorter time. Patients at greater risk are those unable to communicate and/or patients with abnormal circulation to the site of the injection. Injections into more distal sites like the hand or foot are considered venous access risk factors. Use of indwelling catheters in place for more than 24 hours and veins that have been recently punctured are also conditions to be avoided if possible. Extravasated contrast is toxic to the skin and initiates an acute inflammatory response that often peaks in 24 to 48 hours. In rare instances there can be tissue necrosis with skin ulceration. If the volume of extravasated contrast is significant, there may be mechanical compression of adjacent tissues resulting in a compartment syndrome. The best treatment for extravasation is uncertain. Most suggest elevation of the affected extremity above the level of the heart to promote reabsorption by decreasing capillary hydrostatic pressure. Warm or cold compresses may provide symptomatic relief. Clinical follow-up is advised for several hours to determine how the patient will respond. Patients with worsening symptoms, neurologic or vascular symptoms, and skin ulceration require prompt surgical evaluation.

RADIATION SAFETY

An area of active interest in radiology safety is reducing exposure to medical radiation. Much has been written on the topic, yet a great deal remains uncertain. The consensus suggests that there are real and potential risks from medical radiation and radiologists should be actively involved in reducing patient exposure, especially for pediatric populations. The radiology community responded by creating the "Image Gently" campaign. The goals have been to communicate concerns regarding radiation exposure to healthcare professionals, parents, and the public; to create a website highlighting information about medical radiation and dose reduction; and to review and adjust protocols to limit radiation doses to children. The "Image Gently" campaign contributed energy and enthusiasm to launch the "Image Wisely" program, which is focused on optimization of radiation dose in adults. This has raised awareness to lower the dose of radiation in medical exams and to strive to perform only exams that are most appropriate. Similar to "Image Gently," a website has been created with resources to help limit radiation including a Patient Medical Imaging Record that allows patients to track and catalog their imaging exams for future reference. Many radiologists have embraced the concepts of "Image Wisely" and have committed to be consultants regarding imaging and to provide explanations to patients seeking more information about the risks and benefits of medical imaging procedures.

Determining the radiation dose received by a patient having a CT exam is challenging and is affected by many technical parameters and the scan protocol. In order to simplify the radiation dose calculation, medical physicists calculate an estimated dose based on measurement from a phantom. The American College of Radiology (ACR) has developed a Dose Index Registry that allows facilities to compare and benchmark their own data with facilities that are felt to be similar. If a facility notes data that shows higher radiation doses than its peers, it can modify the scanning parameters and tune the equipment to be more in line. Usually, this work is performed under the auspices of a qualified medical physicist.

Radiation dose management and radiation safety in general have been guided by the ALARA principle, which stands for *as low as reasonably achievable*. This means that dose reduction devices are active and used and that periodic radiation exposure is monitored by a trained medical physicist.

The ALARA principle pertains to keeping the radiation dose as low as possible when performing an examination. However, of equal importance is choosing imaging only when appropriate and considering alternative exams that avoid ionizing radiation. To that end, the ACR Appropriateness Criteria and Decision Support assist radiologists and referring physicians in making decisions regarding imaging for specific clinical conditions. The program has continued to expand and become more comprehensive over time, yet not every clinical scenario is covered. The decisions are based on scientific evidence when available and expert consensus when evidence is less robust. The appropriateness of an imaging modality for a given clinical condition is rated on a 1 (low) to 9 (high) scale. Modalities rated 7 to 9 are usually considered appropriate. The process also assigns a *relative radiation level* to a modality so that a provider may also be mindful of patient dose.

IMPROVING RADIOLOGISTS' COMMUNICATION

There is agreement that clear communication is essential to making the patient experience safer. To that end, there has been renewed interest in improving the radiologist's report. The thrust has been to advocate for reports that avoid vague or confusing terminology and to create reports that can be acted upon to improve patient outcomes. The model appears to be based on the Breast Imaging Reporting and Data System, which is used for breast imaging. This model of reporting will decrease variation, which is often an issue in less stable and safe systems.

IMPROVING THE APPROPRIATENESS OF IMAGING UTILIZATION: ACR APPROPRIATENESS CRITERIA

Another campaign designed to decrease radiation dose and enhance safety and quality is the "Choosing Wisely" campaign. This campaign includes guidelines, recommendations, and software to help radiologists and referring providers choose exams for their patients that are most likely to change patient management or improve patient outcomes. For example, information is provided that informs those ordering exams that patients with uncomplicated headaches do not require any special imaging. The recommendations are made by committees composed of a mix of appropriate specialists and are based on peer-reviewed literature. Organizations adopting clinical decision support based on the *ACR Appropriateness Criteria* recommendations (available online) appear to be able to decrease or slow the growth of imaging studies performed, at least with respect to some modalities for some conditions. An example would be reducing MRI exams of the lumbar spine for patients with uncomplicated back pain.

ACR PRACTICE GUIDELINES AND TECHNICAL STANDARDS

In addition to decision support, the ACR provides guidelines regarding radiologic practice in the *ACR Practice Guidelines and Technical Standards*, available online. This document provides radiologists with a roadmap of acceptable approaches for the diagnosis and/or treatment of many diseases or conditions. The guidelines are consensus based and validated by available scientific evidence and they are regularly updated. The guidelines include many useful topics, ranging from how to be an expert witness in a malpractice trial to the safest possible imaging of pregnant patients. Considering the range and depth of topics covered, it is a useful resource to keep in mind and to consult as needed.

PEER REVIEW

Peer review is often required or advised by accrediting groups and hospital administration, such as TJC. Although some view this process as a way to ensure quality, it may also be a method of providing opportunities for learning and improvement. Most peer-review processes randomly sample a small portion (3%–10%) of clinical work done by each radiologist for review with a mechanism for feedback. The standard for peer review is peer consensus, because pathological or surgical proof is often not available. Generally, peer-review data is protected from medical-legal discovery. Ideally, the peer-review process avoids blame and rather presents opportunities for learning and growth. The Joint Commission also requires Ongoing Professional Practice Evaluation and Focused Provider Practice Evaluation in which the qualifications for ongoing practice privileges are monitored and reviewed. The intent is to create opportunities for awareness that the radiologist is performing at a level expected. Although data supporting the value of these evaluations is scarce, the potential for meaningful improvement is real and depends on the details and execution of the processes.

CONCLUSION

The study of safety and quality in healthcare is relatively new and evolving. Improvements in the collection of large volumes of data, data analysis tools, and electronic medical records provide opportunities for rapid advancement. More evidence is needed to validate safety and quality programs and assessment tools on an ongoing basis. There is little doubt that concerns about medical errors impacting patients are real. There is also no doubt that measuring the problem is an essential first step. Dedication to creating better systems to provide safer healthcare and a personal sense of commitment to safety and high-quality care should help to make the experience of being a patient better and safer.

SUGGESTED READINGS

Abujudeh H, Bruno MA. *Quality and Safety in Radiology*. New York, NY: Oxford University Press; 2012.

American College of Radiology. Appropriateness Criteria <http://www.acr.org/quality-safety/appropriateness-criteria>.

American College of Radiology. Practice Parameters and Technical Standards <http://www.acr.org/Quality-Safety/Standards-Guidelines>.

Nijssen EC, Rennenberg RJ, Nelemans PJ, et al. Prophylactic hydration to protect renal function from intravascular iondinated contrast material in patients at high risk of contrast-induced nephropathy (AMACING): a prospective, randomised, phase 3, controlled, open-label, non-inferiority trial. *Lancet*. 2017. Epub ahead of print.

Chapter 6
Quality Improvement in Radiology

Mohammad Mansouri and Hani H. Abujudeh

INTRODUCTION

In 2012, the American Board of Radiology (ABR) implemented a new Maintenance of Certification (MOC) process, known as Continuous Certification, for all participating diplomates. Every year on March 15, the ABR looks back at the previous 3 years for each diplomate to consider if he or she is meeting the MOC requirements.

All diplomates who hold continuous certificates issued in 2012 or after or time-limited certificates are automatically enrolled in the MOC program when they obtain their certification. Diplomates who hold lifetime certificates may voluntarily enroll in the program to enter the MOC process. The MOC program is designed to continuously evaluate the following six essential competencies:
1. Medical knowledge
2. Patient care and procedural skills
3. Interpersonal and communication skills
4. Professionalism
5. Practice-based learning and improvement
6. Systems-based practice
   The MOC program consists of four parts:
1. Professional Standing
2. Lifelong Learning and Self-Assessment
3. Cognitive Expertise
4. Practice Quality Improvement (PQI)

The ABR lists several activities in which diplomates can participate to fulfill the Part 4 requirements. Prior to 2016, completing at least one *PQI project* or activity was mandatory in each 3-year cycle. Currently, a PQI project is one of two activities that demonstrate the diplomate's commitment to and participation in quality improvement, and thus to satisfying the ABR MOC Part 4 requirements. Diplomates who choose to do a PQI project may use any standard quality improvement methodology (including, but not limited to, plan-do-study-act [PDSA], Lean and Six Sigma, failure mode and effects analysis [FMEA], and root cause analysis) to meet the MOC Part 4 requirements. *Participatory Quality Improvement Activities* are also available in which the diplomate engages as a volunteer or by duty during his or her workday. These activities are reasonably expected to contribute directly to or increase the likelihood of advancement or improvement of quality and/or safety in healthcare at the local or national level. This chapter focuses primarily on the elements of a PQI project that satisfy the MOC Part 4 requirements.

TOOLS TO INVESTIGATE QUALITY PROBLEMS IN RADIOLOGY

Several tools can help radiologists find opportunities to improve quality and safety in their practice. These tools include surveys, flowcharts or process maps, safety incident reporting or error reporting systems, chart reviews and investigation of compliance with national patient safety goals, analyzing radiology report addenda, and brainstorming with colleagues.

There are seven basic graphical tools that can be used to depict data: (1) flowcharts, (2) cause-and-effect analysis (Ishikawa or fishbone diagrams), (3) Pareto charts, (4) check or tally sheets, (5) control charts (Shewhart or statistical process charts), (6) histograms, and (7) scatter diagrams. Scorecards and dashboards are the tools to display the data and monitor the results.

PARTICIPATORY QUALITY IMPROVEMENT ACTIVITIES

Candidates must document individual active participation in any of the activities listed in Box 6.1 to fulfill the criteria for MOC Part 4.

PRACTICE QUALITY IMPROVEMENT PROJECTS

The following are examples of PQI project topics:
- Improving report turnaround time
- Improving patient access (next available appointment)
- Optimizing radiation dose/examination or frequency of repeat examinations
- Improving the time-out process for procedures
- Decreasing wrong patient/wrong procedure events
- Standardizing reports
- Reducing magnetic resonance imaging safety events
- Improving critical results notification
- Improving care handoffs

Methodologies to Perform Quality Improvement Projects

Root Cause Analysis

Root cause analysis is an approach that identifies an error, how the error occurred, and why the error occurred to help determine actions to minimize or prevent its recurrence. This approach requires a team of four to 10 investigators who have different roles and

- Participation as a member of an institutional/departmental clinical quality and/or safety review committee. Examples include meaningful participation as a member responsible for creating, reviewing, and/or implementing clinical quality improvement safety activities; service as a radiation safety officer.
- Active participation in a departmental or institutional peer-review process, including participation in data entry and evaluation, the peer-review meeting process, or ongoing professional practice evaluation.
- Participation as a member of a root cause analysis team evaluating a sentinel or other quality- or safety-related event.
- Participation in at least 25 prospective chart rounds every year (peer review of the radiation delivery plans for new cases; radiation oncology and medical physics only).
- Active participation in submitting data to a national registry.
- Publication of a peer-reviewed journal article related to quality improvement or improved safety of the diplomate's practice content area.
- Invited presentation or exhibition at a national meeting of a peer-reviewed poster related to quality improvement or improved safety of the diplomate's practice content area.
- Regular participation (at least 10 per year) in departmental or group conferences focused on patient safety. Examples include regular attendance at tumor boards, morbidity and mortality conferences, diagnostic/therapeutic errors conferences, interprofessional conferences, surgical/pathology correlation conferences, etc.
- Creation or active management of, or participation in, one of the elements of a quality or safety program. Examples include a department dashboard or scorecard, a daily management system to ensure quality and safety, and a daily readiness assessment using a huddle system.
- A local or national leadership role in a national/international quality improvement program, such as "Image Gently," "Image Wisely," "Choosing Wisely," or other similar campaign. Local participation roles include implementation and/or maintenance of, or adherence to, program goals and/or requirements.
- Completion of a peer survey (focused on quality or patient safety) and resulting action plan. The survey should contain at least five quality- or patient safety–related questions and have a minimum of five survey responses.
- Completion of a Patient Experience-of-Care survey with individual patient feedback. The survey should contain at least five quality- or patient safety–related questions and have a minimum of 30 survey responses.
- Active participation in applying for or maintaining accreditation by specialty accreditation programs such as those offered by the American College of Radiology (ACR) or the American Society for Radiation Oncology.
- Annual participation in the required Mammography Quality Standards Act medical audit or ACR Mammography Accreditation Program.
- Completion of a self-directed educational project on a quality- or patient safety–related topic (medical physics only).
- Active participation in a National Cancer Institute cooperative group clinical trial (for diagnostic radiologists, radiation oncologists, and interventional radiologists, entry of five or more patients in a year. For medical physicists, active participation in the credentialing activities).

backgrounds. For example, if the error occurred within a department, the investigators would come from that department and be related to the event that occurred. A fishbone (or cause-and-effect) diagram is usually used, and the *five whys* are asked to identify the root cause of the error. The team first answers the question, "Why did this happen?" After each answer, the question is then repeated at least four more times in an attempt to drill down to the root cause.

Root cause analysis can also be done for sentinel events. The Joint Commission defines a sentinel event as a safety event that affects a patient and results in death or major harm to that patient. Organizations are strongly encouraged to report sentinel events. The Joint Commission recommends 11 steps for performing root cause analysis of sentinel events. These steps are summarized in Fig. 6.1.

Failure Mode and Effects Analysis

This approach aims to prospectively identify and prevent an error before it occurs. Investigators try to identify and understand potential failures in processes, systems, or practices. Because this approach is proactive and thus blame-free, clinicians are more likely to cooperate and accept the process compared with retrospective, potentially blameful approaches like error reporting systems.

Based on The Joint Commission recommendations, a team is organized and chooses a process that can potentially go wrong. The flowchart of the process as it is designed is compared with the flowchart of the process as it is routinely conducted. Discrepancies between the flowcharts are listed as potential failure modes. Each failure mode is assessed for severity of effect, probability of failure, and invisibility of failure. Based on these estimates, a criticality index and risk priority numbers are calculated to rank and prioritize the failure modes. The team creates an action plan and follows up to improve any unacceptable failure mode (Fig. 6.2).

Lean and Six Sigma

Lean and Six Sigma are industrial management techniques that are being increasingly used within the healthcare system. These two techniques focus on eliminating defects. Lean principles come from the Toyota Production System and include a five-step process:

1. Identify value from the customer point of view.
2. Identify the process in the value stream and eliminate steps that do not add value.
3. Tightly sequence the value-creation process so the product will flow smoothly toward the customer.
4. Introduce the new process and let customers pull value from the next upstream activity.
5. Continue the process to create perfect value with no waste (Fig. 6.3).

The Lean technique focuses strongly on customer values and uses a standardized method to solve common problems. However, the Lean method is weak on deployment plans, organizational infrastructure, analytical tools, and quality control management.

The Six Sigma strategy was developed by Motorola and is based on reducing variability within a process and

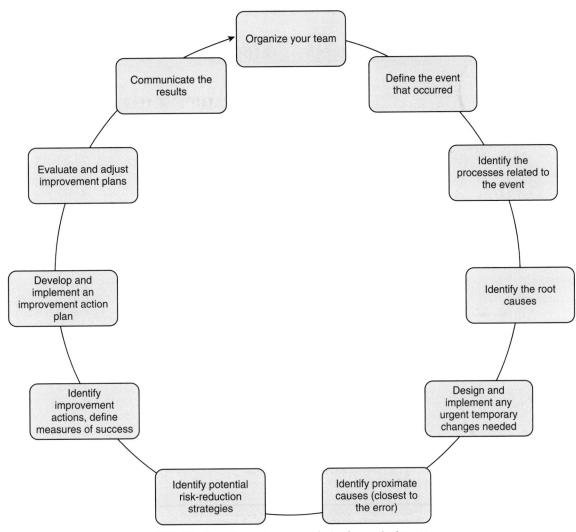

FIG. 6.1 Steps for root cause analysis of a sentinel event.

improving the mean to reach a gold standard. Six Sigma uses a five-step approach called DMAIC (define, measure, analyze, improve, control) to reduce unnecessary variations (Fig. 6.4). Six Sigma is overly complex when applied to solving simple problems that have obvious solutions, which is its main weakness.

Plan-Do-Study-Act

This four-step process is a simple but powerful technique that is commonly used for quality improvement projects. Data is gathered in the initial PDSA cycle, followed by subsequent cycles that assess the effects of quality improvement actions until the goal is reached (Fig. 6.5). Intermittent PDSA cycles help document the stability of achievements.

Plan: Identify an area in need of improvement, the objectives to be attained, and the team. Determine the goal to be achieved and how success will be measured. Create a plan or process for collecting data.

Do: Carry out the plan and collect data.

Study: Compare measures to the desired goal, summarize what was learned, and investigate the root causes.

Act: Make changes to the process based on the results of the analysis and repeat the PDSA cycle.

Individual Practice Quality Improvement Projects

Individual PQI is appropriate when diplomates cannot find colleagues with a similar area of interest. Individuals may choose self-designed projects or preapproved society-sponsored projects, including registries. Table 6.1 compares the differences between self-designed and preapproved society-sponsored projects. The ABR provides a PQI project template for individuals who decide to use the PDSA methodology.

Baseline PDSA Cycle

Select an area of interest and choose a challenging topic. Devise a measure to gauge the issue and set goals. Set the plan in motion and collect data. Analyze the data and compare the results with the desired level. If the target is met, set up a plan to ensure that the gain is sustained and do intermittent PDSA cycles. The diplomate must attest to project completion at the ABR website. If the goal was not achieved, determine the root causes and implement an improvement plan.

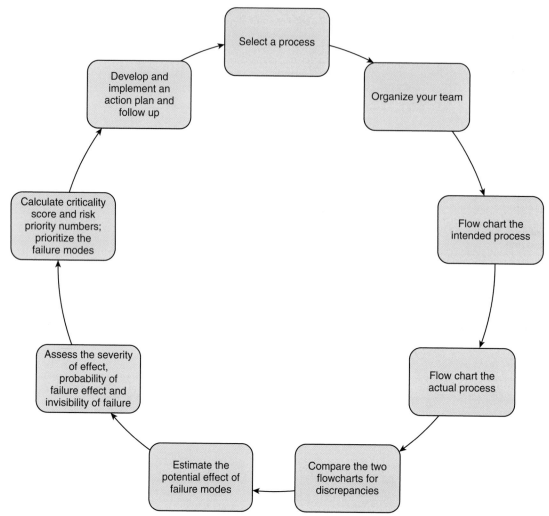

FIG. 6.2 Recommended workflow for failure mode and effects analysis.

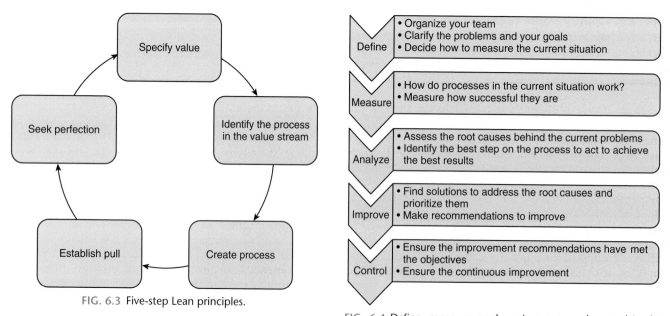

FIG. 6.3 Five-step Lean principles.

FIG. 6.4 Define, measure, analyze, improve, and control in the Six Sigma strategy.

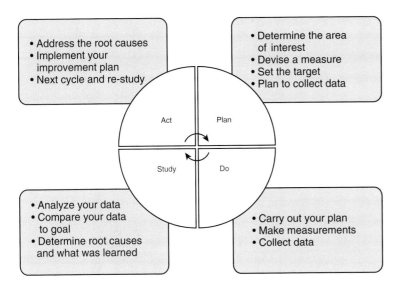

- Address the root causes
- Implement your improvement plan
- Next cycle and re-study

- Determine the area of interest
- Devise a measure
- Set the target
- Plan to collect data

Act   Plan

Study   Do

- Analyze your data
- Compare your data to goal
- Determine root causes and what was learned

- Carry out your plan
- Make measurements
- Collect data

FIG. 6.5 Plan-do-study-act cycle.

TABLE 6.1   Self-Designed Compared With Preapproved Society-Sponsored Projects

Self-Designed Projects	Preapproved Society-Sponsored Projects (Including Registries)
Flexibility in choosing topics	Wide-interest topics; investigators must adapt the projects to local realities
Documentation processes, project design, and data collection should be done by the individual	Time is saved in administrative and documentation processes, project design, and data collection
Approval not required; guidelines and standards must be followed	Approval not required; projects are designed based on guidelines and standards
Documentation and recordkeeping are necessary	Documentation and recordkeeping are necessary

Post-PQI PDSA Cycle

Repeat the PDSA cycle after implementation of the improvement plan. Analyze the data gathered, and consider if the project goals were reached or if additional action and PDSA cycles are required. Repeat the cycle until the goal is reached or the endpoint is determined. Make the improvement plan routine, and perform intermittent PDSA cycles to ensure that the gain will be sustained. Individuals are required to prepare a paragraph of self-reflection, stating how the project improved their practice. Candidates must attest to completing their project at the ABR website.

Group Practice Quality Improvement Projects

A group is defined by the ABR as two or more diagnostic radiologists, radiation oncologists, or medical physicists of the same or different disciplines, sharing a common central organizational structure, who work together to provide patient care, regardless of individual contractual affiliations or relationships. These diagnostic radiologists, radiation oncologists, or medical physicists may provide services at single or multiple facilities or locations in a variety of clinical settings, including hospitals, offices, or patient imaging centers.

Similar to individual PQI projects, groups can perform projects that are designed by the group or preapproved society-sponsored projects (including registries; see Table 6.1). Table 6.2 compares the benefits of individual and group PQI projects. At least four group PQI meetings are required: before the plan, study, and act

phases of the baseline PDSA cycle and before the act phase of the postimprovement PDSA cycle.

Standards for a Group PQI Project

The ABR sets certain standards for group PQI projects to ensure meaningful participation of all candidates:

- The group must identify a radiologist, radiation oncologist, or physicist who is participating in MOC as the group leader. The leader facilitates organizing meetings, taking attendance, and keeping minutes of meetings; coordinating data collection, analysis, and review; and improvement planning and implementation.
- The following information must be documented: each participating radiologist's name, the project title and description, and the start and end dates for the project.
- Individuals are required to attend at least three or more group meetings with minutes taken and attendance documented for each participant.
- Each participant must have access to all project documentation, including meeting minutes and any additional relevant data.
- Each participant must fulfill meaningful participation requirements and prepare a short paragraph of self-reflection when the project is completed.
- The leader must sign off on the project before receiving ABR MOC Part 4 credit.
- Attestation is required for participants through their ABR account (Fig. 6.6).

TABLE 6.2   Individual Compared With Group Practice Quality Improvement Projects

Individual PQI Project	Group PQI Project
Suitable in small or rural areas	Based on The Joint Commission; teamwork is important in QI and patient safety
Suitable for subspecialties with insufficient colleagues in a common area of interest	Teams work smarter and make fewer mistakes than individuals
Projects that are completely administrative or technical	Quality improvement in imaging processes require coordination among individuals with different skills
Projects with outcomes that likely affect only a single radiologist in a practice	Coordination is needed to ensure that changes due to quality improvement projects do not overly disrupt the normal processes
	Staff can be involved in multiple projects based on their experience and knowledge

PQI, Practice Quality Improvement; *QI,* quality improvement.

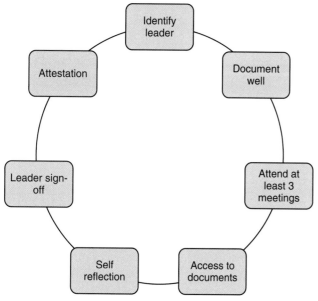

FIG. 6.6 Standards for group practice quality improvement projects.

Institution/Healthcare Organization Practice Quality Improvement Projects

A few leading institutions are approved for MOC credit through the ABR and the American Board of Medical Specialties multidisciplinary portfolio program. Quality improvement programs in these institutions encourage groups of multidisciplinary healthcare providers to participate together in common projects of mutual interest. Radiologists who participate in institutional PQI projects work with the local sponsor to participate in an existing project or to develop and execute a new project. Diplomates are required to attest to PQI activities through the ABR website to receive their MOC Part 4 credits.

HAWTHORNE, LALLI, AND WEBER EFFECTS

Implementing quality improvement projects can change the behavior of subjects. The Hawthorne (observer) effect is a change in human behavior as a result of increased attention on a problem. For example, a study reported an increase in the quality of breast examinations simply due to the clinicians' awareness that exam quality was receiving focused attention. PQI projects can increase awareness of the problem and improve behaviors.

In another example, an initial increase in the rate of reported patient falls was attributed to the Hawthorne effect. This increase was followed by a plateau and finally a sustained decrease in the rate of reported fall incidents. An increase in the rate of adverse events that are noticed in the assessment or analysis section of projects should not stop investigators from following their goals to improve care.

An adverse reaction to contrast media is not always an adverse reaction to the agents. In 1980, Dr. Anthony Lalli correlated reactions to contrast media to patient fear and apprehension. He believed that all the contrast media reactions could be explained through central nervous system mechanisms: administration of contrast media is recognized by the brain, and the brain reacts with potentially fatal responses, including shock. Four years after Lalli's findings, Weber showed that introduction of a new agent or indication can cause a transient increase in the number of reported adverse events; a peak occurs at the end of the second year and then adverse events decline. A transient increase in the number of allergic-like reactions was demonstrated following substitution of gadobenate dimeglumine for gadopentetate dimeglumine. Both Lalli and Weber effects happen frequently after contrast media injection and investigators should be familiar with these phenomena when performing and interpreting PQI projects.

SUGGESTED READINGS

Abujudeh HH, Bruno MA. *Quality and Safety in Radiology.* Oxford, UK: Oxford University Press; 2012.

Brigham LR, Mansouri M, Abujudeh HH. Journal Club: radiology report addenda: a self-report approach to error identification, quantification, and classification. *AJR Am J Roentgenol.* 2015;205(6):1230-1239.

Bruno MA. The "Abujudeh curve" in radiology quality and safety research. *AJR Am J Roentgenol.* 2015;204(5):W606.

Davenport MS, Dillman JR, Cohan RH, et al. Effect of abrupt substitution of gadobenate dimeglumine for gadopentetate dimeglumine on rate of allergic-like reactions. *Radiology.* 2013;266(3):773-782.

Goodson WH 3rd, Hunt TK, Plotnik JN, Moore DH 2nd. Optimization of clinical breast examination. *Am J Med.* 2010;123(4):329-334.

Kelly AM, Cronin P. Practical approaches to quality improvement for radiologists. *Radiographics.* 2015;35:1630-1642.

Kruskal JB, Anderson S, Yam CS, Sosna J. Strategies for establishing a comprehensive quality and performance improvement program in a radiology department. *Radiographics.* 2009;29(2):315-329.

Kruskal JB, Eisenberg R, Sosna J, Yam CS, Kruskal JD, Boiselle PM. Quality initiatives: quality improvement in radiology—basic principles and tools required to achieve success. *Radiographics.* 2011;31(6):1499-1509.

Kruskal JB, Siewert B, Anderson SW, Eisenberg RL, Sosna J. Managing an acute adverse event in a radiology department. *Radiographics.* 2008;28(5):1237-1250.

Lalli AF. Contrast media reactions: data analysis and hypothesis. *Radiology.* 1980;134(1):1–12.

Lee CS, Wadhwa V, Kruskal JB, Larson DB. Conducting a successful practice quality improvement project for American Board of Radiology Certification. *Radiographics.* 2015;35(6):1643–1651.

Mansouri M, Aran S, Shaqdan KW, Abujudeh HH. Rating and classification of incident reporting in radiology in a large academic medical center. *Curr Probl Diagn Radiol.* 2016;45(4):247–252.

Mansouri M, Shaqdan KW, Aran S, Raja AS, Lev MH, Abujudeh HH. Safety incident reporting in emergency radiology: analysis of 1717 safety incident reports. *Emerg Radiol.* 2015;22(6):623–630.

Mansouri M, Abujudeh HH. Practice Quality Improvement (PQI) project. In: Kandarpa K, ed. *Handbook of Interventional Radiologic Procedures.* Philadelphia, PA: Lippincott Williams & Wilkins; 2015:855–863.

American Board of Radiology. Maintenance of Certification. <http://www.theabr.org/moc-gen-landing>.

American Board of Radiology. Maintenance of Certification Part 4: ABR Guide to Practice Quality Improvement (PQI) Projects. < http://www.theabr.org/sites/all/themes/abr-media/pdf/ABR-PQI-Guide.pdf>; 2015.

The Joint Commission. Failure Mode, Effect, and Criticality Analysis (FMECA) Worksheet. <http://www.jointcommission.org/assets/1/18/fmeca.pdf>.

The Joint Commission. Sentinel Event Policy and Procedures. <http://www.jointcommission.org/sentinel_event_policy_and_procedures/>.

Chapter 7
Radiology-Related Quality Programs and Organizations

Behrang Litkouhi and Zachary Masi

In recent years there have been several initiatives dedicated to improving radiologic standards of practice. Many of these programs, such as "Image Gently," "Image Wisely," "Step Lightly," and the Dose Index Registry, address growing concerns over patient exposure to high levels of ionizing radiation from radiologic exams and raise awareness in both the medical community and public to these trends while taking steps to curtail radiation dose where reasonably achievable. Other programs, such as "Choosing Wisely," were initiated in recognition of the frequent overuse of medical tests and procedures—including radiologic exams—and aim to eliminate unnecessary tests through improved screening methods, clinician education, and systemic checks and balances. This chapter summarizes these programs and comments briefly on several additional national programs and organizations that contribute to improving medical and radiologic practice quality.

IMAGE GENTLY

Several studies have documented a rapid growth in computed tomography (CT) use in children since the advent of helical CT scanning, especially in the emergency department (ED) setting. From 1995 to 2008, there was a fivefold increase in CT exams in children visiting the ED. Over this time, the annual growth rate of CT use in pediatric ED visits was 13.2%. There are several reasons for this dramatic increase in CT in pediatric ED settings; most significantly, it paralleled technological advancements that allowed high-quality CT exams to be performed in a matter of seconds, which in turn usually obviated the need for sedation. Other proposed factors include the ability of CT to improve ED throughput, cost savings due to more accurate diagnoses, fear of malpractice, and repeat imaging due to breakdowns in communication.

The main concern over the increased use of CT in children is the risk of radiation-induced cancers. It is generally accepted that children are more susceptible to the effects of ionizing radiation from CT exams, due to a larger number of dividing cells and because they have more years of life for cancer induction to occur. A landmark paper by Brenner et al. in 2000 estimated that of 600,000 annual CT exams performed on children, an estimated 500 will ultimately die of radiation-induced cancer from the CT exam. A more recent study from the United Kingdom in 2012 estimated a 3.2 times greater risk of leukemia and a 2.8 times greater risk of brain cancer in children receiving effective doses currently in use.

In recognition of these trends and public health concerns, in 2006 the Society of Pediatric Radiologists (SPR) formed a committee to raise awareness within the medical community to the harmful effects of ionizing radiation exposure in children. In 2007, the SPR collaborated with the American College of Radiology (ACR), the American Society for Radiologic Technologists (ASRT), and the American Association of Physicists in Medicine (AAPM), to form the Alliance for Radiation Safety in Pediatric Imaging (ARSPI). The main purpose of the Alliance was to improve awareness in the imaging community and among pediatricians of the increasing use of CT in children and the potential harmful effects of ionizing radiation. The ultimate goal was to improve practice by reducing CT dose in children. One of the early actions of the campaign was to encourage imaging professionals to take a pledge to image gently. The pledge included the following:

1. Spreading the Image Gently message among staff
2. Evaluating protocols and making adjustments where appropriate to reduce dose
3. Respecting and listening to suggestions from every member of the imaging team
4. Communicating openly with parents

Much of the Alliance's initial efforts went to educating imaging professionals in primarily adult hospital settings. In a 2008 article in the *American Journal of Radiology* (AJR), the core principles of the Image Gently campaign were outlined as follows:

1. *Reduce or "child size" the radiation dose.* The radiologist, technologist, and medical physicist should work together to adjust the kVp and mAs according to the size of the patient. Protocols for children are listed on the Image Gently website.
2. *Scan only when necessary.* For each proposed CT exam, the expected benefit of the exam must outweigh the risk of ionizing radiation exposure. This requires a discussion between the radiologist consultant and the referring physician.
3. *Scan only the indicated region.* Every attempt should be made to limit radiation exposure to the area of clinical concern. For example, if an incidental lung nodule is being monitored, it is unnecessary to scan the entire chest.
4. *Scan once.* Multiphase exams needlessly double or triple radiation dose and rarely provide more clinically relevant information.

Understandably, the first phase of the campaign focused on spreading their message to imaging professionals, including radiologists, technologists, and medical physicists. The next phase targeted referring physicians—pediatricians, emergency physicians, surgeons, and oncologists. Finally, the third phase focused on parents and the general public. The campaign effectively used social marketing to spread their message, including an Image Gently website, press releases, public service announcements, and healthcare blogs.

Studies performed more recently have suggested that CT use in children has stabilized or begun to decrease. A study in 2013 analyzing data from six major national health organizations showed stabilization followed by a slight decline in pediatric CT since 2007. The reasons for this trend are not entirely clear, but are likely due in part to efforts of the Image Gently campaign to raise awareness in the medical community to the harmful effects of ionizing radiation in children. However, the paper also made clear that there is still much room for improvement. For example, the authors estimated that applying the ALARA (as low as reasonably achievable) principles to reduce the highest 25% of doses to the median level would result in a 43% reduction in radiation-induced cancer in the future.

As of 2015, 91 organizations joined the Image Gently campaign and there have been more than 35,000 pledges. The Image Gently website serves as an excellent resource on radiation exposure from radiologic exams for imaging professionals, pediatricians, and parents. Although there is an emphasis on CT, radiation exposure from other radiologic exams, such as radiography, fluoroscopy, and nuclear medicine studies, is also addressed. The website also makes available appropriate CT protocols for children, a feature that several institutions have used. The protocols listed are a good starting point from which facilities may adjust techniques to further reduce dose while maintaining diagnostic quality.

STEP LIGHTLY

With the well-documented risk of malignancy for children exposed to increased radiation levels since the 1980s, the medical community has made great leaps in the effort to reduce the number of CT exams in children and to create pediatric protocols that reduce CT dose. Often overlooked, however, are other radiation-intensive exams and procedures. Encouraged by the success of the Image Gently campaign, in 2009 the Alliance for Radiation Safety in Pediatrics launched a similar initiative directed specifically at interventional radiology. This new program was titled Step Lightly, in reference to the idea that interventionalists should tread lightly on the foot-pedal by which images are obtained in the interventional suite.

A team of interventional radiologists, medical physicists, and radiation technologists developed a set of recommendations to inform the actions of the medical professionals ordering and performing interventional procedures. A checklist of important steps for reducing radiation dose to pediatric patients undergoing image-guided procedures now serves as a reminder to the treatment team, which is especially critical in facilities that are more accustomed to treating adult patients. The checklist highlights using alternatives to ionizing radiation such as ultrasound, and to use child-sized doses by adjusting acquisition parameters and collimating when using fluoroscopy. Advice and explanations for parents of patients are also provided via the Step Lightly section of the Image Gently website.

In the quest for achieving lower all-around radiation doses in children, certain steps are critical to the use of fluoroscopy. These are generally outlined in the checklist but should be addressed in depth for all interventional radiology staff at facilities that treat children. Some of the steps involve knowledge of equipment. There is a grid that is part of the fluoroscopy unit that reduces scatter and thereby sharpens the final image and increases contrast. Eliminating part of the beam, however, necessitates increasing the dose. Removing the grid results in a dose reduction of one-third to one-half, and there is now a wide consensus that grids should be removed for pediatric cases unless extenuating circumstances are present. In addition, newer fluoroscopy machines have the option to use pulse rather than continuous image acquisition. The x-ray tube emits pulses, lowering the dose in most cases by 25% to 28%. This can result in a *choppy* appearance when imaging a structure with rapid motion, such as the heart, but for most procedures the image quality is absolutely adequate and easily justified by the reduced levels of radiation. All members of the interventional radiology team should be aware of pulse fluoroscopy, and continuous fluoroscopy should be employed in the pediatric patient only under special circumstances. Finally, collimating the x-ray beam, as in adult fluoroscopy, limits patient and operator exposure by passing the beam only through the selected anatomic region.

Another factor in lowering the radiation dose to safer levels for children relates to operator technique. As indicated by the name Step Lightly, physicians and technicians should press on the fluoroscopy pedal only intermittently. Operators are reminded of this by placing an adhesive with the Step Lightly butterfly icon on the pedal itself. The last image saved should be used instead of obtaining a standard radiograph and can be used by the interventional radiology physician to take stock of the relevant anatomy with the x-ray beam off. Collimation, itself an essential dose reduction technique, should be performed with the beam off. This avoids obtaining unnecessary images while the collimator blades move into place. Many modern units have electronic collimation, whereby the operator can view the blades moving in or out on a last image save, instead of a live image. Operators must also keep in mind that both geometric and electronic magnification increases patient radiation dose and should be used sparingly in the pediatric population.

A final method of reducing ionizing radiation when a pediatric patient is on the fluoroscopy table is by adjusting patient positioning. Having the patient as close as possible to the image intensifier and as far away from the x-ray tube as possible minimizes radiation exposure and also minimizes image blurring. In the pediatric population it is also necessary to consider the vulnerability of developing organ systems. The male and female reproductive organs should be covered with lead shields at all times during fluoroscopy unless imaging these structures is essential for the procedure. In instances where a particular body part must be under fluoroscopy for an extended time period, rotating the patient or the c-arm of the fluoroscopy unit can achieve dose spreading, or distribution of the dose over a larger region of the patient's skin, with a less concentrated dose to any one area.

Following a procedure, the dose administered to the pediatric patient should be reviewed and recorded. Reviewing the dose creates increased awareness among the members of the treatment team of how much exposure patients are receiving and can alert them to potential problem areas in complying with their checklist. Recording the dose helps the patient's family and the medical community keep track of how much radiation the patient is receiving over time, which can influence future decisions about imaging and procedures. Using these methods, the interventional radiologist and technologist play a major role in reducing the risk of malignancy and other negative sequelae of radiation in child patients.

IMAGE WISELY

From 1995 to 2006 the volume of CT scans in the United States increased from 20 million to 60 million. Much of this increase was concentrated in at-risk populations who were subjected to repeated imaging for chronic illnesses. It was hypothesized for decades that high-dose radiation exposure from multiple CT scans, interventional radiologic procedures, and barium fluoroscopic studies might lead to an increased incidence of malignancy. These conclusions were largely extrapolated from data on Japanese survivors of atomic bombs and the survivors of the Chernobyl disaster. At the turn of the millennium, reliable data on the increased cancer risk to pediatric populations was available and has been widely disseminated through the Image Gently campaign.

The health effects of ionizing radiation on adult patients are poorly delineated by comparison, and concerns over radiation exposure are all too often ignored. To address these challenges, in 2009 the ACR and the Radiological Society of North America (RSNA) established the Joint Task Force on Adult Radiation Protection. In 2010 the Joint Task Force rolled out Image Wisely, a comprehensive campaign to eliminate unnecessary radiation exposure and minimize radiation exposure when performing necessary studies.

The two main goals of Image Wisely are eliminating superfluous studies and completing necessary exams using lower radiation doses. To address the first goal, radiologists, referring physicians, CT technicians, medical physicists, and patients were targeted in a multifaceted awareness campaign designed to inform each group of their responsibilities in reducing overuse of ionizing radiation. Due to the heavy use of CT in the emergency setting and the relatively high dose associated with CT as compared to other imaging modalities, the Image Wisely campaign is focused largely on the use of CT. Resources are now available through the Image Wisely website, including links to the ACR appropriateness criteria (AC). The ACR AC provide official recommendations for the most suitable imaging modality in hundreds of different clinical scenarios and list the relative radiation doses for each study. This information helps ordering clinicians decide whether the risk of radiation exposure outweighs the benefits, and whether a less radiation intensive study may be equivalent or preferable to CT. Another tool in the fight against unwarranted CT scans is the Patient Medical Imaging Record. This allows providers to see what studies a patient has already had and, in many nonemergent situations, can prevent a repeat examination. Available on the Image Wisely website, this tool

also allows patients to be more involved in their own care. A third branch of outreach to referring clinicians is a Q&A on radiation safety, covering the most common dilemmas that arise when considering an imaging test. Additional resources for patients are available at Radiologyinfo.org, including a basic explanation of the risks of ionizing radiation from CT scans. The site receives over 25,000 visits a day from an average of 4455 individuals.

Even with improved competency among ordering physicians, the radiologist is still the gatekeeper of patient safety when it comes to radiation dose. Despite this, multiple surveys have demonstrated that many radiologists and radiology residents are unaware of the resources available to them. Image Wisely has therefore provided tools for radiologists (and the medical physicists and CT technicians on whom they rely) to protect patients and guarantee quality of care. These tools include CT protocols that are structured to minimize radiation dose to patients, and information on CT equipment with specific parameters for use on all major brands of scanners. This effort has been further facilitated by the release of Dose Check, a feature of newer CT scanners that was developed in response to a request by the US Food and Drug Administration in 2009 that industry leaders help avoid operator-dependent incidents of unnecessarily high radiation exposure. Guidelines are also available for using adaptive iterative reconstruction, an algorithm that allows reduction of image noise without loss of spatial or contrast resolution; this ultimately allows the operator to reduce the radiation dose without sacrificing image quality.

The underpinnings of the Image Wisely campaign are summarized in the Image Wisely pledge. The pledge is a commitment by radiologists to protect patients from harm by limiting use of radiation. The pledge has four components: using only the necessary level of radiation to obtain diagnostic quality images, conveying principles of radiation safety to the imaging team, communicating imaging strategies to referring physicians, and routinely reviewing imaging protocols to minimize patient radiation exposure. An additional pledge for facilities was also developed. This consists of three separate levels of commitment, the first of which is simply taking the Image Wisely pledge. The second level of commitment allows the facility to earn accreditation and involves maintaining radiation dose indices in compliance with thresholds, maintaining peer-reviewed image quality standards, physicist-reviewed phantom image quality standards, and personnel requirements. The third level of commitment is participation in the DIR.

Moving forward, the Image Wisely campaign aims to expand beyond CT safety, applying their principles to dental imaging, fluoroscopy, and imaging in pediatric head trauma, while also complying with The Joint Commission's standards for radiation doses. These goals will add to the impact of the Image Wisely campaign in lowering radiation doses, and in doing so reduce the risks of imaging-related radiation-induced malignancy in adult patient populations.

DOSE INDEX REGISTRY

The Dose Index Registry (DIR) was initiated due to concerns over increasing exposure to ionizing radiation from radiologic exams, with a particular emphasis on CT. Initial efforts began in 2005, at a time when radiation exposure from CT was gaining much media attention, and scanners did not routinely record the now standard radiation exposure parameters of the CT dose index (CTDI) and dose length product (DLP). After two pilot runs, the DIR opened to all facilities in May 2011. As of August 2013, more than 750 facilities participate in the DIR, and 465 actively contribute data.

The purpose of the DIR is to provide participating institutions with an analysis of their dose index data and to compare their data to regional and national institutions. By doing so, the DIR aims to raise institutional self-awareness of dose data and encourage users to undertake quality assurance measures to improve their dose profile.

Enrolling in the DIR is a joint effort that requires the collaboration of the information technology (IT) staff, a site physicist, and a site radiologist. Participating facilities install TRIAD, the dose data gathering software developed by the ACR, on a PC. TRIAD can be set up to gather data directly from scanners or from the picture archiving and communication system (PACS). This data typically comes in the form of a Radiation Dose Structured Report (RDSR). Some older scanners do not generate RDSRs; in these instances, TRIAD converts dose information into RDSR format. TRIAD is also responsible for anonymizing data and eliminating superfluous information before securely submitting data to the DIR.

Participating facilities receive semiannual reports of their dose indices. Adult and pediatric data are reported separately. Moreover, pediatric reports are subdivided into five age groups to account for the variability in patient size. The specific dose parameters listed in the report are the CTDI, DLP, and, for body exams, a size-specific dose estimate (SSDE). The CTDI is an estimate of radiation energy absorbed per unit mass as determined by a phantom, not a patient, and is reported in milligrays (mGy). DLP is the absorbed dose multiplied by the length of exposure as determined by a phantom and is reported in milligray-centimeters (mGy-cm). The SSDE takes into account patient size to better estimate the patient dose and is reported in mGy.

Users are encouraged to participate in webinars with other participating facilities and DIR committee members. These sessions assist users in understanding their report and may facilitate appropriate quality improvement measures aimed at reducing dose.

One challenge faced by the DIR is the variability in procedure names across various facilities. To this end, the DIR implemented the RadLex playbook, which lists and describes various procedures and assigns a RadLex playbook ID (RPID). The DIR has a mapping tool that assists users in selecting the appropriate matching RPID. If no matching RPID can be found, users can select descriptors for a given procedure and request an RPID from RadLex. This can be a time-consuming process, especially at larger facilities that have several different procedure names. For example, in a paper on the implementation of the DIR at the University of Washington, the authors reported that one of their facilities had 19 different exam names for a noncontrast head CT.

There are currently many facilities participating in the DIR, including large multisite institutions and small facilities with a single scanner. Participation in the DIR is voluntary. An annual nominal fee is determined based on the number of facilities and radiologists at the participating institution.

The early impact of the DIR in increasing awareness and motivating facilities to implement dose reduction measures has been promising. In the largest such study to date, a large academic institution used dose data from the DIR to plan and implement dose reduction measures. The results of their quality improvement initiative was a substantial decrease in dose in the four most commonly ordered CT exams—CT head without contrast, CT chest with contrast, CT chest without contrast, and CT abdomen and pelvis with contrast. As more facilities join the DIR and more data are acquired, more such quality improvement initiatives will likely be undertaken.

CHOOSING WISELY

The Choosing Wisely campaign is an initiative begun in 2012 by the American Board of Internal Medicine (ABIM) in recognition of the often excessive and unnecessary use of medical procedures and tests. The stated goal of the campaign at the time was to "spark conversation" among the medical community and patients with regard to the necessity for medical tests. At its core, the campaign advocated that medical testing should (1) be supported by evidence, (2) not be a duplicate of other tests already performed, (3) not result in patient harm, and (4) be truly necessary.

Medical imaging has long been recognized as one of the large subsets of medical tests that are overused. A 2005 study by the Center for Information Technology Leadership at Harvard University estimated that 20% of imaging tests are "duplicate" studies. In 2008, America's Health Insurance Plans reported that 20% to 50% of advanced imaging tests are unnecessary. Moreover, radiologists have faced criticism within their own community for not doing enough to limit medical imaging overuse. Swenson et al. reported in 2010 that "30% of radiologic exams do not meet standard appropriateness criteria" and that the radiologists are at fault for not effectively screening for appropriateness.

In 2012, the ABIM foundation, in collaboration with *Consumer Reports*, requested each of its nine national medical organization partners—including the ACR—to create a list of five procedures that are often unnecessarily performed. Not surprisingly, all five of the procedures chosen by the ACR were imaging tests. However, several other specialties also chose medical imaging tests in their lists, and together, a total of 24 of the 45 tests listed were imaging related. These reports gained much media attention, and soon thereafter the Choosing Wisely campaign was covered on the front page of the *New York Times*. Interestingly, although medical imaging as a whole was seen as one of the main offenders of medical overuse, radiologists were also among groups that were commended for showing "admirable statesmanship by proposing cuts that would affect their incomes."

Over the next several months, the Choosing Wisely campaign gained more momentum, and by February 2013, 17 additional medical organizations had joined. The collective list of overused medical tests chosen by these 26 medical organizations revealed a total of 43 tests that are typically performed by radiologists.

The ACR has collaborated with the ABIM to educate the medical community and the general public on the appropriate use of radiologic tests. Several press releases have questioned the utility and the potential negative impact of tests classically ordered as a knee-jerk reaction, among them, preoperative chest x-rays in otherwise healthy patients, CT and MRI exams of the brain for headaches, and CT angiography of the chest for evaluation of pulmonary embolism in patients with a low pretest probability. The ACR AC are established for all available imaging tests, and are constantly updated on the ACR website. The imaging community faces the challenge of applying these criteria on a day-to-day basis, by continuing to educate its clinical colleagues and striving to act as appropriateness gatekeepers.

The early impact of the Choosing Wisely campaign in curtailing unnecessary use of imaging tests has been mixed. In a recent article published in *JAMA Internal Medicine*, investigators analyzed the use of seven of the commonly overused tests, four of which were imaging related, and found that two of the four—cardiac stress imaging for low-risk patients without symptoms and imaging for uncomplicated headaches—showed a significant decrease in use since the Choosing Wisely campaign. The other two investigated radiologic tests—preoperative chest x-rays in low-risk patients and imaging for lower back pain—showed no significant change. The results signify that raising awareness and sparking conversation, while a good first step, can only go so far to change deep-rooted exam ordering habits of physicians. For substantial change to occur, there must be a concerted effort by physicians and data delivery systems to implement checks and balances such as data feedback, system interventions, and clinician scorecards. Because many institutions are now beginning to experiment with these types of measures, the next few years will be crucial in defining the success of the campaign.

ADDITIONAL QUALITY PROGRAMS AND ORGANIZATIONS

The *Joint Commission* (JC) is a nonprofit organization responsible for accrediting over 21,000 healthcare organizations in the United States. Accreditation by the JC ensures that certain minimum standards of quality are met.

The *Center for Medicare and Medicaid Services* (CMS) is the federal agency that runs the Medicare program and works with state governments to administer Medicaid, the State Children's Health Insurance Program, and health insurance portability standards. Other responsibilities include maintaining quality standards of nursing homes, maintaining the Health Insurance Portability and Accountability Act standards of practice, and overseeing the healthcare.gov site.

The *Physician Quality Reporting System* (PQRS) is a federal program that requires providers to submit quality measures to the CMS. Reporting may be performed on an individual basis by an eligible professional or as a group practice. Because PQRS is a Medicare-sponsored program, only providers who care for Medicare patients qualify to participate. PQRS is an incentive-based program. As such, successful reporting of PQRS measures will improve reimbursement for CMS patients, whereas failure to report

will result in a loss of reimbursement. There are a total of 281 quality measures for 2016, of which 30 are imaging related. Providers are required to provide nine measures across three domains. Examples of imaging-related PQRS measures include use of radiation dose-reduction techniques and appropriate follow-up for incidental abdominal lesions.

Multiple Procedure Payment Reduction (MPPR) is a federal policy with the goal of avoiding duplicate payments when multiple procedures are performed on the same patient during a single visit. After reimbursing the most expensive procedure, additional related procedures are reimbursed at a lower rate. CMS has applied various reductions in multiple payments over the years.

The ACR is a nonprofit organization, founded in 1922, that serves as the major governing board for radiologic standards of practice. It is composed of diagnostic and interventional radiologists, radiation oncologists, nuclear medicine physicians, and medical physicists. In the 1990s the ACR began a large initiative, the AC, with the goal of providing guidelines for appropriate use of imaging studies by ordering physicians. Since its initiation, the AC have undergone several updates. ACR initiative 3.0 started in 2013, largely in response to long-standing overutilization of radiologic studies and a fragmented delivery system. The goals of the initiative are to make imaging a more valuable service by focusing on patient-centered care. By advocating patient safety, application of AC, and development of a robust medical imaging support system, the initiative hopes to achieve a paradigm shift in the way radiology is practiced, to one that is transparent, efficient, and ultimately better for patient care.

Clinical Decision Support (CDS) software analyzes and ranks the appropriateness of an ordered test. Appropriate use criteria (AUC) are implemented in the software according to guidelines from several medical societies, including the ACR. In June 2016, the CMS approved the ACR AUC as a guide for ordering advanced imaging tests for Medicare patients. The ACR AUC has a digital format, licensed by the National Decision Support Company, which can be integrated with all major electronic health record (EHR) systems. Starting January 1, 2017, ordering physicians must use criteria established by a government-approved CDS system when ordering advanced imaging studies.

The *Leapfrog* group is a nonprofit organization that was formed in 2000 by several large US companies that were concerned about the rising cost of healthcare insurance for their employees. The goal of the group was to use their purchasing power to ensure safe and high-quality healthcare, and ultimately lower healthcare costs. Hospitals are evaluated based on several safety and quality standards, and this information is made public to create transparency and encourage accountability and self-improvement. Currently, Leapfrog includes of more than 170 public and private purchasers that provide health insurance to more than 37 million employees and retirees.

The *American Board of Radiology* (ABR) is a nonprofit organization established in 1934, which oversees board certification and maintenance of certification (MOC) for diagnostic and interventional radiologists, radiation oncologists, and medical physicists. The minimum criteria for initial board certification and MOC are established by ABR's oversight organization, the American Board of Medical Specialties (ABMS). The ABMS is a nonprofit organization that oversees the activity of 24 medical specialties and is the largest physician-led specialization certification organization in the United States.

The *National Institute of Biomedical Imaging and Bioengineering* (NIBIB) is the most recent research organization established by the National Institutes of Health and was signed and approved by President Clinton in 2000. The goal of this federal institute is to improve human health through the development of imaging technologies aimed at preventing and detecting disease processes. Its establishment was largely due to efforts led by the Academy of Radiology Research, an alliance of 25 professional imaging societies. The NIBIB funds research to investigate cutting-edge imaging technologies such as magnetic resonance elastography, phase contrast CT, and chemical exchange saturation transfer.

The *Agency for Healthcare Research and Quality (AHRQ)* is a federal agency operating as the research arm of the US Department of Health and Human Services, with the task of improving healthcare quality and safety in the United States. The AHRQ emphasizes that medical practice guidelines should be based on scientific evidence, and when such evidence is insufficient, expert consensus measures should be used. Acceptable medical practice guidelines developed by the AHRQ have been incorporated into the ACR AC. ACR AC topics are listed on the National Guidelines Clearinghouse website, an initiative of the AHRQ that functions as a public resource for evidence-based practice guidelines.

The Patient Protection and Affordable Care Act, also known as the Affordable Care Act and colloquially as Obamacare, was signed by Barack Obama on March 23, 2010. The goals of this federal statute are to provide more affordable and higher-quality healthcare insurance and to reduce the uninsured population. Health insurance companies were given new minimum standards of coverage and were prohibited from limiting healthcare coverage due to preexisting conditions. The act includes a mandate that requires individuals who are not insured by employers, Medicaid, or Medicare to purchase health insurance or pay a penalty. Moreover, the act includes a restructuring of Medicare payments, shifting from a fee-for-service to a bundled payment model, in an attempt to make healthcare delivery more efficient.

The *Medicare Access and CHIP Reauthorization Act of 2015* is colloquially known as the Permanent Doc Fix. Under this federal act, the sustainable growth rate formula for determining Medicare payments, which threatened physician payment cuts annually, has been eliminated. Medicare payments are stabilized by offering an annual increase in reimbursements through 2019. Moreover, physicians have the choice of enrolling in one of two payment programs: a merit-based incentive payment system (MIPS) or an alternate payment model (APM). It is expected that the majority of physicians will at least initially enroll in MIPS. Under MIPS, physicians report activities in four performance categories: quality, advanced care information, clinical practice improvement activities, and cost. Through APMs, physicians who partake in new payment and delivery models approved by CMS are supported and exempt from MIPS.

SUGGESTED READINGS

ACR appropriateness criteria now satisfy federal AUC requirements. <https://www.acr.org/About-Us/Media-Center/Press-Releases/2016-Press-Releases/20160620-ACR-Appropriateness-Criteria-Now-Satisfy-Federal-AUC-Requirements>.

Agency for Healthcare Research and Quality. www.ahrq.gov.

Agency for Healthcare Research and Quality. National Guideline Clearinghouse. www.guideline.gov.

American College of Radiology website. http://www.acr.org.

American Medical Association. Understanding Medicare Payment Reform (MACRA). www.ama-assn.org/ama/pub/advocacy/topics/medicare-physician-payment-reform.page.

America's Health Insurance Plans (AHIP). *Ensuring Quality Through Appropriate Use of Diagnostic Imaging.* Washington, DC: AHIP; 2008.

Brenner DJ, Elliston CD, Hall EJ, et al. Estimated risks of radiation-induced fatal cancer from pediatric CT. *AJR Am J Roentgenol.* 2001;176:289–296.

Brenner DJ, Hall EJ. Computed tomography—an increasing source of radiation exposure. *N Engl J Med.* 2007;357:2277–2284.

Brink JA, Amis ES. Image Wisely: a campaign to increase awareness about adult radiation protection. *Radiology.* 2010;257:601–602.

Broder J, Fordham LA, Warshauer DM. Increased utilization of computed tomography in the pediatric emergency department, 2000–2006. *Emerg Radiol.* 2007;14:227–232.

Bushberg J, Seibert J, Leidholdt E, Boone J. *The Essential Physics of Medical Imaging.* 3rd ed. Philadelphia, PA: Lippincott Williams and Wilkins; 2001.

Casey B. Choosing wisely drives down imaging use—sometimes. <http://www.auntminnie.com/index.aspx?sec=scr&sub=def&pag=dis&ItemID=112087>.

Chatfield MB, Morin RL. The ACR computed tomography dose index registry: the 5 million examination update. *J Am Coll Radiol.* 2013;10:980–983.

Choosing Wisely. www.choosingwisely.org.

Drury P, Robinson A. Fluoroscopy without the grid: a method of reducing the radiation dose. *Br J Radiol.* 1980;53(626):93–99.

Fornell D. An intro to clinical decision support for radiology. <https://www.itnonline.com/article/intro-clinical-decision-support-radiology>.

Goske MJ, Applegate KE, Boylan J, et al. The Image Gently campaign: working together to change practice. *AJR Am J Roentgenol.* 2008;190:273–274.

Haines B. The big questions: what is imaging 3.0? Health imaging. <http://www.healthimaging.com/topics/practice-management/big-question-what-imaging-30>.

Hall EJ, Brenner DJ. Cancer risk from diagnostic radiology. *Br J Radiol.* 2008;965:362–378.

Image Gently Alliance. Interventional Radiology—Step lightly Resources. <http://www.imagegently.org/Procedures/Interventional-Radiology/Image-Safely-Resources>.

Image Wisely. Radiation Safety in Adult Medical Imaging. www.imagewisely.org.

IMV 2006 CT Market Summary Report. <http://www.imvinfo.com/user/documents/content_documents/nws_rad/MS_CT_DSandTOC.pdf>.

Keen CE. The clinical decision mandate: now what? <http://www.radiology-business.com/topics/policy/clinical-decision-support-mandate-now-what>.

Larson DB, Johnson LW, Schnell BM, Salisbury SR, Forman HP. National trends in CT use in the emergency department: 1995–2007. *Radiology.* 2010;258(1):164–173.

Larson DB, Johnson W, Schnell BM, Goske MJ, Salisbury SR, Forman HP. Rising use of CT in child visits to the emergency department in the United States, 1995–2008. *Radiology.* 2011;259(3):793–801.

Latest version of ACR appropriateness criteria expands clinical indications. <https://www.itnonline.com/content/latest-version-acr-appropriateness-criteria-expands-clinical-indications>.

Little BP, Duong P, Knighton J. A comprehensive CT dose reduction program using the ACR dose index registry. *J Am Coll Radiol.* 2015;12:1257–1265.

Mahesh M, Morin R. What is the CT dose check standard, and why do CT scanners need to be in compliance? *J Am Coll Radiol.* 2016;13:64–66.

Mahesh M. Fluoroscopy: patient radiation safety issues. *Radiographics.* 2001;4:1033–1045.

Maynard CD. The National Institute of Biomedical Imaging and Bioengineering: vision, current status, and future directions. *J Magn Reson Imaging.* 2001;14:201–202.

Migloretti DL, Johnson E, Williams A. The use of computed tomography in pediatrics and the associated radiation exposure and estimated cancer risk. *J Am Med Assoc Pediatr.* 2013;167(8):700–707.

Miller DL, Bharghavan-Chatfield M, Armstrong MR, Butler PF. Clinical implementation of National Electrical Manufacturers Association CT dose check standard at ACR dose index registry sites. *J Am Coll Radiol.* 2014;11:989–994.

Morin RL, Coombs LP, Chatfield MB. ACR Dose Index Registry. *J Am Coll Radiol.* 2011;8:288–291.

Pearce MS, Salotti JA, Little MP. Radiation exposures from CT scans in childhood and subsequent risk of leukaemia and brain tumors: a retrospective cohort study. *Lancet.* 2012;380(9840):499–505.

Rao VM, Levin DC. The choosing wisely initiative of the American Board of Internal Medicine: what will its impact be on radiology practice? *AJR Am J Roentgenol.* 2014;202:358–361.

Robinson TJ, Robinson JD, Kanal KM. Implementation of the ACR Dose Index Registry at a large academic institution: early experience. *J Digit Imaging.* 2013;26:309–315.

Rogers LF. NIBIB: Radiology achieves a toehold in the federal research establishment. *AJR Am J Roentgenol.* 2002;178(2):273.

Shah NB, Platt SL. ALARA: is there a concern for alarm? Reducing radiation risks from computed tomography scanning in children. *Curr Opin Pediatr.* 2008;20:243–247.

Sidhu M, Goske M, Connolly B, et al. Image Gently, Step Lightly: promoting radiation safety in pediatric interventional radiology. *AJR Am J Roentgenol.* 2010;95(4):299–301.

Silva AC, Lawder HJ, Hara A, Kujak J, Pavlicek W. Innovation in CT dose reduction strategy: application of the adaptive statistical iterative reconstruction algorithm. *AJR Am J Roentgenol.* 2010;194:191–199.

Strauss K, Kaste S, The ALARA (as low as reasonably achievable) concept in pediatric interventional and fluoroscopic imaging: striving to keep radiation doses as low as possible during fluoroscopy of pediatric patients—a white paper executive summary. *Pediatr Radiol.* 2006;36:110–112.

Swenson SJ, Johnson DC. Flying in the plane you service: patient-centered radiology. *J Am Coll Radiol.* 2010;7:216–221.

The Image Gently Alliance. www.imagegently.org.

Townsend BA, Callahan MJ, Zurakowski D, Taylor GA. Has pediatric CT at children's hospitals reached its peak? *AJR Am J Roentgenol.* 2010;194(5):1194–1196.

US Department of Health and Human Services. Administration Takes First Step to Implement Legislation Modernizing How Medicare Pays Physicians for Quality. www.hhs.gov/about/news/2016/04/27/administration-takes-first-step-implement-legislation-modernizing-how-medicare-pays-physicians.html.

Chapter 8

Highly Reliable Organizations/Systems in Healthcare and Radiology

Adam Danielson and Hani H. Abujudeh

INTRODUCTION

The Institute of Medicine's reports, *Crossing the Quality Chasm* and *To Err Is Human*, created an awareness within the American healthcare system that change and redesign are necessary to improve patient safety and quality of care. This is exemplified by studies performed by RAND Health that found Americans with common health problems receive only 50% of recommended care. These needed changes clearly include healthcare professionals and organizations, but they also extend to the systems and processes within the healthcare environment. To address the inconsistencies seen in the delivery of high-quality healthcare, organizations have examined reliability principles from other industries such as nuclear power, the airline industry, and the military (Fig. 8.1). Organizations in these industries must be highly reliable and perform highly predictable and effective operations in settings where hazards could result in harm to hundreds or thousands of people.

Reliability is defined as failure-free operation over time and is a measure of how consistently a system operates as intended. Reliability can be measured as the number of actions that achieve the intended result among the total number of actions taken. One can also measure the failure rate, which is calculated as 1 minus the reliability or the unreliability of a system. The unreliability of a system is frequently measured and is expressed as an order of magnitude where a system with a defect rate of one in 10, or 10%, performs at a level of 10^{-1}. Studies suggest that the 10^{-1} level is where most US healthcare organizations currently perform. This is far below the performance of the aviation and nuclear power industries, which perform at a defect rate of 10^{-6}.

To move toward a high-reliability system, healthcare organizations, including radiology groups, need to adopt a culture of quality and safety. A culture is the attitudes, values, and behaviors of individuals when acting in a group or environment where they are encouraged to work proactively as a team. This culture should empower individuals to speak up and look beyond their own boundaries to ensure patient safety. Organizations should develop a shared vision with mutual accountability and frequent constructive communication centered around common principles of teamwork, especially when there are system failures. High-reliability systems must be flexible to respond to complex problems without error. This requires adherence to certain fundamental principles of high reliability.

FIVE FUNDAMENTAL PRINCIPLES OF HIGHLY RELIABLE ORGANIZATIONS/SYSTEMS

Weick and Sutcliffe devised five fundamental principles that are essential elements of all high-reliability organizations. Radiology groups and other healthcare organizations should work to incorporate these principles into their systems and practices to achieve higher levels of reliability. These principles include a preoccupation with failure, reluctance to oversimplify, sensitivity to operations, a commitment to resilience, and deference to local expertise.

Preoccupation With Failure

A preoccupation with failure is a proactive approach to prevent failures from occurring. In a high-reliability system, all employees at all levels are encouraged to think of ways in which work processes might break down or accidents occur. This shared mindfulness includes the full spectrum of failures, from small inefficiencies to catastrophic system failures, and allows for development of best practices within organizations. Errors that are detected are ideally corrected before any harm occurs, and employees are encouraged to report any near misses to further safe-proof systems and practices. It is important to destigmatize failure and see it as an opportunity for improvement. Evaluating and addressing the root causes of near misses throughout the chain of steps that lead to a potential failure are critical for increasing the reliability of a system. High-reliability organizations must also combat complacency with the status quo and embrace aggressive troubleshooting and continuous improvement.

Within radiology, the staff needs to be well prepared prior to beginning examinations or procedures. All necessary supplies should be readily available with extra supplies if necessary. Care providers should take ownership of their processes and actions and be prepared for potential complications. Radiology leadership should be committed to long-term process improvement and lead employees to see that success is attainable and borrow best practices from other successful operations within their department or others within the healthcare system.

Reluctance to Oversimplify

A reluctance to oversimplify is a principle of high-reliability organizations and systems that ensures problems and processes are deeply examined and appropriately managed. Although it is advantageous to simplify work processes

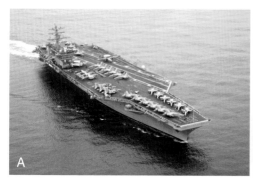
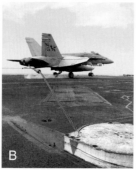
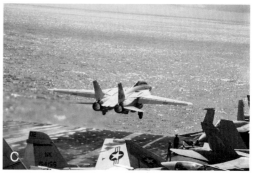

FIG. 8.1 An aircraft carrier is a high-reliability organization. It has high-risk operations, errors are disastrous when they occur, and the operator is the victim. (A) The *USS Nimitz* aircraft carrier. (B) An F/A-18C Hornet catches an arresting wire on the *USS Nimitz*. (C) An F-14 Tomcat takes off from an aircraft carrier. (**A,** Courtesy US Navy. **B–C,** Courtesy US Department of Defense.)

whenever possible, high-reliability organizations see the risks inherent in a superficial approach. It is critical to respect the complexity of processes and problems and to explore problems deeply to find the root cause or true source of a problem so a meaningful solution can be formulated. Leaders of high-reliability organizations should constantly seek information that challenges their current beliefs as to why problems exist. They should also question explanations that may seem reasonable or obvious unless they are backed by data. This principle is applicable to radiology, which is a very complex field involving different types of imaging studies, techniques and protocols, acuity of examinations/procedures, reporting structures, and a wide range of diseases. A respect for these nuances is required when solving problems or redesigning radiologic systems or procedures.

Sensitivity to Operations

High-reliability organizations and systems are sensitive to their own operations and processes. Although it is common for organizations to have standard operating procedures, a highly reliable organization must be constantly aware of written procedures and policies and also what truly happens in the workplace. Certainly there is some level of disparity between what is official policy and what occurs in the real-time work environment, and highly reliable organizations are attune to this phenomenon. These discrepancies are both a potential occupational hazard and an opportunity for system improvement. In high-reliability systems, every employee needs to pay close attention to processes and operations to be aware of what is or is not working. This is particularly important in a field like radiology where there are numerous protocols and clinical scenarios that are routinely encountered.

Sensitivity to operations can be improved by increasing transparency, conducting leadership rounds, and using computer-generated analytics tools. Increasing intraorganizational transparency with improved communication and sharing of data regarding processes and problems engages employees and encourages them to pay closer attention. Hospitals or radiology groups might share patient safety or satisfaction data. Leaders in high-reliability organizations should also make workplace rounds to directly observe operations and have open communication with staff. Rounding improves leaders' understanding of processes and allows an opportunity for staff to voice concerns or suggestions for improvement. Computer-generated analytics tools are also helpful in collecting process data and comparing documentation across multiple systems like the radiology information system (RIS), picture archiving and communication system (PACS), and electronic medical records. Analytics tools can be used to assist in regular internal auditing, which can uncover potentially dangerous discrepancies in process and sources of error. This should improve documentation, attention to detail, and process accuracy.

Commitment to Resilience

A commitment to resilience is a hallmark of highly reliable systems. High-reliability systems account for failures and are prepared to respond when they occur. Flexibility in a system is essential in mitigating failures and potential harm. According to Ashby's law of requisite variety, a system must be more complex than its set of inputs to adapt appropriately to changes. Some level of redundancy should be built into a high-reliability system to provide flexibility during unexpected events or larger system failures. Radiology groups may have a backup physician or technologist available to cover for another's unexpected absence. Radiology groups should develop a backup process when there are RIS or PACS failures for emergency interpretation and reporting. Large system redundancies are inefficient, but small redundancies are critical for resilience in times of failure. Highly reliable organizations are resilient and will bend without breaking when a large problem occurs.

Highly reliable organizations also see failures as critical learning opportunities. System failures occur within a matrix of processes and the causes are not always readily apparent. Once the immediate threats of a failure are neutralized, a longer-term analysis can begin. System failures are an opportunity to closely examine problems and processes to improve or replace them if necessary and increase future reliability. It is also important to evaluate how leadership responds to problems to drive future improvement and create a shared sense of resilience throughout an organization.

Deference to Local Expertise

Deference to local expertise is a fundamental principle of high reliability. It acknowledges that those in management and authority roles within an organization are not always the most experienced or knowledgeable. This is important when considering highly reliable performance in complex situations and settings. Although leaders will determine the overall organizational strategy for improvement, the front-line staff possesses vital knowledge about their work. Highly reliable systems encourage staff feedback and minimize the power distance between employees and management. For example, a first-year resident may have a more advanced degree and perceived rank than a senior ultrasound technologist; however, the experience of the technologist brings more value to the team. Deferring to the expertise of the most qualified individual regardless of title demonstrates respect, builds an environment of trust, and improves patient care. When working in healthcare and radiology, the vast and varying expertise of staff and complexity of clinical scenarios necessitates the empowerment of all staff members to improve care. Another important source of expertise is the prior work experience of all staff. Many healthcare workers have experience in other systems and leaders in high-reliability organizations encourage employees to share their prior experiences and incorporate foreign successful processes and systems whenever possible.

HOW TO APPLY RELIABILITY TO HEALTHCARE: THE INSTITUTE FOR HEALTHCARE IMPROVEMENT MODEL

The Institute for Healthcare Improvement has developed a three-tiered strategy for designing reliable care systems. This system is designed to take the unreliability of healthcare delivery from the 10^{-1} level (90% reliable) to the 10^{-3} level (99.9% reliable). The three-tiered approach includes three stages: preventing failure, identifying and mitigating failure, and redesign. Each stage of design allows a system to reach the next order of reliability where a cumulative adaptation of lower- and higher-reliability strategies is necessary to achieve high reliability.

Prevent Failure

The first stage of designing a reliable care system is to prevent failures or breakdowns in operations or functions. This stage is designed to create 10^{-1} level (90% reliable) performance and involves the creation and application of standardized approaches to care whenever possible. The emphasis is on creating uniform processes and guidelines and ensuring that doctors, nurses, and technologists adhere to them. This stage includes the standardization of processes and procedures, equipment and order sheets, and the creation of memory aids like checklists. Organizations will also raise employee awareness of their guidelines and standards and train staff to incorporate them into their care.

Identify and Mitigate Failure

The second stage of design for a reliable care system is to identify system failures and intervene before there is harm or mitigate the harm caused by undetected failures. This stage is designed to create 10^{-2} level (99% reliable) performance. Strategies in this stage of design focus on the identification of instances when the standardized approach is not used and the reduction of opportunities for humans to make mistakes. This involves the development of error-proofing systems that eliminate ambiguities or nonstandard ways of performing tasks. Organizations can use reminders for patients regarding appointments and checklists and alarms for staff. Similar equipment can be differentiated by using different colors, sizes, or shapes so they cannot be mistakenly combined and result in error. Constraints can be placed on machines and electronic systems, like the electronic medical record, that prevent a contraindicated medication from being ordered. Affordances, visual and other sensory clues that lead a person to properly use a product or tool, can also be adapted, like a push plate on an outward swinging door. Organizations can also develop decision-aid software and make the desired action the default action.

Redesign

The third stage for increasing system reliability is periodic system redesign, which is based on the failure modes of the system and standardized processes. Two important tools for system redesign include root cause analysis and failure modes and effects analysis (FMEA). Using these processes allows reliability to progress from 10^{-2} (99.0% reliable) to the 10^{-3} level (99.9% reliable) and tackles the remaining weaknesses in the design of the standardized processes, which have led or may lead to failure. The focus must be on processes and the structure in which a process operates. This can be a complicating factor in healthcare with various care teams, subspecialties, and locations of care.

A root cause analysis (RCA) is a reactive examination of problems, defects, or system failures that have already occurred to discover the root causes. The root causes of error are the highest level, specific, underlying causes of a problem that can be identified and managed. Addressing nonroot causes of errors may only temporarily or incompletely prevent further occurrences, so it is essential to conduct RCA for lasting improvement and reliability. RCA can also be performed to evaluate near-miss events or patterns of events. The RCA is a structured process that is typically carried out by small teams. These teams include individuals from all levels of an organization associated with an error or event and meet at least weekly for approximately 2 months. Once the event and related processes are defined, immediate and proximate causes are addressed to temporarily mitigate errors. The RCA will then identify the root causes and generate risk reduction strategies and improvement action plans. A pilot test of the solutions on a small scale is helpful to monitor unintended consequences and define measures of success for the solutions. These measures should be clear and quantifiable and must show the impact of actions on the root causes.

FMEA is a proactive tool for systems redesign that is essential to reach the 10^{-3} level of reliability (99.9% reliable). FMEA is a standardized way to evaluate processes to identify potential weak points or methods of failure and to rate the relative impact and severity of different types of failures. This allows an organization to prioritize the parts of a process in greatest need of improvement. FMEA evaluates each step in a process to determine what could go wrong (failure modes), why the failure would occur (failure causes), and what the consequences of failure would be (failure effects). Frequently occurring failure modes should be addressed by amending the process design itself, while infrequent failure modes can be addressed by many of the methods used throughout the three-stage high-reliability design process. A typical healthcare FMEA is a five-step process including: topic selection, team assembly, process mapping, hazard analysis, and finally an action plan with outcome measures for each failure mode cause. The topic should be in a high-risk area where failures are highly severe, highly probable, or both. FMEA teams should be diverse and include subject matter experts, advisors, and a team leader. In a traditional FMEA, failure modes are scored and prioritized based on their frequency and severity during the hazard analysis. However, in healthcare FMEA, it is important not to neglect failure modes that may be severe, even if they rarely occur, because the potential harm to patients is unacceptable.

ROBUST PROCESS IMPROVEMENT

Healthcare systems and organizations need process improvement tools and methodologies to achieve higher reliability. These methods have evolved over time. In the 1980s many healthcare systems adopted total quality management and continuous quality improvement from other industries, but more recently have employed Lean and/or Six Sigma methodologies for efficiency and quality improvement. Lean is a set of principles and techniques that add value to production by enhancing necessary, relevant, and valuable steps and eliminating wasteful steps that do not add value. These methods improve quality while reducing time and costs. Six Sigma is a process improvement strategy that focuses on removing the causes of error and minimizing variability in a process. Six Sigma is an organized process of data analysis that uses a five-step approach: define, measure, analyze, improve, and control (DMAIC). In 2008, The Joint Commission Center for Transforming Healthcare created the robust process improvement toolset, which is a combination of Lean, Six Sigma, and change management designed for use in the healthcare environment. This comprehensive methodology has been shown to significantly improve hand hygiene compliance, ineffective handoffs at care transitions, and risk of wrong-site surgery and reduce cases of surgical site infections. The combination of Lean and Six Sigma is complementary because Lean improves process speed and optimizes flow while Six Sigma improves reliability through reduction of variation. Robust process improvement also includes change management as a systemic approach to prepare an organization to accept, implement, and sustain improved processes.

SYSTEMS THINKING

Healthcare systems are complex and dynamic in nature, with care provided by increasingly specialized individuals and organizations that employ specialized methods and technologies. In such systems, any single process within a system can be influenced by unseen variables, and properties that exist in larger systems may not exist when systems are separated into smaller parts. Achieving reliability in this sort of system requires a way of approaching problems that considers the nature of complex systems or systems thinking. Within the healthcare system, there are several layers of care including a macrosystem, consisting of senior leadership, a mesosystem, which includes major divisions of care like oncology or radiology, and a microsystem, which consists of the small functional units that directly provide care. Communication among these layers and a conceptually broader approach to problems as they arise are critical elements to systems thinking in healthcare. To adopt systems thinking, organizations should consider framing a problem as a pattern of behavior over time; look beyond external causes for problems and consider internal causes from within different parts of the system; try to understand the context of relationships among different parts of a system; concentrate on causality and understanding how a behavior is generated; and conceptualize causality as an ongoing process with effect influencing the causes and the causes affecting each other.

DAILY MANAGEMENT SYSTEMS

High-reliability organizations understand that the law of entropy and human behavior lead to eventual deviation from standards over time. Healthcare organizations are complex adaptive systems with many nuanced and interdependent connections between individuals that require a method to maintain reliable, standardized work. High-reliability healthcare organizations must implement a daily management system like those used by high-reliability organizations in other industries. A daily management system is a continuous process that ensures work is done in the right way and in the right time according to an organization's set objectives and priorities. Daily management systems are designed for rapid problem identification and problem solution by frontline staff whenever possible. If solutions exceed the capabilities of frontline staff, problems are quickly escalated to leadership for the creation of appropriate countermeasures.

Key components of a daily management system include leadership standard work, visual controls, and a daily accountability process. Leadership standard work typically includes checklists and standard processes that focus on assuring that a system runs as designed and emphasize continuous improvement of a system's performance. Visual controls include dashboards for important metrics and visibility boards that simply indicate whether daily performance is on target. These visual controls should be strategically designed and customized for individual departments or work cells. A daily accountability process is a standardized means of identifying problems, assigning ownership of problems, and establishing expectations for follow-up and implementation of a solution or countermeasure. In many highly reliable and lean institutions, the daily accountability process is accomplished through tiered meetings or huddles. Countermeasure tracker forms and task accountability boards may also be used to capture countermeasures, including ownership, countermeasure status, and when countermeasures should be completed.

HEALTHCARE HUDDLES FOR HIGH RELIABILITY

High-reliability organizations require continuous sharing of information among employees of all levels and roles, as well as mindfulness of the current state of their systems and processes. A common mechanism to achieve these aims is the huddle, a brief daily meeting of functional groups built into the workplace routine. Huddles are already used by healthcare organizations and have been linked to improvements in patient safety and operational and teamwork benefits. Huddles can be an important mechanism for active daily management and have also been found to create time and space for conversations, enhance relationships, and strengthen a culture of safety. The huddle is an opportunity to engage employees throughout an organization, encourage all staff to voice concerns or potential opportunities for improvement, and to build alignment across units. There is also a potential to reinforce a high-reliability culture including the five key principles of high reliability: a preoccupation with failure, reluctance to oversimplify, sensitivity to operations, a commitment to resilience, and deference to local expertise. A standardized agenda for a huddle may include a review of metrics and goals, a daily readiness assessment for the day's anticipated work including supplies and staffing, and a problem management accountability cycle to identify and resolve problems. Many organizations use a tiered huddle system, including a first tier of frontline staff and local leaders and higher-level tiers that consist of lower-tiered huddle representatives and higher levels of management. Within a radiology department, a tiered huddle structure may consist of modality-oriented huddles (computed tomography, ultrasound, magnetic resonance imaging, etc.) or organ-based divisions (neuroimaging, body imaging, musculoskeletal). Each of these huddles could send representatives to a second-tier department-wide huddle. This second huddle could then send representatives to a third-tier hospital-wide huddle.

CULPABILITY DECISION TREE

Whenever there are problems or errors within a system, a reliable organization needs to be able to discern whether those errors are the result of the system or the result of human error. When there is human error, an organization must be able to determine whether the erring employee intended harm, is significantly culpable for the error, or if a blameless error has occurred. This is important because assigning individual blame in an adverse event where there was no intent to harm is both ineffective in decreasing future adverse events and discourages future reporting of adverse events, contributing to an unsafe environment.

To create a just culture that balances individual accountability with accommodation for unavoidable human and system errors, James Reason created a culpability decision tree (Fig. 8.2). The culpability decision tree is a tool that can be used whenever there is an adverse event with a potentially culpable individual. The decision tree places individuals within a spectrum of culpability based on intent, substance abuse, violation of procedures, and history of unsafe acts and extends from blameless error to criminal activity. Another tool that can be used when assigning culpability is the substitution test, which considers whether an average equally trained individual would likely behave in the same way. These tools are important for maintaining a just culture and deciding whether system redesign/modification, further employee training/coaching, or punitive action is required.

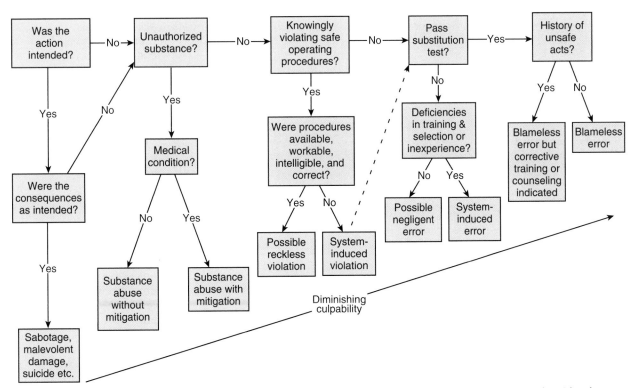

FIG. 8.2 A decision tree for determining the culpability for unsafe acts. (From Reason J. *Managing the Risks of Organizational Accidents*. Farnham, UK: Ashgate; 1997:209.)

SUGGESTED READINGS

Abujudeh H, Kaewlai R. Radiology failure mode and effect analysis: what is it? *Radiology*. 2009;252(2):544–550.

Batalden PB, Nelson EC, Gardent PB, Godfrey MM. Leading macrosystems and meso-systems for microsystem peak performance. In: Nelson EC, Batalden PG, Godfrey MM, eds. *Quality By Design: A Clinical Microsystems Approach*. San Francisco, CA: Jossey Bass; 2007:69–105.

Carroll JS, Rudoph JW. Design of high reliability organizations in health care. *Qual Saf Health Care*. 2006;15(suppl I):i4–i9.

Chassin M, Loeb J. High-reliability health care: getting there from here. *Milbank Q*. 2013;91(3):459–490.

Committee on Quality of Health Care in America, Institute of Medicine. *Crossing the Quality Chasm: A New Health System for the 21st Century*. Washington, DC: National Academy Press; 2001.

Dingley C, Daugherty R, Derieg MD, Persing R. Improving patient safety through provider communication strategy enhancements. In: Henriksen K, Battles JB, Keyes MA, Grady ML, eds. *Advances in Patient Safety: New Directions and Alternative Approaches: Performance and Tools*. Rockville, MD: Agency for Healthcare Research and Quality (US); 2008 vol.3.

Donnelly L. Practice policy and quality initiatives daily management systems in medicine. *Radiographics*. 2014;34(2):549–556.

Ferro J, Gouveia R. Strategy-driven daily management. *Planet Lean*; 7 July 2015. Available at http://planet-lean.com/how-to-create-an-effective-daily-management-system.

Gamble M. 5 traits of high reliability organizations: how to hardwire each in your organization. Becker's Hospital Review. <http://www.beckershospitalreview.com/hospital-management-administration/5-traits-of-high-reliability-organizations-how-to-hardwire-each-in-your-organization.html>.

Institute of Medicine. *To Err Is Human: Building a Safer Health System*. Washington, DC: National Academy Press; 1999.

Jamlik-Omari Johnson. Six Sigma and Lean opportunities for health care to do more and better with less. In: Abujudeh H, Bruno M, eds. *Quality and Safety in Radiology*. Cary: Oxford University Press; 2012.

Joint Commission. Root cause analysis practical tips for implementing the results of an RCA. *Jt Comm Perspect Patient Saf*. 2003:3.

Kaewlai R, Abujudeh H. Root Cause Analysis (RCA) and Health Care Failure Mode and Effect Analysis (HFEMA). In: Abujudeh H, Bruno M, eds. *Quality and Safety in Radiology*. Cary: Oxford University Press; 2012.

Kerr EA, McGlynn EA, Adams J, Keesey J, Asch SM. Profiling the quality of care in twelve communities: results from the CQI study. *Health Affairs*. 2004;23(3):247–256.

Larson D, Jonathan K, Karl K, Lane D. Key concepts in patient safety in radiology. *Radiographics*. 2015;35(6):1677–1693.

Lisa L. Safety and high reliability in the hospital radiology department. Radiology Business. <http://www.radiologybusiness.com/topics/practice-management/quality/safety-and-high-reliability-hospital-radiology-department?nopaging=1>.

Leape L. Errors in medicine. *Clin Chim Acta*. 2009;404:2–5.

Leonard M, Graham S, Bonacum D. The human factor: the critical importance of effective teamwork and communication in providing safe care. *BMJ Qual Saf Health Care*. 2004;13:85–90.

Leonard M, Graham S, Bonacum D. The human factor: the critical importance of effective teamwork and communication in providing safe care. *Qual Saf Health Care*. 2004;13(suppl):85–90.

Liker JK, Covnis GL. *The Toyota Way to Lean Leadership: Achieving and Sustaining Excellence Through Leadership Development*. New York, NY: McGraw Hill; 2012:121–143.

McGlynn EA, Asch SM, Adams J, et al. The quality of health care delivered to adults in the United States. *N Engl J Med*. 2003;348(26):2635–2645.

Nolan T, Resar R, Haraden C, Griffin FA. *Improving the Reliability of Health Care: IHI Innovation Series White Paper*. Boston, MA: Institute for Healthcare Improvement; 2004.

Prasanth P, Paul N. Learning from high-reliability organizations. *J Am Coll Radiol*. 2011;8(10):725–726.

Provost S, Lanham H, Leykum L, McDaniel R, Pugh J. Health care huddles: managing complexity to achieve high reliability. *Health Care Manage Rev*. 2015;40(1):2Y12.

Reason J. Engineering a safety culture. In: Reason JT, ed. *Managing the Risks of Organizational Accidents*. Farnham, Surrey, England: Ashgate; 1997: 191–222.

Richmond B. *The "Thinking" in Systems Thinking: Seven Essential Skills*. Waltham, MA: Pegasus Communications; 2000.

Rooney JJ, Vanden Heuvel LN. Root cause analysis for beginners. *Quality Progr*. 2004;37:45–53.

Rubenstein-Montano B, Liebowitz J, Buchwalter J, McCaw D, Newman B, Rebeck K. A systems thinking framework for knowledge management. *Decis Support Syst*. 2001;31(1):5–16.

Weick KE, Sutcliffe KM. *Managing the Unexpected: Assuring High Performance in an Age of Complexity*. San Francisco, CA: Jossey-Bass; 2007.

Chapter 9
Future of Quality Assurance

Aine M. Kelly and Paul Cronin

INTRODUCTION

Quality assurance, quality improvement, and total quality Management initiatives and programs have been used, to different degrees, in business, management, and healthcare settings for decades now. However, despite the obvious positive impact on all healthcare outcomes, diffusion and integration of these methodologies have been inconsistent across health systems, subspecialty disciplines, and programs. There are many causes and contributing factors to this lack of penetration, which include ongoing disparities in healthcare, a lack of accountability, the existence of diffuse and nonspecific goals, the use of measurements or metrics that did not always impact patient outcomes, and systems that encouraged volume over value.

At the same time, current healthcare costs are not sustainable, and we are moving toward healthcare coverage and regulations that incentivize and reward quality rather than quantity. The landscape of quality assurance is also set to change due to new managed healthcare plans (bundling of care, capitation, and accountable care organizations [ACOs]), federal and state regulatory requirements (increased reporting and accountability), technological advances (electronic medical records and systems, clinical decision support [CDS] at order entry, electronic closed-loop communication systems), the increased emphasis on preventative medicine (more screening rather than diagnosis and follow up), changes in patient attitudes (patient-centered imaging, patients as partners in healthcare), and globalization (telemedicine and teleradiology).

This chapter outlines the main influences (external and internal) that have governed quality assurance in the past and today and looks into the future of healthcare and the challenges that we will face. We outline the opportunities that we believe exist for diagnostic imagers to enhance the quality of imaging locally and nationally and make suggestions for overcoming barriers.

CHANGING HEALTHCARE LANDSCAPE INFLUENCES

Alternative Care Models

The cost of healthcare (and imaging) has been spiraling upward over the past couple of decades, such that payers, state and federal agencies/regulators, and government have taken major steps to contain it. These include the establishment of the federal government's Medicare Shared Savings Program (Section 3022 of the Patient Protection and Affordable Care Act [PPACA]), which set the structural foundation for ACOs and established certain quality performance standards that ACOs must meet to receive payments for shared savings.

Accountable Care Organizations

The ACO framework encourages cost control by guiding healthcare providers and hospitals toward more coordinated, higher-quality, patient-centered care for Medicare patients, and to replace the sometimes fragmented care received under the single payment, single provider system under the fee-for-service payment system. The ACO concept increases quality and access by tying participation in economic incentive programs to meeting certain quality performance goals. Under the PPACA, ACOs are accountable for the quality, cost, and overall care of the Medicare fee-for-service beneficiaries assigned to it and have processes in place to promote evidence-based medicine, coordinated care, and transparency.

Under ACOs, a capitated model of payment is intended to encourage better coordination of care and minimize duplication and inappropriate use of services. With capitated payment systems, physicians and other providers must assume considerable risk but are potentially rewarded by returning savings achieved beyond predetermined targets. This payment system shift (from fee for service to capitation) is converting specialty services such as diagnostic imaging from a profit center to a cost center. This gives health systems an economic incentive to further reduce the use of diagnostic imaging and encourage the use of potentially less efficacious alternatives.

ACOs potentially pose threats to radiology under fee-per-service (with decreased reimbursement per study, decreased utilization, and a shift toward less expensive imaging under cost containment initiatives, and by participation in ACO *shared savings* bonuses and penalties); under capitation (with potential financial risk to radiology for imaging utilization by other providers, mixed incentives for radiologists serving both fee-for-service and capitated patient pools); under health system integration (with reduced bargaining leverage for radiology groups, especially smaller ones); and increased malpractice risk for radiologists who are under pressure to decline imaging for financial reasons.

Given that imaging is critical to effective and efficient diagnosis and treatment of most patients with serious or chronic illnesses, radiologists should play an integral role in ACOs. In conjunction with primary care providers, radiologists can play an important role in screening programs and in the management of a variety of medical conditions by helping to provide the most effective care. Radiologists' roles in patient care include recommending the appropriate use of imaging studies, which, if normal or negative, could limit unnecessary referrals to specialists or additional procedures by having the right test done initially. Functioning as imaging experts or consultants is critical, particularly with physician extenders such as physician assistants and nurse practitioners, who are providing an increasing amount of healthcare.

Although healthcare reform brings challenges, these may be the catalyst for radiology to show its value proposition, transform the existing service delivery model, and assume a central role in healthcare organizations. To decrease the risk of becoming increasingly marginalized and vulnerable with market forces threatening to cast radiology as a commodity, radiology groups need to safeguard and promote their position within healthcare systems. Accountable care provides opportunities for radiology groups by emphasizing the need for physician leadership with the clinical, technical, and operational areas to direct and promote cost-control initiatives while preserving quality of care. Radiologists are well equipped to assume these leadership positions by virtue of our whole-body clinical knowledge base; our broad interfaces with the complete spectrum of primary care and specialty physicians; our long history of innovation in information technology (IT), especially electronic image data management and processing of large volumes of patient encounters; our experience with the development and deployment of sophisticated and expensive diagnostic equipment; and our extensive involvement in hospital operations, including education, supervision, and management of technologists and nurses.

To capitalize on this opportunity, radiologists must alter their fundamental image of themselves. Radiologists are the imaging experts or consultants, just like any other subspecialist, and not just image readers. Physician-to-physician consultation (with a discussion of relevant patient history, symptoms, and signs) is essential in optimizing the appropriate imaging for a specific patient at the right time. This is challenging under the current model, which emphasizes throughput (scheduling and performing examinations and finalizing their reports) and provides less time to stop and think about what is better for the patient. The current metrics, which focus on turnaround times, are not always the best for the individual patient or the health system.

Accountable Care Organizations and Program Performance Indicators

The Deficit Reduction Act (DRA) of 2005 directed the Agency for Healthcare Research and Quality (AHRQ) to develop program performance indicators and measures of client satisfaction for Medicaid beneficiaries receiving home- and community-based services. The AHRQ and its contractors analyzed promising claims-based quality measures, including adaptation of prevention quality indicators and recommended two sets of outcome measures: serious reportable events and potentially avoidable hospitalizations due to ambulatory care–sensitive conditions.

The DRA also delineated that for ACOs to share in any savings created, they had to prove they met various defined quality performance measures. These process and outcome measures span five quality domains: patient experience of care, care coordination, patient safety, preventive health, and at-risk population/frail health of older adults. Many of the proposed quality measures align with those used in other Centers for Medicare and Medicaid Services (CMS) quality programs, such as the Physician

Quality Reporting System (PQRS), the Electronic Health Record (EHR) incentive program, and the Hospital Inpatient Quality Reporting (Hospital IQR) program. To date, most of the measures relate to medical conditions or surgical/procedural/iatrogenic complications and readmission rates. Rather than wait for nonradiologists and administrators to determine relevant metrics applicable to diagnostic imaging, this offers an opportunity for radiologists to get involved in defining measures pertinent to patient imaging. These metrics could focus on a variety of measures, for example, screening uptake rates, scheduling time for oncology patients, imaging appropriateness (particularly for areas with society guidelines, such as in the setting of suspected pulmonary embolism), waiting time, complication rates, and patient and physician satisfaction with report issuance.

Pay for Performance

Authorized by the 2003 Medicare Prescription Drug, Improvement, and Modernization Act (also called the Medicare Modernization Act) and the 2005 DRA, the Hospital IQR program requires hospitals to report on quality measures to receive full annual payment updates. Under Section 3001 of the PPACA, the CMS Hospital Value-Based Purchasing program was designed to improve quality, reduce inappropriate care, and promote better health outcomes and patient experiences during hospital stays through a system of financial incentives and penalties. These pay-for-performance (P4P) programs reduce Medicare reimbursement to hospitals and physicians who score below national performance benchmarks on selected quality measures. For hospitals, some of the areas measured include readmissions, hospital-acquired conditions, mortality, patient experience of care, and clinical process measures of heart attack, heart failure, and pneumonia.

Under this program, a hospital's payments are adjusted based on its performance in four domains that reflect hospital quality: the clinical process of care domain, the patient experience of care domain, the outcome domain, and the efficiency domain. The Total Performance Score (TPS) comprises the clinical process of care domain score (weighted as 10% of the TPS), the patient experience of care domain (weighted as 25% of the TPS), the outcome domain score (weighted as 40% of the TPS), and the efficiency domain score (weighted as 25% of the TPS). Some of these are relevant to radiology, particularly the patient experience of care domain, the outcome domain, and the efficiency domain.

In the patient experience of care domain, patients are asked to rate hospital quality in eight areas including: nurses' communication, doctors' communication, responsiveness of hospital staff to their needs, controlled pain management, cleanliness and quietness of hospital environment, adequate communication about medicines, discharge and expected recovery information, and their overall rating of the hospital.

In the outcomes domain, metrics include inpatient measures (occurrence of hospital-acquired infections and other patient safety breaches such as falls and complications from procedures), outpatient measures (imaging efficiency patterns, emergency department [ED] throughput efficiency, use of health information technology [HIT],

TABLE 9.1 Hospital Outpatient Quality Reporting Program Imaging Efficiency Measures for 2016

Imaging Modality	Measurement
MRI lumbar spine for low back pain (OP-8)	Number of MRIs without antecedent conservative therapy
Mammography follow-up rates (OP-9)	Number of follow-up diagnostic mammograms, ultrasounds, or MRI within 45 days of screening mammogram
Abdomen CT—use of contrast material (OP-10)	The number of combined studies (with and without contrast)
Thorax CT—use of contrast material (OP-11)	The number of combined studies (with and without contrast).
Cardiac imaging for preoperative risk assessment for noncardiac low-risk surgery (OP-13)	The number of stress echocardiography, SPECT MPI, and stress MRI studies performed at the hospital outpatient department within 30 days of noncardiac, low-risk surgery performed at any location
Simultaneous use of brain CT and sinus CT (OP-14)	Number of studies with a simultaneous sinus CT study (i.e., on the same date, at the same facility as the brain CT) (Medicare OIE measures)

CT, Computed tomography; *MPI*, myocardial perfusion imaging; *MRI*, magnetic resonance imaging; *OIE*, outpatient imaging efficiency; *SPECT*, single-photon emission computed tomography.

care coordination, patient safety, and volume), and measures related to physician offices (prevention of avoidable conditions, supporting physicians in providing treatment).

Within many of the domains, outcome measures related to imaging are not specified, which provides radiologists with an opportunity to participate in determining which quality metrics or measures they deem relevant. For example, under care coordination, imagers could base themselves within the oncology clinic unit and be available for reporting of studies and consultation, including direct face-to-face patient consultation. Radiology organizations such as the American College of Radiology (ACR) and the national radiology societies should use their collective expertise and be proactive in defining and constantly updating relevant outcomes within the TPS domains of the. Initiatives such as the National Oncology Positron-Emission Tomography (PET) Registry are collaborations among radiology organizations. These initiatives collect data, including the impact of PET imaging, to justify Medicare reimbursement for imaging. Similar initiatives and programs could be applied to other imaging modalities to provide evidence of their impact on patient care quality and outcomes to justify reimbursement. Imaging organizations should form study subgroups of experts in the various fields.

In the efficiency domain, hospitals that provide efficient care at a lower cost to Medicare are recognized. Radiology departments can easily demonstrate efficiency in imaging and patient pathways because they comprise various processes and pathways. This is an opportunity for radiology departments with excellent IT infrastructure, integrated with electronic medical record systems, to document, illustrate, and demonstrate efficiency and continued improvement of the processes and pathways. The publicly reported Hospital Outpatient Quality Reporting (Hospital OQR) program outpatient imaging efficiency measures payment determinations for the calendar year 2016 are depicted in Table 9.1.

Radiologists can also increase efficiency and reduce the volume of costly high-end imaging through a consultation and review model. If a consult with imaging experts (radiologists) became a requirement for advanced imaging requests such as cross-sectional imaging (computed tomography [CT], magnetic resonance imaging [MRI], nuclear medicine) and procedures, as would happen for other subspecialties, relationships between radiology and

other subspecialty departments would improve, as well as the perception of radiology as a specialty.

Although desirable, there are significant challenges to applying P4P to radiology because of a lack of standardized radiology performance metrics and the difficulty of linking imaging with patient outcomes. The ACR has proposed several performance goals and activities (Box 9.1).

Diagnostic radiologists must look at the P4P systems that are in place in hospital systems, determine what part diagnostic imaging plays in meeting the hospital's requirements, and participate in achieving the hospital's goals. If radiologists do not do this, other stakeholders and specialists will determine radiology's role, and imaging departments risk being undervalued or left out of the equation altogether.

The existing metrics for diagnostic imaging departments are not always relevant to patient outcomes or aligned with outcomes in the current value-based system. Current process and outcome metrics include turnaround times and percentage of fall incidents while the patient is in the radiology department. Additional metrics proposed by regulatory agencies and reported in the Hospital Consumer Assessment of Healthcare Providers and Systems survey include the use of intravenous contrast material in body (chest, abdomen, and pelvis) CT and early MRI in low back pain. Suggested metrics for radiologists to use in the future include value metrics such as imaging impact on prevention of complications (detecting appendicitis before rupture) and impact on prognosis (detecting a breast carcinoma while it is small and completely surgically resectable). Table 9.2 provides examples of current process and outcome metrics and proposed metrics for the value-based system.

Physician Quality Reporting System

Within the CMS PQRS, providers are encouraged to report information on quality of care to CMS and reimbursements are linked to this reported information. This allows providers to assess the quality of the care they provide and to quantify how often they meet particular quality metrics. Participation in PQRS was initially voluntary, but since 2015, all providers eligible for incentive payments who fail to participate are subject to penalties. Since 2016, the penalty for those who fail to report on the minimum measure set is a 2% reduction in reimbursement. The goal of PQRS is to incentivize discussion of quality-oriented

- Create a set of radiology performance measures and objectively measure the quality of radiology practices.
- Create outcome and process metrics that have target benchmarks for performance.
- Identify metrics that emphasize the added value of radiology and are useful in continuous quality improvement within radiology practices.
- Promote the widespread use of registries such as the National Radiology Data Registry.
- Continue to promote the use of the appropriateness criteria or other forms of Decision Support in Computerized Physician Order Entry as a tool to reduce inappropriate imaging.
- Develop specific performance measures as part of program accreditation.

TABLE 9.2   Current and Proposed Metrics for Radiologists in a Value-Based Healthcare System

Pathological Condition	Volume Metrics	Value Metrics
Abdominal pain	Turnaround time	Prevention of complications (e.g., perforation)
	Adverse events (e.g., contrast-induced nephropathy or extravasation)	Effect of imaging on length of stay in hospital or emergency room
Breast cancer	Access times	Percentage of patients diagnosed while cancer is surgically resectable
	Percentage of BIRADS type 3 reports	Percentage of patients requiring repeat imaging or biopsy
Stroke	Access times	Cost vs. outcomes of imaging (CT perfusion vs. MRI) in triage to therapy
	Stroke-to-revascularization time	Stroke-to-revascularization time

BIRADS, Breast Imaging Reporting and Data System; *CT*, computed tomography; *MRI*, magnetic resonance imaging.

questions between patients and providers, and to promote awareness among providers of opportunities for quality improvement in daily care. Examples of measures to be reported in 2016 include the percentage of CT or MRI reports for chest or neck and neck ultrasound for adult patients without known thyroid disease with a less than 1.0 cm thyroid nodule noted incidentally with follow-up imaging recommendations.

Radiology Benefits Management

Radiology benefits managers (RBMs) are companies that are employed by third-party payers (insurance companies) to provide preauthorization for imaging using society guidelines and evidence or propriety algorithms. Some RBMs merely consult and advise; others may impose small consequences on the referring physician, and others may deny coverage if the patient actually receives the imaging as requested at the specific location. The process by which the RBM decides where patients can go for imaging should be based on evidence or quality factors, rather than on other factors such as lower cost, nearby location, or convenience. Some view the formation of RBM companies as a challenge to maintaining good relationships between radiologists and referring physicians, whereas others have criticized preauthorization programs for not always being transparent or evidence based, or because of perceived increased workflow or intrusions that could delay patient care. It is critical that doctors and nurses are involved in the authorization process, and radiologists should get involved so that they can participate in determining the structure and operation of RBMs in their health systems.

Utilization Management

Utilization management requires that radiologists use their expertise in imaging to ensure that imaging studies are performed appropriately. Radiologists are being encouraged to align with primary care practitioners to guide the appropriate use of imaging and referral to subspecialists through meetings and education. These measures may decrease inappropriate utilization by requiring peer-to-peer consultation with a radiologist for low-yield examinations and offering a means of comparing utilization rates of individual providers to established benchmarks. Combining utilization management with decision support in the context of computerized order entry would enable tracking of appropriate and inappropriate utilization rates. This approach would be a natural expansion of the *reading room consultation* model and would help counteract potential commoditization of radiology by nonphysician resource management groups and improve the *face* of radiology and its relationships with other departments.

Bundled or Capitated Payments

Specific interventions addressing the cost of imaging, including reducing fee-for-service reimbursement rates (Section 5102 of the DRA of 2005), may not necessarily improve quality because providers might try to increase quantity at the expense of quality. As part of the national and regional healthcare reform debates, many leading policy makers have advocated a major shift in the method of payment for medical services, moving away from fee-for-service care to bundled or capitated payments to hospitals and physicians for managing the health of a defined population of patients. Bundled payments are implemented through the ACO, based on a bundled episode of care or global (capitated) payments. Within episodes of care, a fixed payment is provided that is based on the diagnosis-related group (DRG), regardless of the number and complexity of diagnostic and other testing that might take place. Bundling is now occurring for inpatient episodes and will likely be extended to other care venues, so it is critical for radiologists to pay close attention to the parts of their work that are bundled, how the bundling is done, and the rules that govern the bundling. Radiologists must participate in deciding how and when to parcel episodes for bundling of payments by knowing what and when imaging is appropriate.

LEGAL AND REGULATORY INFLUENCES

External Review/Oversight Agencies

In addition to being subject to healthcare changes at the government level, there are multiple external agencies and reviewers who oversee quality in American healthcare. These include the Department of Health and Human Services (DHSS), the CMS, The Joint Commission (TJC), the Institute of Medicine (IOM), the AHRQ, the National Committee for Quality Assurance (NCQA), and the National Quality Forum (NQF).

The law directs the DHSS to create a strategic plan that identifies critically important areas for improvement, sets goals, and selects measures to be used in federal programs. This plan relies on input from affected stakeholders, including hospitals, patients, purchasers, insurers, and public policy experts.

TJC is a government nonprofit organization with the intended function of providing voluntary accreditation of hospitals based on a rubric of defined minimum quality standards. Its objective is to improve the quality of healthcare by evaluating healthcare organizations and providing guidance on the elements necessary to deliver care that optimizes quality and value. TJC performs regular reviews of health systems and hospitals, and radiologists can get involved in their local quality improvement committees to ensure that accreditation efforts are being met.

In 1970, the National Academies of Science established the IOM, which has since launched numerous concerted efforts focused on evaluating, informing, and improving the quality of healthcare delivery. The IOM has issued landmark reports, several of which have focused on quality concerns in healthcare (including *To Err Is Human* and *Crossing the Quality Chasm*), with their most recent report in 2015, *Improving Diagnosis in Healthcare*, focused on diagnostic errors in healthcare. The recommendations from their 2015 report include promoting more effective teamwork, enhancing professional education, encouraging HIT support of the diagnostic process, developing approaches to identify and learn from diagnostic error, establishing nonpunitive work cultures that support improving the diagnostic system, developing an environment to enable learning from diagnostic errors and near misses, designing a payment system that rewards diagnostic process, and providing dedicated funding to improve the diagnostic process. Given that diagnostic imaging is a large component of most patient care pathways, radiologists are ideally poised to improve upon and refine the diagnostic process.

The precursor to the current-day AHRQ was established in 1979 in response to reports of wide geographic variations in practice patterns without supporting clinical evidence, with reports of misuse and overuse of procedural treatments. Its roles include investing in clinical effectiveness, treatment outcomes, and evidence-based practice guidelines. The AHRQ's initiatives include the US Preventative Services Task Force and the National Guidelines Clearinghouse. Many guidelines relate to screening and diagnosis, in which imaging plays a central role. There have

been recent revisions to the guidelines for breast cancer screening with mammography and some confusion exists within the community and the medical profession. Radiologists have an opportunity to get involved and contribute to researching and developing revisions of the screening and diagnostic guidelines.

The NCQA is a private nonprofit organization established in 1990 with the objective of improving healthcare quality by managing accreditation programs for individual physicians, health plans, and medical groups. It measures accreditation performance through the administration of the Healthcare Effectiveness Data and Information Set and the submission of the Consumer Assessment of Healthcare Providers and Systems survey. Radiologists can get involved in ensuring that their health systems meet the standards required to be accredited by the NCQA or by participating as a member.

In 1999, the NQF, a nonprofit organization, was set up with its mission to improve the quality of US healthcare. The forum works to define national goals and priorities for healthcare quality improvement, to build national consensus around these goals, and to endorse standardized performance metrics for quantifying and reporting on national healthcare quality efforts. The NQF's endorsement of programs has become the gold standard for healthcare performance measures and is relied upon by healthcare purchasers including the CMS. The forum's membership includes a wide variety of stakeholders including hospitals, healthcare providers, consumer groups, purchasers, accrediting bodies, and research and healthcare quality improvement organizations.

Patient-Centered Outcomes Research Institute

One of the key provisions of the PPACA centered on quality was the creation of a nonprofit Patient-Centered Outcomes Research Institute (PCORI) to conduct comparative effectiveness research (CER) in clinical care to inform decision making. This research will determine which interventions are most effective for different patient populations under various circumstances, and findings will be used to guide treatment pathways that support patient-centered, evidence-based, high-quality care. Gazelle and colleagues have proposed a framework for assessing the value of imaging on outcomes of interest to assist PCORI in selecting imaging for CER. They suggested that imaging technologies that could affect larger numbers of patients with smaller expected anticipated clinical benefits should require higher levels of outcomes data (Fryback and Thornbury's diagnostic imaging efficacy hierarchy). If these imaging technologies also have the potential to substantially increase costs or not be cost-effective, the need for higher-level outcomes evidence is reinforced. Alternatively, if imaging technologies that would potentially affect a smaller number of patients, with higher anticipated clinical benefits, have a lower impact on overall costs and are likely to be cost-effective, then lower levels of outcomes data would be required.

In imaging, patient-centered outcomes extend beyond the traditional metrics of patient satisfaction. Instead, these outcomes should encompass all potential benefits and harms, focus on outcomes that are relevant to patients, and provide information to inform decision making. Therefore, it is important that radiologists be involved and participating on key committees that will set national agendas for patient-centered outcomes research, determine funding priorities, and communicate and disseminate evidence leading to integration of the best imaging evidence into policy.

Getting Imaging Into Comparative Effectiveness Research

In addition to enhancing their role in population screening, radiologists need to be at the forefront of CER, using their human capital, from the beginning of residency training, to pursue studies that demonstrate radiology's value in affecting population-based health outcomes. Radiology organizations and societies should be contributing to discussions on the value of imaging and imaging-based interventions. Current and future efforts at improving population health will benefit from the collection of pooled data and the creation of robust registries, and radiology should be at the forefront of managing these large databases. The diagnostic work of radiologists benefits patients predominantly through directing care pathways. Decisions as to whether to treat, and how to treat, are often based on the results of a diagnostic imaging exam. The cognitive work of radiologists therefore plays a role in managing care and affects the costs of care. In an era in which population health will become a greater focus of policymakers, it is critical for radiology to stress the importance of its care management roles and to be reimbursed for its services. The explosion in imaging that has occurred over the past 20 years underlines the greater need for radiologists to act as stewards of appropriate imaging resources. The growth in imaging has resulted in an increase in incidental findings. Managing these findings consistently, to optimize patient health and effectively use imaging and healthcare resources for the population, is an important goal for radiology to pursue.

TRADITIONAL AND FUTURE QUALITY ASSURANCE APPROACHES/METRICS

Currently, many physician quality incentives are oriented toward process metrics (such as door-to-balloon/thrombolysis time) rather than outcomes. This might not be optimal because we do not know if strict adherence to prescribed processes ensures the best quality. Following guidelines could undermine outcomes, if the guidelines are not well grounded in evidence or are outdated. We need to determine which quality metrics are meaningful and important to patients and society. A challenge is that many quality metrics are difficult to quantify and it is therefore impossible to track progress toward goals. For example, misdiagnosis does not have any measures or standards. There are many reports with information on measures and metrics, but often there is not sufficient overlap between them to allow valid comparisons. Traditional quality metrics have focused on diagnosis and treatment, and less on preventative care and screening.

In addition, high quality is often invisible or not obvious, making it difficult to set targets and assess progress. Furthermore, not all of the quality metrics that will become important in the future are known today. Important quality measures will include out-of-network costs, access rates/issues, ease of getting services, claims denied by insurance, and comparisons of quantity to quality. It will become important to develop measures that incorporate patient feedback on care received and on their outcomes. Patients and healthcare providers will need to become contributors to the value-based systems of the future.

From Individual Health to Population Health

With few exceptions, such as the Veterans Health Administration, the focus of healthcare in the United States for the past century has been on the health of individuals. To expand healthcare coverage in the United States, the healthcare system must maintain reasonable equity and access at affordable costs and realign so that stakeholders are incentivized to improve both public health and the health of individuals. Radiologists have a role to play in population and public health, through the development and refinement of imaging screening tests and imaging biomarkers. Examples of radiologists' impact on cancer screening include mammography for breast cancer, CT colonography for colon cancer, and low-dose CT for lung cancer. For us to build on this foundation, we must continue to more specifically define target populations for screening programs, tailor follow-up protocols based on both the initial screening results and updated relative risk, and assign resources based on expected benefits. Imagers need to be greater stakeholders in research involving the use of imaging biomarkers and be integral in the development of precision medicine as part of customized care of individual patients.

Increased Emphasis on Prevention and Screening

Current quality metrics often focus on diagnosis and treatment, in which imaging plays a central role. Examples include diagnostic accuracy (sensitivity and specificity), access to imaging, scheduling time, turnaround time (from initiation of imaging request to final report signing and communication), treatment effects, and complication rates. Governments and health systems have realized that the key to helping the healthcare system is removing the burden of chronic care and reducing preventable disease. The emphasis is now switching to preventive care and screening. Diagnostic imaging already plays a major role in screening efforts and this role will increase. Other opportunities include teachable moments, whereby candidates for screening examinations can receive advice and counseling on additional lifestyle changes or other screening options. For example, women presenting for breast screening examinations could meet with a radiologist and discuss their risks for colon cancer and screening options. Other potential roles for radiologists are in preventative medicine where, for example, radiologists review coronary calcium screening exams with patients and discussing calcium scores and their implications for coronary artery disease and future events. The metrics that doctors believe are important are probably not important to patients. It will become important for radiologists to talk to patients and pay attention to patient satisfaction surveys, to direct future quality efforts.

Managing Incidental Findings

Imaging technology continues to advance with the result that radiologists are diagnosing disease sooner and cancers at earlier stages. Radiologists continue to work on improving image quality, driving down radiation dose and making imaging available to more patients and screening subjects. A downside to improved detection is the discovery of more pseudo-disease and incidental findings. There are many large-scale trials that support larger-scale screening efforts including, for example, lung cancer screening. A side effect of diagnostic imaging and screening examinations is an increasing number of incidental lesions in solid organs or nodules in the lungs. Studies are under way to evaluate this situation, with radiologists involved. More good-quality imaging research is needed, including meta-analyses to evaluate the outcomes and the most appropriate follow-up and management. This information can be used to derive evidence-based follow-up guidelines and white papers with radiologists playing a central role in their development.

Addressing Healthcare Disparities

Steps have been taken to make healthcare available to patients of all ages and socioeconomic groups. The government is working toward universal healthcare, but unfortunately a significant proportion of adults are underinsured or have no health insurance. Similarly, access and availability of screening and diagnostic tests is not uniform across the population. Some of the underlying factors involve remote geographic locations or economic issues such as local availability of subspecialty expertise. Occasionally, the drivers for disparities in use of screening programs have origins in cultural beliefs and preferences. Radiologists and practices have taken steps to address barriers with telemedicine (teleradiology) and remote conferencing (image viewing and reporting). Radiology subspecialty expertise may cross boundaries and borders, allowing high-quality care for more patients. Similarly, radiologists and other specialists may be able to participate in multidisciplinary clinical radiological meetings at remote far away locations.

Value-Based Insurance Design

Several healthcare systems have engaged in value-based insurance design (VBID), in which high-value services and treatments are associated with low or no copays from patients. For example, diabetic care such as insulin treatment or foot and eye checkups are covered in some health systems, because good diabetic sugar control and checkups can prevent disease complications that will cost more healthcare dollars downstream. Extending such initiatives into imaging will involve evaluating what constitutes high-value imaging for patient DRGs or for individual patients. Decisions will have to be made by insurance companies regarding the imaging tests that are covered or affected by VBID. If radiologists do not take their place at the table during discussions, they run the risk of other stakeholders influencing whether imaging is viewed as a high-value service or not, which could negatively impact the quality of patient care received.

Peer Review

For radiologists in practice, participating in local or national quality control committees are ways to learn about quality improvement. Similarly, being enrolled in maintenance of certification programs encourages them to engage in practice quality improvement, part of which involves peer review by colleagues. Despite the best of efforts, the peer-review process is not completely free of blame and is a challenge to maximizing its benefits (improving quality in diagnostic imaging reporting). On the other side, there can be a reluctance of radiologists to report a misdiagnosis for fear of causing punishment of a colleague. There is a need to detoxify peer review, which starts with eliminating the culture of blame and making a more collaborative culture.

These are obstacles that many have not been able to overcome to date. Having electronic systems where colleagues could anonymously flag reports and insert free-text comments is one solution. There are no proprietary electronic peer-review systems available at present for individual radiologists to use locally in their practices. Another challenge is the lack of standardization of error type or severity. The ACR's RADPEER program is a centralized system through which subscribers can have their data benchmarked to peer radiology practices; it has some standardization with four grades or levels of error that can be applied. Some authors have introduced (and tested for feasibility) consensus-oriented peer review to foster a better atmosphere for peer review. In these systems, reports (from conference participants only) are randomly selected, reviewed for consensus, and the consensus results are distributed to all conference participants. Some institutions have incorporated scorecards into systems such as RADPEER to increase transparency and feedback. Software programs that are incorporated into workstations can be used to enable individual peer review, and have been tested with radiologists increasingly engaged in the peer-review process.

TECHNOLOGY

Clinical Decision Support at Order Entry/ Utilization Management

Section 218 of the Protecting Access to Medicare Act (2014) mandates that by 2017 physicians must reference appropriateness guidelines from provider organizations when ordering advanced imaging for Medicare beneficiaries. The use of imaging CDS for targeted ambulatory imaging services, where high-quality evidence exists, will be a requirement for payment for performing such imaging services beginning January 1, 2017. Although practical aspects of the law's implementation still need to be clarified, many health systems are incorporating CDS systems at order entry to help providers select the most appropriate form of imaging in an effort to limit overutilization. This trend reflects the move from volume- to value-based care. The law also calls for identification of ordering providers with low adherence to evidence presented in CDS beginning in 2017, with the expectation that outliers may be subject to preauthorization beginning in 2020. The stage II meaningful-use criteria of HIT, part of the Economic and Clinical Health Act of 2009, promotes the use of imaging CDS through modest near-term financial incentives and subsequent long-term financial penalties. Radiologists will have to partner with these new integrated delivery systems (accountable care, P4P, and bundled payments) to effectively manage radiology utilization and cost. This provides an opportunity for radiologists to work within these systems to increase quality while containing costs.

Radiologists could oversee the content and implementation of CDS systems that can be delivered electronically at the point of imaging test requisition. These systems would provide information on whether imaging is indicated; the likely benefits associated with different imaging options, including which imaging study is likely to be most beneficial; and the relative costs, risks, and radiation exposures associated with different imaging options. Although best practices for implementation and adoption of evidence through CDS are still debated, there is a growing body of evidence for its effectiveness and impact. It is uncertain if large-scale implementation of imaging CDS will lead to improved healthcare quality, as seen in smaller settings, or to improved patient outcomes. However, imaging CDS enables the correlation of existing imaging evidence with outcome measures, including morbidity, mortality, and short-term imaging-relevant management outcomes (e.g., biopsy, chemotherapy).

Components of effective CDS systems are listed in Box 9.2. In addition, radiologists should consult on the appropriate use of imaging and the clinical implications of the imaging findings, profile the use of imaging tests at the referrer level to provide feedback and education to providers regarding their patterns of imaging use, and leverage lower-cost community offsite locations within integrated delivery systems to provide high-quality care where and when it is needed.

Meaningful Use

The American Recovery and Reinvestment Act (ARRA) has expedited the adoption of computerized physician order entry and CDS systems in healthcare through the creation of financial incentives and penalties to promote the *meaningful use* of HIT. Meaningful use is a collection of government-sponsored initiatives designed to encourage providers to use healthcare IT solutions to improve the quality of care while lowering costs. The Medicare and Medicaid EHR incentive program provides incentive payments to eligible professionals, eligible hospitals, and critical access hospitals as they adopt, implement, upgrade, or demonstrate meaningful use of certified EHR technology. The desired endpoint includes a fully integrated electronic medical record (EMR), radiology information system (RIS), and picture archiving and communications (PACS) systems using Digital Image Communications in Medicine for storage and Health Level 7 for transfer of information.

Full integration is still a challenge in many health and hospital systems. Currently, there remain several opportunities for improvement. These include the need to reduce the reimaging of transferred patients, which is still an issue in many hospitals and departments. Even with seamless EHR systems, there is a need for consistency in protocols and a requirement for secondary interpretation.

BOX 9.2   Essentials for Effective Clinical Decision Support (CDS)

- CDS is a multidisciplinary clinical program and not an information technology initiative.
- Evidence supporting clinical actions and recommendations embedded in imaging CDS is transparent to users at order entry.
- Evidence sources embedded in imaging CDS are diverse.
- Evidence is up to date.
- Clinical recommendations and assessments embedded in imaging CDS are brief, unambiguous, and achievable.
- CDS systems are user friendly and respect provider workflow.
- Establishing consequences for ignoring CDS recommendations will enhance the impact of imaging CDS as education alone.
- Imaging CDS initiatives targeting well-defined clinical performance deficiencies are more effective.
- Imaging CDS should enable measurement of its impact.
- CDS is positioned to increase workflow efficiency for all stakeholders.

Modified from Khorasani R, Hentel K, Darer J, et al. Ten commandments for effective clinical decision support for imaging: enabling evidence-based practice to improve quality and reduce waste. *AJR Am J Roentgenol.* 2014;203(5):945-951.

In addition to the provision of efficient primary care and shared savings, successful ACO model principles include an IT infrastructure. Such information systems should exist as data warehouses and not be proprietary. The optimal use of HIT should extend beyond the storage and transfer of image data to include the promotion of direct patient communication outside of office visits, making available up-to-the minute performance data for doctors, simplifying the task of doing the right thing at every patient contact, supporting disease registries, and saving money, including presenting value propositions to care providers at the point of care.

Closed-Loop Communication Systems

Accurate and timely communication of patient care–related information among medical professionals is a major challenge in prevailing healthcare delivery systems, with the current emphasis on patient throughput and efficiency. Communication lapses, omissions, and errors are also frequently implicated in medicolegal cases. To enable further patient management or *disposition*, radiologists are under pressure to finalize their reports and communicate significant, urgent, or unexpected findings. It is essential for radiologists to know that report information has been successfully received and understood by the relevant party. Confirmation of receipt and understanding is easy in synchronous communications such as face-to-face interactions, phone conversations, or online meetings. When communication is asynchronous, such as text messages, wireless pager messages, or emails, confirmation of receipt is more difficult. Today, there are multiple electronic systems, integrated with PACS, RIS, and EMR, that enable closure of this communication loop (radiologist to referrer). With closed-loop communication, information is sent to its intended recipient to start the cycle and a message comes back to the originator confirming that the information was received to close the loop. Radiologists can fail to confirm that the referrer received the report information, and the responsibility for communicating findings rests more with the radiologist, as evidenced by multiple legal cases, many of which cite the ACR practice guideline for communication. However, with integrated electronic systems, effective closed-loop communication of urgent and nonurgent imaging findings can be achieved while minimizing interruptions in daily workflow.

QUALITY APPROACHES ADAPTED FROM THE BUSINESS WORLD

Traditional quality improvement methodologies have been adapted from business and management by healthcare, including the Lean approach. Additional modern management science approaches to quality that healthcare organizations could incorporate include the Baldridge criteria, the International Standardization Organization (ISO), and Six Sigma.

Lean Management

Lean derives from the Japanese Toyota Production System management and manufacturing policies and was designed to allow personnel and organizations to become more efficient while eliminating waste. Continuous incremental improvements in performance are made with the goals of adding value to services provided while maintaining the highest possible customer satisfaction. Expenditure for resources, other than those that create value for the customer, is regarded as wasteful and targeted for elimination. As waste is eliminated, production times and costs decrease. Lean emphasizes process analysis and is particularly relevant to radiology departments, which depend on a smooth flow of patients and uninterrupted equipment function for efficient operation. The principles of Lean are summarized in Box 9.3. In any part of Lean processes, one must not lose focus on the customer and ensure that value is being added from the customer's perspective. Within radiology, *customers* include referring physicians and patients. One must solicit feedback from these groups, because our perception of their values may not be accurate. Referring physicians rely heavily on imaging and often value timeliness of report finalization, whereas patients value aspects like ease and speed of procedure scheduling or comfort in the reception area.

International Standardization Organization

The ISO has developed and published a series of standards, including the ISO 9000 family of standards (quality management), that define, establish, and maintain an effective quality assurance system for manufacturing and service industries. The ISO 9000 standards include subcategories pertaining to basic concepts and language (ISO 9000); the requirements for a quality management system (ISO 9001); how to make a quality management system more efficient and effective (ISO 9004); and guidance on internal and external audits of quality management systems (ISO 19011).

ISO quality standards are based on a number of quality management principles including a strong customer focus, the motivation and implication of top management, the process approach, and continual improvement. The

---

BOX 9.3 Lean Principles

- Respect all staff and involve them equally.
- Observe and analyze processes where they occur; *go to the gemba* ("go to the real work place").
- Eliminate all forms of waste or steps in a process that do not add value.
- Standardize work processes to minimize variation.
- Improve flow of all processes in the system.
- Use visual cues to communicate and inform.
- Add value for the customer.
- Apply Lean (graphical) tools.

---

seven quality management principles are: customer focus, leadership, engagement of people, the process approach, improvement, evidence-based decision making, and relationship management.

Baldridge Criteria for Performance Excellence

The Baldridge program is a public-private partnership between the United States Department of Commerce, the National Institute of Standards and Technology, and the Foundation for the Malcolm Baldrige National Quality Award (funded by the American Society for Quality, a nonprofit professional agency and the Alliance for Performance Excellence, a nonprofit national network). Named after the US secretary of commerce, Malcom Baldridge, the Baldridge standards (or criteria) were established in 1987 to help US manufacturers compete in a global economy. The Baldridge program's main mission is to promote quality excellence in all US professional organizations through education, with an award component. In fact, most winners of the 102 annual Malcolm Baldridge National Quality Awards represent the business sector, whereas health systems won only 17 awards with only one entity, the North Mississippi Health System, winning it twice. Applicants are evaluated rigorously by an independent board of examiners in seven areas defined by the Baldrige Criteria for Performance Excellence: leadership; strategic planning; customer focus; measurement, analysis, and knowledge management; workforce focus; operations focus; and results.

Six Sigma

Six Sigma has been around for about a century and was popularized by Motorola in the 1980s. In manufacturing, Six Sigma is a quality standard based on reducing variability within processes or products to move the mean toward a gold standard. Six Sigma indicates six standard deviations from the arithmetic mean, which equates to having only 3.4 defects per million. By measuring the number of defects, identifying the sources of error, and systematically determining how to avoid them, one aims to achieve nearly zero defects. Six Sigma involves complex statistical methods and starts with identifying the process and key customers, which requires a team of individuals that understand the problem and are familiar with the institution. The five steps of the Six Sigma process are: defining customer needs, measuring performance, analyzing data, setting priorities and launching improvements, and checking for change compared to the baseline to control the future process (define, measure, analyze, improve, and control, or DMAIC).The elements of Six Sigma are similar to plan-do-study-act (PDSA) and other quality improvement tools, and align with good medical practice. A criticism of Six Sigma is its complexity, with rigorous adherence to problem solving potentially resulting in overanalysis of simple problems that might have more obvious solutions.

QUALITY APPROACHES FROM MANUFACTURING AND AVIATION

Systems Engineering

A 2010 report from the IOM (*For the Public's Health: The Role of Measurement in Action and Accountability*) made key recommendations to improve health data analysis and reporting.This report proposed that the DHSS should coordinate the development, evaluation, and advancement of predictive and system-based simulation models to understand the consequences of underlying determinants of health. The report also suggested that DHSS should use modeling to assess intended and unintended outcomes associated with policy, funding, investment, and resource options.

The Presidents' Council of Advisors on Science and Technology issued a report in 2014 entitled *Better Healthcare and Lower Costs: Accelerating Improvements Through Systems Engineering*, in which it recommended that the DHSS and the Department of Commerce recognize healthcare providers that successfully apply systems engineering approaches. The council made these seven recommendations for healthcare: (1) align payment incentives and reported information with improved patient and population outcomes; (2) accelerate efforts to improve the nation's health data infrastructure; increasing technical assistance to healthcare systems and communities that are applying systems engineering approaches; (3) support efforts to engage communities in systematic healthcare improvement; (4) establish awards, challenges, and grants to promote use of healthcare systems tools and methods; (5) build competencies and workforce to redesign healthcare; and (6) provide leadership in systems engineering through increasing data available to benchmark performance, understand community health, and examine broader regional and national trends.

Policies from the Affordable Care Act and the ARRA have laid the groundwork for wider use of systems engineering through new care models that promote integrated care and rapid adoption of EHRs. In addition, the National Quality Strategy identifies areas for improvement in healthcare quality and outcomes that systems-engineering initiatives should address. A recently published joint report from the National Academy of Engineering and the IOM advocated the widespread application of systems-engineering tools to improve healthcare delivery.

Systems engineering focuses on coordinating, synchronizing, and integrating complex systems of personnel, materials, information, and financial resources. This is achieved through the application of mathematical modeling and analysis techniques. Over recent decades, the continuing development and application of systems-engineering methods have allowed unprecedented growth in the manufacturing, logistics, distribution, and transportation sectors of the economy.Although direct comparisons between other economic sectors and healthcare delivery are not possible, many functions common to both have been significantly improved in other sectors through engineering analysis. Systems engineering can be applied to inventory control and logistics, scheduling, operations management, project planning, facilities design, process flow analysis, resource synchronization, engineering economic analysis, and many other areas.

Systems engineering focuses on the design, control, and orchestration of system activities to meet performance objectives.A healthcare system (or radiology department) is a set of possibly diverse entities (patients, nurses, physicians, technologists, etc.), each performing some set of functions.The interaction of these entities as they perform their various functions gives rise to a global system behavior. The state of a system is a real-time snapshot of its status with different components being occupied or in use, free or idle, or not available or on a break. As the system operates, it moves from one state to the next through the occurrence of enabled events. An event is enabled when the preconditions for its occurrence are met and it occurs when its associated actions are performed. For example, if the CT scan suite has seven scanners, with six occupied and one open, and there is a patient in the ED requiring an emergency trauma CT, then a CT scan slot allocation event is enabled and can be performed.This event is performed when the CT time slot is assigned to the patient. If another patient arrives needing an urgent CT, the CT slot allocation event is not enabled until a time slot becomes available.

The sequence of states that the system traverses over some time horizon is referred to as the state trace of the system. There are many system state traces that might possibly evolve, and because of the presence of uncontrollable events such as walk-in or ambulance arrivals, the future state trace is not always predictable or controllable. System performance measures are statistics computed from information in a given system trace. Examples of performance measures could be the number of outpatient CT scans delayed by at least 20 minutes, the number of coronary CT angiography patients with optimal heart rates, or the turnaround time (from CT request to final report) for the ED and inpatients during peak hours.

Systems-Engineering Modeling Approaches

Systems modeling involves identifying the most relevant system characteristics and representing them in a mathematical model. The model is then analyzed to learn about and improve the behavior of the original system. This process is significantly different from the hypothesis-based clinical trial mode of research prevalent in medical research. There are six steps in the process, as shown in Box 9.4.

Challenges to the implementation of systems-engineering approaches include the extensive data requirements and the fact that reimbursement models do not incentivize practices to use these models or approaches, so managerial support might be difficult to obtain. Healthcare also has a traditional culture of rigid division of labor, and it might be difficult to erode these traditional boundaries. In addition, the presence of engineers may spark skepticism or fear; very few healthcare workers are trained to think

1. Define system purpose and scope, specify required functions and resource types, and develop relevant performance measures.
2. Specify, collect, and develop required data.
3. Design, validate, and verify appropriate system models.
4. Use the model to learn about system behavior to find the best design alternative.
5. Using results of the previous step, determine how to configure the system for best performance.
6. Develop implementation and evaluation plans and coordinate their performance.

analytically about healthcare delivery, and, conversely, engineers have little education in healthcare delivery.

Complexity Science

There has been an explosion in the amount of information available (thanks to the worldwide web and the Internet), and new (and sometimes imprecise, equivocal, or conflicting) evidence emerges every day. At the same time, healthcare has become much more complex, and technology makes health systems more integrated and automated. In the past, public health was concerned with containing or eradicating largely infectious diseases, whereas the focus has now shifted toward disease entities with fuzzier boundaries, which are often the result of the interplay among genetics, the environment, and lifestyle choices. There is increased emphasis on prevention and screening, which comes alongside more sophisticated and complex diagnostic tools, more integrated follow-up, and ever more advanced and complex treatments. Today, patient values or preferences are increasingly taken into account with shared decision making. Treatment decisions are now made with the help of multidisciplinary teams. New integrated healthcare plans and managed healthcare systems have emerged that impact screening, diagnostic, and treatment decisions. Healthcare is inextricably linked to the legal and regulatory system and is also influenced by politics, climate, geography, and the economy. Healthcare systems have become very large, unpredictable, and sometimes chaotic. We can attempt to break the systems down into component parts or processes to analyze and fix them, like a machine, but in healthcare, no part of the equation is constant, independent, or predictable.

A complex adaptive system is a collection of individual agents with the ability to act in ways that are not always totally predictable, and whose actions are interconnected such that one agent's actions affect other agents. Complex adaptive systems have processes and parts with overlapping or indistinct boundaries, with some elements belonging to multiple different systems at any one time. The actions of the various working parts of complex systems, like healthcare, are based on instinct, informal theories, and mental models of human thinking and reasoning. Because the components or agents within the system can change, the overall system is also adaptive, which can be for better or worse. Systems are embedded within other systems and as each evolves or adapts, any systems within which it is nested will also change. Understanding complexity science includes accepting that tensions and paradoxes will occur and that not everything can be rationalized or resolved. The behavior of a complex system emerges as a result of the interactions among its elements and the outcomes are often more than the sum of the parts. Having multiple different components can lead to some novel or innovative outcomes. Furthermore, the various processes and pathways do not follow the rules of linear dynamics; a small initial change can have large effects. Some effects can also be unpredictable in complex systems, even if a main theme is apparent. Complexity thinking suggests that relationships between parts are more important than the parts themselves, and that minimum specifications yield more creativity than detailed plans.

Interdisciplinary Team Training

Modern forms of healthcare, such as managed care, will increase the need for interdisciplinary teamwork. Radiologists will be competing with other subspecialists for limited resources. We will also have to work alongside disciplines with a different way of thinking, such as nursing, pharmacy, or social work. We will need to understand their way of thinking and the challenges that face them to understand how we can thrive together. Ultimately, if radiologists are to take their place in policy debates, we will need to understand management in organizations and interdisciplinary teamwork principles.

Diagnostic imaging lies at the intersections of patient care, and most patients interact with radiology departments and radiologists during their course of care. As a specialty, we are primarily hospital based, but we intersect with most specialties. Understanding systems-based practice and our place in the system would benefit us and the system as a whole. Radiologists should undergo management training to allow them to manage the entire organization's imaging enterprise. Integrated relationships with hospitals (administration and leadership) would create opportunities for radiologists to ensure appropriate reimbursement for participation in nonclinical activities such as enterprise administration, utilization management, quality control, radiation safety, technologist supervision and education, equipment selection and optimization, and educational and regulatory oversight.

Reducing Errors in Aviation

Pilots and doctors operate in complex environments where teams interact with technology. In both domains, risk varies from low to high with threats coming from a variety of sources in the environment. Safety is paramount for both professions, but cost issues can influence the commitment of resources for safety efforts. Aircraft accidents are infrequent, but highly visible, often involving massive loss of life, and resulting in exhaustive investigation into causal factors, public reports, and remedial action. Research by the National Aeronautics and Space Administration into aviation accidents has found that 70% involve human error.

In both aviation and medicine, teamwork is required, and team error can be defined as action or inaction leading to deviation from team or organizational intentions.

Aviation increasingly uses error management strategies to improve safety. Error management is based on understanding the nature and extent of error, changing the conditions that induce error, determining behaviors that prevent or mitigate error, and training personnel in their use.

Cockpit observations made by experts during the line operations safety audit reveal that threat and error are ubiquitous in the aviation environment, with an average of two threats and two errors observed per flight. Some errors, such as proficiency errors, suggest the need for technical training, whereas communications and decision errors require team training. Procedural errors may result from human limitations or from inadequate procedures that need to be improved.

Crew Resource Management

Given the extent of threats and errors, crew resource management (CRM) is a large focus in aviation today and covers human performance limitations (such as fatigue and stress) and the nature of human error, and not just technical aspects. It emphasizes habits and behaviors that are countermeasures to error, such as leadership, briefings, monitoring and cross checking, decision making, and review and modification of plans. CRM is now required for flight crews worldwide, and there is evidence that it is effective in enhancing safety and changing attitudes and behavior. The program employs simulation, team training, interactive group briefings, and a performance improvement process, with the focus on how human factors interact with high-risk and high-stress environments. Participants develop an understanding of how cognitive errors may result when stressors like fatigue, overwork, and emergencies occur. The components of CRM are depicted in Table 9.3.

Evaluators of CRM training have concluded that such training needs to be ongoing, because without repeat training and reinforcement, the effects decrease; it also needs to be tailored to the particular organization's conditions and experience. Simulators and models are used in training and learning. In aviation, threat and error models can be built to analyze causes of errors and to uncover latent threats and risks. Models usually reveal multiple causes and the aim is to uncover latent threats that can interact with present conditions to precipitate error. In healthcare, large team size and the heterogeneity of personnel decrease team efficiency and may hinder establishment of leadership under adverse circumstances. Aviation has a straightforward and clear hierarchy, whereas healthcare does not, and this particularly comes into play in emergencies. Communication is relatively standardized in aviation but is much more complex in medicine. Flight processes lend themselves to checklists, but standards in medicine do not always conform to checklists.

In medicine as in aviation, the barriers to disclosure of error need to be addressed with a change in the culture toward accountability and openness. Training efforts need to focus on the culture of underreporting to capitalize on learning opportunities. *Light touch* mechanisms have been suggested to increase peer-to-peer accountability, in which coworkers look out for each other, like a wingman in aviation. This involves approaching the colleague who might be compromising safety and quality in a nonthreatening, respectful way at first, before following up the chain of command to raise the concern. Like

TABLE 9.3   **Critical Components of Crew Resource Management**

Component	Explanation
Situational awareness	Actively involve all team members; shared model to visualize the field
Problem identification	Voluntary, active, and open communication to share concerns
Decision making	Generate alternative acceptable solutions through active anticipation and accurate diagnosis of problems.
Workload distribution	Reasonable assignment of tasks so no team member is unduly overloaded
Time management	Appropriate use of resources to solve time-critical problems
Conflict resolution	Gaining consensus through active listening, focus on issues and respect

aviation, healthcare needs to develop an infrastructure for the responsible reporting of safety concerns, without fear of retaliation or intimidation. In the AHRQ 2016 Hospital Survey on Patient Safety Culture, many respondents reported that their organizations response to errors was nonpunitive, which is a step in the right direction. TJC Center for Transforming Healthcare Oro 2.0 is an online assessment tool to guide leaders in the areas of leadership commitment, safety culture, and performance improvement. This service is complimentary to JC domestic customers and is separate from accreditation.

Human Factors Science

Human factors engineering is used to ensure safety in several industries including aviation, automobiles, and in nuclear power plants. Its use in healthcare is relatively recent; pioneering studies of human factors in anesthesia were integral to the redesign of anesthesia equipment, significantly reducing the risk of injury or death in operating rooms.

Human factors engineers evaluate human strengths and limitations in the design of systems in which humans and technology interact. Activities are analyzed, breaking them down into multiple parts, and assessed for physical demands, skill demands, mental workload, team dynamics, work environment, and device design necessary to complete the task optimally.

Human factors engineering studies show systems actually work in real practice, with human beings as the controls and attempts to design systems to optimize safety and reduce the risk of error in complex environments. Several techniques or tools are used in human factors engineering approaches to quality and safety. These are listed with examples in Table 9.4.

Making Healthcare Systems Resilient

Resiliency refers to detection of adverse effects before they occur or early in their course, to minimize effects. In addition to studying error and designing measures to prevent it, resiliency approaches tap into the dynamic aspects of risk management and explore how organizations anticipate and adapt to changing conditions and recover from system anomalies. Resilient systems can adjust their functioning before, during, and after events that threaten

TABLE 9.4 Tools Used in Human Factors Engineering

Tool	Example
Usability testing: testing new systems and equipment using real-world conditions	Testing a clinical decision support system in one work area before implementing it hospital-wide
Forcing functions: designs prevent certain actions from taking place or design forces user to perform another action beforehand	Biopsy needles: it is necessary to engage (load) the cutting needle before inserting the biopsy apparatus, which ensures that the cutting needle will extend across the lesion when the biopsy gun is inserted.
Standardizing: standardize equipment and processes to be reliable, improve information flow	Color coding of different lengths or sizes of catheters
Resilience: detection of adverse effects before they occur or early in their course, to minimize effects	Carrying out failure modes and effects analysis on a process, such as scheduling for coronary computed tomography angiography
Discrete event simulation: using computer decision models to test initiatives	Modeling a screening program in a population to assess if it has an effect on patient outcome

them, and still remain operational. These systems demonstrate qualitative shifts in performance in response to varying demands; exhibit purposeful, meaningful responses reflected by goal trade-offs; and show tenacity of effort to effectively respond, even when confronted by escalating demands or threats to their existence. Having alternative options and the ability to critically assess situations allow resilient systems to direct resources to achieve meaningful, high-priority goals. These factors come into play when contemplating and planning quality assurance initiatives.

The application of resilience engineering to healthcare is essential to ensure patient safety. Resilience is necessary when systems are subjected to usual and unusual demands, exposed to catastrophes or disasters in the environment (e.g., political, financial, legal), and experience variations in staffing or other resources. Systems with high stakes and substantial risks, changes in workload and tempo, and that employ complex technology that is controlled by humans need to be resilient.

Resilience engineering theorists have identified four aspects of resilient systems: (1) monitoring or exploring the system's function and performance, (2) responding or reacting to new events or current conditions, (3) anticipating or foreseeing future events and conditions, and (4) learning or reorganizing system knowledge (for similar repeat events). An example in radiology is the unexpected influx of several emergency cases following a multiple motor vehicle trauma. This requires flexibility on the part of workers, and the willingness to do different tasks, occasionally outside of their usual duty or comfort zone. Supervisors and organizers need to ensure that workers feel empowered to trade off less urgent duties in the face of an emergency.

Workers at the frontline, including radiographic technologists and nurses, use their knowledge and experience to monitor the clinical situation and assess the immediate demands, the systems technical and organizational features capability, the available resources, and the consequences of reallocating resources. The response might result in reassignment of technologists, patients, and helpers to other CT scanners, and the attendance of a fellow to oversee some of the trauma cases being scanned and issue preliminary reports to expedite appropriate next management. Having knowledge of the appropriate imaging and specific imaging protocols allows workers to anticipate worklists and to prioritize the scanning order of the trauma patients. Reviewing how things went in the acute situation will help all to learn and to reorganize system

knowledge. These resilience efforts might be applied at a later date if a CT or MRI scanner malfunctions and is out of action for a period of time. Many of these principles are embodied in the proactive healthcare failure modes and effects analysis approach.

High-Reliability Organizations

High-reliability organizations (HROs) operate in unforgiving social and political environments. Their technologies may be risky and present the potential for error, with the scale of possible consequences from mistakes precluding learning through experimentation. To avoid failures these organizations must use complex processes to manage complex technologies and complex work. These organizations have properties that are similar to other high-performing organizations including highly trained personnel, continuous training, effective reward systems, frequent process audits, and continuous improvement efforts. At the same time, there is a distinct sense of vulnerability; a widely distributed sense of responsibility and accountability for reliability; widespread concern about misperception, misconception, and misunderstanding that is generalized across all tasks, operations, and assumptions; pessimism about possible failures; redundancy; and a variety of checks and counterchecks as a precaution against potential mistakes.

HROs are a subset of organizations that function in risky environments that have enjoyed a record of exceptional safety over long periods of time, and that have resisted multiple threats of failure with catastrophic consequences. These organizations constantly seek to improve reliability, intervene to prevent errors and failures, and cope and recover quickly in a dynamic fashion, should errors become manifest. They are reliability-seeking rather than reliability-achieving. These organizations are not distinguished by their absolute error or accident rates, but more by effective management of innately risky technologies through organizational control of both hazards and probability. As a result, the term *high reliability* has generally come to mean that high risk and high effectiveness coexist, that some organizations must perform well under very trying conditions, and that it takes intensive effort to do so.

The infrastructure of high reliability is grounded in processes of *collective mindfulness*, which includes a preoccupation with failure, reluctance to simplify interpretations, sensitivity to operations, commitment to resilience,

TABLE 9.5 Planned Change Theories Compared

Lewin	Bullock and Batten	Kotter	Lippitt
1. Unfreezing	1. Exploration: make decision on need for change	1. Establish a sense of urgency	1. Diagnose the problem
			2. Assess motivation and capacity for change
	2. Planning: understand the problem	2. Create a guiding coalition	3. Assess change agents' motivation and resources
		3. Develop a vision and strategy	
2. Moving	3. Action: identify, agree upon, and implement changes	4. Communicate the change vision	4. Select a progressive change objective
		5. Empower employees for broad-based action	
		6. Generate short-term wins	5. Choose an appropriate role for the change agent
		7. Consolidate gains and produce more change	
3. Refreezing	4. Integration: stabilize and embed change	8. Anchor new approaches in the culture	6. Maintain the change
			7. Terminate the helping relationship

and deference to expertise. In other words, HROs are distinctive because of their efforts to organize in ways that increase the quality of attention across the organization, thereby enhancing people's alertness and awareness of details so that they can detect subtle ways in which contexts vary and call for contingent responses (i.e., collective mindfulness). This *mindful organizing* forms a basis for individuals to interact continuously as they develop, refine, and update a shared understanding of the situation they face and their capabilities to act on that understanding. With mindful organizing, actions that forestall and contain errors and crises are proactively triggered. Leaders and organizational members need to pay close attention to shaping the social and relational infrastructure of the organization, and to establishing a set of interrelated organizing processes and practices, which jointly contribute to the system's overall culture of safety.

Applying the principles of HROs like aviation (nuclear energy and amusement parks) to healthcare will be challenging, but will involve three major domains of change, each with four increments of maturity as outlined by Chassin and Loeb in their study in conjunction with the TJC. Leadership needs to be committed to the goal of zero patient harm, all principles of a safety culture need to be incorporated across the entire system, and the most effective process improvement tools and methods need to be adopted widely and deployed. The four stages of maturity (beginning, developing, advancing, and approaching) are applied and assessed in the three domains of leadership, safety culture, and robust process improvement. Robust process improvement includes Lean, Six Sigma, and Change Management (discussed below), which are process management tools developed in industry and imported into healthcare.

Change Management

This is a systematic approach that is used alongside Lean and Six Sigma and prepares an organization to accept, implement, and sustain improved processes that result from the application of Lean and Six Sigma tools. These three sets of tools are complementary, and together provide the best available methods for hospitals to achieve major improvements in faulty processes. The two change management models include planned change management and emergent change management.

Planned change management dominates the academic literature and owes much to the work of Kurt Lewin. The planned change approach views change as a transitional process between fixed states. Under this model, to successfully adopt new behaviors within the organization, old behaviors must be relinquished. Planned change assumes that the overall change targets within an organization align with management's vision of change and the steps designed to transition to the changed state. In practice, workers within an organization come from different backgrounds and have varying attitudes, beliefs, and needs, making complete agreement on a course of action virtually impossible. Planned change places much emphasis on managers' roles and may overlook employees' contributions to the change process. By emphasizing preplanned processes, timetables, and objectives, all of which are developed by management, this approach overlooks the impacts that employees have on change initiatives.

Other planned change theories created are extensions of Lewin's three-step model and include Lippitt et al.'s seven-phase model, Kotter's eight-step change model, and Bullock and Batten's four-phase model. These models have several elements in common and are summarized in Table 9.5.

Emergent change is a newer concept and consists of many unrelated theories presenting different approaches to change management. This approach views change as a less prescriptive and more analytical undertaking. Although change will ultimately transition an organization from one state to another, the emergent change approach places less emphasis on plans and projections and focuses on understanding the complexity of the environment and developing a range of alternatives to guide decision making. The emergent change approach recognizes that change must be linked to market forces, work organizations, systems of management control, and the ever-changing nature of organizational boundaries and relationships. In contrast to planned change, emergent change emphasizes a bottom-up approach to change management. The planned change model emphasizes preplanned processes and objectives that underscore the role of management, whereas the emergent change approach acknowledges that the pace and nature of change is so rapid and complex that senior managers may have difficulty identifying changes and devising

TABLE 9.6   Emergent Change Theories Compared

Hinings and Greenwood	Kanter's Big 3 Model of Organizational Change	Pettigrew's Process Context Content Model
Change occurs through the interplay of five factors: 1. Situational constraints (environment, technology, labor force) 2. Interpretive schemes (ideas, beliefs, and values) 3. Interests (of organizational subunits) 4. Dependencies of power (relations and distribution of power) 5. Organizational capacity (the ability of leadership to be transformative and to construct and communicate visions for change)	**Five acknowledgments:** 1. It is hard to make changes stick. 2. There are clear limitations to managerial action in making change. 3. Attempts to carry out programmatic continuing change through isolated single efforts are likely to fail because of the effects of system context. 4. The need for change may make it harder for change to occur. 5. Some of those best at new practices in one realm may show limitations in others. **Three kinds of motion:** 1. Organization-environment 2. Organizational components 3. Individuals **Three forms of change:** 1. Identity changes 2. Coordination changes 3. Control changes **Three roles in change process:** 1. Change strategists 2. Implementers 3. Recipients	• Acknowledges complexity and continuity of change. • Change is purposive because it is undertaken in search of a competitive advantage and not just to keep up with the external environment. • Change should be analyzed based on three dimensions: context, content, and process. • Context includes the internal (structures, culture, power distributions, skill base, resources) and external (economic, legal, and social circumstances) environment in which the organization operates. • Components of change should respond to external environment factors (e.g., market forces) and internal organization factors (e.g., improving operational efficiency). • Process of change includes operational activities undertaken to materialize change. Three factors managers must address: (1) development of the logic of change implementation, (2) managing change transition, (3) and curtailing resistance to change.

TABLE 9.7   Change Management Models Used in Healthcare

Lukas Organizational Model	IHI Triple Aim Framework	Canadian Health Services Research Foundation Evidence-Informed Change Management Approach	NHS Change Management Guidelines
Four components of healthcare organizations: 1. Mission, vision, and strategies, which set direction and priorities 2. Culture, which is determined by values and norms 3. Operational functions and processes, which are embodied by work done in patient care 4. Infrastructure **Five elements of change:** 1. Impetus to transform 2. Leadership commitment to quality 3. Improvement initiatives that actively engage staff in meaningful problem solving 4. Alignment to achieve consistency of organization-wide goals with resource allocation and actions at all levels of the organization 5. Integration to bridge traditional intraorganizational boundaries between individual components	**Triple aim concept:** 1. Improving health of populations 2. Improving patient experience of care 3. Reducing per capita cost of healthcare **Steps enclosed within five domains:** 1. Individuals and families 2. Redesign of primary care services and structures 3. Prevention and health promotion 4. Cost control 5. System integration	**Four stages:** 1. Planning (understand context and dynamics of change) 2. Implementing (take action based on planned approach) 3. Spreading (propagate change beyond initial concept) 4. Sustaining change (monitoring and adjusting change process as experience is gained)	**Six-step approach to successfully implementing change:** 1. Know where you are going and why (develop business case) 2. Analyze and design (consult all stakeholders, develop delivery strategy) 3. Gain commitment (prepare for implementation, ensure all stakeholders are ready for change) 4. Deliver it (ensure staff is trained to execute change) 5. Reinforce it (review and embed work processes and elicit feedback) 6. Sustain it (measure change against goals and develop continuous quality improvement)

IHI, Institute for Healthcare Improvement; *NHS*, National Health Service.

strategies to address them in a timely fashion. As a result, managers must relinquish some of the decision making to employees and act as facilitators of change as opposed to controlling it.

The emergent approach to change management is relatively new and does not have a main theoretical foundation. The most commonly cited current models of emergent change management include Hinings and Greenwood's model of change dynamics, Kanter et al.'s Big Three model of organizational change, and Pettigrew's process/content/context model. These models and their components/stages are summarized in Table 9.6.

The planned and emergent change theoretical approaches can coexist and should be drawn upon for guidance. Change agents and change targets alike must recognize that to achieve successful change, an interplay of factors will need to be considered, including the organizational (internal) and environmental (external) circumstances driving the change.

Change Management Models in Healthcare

In addition to the planned and emergent change management approaches, which arose largely from business literature, several other change management models have recently developed from a healthcare context. Three such models are Lukas et al.'s Organizational Model for Transformational Change in Healthcare Systems, the Canadian Health Services Research Foundation Evidence-Informed Change Management Approach, the National Health Service change management guidelines, and the Institute for Healthcare Improvement Triple Aim Framework. A summary of these models' elements are provided in Table 9.7.

Although healthcare leaders should make attempts to incorporate the core elements of change management into their approach, no singular element or combination of elements is sufficient to successfully achieve change. Healthcare leaders must tailor their change management approach to the unique circumstances of their organization and the external environment. In practice, change efforts will vary in complexity and might be difficult to achieve. For example, buy-in from all relevant stakeholders that can influence outcomes in an organization may be impossible at times due to divergent interests among senior management. However, if healthcare leaders are shrewd in the development of their change management approach, they may still be able to successfully achieve change in light of unfavorable circumstances.

CONCLUSION

Quality improvement is essential now more than ever, given the current era of healthcare delivery, with the emphasis on quality over quantity. Radiology is essential to most patient care, including diagnosis, treatment monitoring, and follow-up. However, diagnostic imaging is costly and has become the focus of some cost containment initiatives. Radiologists need to add value and be able to demonstrate value to payers, government, patients, and all stakeholders. This will require radiologists to learn management skills and interact in our healthcare systems as members of interdisciplinary teams. Departments of diagnostic imaging will have to become responsive to change in the external healthcare environment and be resilient and effective. Quality improvement initiatives and programs are an essential part of radiologists' value and are necessary for many reasons, including regulatory, legal, and ethical concerns and for financial survival. Industries, including manufacturing and aviation, have successfully adopted quality improvement approaches, some of which are being adapted to healthcare. In healthcare, we need to adopt and adapt these approaches to deliver the best possible patient care and outcomes. We hope that this chapter outlined some of the current quality improvement approaches that will be around for the next few years.

SUGGESTED READINGS

Abramson RG, Berger PE, Brant-Zawadzki MN. Accountable care organizations and radiology: threat or opportunity? *J Am Coll Radiol*. 2012;9(12):900–906.

Alkasab TK, Harvey HB, Gowda V, Thrall JH, Rosenthal DI, Gazelle GS. Consensus-oriented group peer review: a new process to review radiologist work output. *J Am Coll Radiol*. 2014;11(2):131–138.

Allen B Jr, Levin DC, Brant-Zawadzki M, Lexa FJ, Duszak Jr R. ACR white paper: strategies for radiologists in the era of health care reform and accountable care organizations: a report from the ACR Future Trends Committee. *J Am Coll Radiol*. 2011;8:309–317.

American Recovery and Reinvestment Act (ARRA) of 2009, Pub. L. No. 111-115, 123 Stat. 115.

Antwi M, Kale M. *Change Management in Healthcare. Literature Review*. Queens School of Business and The Monieson Centre for Business Research in Healthcare. <https://smith.queensu.ca/centres/monieson/knowledge_articles/files/Change%20Management%20in%20Healthcare%20-%20Lit%20Review%20-%20AP%20FINAL.pdf>.

Bamford D, Daniel S. A case study of change management effectiveness within the NHS. *J Change Manage*. 2005;5(4):391–406.

Beasley C. The Institute for Healthcare Improvement (IHI). The Triple Aim. Optimizing health, care and cost. *Healthc Exec*. 2009;24(1):64–65. <http://www.ihi.org/engage/initiatives/TripleAim/Documents/BeasleyTripleAim_ACHEJan09.pdf>.

Birk S. Accelerating the adoption of a safety culture. *Healthc Exec*. 2015;30:19–20. 22–26.

Breslau J, Lexa FJ. A radiologist's primer on accountable care organizations. *J Am Coll Radiol*. 2011;8(3):164–168.

Bright TJ, Wong A, Dhurjati R, et al. Effect of clinical decision-support systems: a systematic review. *Ann Intern Med*. 2012;157:29–43.

Burleson J. Quality and the physician value-based payment program. *Radiol Manage*. 2014;36(1):14–20. quiz 22–23.

Burnes B. Kurt Lewin and the planned approach to change: a re-appraisal. *J Manage Stud*. 2004;41(6):977–1002.

Carthey J, de Leval MR, Reason JT. Institutional resilience in healthcare systems. *Qual Health Care*. 2001;10(1):29–32.

Chassin MR, Loeb JM. High-reliability health care: getting there from here. *Milbank Q*. 2013;91(3):459–490.

Fairbanks RJ, Wears RL, Woods DD, Hollnagel E, Plsek P, Cook RI. Resilience and resilience engineering in health care. *Jt Comm J Qual Patient Saf*. 2014;40(8):376–383.

Fryback DG, Thornbury JR. The efficacy of diagnostic imaging. *Med Decis Making*. 1991;11(2):88–94.

Gazelle GS, Kessler L, Lee DW, et al. A framework for assessing the value of diagnostic imaging in the era of comparative effectiveness research. *Radiology*. 2011;261(3):692–698.

Gunderman RB, Patti JA, Lexa F, et al. The 2009 ACR Forum: health care payment models. *J Am Coll Radiol*. 2010;7(2):103–108.

Harvey HB, Alkasab TK, Prabhakar AM, et al. Radiologist Peer Review by Group Consensus. *J Am Coll Radiol*. 2016;13(6):656–662.

Helmreich RL. On error management: lessons from aviation. *BMJ*. 2000;320(7237):781–785.

Hickner-Cruz K, Dresevic A. The Medicare hospital value-based purchasing program and imaging's role. *Radiol Manage*. 2012;34(1):36–38.

Inventory of Human Factors Tools and Methods. A Work-System Design Perspective. <http://www.ryerson.ca/hfe/documents/hf-tools-beta200.pdf>.

Iglehart JK. The ACO regulations—some answers, more questions. *N Engl J Med*. 2011;364. e35.

Ingraham B, Miller K, Iaia A, et al. Reductions in high-end imaging utilization with radiology review and consultation. *J Am Coll Radiol*. 2016;13(9):1079–1082.

Institute of Medicine (IOM) Report. For the Public's Health: The Role of Measurement in Action and Accountability. <http://www.nap.edu/catalog/13005/for-the-publics-health-the-role-of-measurement-in-action>.

Institute of Medicine (IOM) Report. Improving Diagnosis in Healthcare. <http://www.nationalacademies.org/hmd/Reports/2015/Improving-Diagnosis-in-Healthcare.aspx>.

International Standardization Organization. Quality Management Principles. <http://www.iso.org/iso/pub100080.pdf>.

Iyer RS, Munsell A, Weinberger E. Radiology peer-review feedback scorecards: optimizing transparency, accessibility, and education in a children's hospital. *Curr Probl Diagn Radiol*. 2014;43(4):169–174.

Johnson JO. Six sigma and Lean: opportunities for health care to do more and better with less. In: Abujudeh HH, Bruno MA, eds. *Quality and Safety in Radiology*. Cary, NC: Oxford University Press; 2012.

Kelly AM, Cronin P. Practical approaches to quality improvement for radiologists. *Radiographics*. 2015;35(6):1630–1642.

Khorasani R, Hentel K, Darer J, et al. Ten commandments for effective clinical decision support for imaging: enabling evidence-based practice to improve quality and reduce waste. *AJR Am J Roentgenol*. 2014;203(5):945–951.

Kopach-Konrad R, Lawley M, Criswell M, et al. Applying systems engineering principles in improving health care delivery. *J Gen Intern Med.* 2007;22(suppl 3):431–437.

Krishnaraj A, Norbash A, Allen B Jr, et al. The impact of the Patient Protection and Affordable Care Act on radiology: beyond reimbursement. *J Am Coll Radiol.* 2015;12(1):29–33.

Kruskal JB, Reedy A, Pascal L, Rosen MP, Boiselle PM. Quality initiatives: Lean approach to improving performance and efficiency in a radiology department. *Radiographics.* 2012;32(2):573–587.

Kurt Lewin's Change Model. Strategies for Managing Change. <http://www.strategies-for-managing-change.com/kurt-lewin.html>.

Lacson R, Prevedello LM, Andriole KP, et al. Four-year impact of an alert notification system on closed-loop communication of critical test results. *AJR Am J Roentgenol.* 2014;203(5):933–938.

Lee DW, Rawson JV, Wade SW. Radiology benefit managers: cost saving or cost shifting? *J Am Coll Radiol.* 2011;8(6):393–401.

Li Y, Kong N, Lawley M, Weiss L, Pagán JA. Advancing the use of evidence-based decision-making in local health departments with systems science methodologies. *Am J Public Health.* 2015;105(suppl 2):S217–S222.

Lukas CV, Holmes SK, Cohen AB, et al. Transformational change in health care systems: an organizational model. *Health Care Manage Rev.* 2007;32(4):309–320.

Marjoua Y, Bozic KJ. Brief history of quality movement in US healthcare. *Curr Rev Musculoskelet Med.* 2012;5:265–273.

Martin CM. Complexity in dynamical health systems—transforming science and theory, and knowledge and practice. *J Eval Clin Pract.* 2010;16(1):209–210.

Medicare Hospital Value Based Purchasing Program. <https://www.medicare.gov/hospitalcompare/data/hospital-vbp.html>.

Medicare Outpatient Imaging Efficiency Measures. <https://www.medicare.gov/hospitalcompare/Data/Outpatient-Measures.html> and <http://www.qualitynet.org/dcs/ContentServer?c=Page&pagename=QnetPublic%2FPage%2FQnetTier2&cid=1228695266120>.

Medicare Value Based Purchasing (VBP) Program and Imaging's Role. <http://www.thehealthlawpartners.com/files/rm341_p36-38_features.pdf>.

Merry MD, Crago MG. The past, present and future of health care quality. The physician executive. *Physician Exec.* 2001;27(5):30–35.

Mukherji SK. The potential impact of accountable care organizations with respect to cost and quality with special attention to imaging. *J Am Coll Radiol.* 2014;11(4):391–396.

O'Connor SD, Dalal AK, Sahni VA, Lacson R, Khorasani R. Does integrating nonurgent, clinically significant radiology alerts within the electronic health record impact closed-loop communication and follow-up? *J Am Med Inform Assoc.* 2016;23(2):333–338.

O'Keeffe MM, Davis TM, Siminoski K. A workstation-integrated peer review quality assurance program: pilot study. *BMC Med Imaging.* 2013;13:19.

O'Keeffe MM, Davis TM, Siminoski K. Performance results for a workstation-integrated radiology peer review quality assurance program. *Int J Qual Health Care.* 2016;28(3):294–298.

Oriol MD. Crew resource management: applications in healthcare organizations. *J Nurs Adm.* 2006;36(9):402–406.

Plsek PE, Greenhalgh T. Complexity science: the challenge of complexity in health care. *BMJ.* 2001;323(7313):625–628.

Plsek PE, Wilson T. Complexity, leadership, and management in healthcare organisations. *BMJ.* 2001;323(7315):746–749.

Presidents' Council of Advisors on Science and Technology (PCAST) 2014 Report. Better Health Care and Lower Costs: Accelerating Improvements Through Systems Engineering. <https://www.whitehouse.gov/sites/default/files/microsites/ostp/PCAST/pcast_systems_engineering_in_healthcare_-_may_2014.pdf>.

Qayyum A, Yu JP, Kansagra AP, et al. Academic radiology in the new health care delivery environment. *Acad Radiol.* 2013;20(12):1511–1520.

Sarwar A, Boland G, Monks A, Kruskal JB. Metrics for radiologists in the era of value-based health care delivery. *Radiographics.* 2015;35(3):866–876.

Seltzer SE, Lee TH. The transformation of diagnostic radiology in the ACO era. *JAMA.* 2014;312(3):227–228.

Strickland NH. Quality assurance in radiology: peer review and peer feedback. *Clin Radiol.* 2015;70(11):1158–1164.

The Agency for Healthcare Research and Quality (AHRQ) 2016 Hospital Survey on Patient Safety Culture. <http://www.ahrq.gov/sites/default/files/wysiwyg/professionals/quality-patient-safety/patientsafetyculture/hospital/2016/2016_hospitalsops_report_pt1.pdf>.

The Agency for Healthcare Research and Quality (AHRQ). Clinical Guidelines and Recommendations. <http://www.ahrq.gov/professionals/clinicians-providers/guidelines-recommendations/index.html>.

The Agency for Healthcare Research and Quality (AHRQ). Human Factors Engineering. <https://psnet.ahrq.gov/primers/primer/20/human-factors-engineering>.

The American College of Radiology (ACR) Communication Guideline. <http://www.acr.org/~/media/ACR/Documents/PGTS/guidelines/Comm_Diag_Imaging.pdf>.

The American College of Radiology (ACR). Physician Quality Reporting System (PQRS). Diagnostic Radiology Measure Specifications. <http://www.acr.org/~/media/ACR/Documents/P4P/2016%20PQRS/DX/Diagnostic%20Radiology%20Measure%20Specifications_Table.pdf>.

The Baldridge Criteria for Performance Excellence. <http://www.nist.gov/baldrige/>.

The Deficit Reduction Act of 2005. <https://www.cms.gov/Regulations-and-Guidance/Legislation/DeficitReductionAct/index.html?redirect=/deficitreductionact>.

The International Standardization Organization. <http://www.iso.org/iso/home/standards/management-standards/iso_9000.htm>.

The Joint Commission Center for Transforming Healthcare Oro 2.0. <http://www.centerfortransforminghealthcare.org/oro.aspx>.

The National Academy of Engineering (NAE) and Institute of Medicine (IOM). <http://nationalacademies.org/onpi/030909643X.pdf>.

The National Association for Healthcare Quality (NAHQ). Call to Action. Safeguarding the Integrity of Healthcare Quality and Safety Systems. <http://news-quality.com/2012/10/call-to-action-safeguarding-the-integrity-of-healthcare-quality-and-safety-systems-102812/>.

The National Committee for Quality Assurance. <http://www.ncqa.org/AboutNCQA.aspx>.

The National Oncology PET Registry. <https://www.cancerpetregistry.org/index.htm>.

The National Quality Forum. <http://www.qualityforum.org/About_NQF/>.

The National Quality Strategy. <http://www.ahrq.gov/workingforquality>.

The Patient-Centered Outcomes Research Institute. <http://www.pcori.org/>.

The Patient Protection and Affordable Care Act, Pub L No. 111–148, 124 Stat 119 (March 23, 2010).

Thornton E, Brook OR, Mendiratta-Lala M, Hallett DT, Kruskal JB. Application of failure mode and effect analysis in a radiology department. *Radiographics.* 2011;31(1):281–293.

Value-Based Insurance Design. <http://www.ncsl.org/research/health/value-based-insurance-design.aspx>.

Weick K, Sutcliffe K. *Managing the Unexpected.* <http://high-reliability.org/Managing_the_Unexpected.pdf>.

Weiss DL, Kim W, Branstetter BF 4th, Prevedello LM. Radiology reporting: a closed-loop cycle from order entry to results communication. *J Am Coll Radiol.* 2014;11(12 Pt B):1226–1237.

Zafar HM, Mills AM, Khorasani R, Langlotz CP. Clinical decision support for imaging in the era of the Patient Protection and Affordable Care Act. *J Am Coll Radiol.* 2012;9:907–918. e4.

Core Concepts in Radiology Noninterpretive Skills

Chapter 10

Evidence-Based Imaging

C. Craig Blackmore

INTRODUCTION

Over the past 2 decades, evidence-based medicine has become a dominant paradigm for understanding best practices in medicine. Simply put, evidence-based medicine is the explicit incorporation of the best research evidence into the care decision-making process. More formally, evidence-based medicine has been defined by Sackett and others as the incorporation of the best available evidence with physician judgment and experience and patient values and preferences. Evidence-based medicine should be distinguished from eminence-based medicine, typified by the seasoned professional using his or her best judgment and knowledge, without explicit review and incorporation of medical evidence. Implicit within evidence-based medicine is a process of identifying relevant evidence, critically appraising the evidence to identify and weight most heavily that which is methodologically most valid, and incorporating the best evidence into clinical care.

In the therapeutic arena, evidence-based medicine is generally focused on the choice between competing drugs or procedures to treat specific diseases. In this realm, randomized clinical trials are supreme as the research approach most likely to lead to unbiased estimates of the effectiveness of the various treatments. However, in diagnostics, including imaging, the process is more complex. Diagnostic tests do not directly affect clinical outcome, but rather that effect is mediated by treatment. In addition, randomized clinical trials are an inefficient means of understanding the performance of diagnostic tests. More commonly, diagnostic tests are evaluated based on cohort studies, where all patients get one or more imaging studies. However, as discussed in this chapter, such cohort studies are susceptible to a number of different biases, emphasizing the need for critical analysis. Screening introduces an additional set of biases that are difficult to avoid, compelling the use of randomized clinical trials to evaluate screening studies despite their relative inefficiency and large sample size requirement. Accordingly, evidence-based medicine applied to imaging, known as evidence-based imaging, has particular challenges in its application. However, despite its limitations, incorporation of evidence into imaging practice remains essential for the highest-quality clinical care.

Evidence-based imaging consists of identifying the relevant imaging literature for a specific clinical question, understanding the strengths and limitations of the existing evidence, and then incorporating that evidence into clinical care. The strength of evidence is based on the quality of the published studies, including the study size and potential for bias. Grading schemes are often used to categorize the strength of evidence as low or high. Because most radiologists do not directly order imaging studies, evidence-based imaging is, by nature, a collaborative process between radiologists and referring clinicians, incorporating the best evidence with patient values, and the experience of radiologist and clinician alike.

In this chapter, we discuss the critical analysis of the radiology literature to understand the methodological rigor of the published information. Second, we define how to incorporate evidence from the literature into an understanding of whether imaging will have value. Finally, in the third section, we explore how to apply evidence-based imaging in clinical practice and answer the critical question of whether imaging should be performed.

CRITICAL ANALYSIS OF IMAGING RESEARCH

There is abundant literature evaluating radiology tests. As of 2015, there were over 100 journals devoted to imaging, with additional publication of imaging research in other nonimaging journals as well. This massive body of research is comprehensive in breadth, but unfortunately limited in depth, with most research pertaining only to new experimental imaging techniques and accuracy of existing imaging tests. Further, methodological flaws are common in the imaging literature (as in the rest of medicine). Intrinsic to evidence-based imaging is that medical evidence or research undergoes a critical evaluation process. In the radiology literature, there are several consistent pitfalls that decrease the validity of the published information (Table 10.1). Often these biases cannot be completely excluded even with careful research design, but it is critical for the

TABLE 10.1   **Biases in Imaging Research**

BIASES IN INCLUSION OF SUBJECTS	
Selection bias	Selection only of subjects in whom an imaging study will perform well, nonrandom, or nonconsecutive selection
Spectrum bias	Selection of only subjects with severe disease
Case-mix bias	Comparison subjects selected who are completely normal (rather than representing the clinical spectrum of those who would be imaged)
Imaging-based selection	Including only those who undergo the two different tests being compared
BIASED REFERENCE STANDARD	
Indeterminate reference standard	Reference standard itself is not accurate in identifying the presence of disease
Verification bias	Not all subjects undergo the same reference standard
Differential verification bias	Different reference standards, and the choice of reference standard is determined by the imaging study
BLINDING	
Unblinded interpretation	Interpreting radiologist has knowledge of the reference standard
Unblinded reference standard	Individuals determining the reference standard have knowledge of the imaging test results
SCREENING BIASES	
Lead time bias	The time of survival from diagnosis is increased by early detection even without a decrease in actual time of death.
Length bias	Less aggressive lesions will have a longer time in the screen-detectable preclinical interval, causing screening to have a higher probability of detecting such less aggressive lesions.
Overdiagnosis	Earlier detection leads to identification of some lesions that would never have been clinically known, leading to treatment without benefit.

user of literature to understand the presence and magnitude of such concerns.

Selection bias occurs when a research study is conducted on only a portion of the population; such bias means that the results do not reflect the population as a whole. Selection bias can take on many forms. Restricting selection to study subjects in whom the imaging study will perform well will make the test look better than it actually is. For example, ultrasound is known to perform better in thinner subjects. So, an ultrasound study limited to those with low body mass index will have questionable relevance for the broader population. Similarly, imaging tends to be more accurate in more severe disease. Hence, including only advanced cases in an accuracy study will lead to overestimation of accuracy, also known as spectrum bias. For example, the accuracy of computed tomography (CT) for detection of hepatoma in patients with clinical symptoms and abnormal liver function tests might differ from the accuracy for screening in clinically normal but at-risk patients. Finally, an extreme form of spectrum bias occurs when accuracy is evaluated on a mix of clinically normal subjects and those with advanced disease. This design, sometimes erroneously referred to as a case-control study, may lead to the largest overestimation of both sensitivity and specificity. To avoid this bias, subjects should be selected from the clinically relevant group, representing both the spectrum of disease and normal that would be encountered in clinical practice. At a minimum, users of the imaging literature can often get a quick estimate of the potential for selection bias by closely examining the relative number of enrolled subjects versus the number of subjects who were not included in the study. Though not always clearly reported in many papers, readers can infer from the number of subjects recruited over the time frame of the study if the sample is consecutive or sporadic.

Sporadic or convenience samples are obviously much more susceptible to selection bias.

A particularly insidious form of selection bias in imaging is imaging-based selection. Often in the comparison of competing imaging modalities, individuals are selected for inclusion because they have undergone both studies. This can be unbiased if all individuals are selected a priori to undergo both studies as part of the research protocol. However, more commonly, retrospective studies are performed selecting only those individuals who underwent both studies based on clinical indications rather than on a consecutive research protocol. In the latter design, it must be understood that individuals who undergo both imaging studies are unlikely to be representative of the more general population. Usually, individuals undergo both studies because the initial study is for some reason inadequate or not definitive. Obviously this creates a bias against the initial study. As a hypothetical example, one could compare the accuracy of ultrasound and CT scan for severe splenic injury in hemodynamically unstable trauma patients who underwent both studies. If the protocol was for patients to undergo ultrasound initially, with CT as a secondary study, the comparison would be biased because those patients with clearly positive ultrasound studies might be expected to go to the operating room or to angiography for definitive treatment without CT. Thus, the study would be composed of those in whom the ultrasound for some reason was not definitive.

This same example also highlights an additional challenge with imaging research, the selection of an appropriate reference standard. A reference standard should be definitive for the presence of pathology, should be the same for all individuals, and should be independent of the imaging studies being compared. In the ultrasound versus CT for splenic rupture example, pathology of the spleen in the operating room would be an appropriate reference standard as it is definitive and not affected by imaging modality. However, it is likely that not all patients will go to the operating room, so a secondary reference standard would also have to be employed. If CT is used as a reference standard for ultrasound, then the results will be biased in favor of CT. In addition, differential verification bias occurs when the imaging modality itself determines what reference standard will be performed. For example, if operative findings are used as a reference standard in some individuals, and imaging findings in others, then the imaging findings themselves will likely drive the determination of who goes to the operating room and will have the potential to affect the reference standard. For example, if ultrasound identifies some splenic ruptures but not others, the ones identified by ultrasound will be considered true positive diagnoses in the operating room. However, those that are missed by ultrasound might undergo conservative treatment, and because the patient may recover clinically, may not be considered as ruptured spleen based on the clinical reference standard (true negatives). In truth, these are missed diagnoses (false negatives) but with good clinical outcome because conservative treatment may sometimes be effective.

An additional bias in imaging is blinding of the imaging interpretation. This can be a particular problem with retrospective studies. The interpreting radiologists, if aware of the final diagnosis will, even without intending to, almost certainly change their subjective assessments to match the known diagnosis. This may be particularly problematic with new imaging tests in rare diseases, where the findings on imaging study may be remembered by the radiologist even for some time afterward. Blinding is also important for the reference standard. Though we tend to think of pathology and surgical findings as objective outcomes, they do have a subjective component that may be biased by knowledge of the imaging findings. For example, consider CT for the detection of ischemic bowel. We tend to think of bowel ischemia as a binary diagnosis. However, in reality, ischemia, like many diseases, runs a spectrum from mild (which may be hard to differentiate from normal) to severe, which is more unequivocal. Knowledge of the CT findings may certainly influence the surgeon's decision to remove a segment of bowel and therefore determine the reference standard.

Screening carries an additional set of challenges. The premise underlying screening is that through performance of imaging, we will identify disease earlier and that earlier identification will enable more effective therapy and better outcomes. These are simple and appealing concepts, but in practice, measurement of the effectiveness of screening is challenged by several biases. The first of these is lead time. Lead time as a bias is an artifact of our reliance on survival as a metric for assessing screening. Survival is generally thought of as the time from diagnosis to death or some other adverse outcome, as in 5-year survival or mean survival. However, if a diagnosis is made earlier, then even if death occurs at the same time, the time from diagnosis to death is increased. The patient may not actually live longer, but he or she will live longer from the time of diagnosis and with knowledge of disease. Simply by detecting disease earlier, measured survival must be increased, even without any true effect on outcome. Increased survival in

effect means earlier detection but provides no real information about clinical outcome.

A second challenge with screening is length bias. Length bias is due to the reality that the conditions for which screening is done (e.g., tumors or disease) are not homogeneous but will progress at different rates in different individuals. Screening only has potential value from the time that lesions reach a certain size threshold when they can be found by screening, known as the screen-detectable threshold, to the time when such lesions become clinically apparent. This time period is known as the preclinical screen-detectable interval. However, different tumors will exist in the preclinical screen-detectable interval for different lengths of time, depending on how aggressively they are growing. More aggressive tumors will rapidly grow through this screen-detectable preclinical interval, achieving clinical detectability after only a brief period of time. A more indolent tumor, on the other hand, because of its slow growth, will have a longer period of time in the screen-detectable preclinical interval. Thus, there is a longer time period when screening can detect slower growing lesions, and screening will be more likely to detect these less aggressive lesions. Screen-detected lesions will therefore be less aggressive than those detected on clinical grounds. Unfortunately, pathologic examination may not be able to differentiate these slower growing lesions from those that are more aggressive.

Finally, in screening, there is the construct of pseudo-disease, also called overdiagnosis. Simply put, early detection means that some tumors will be found years sooner than they would have become clinically manifest. If an individual dies after a tumor is detected by screening but before the tumor would have become clinically evident, then the screening has assigned that individual a diagnosis that he or she would never have known about otherwise. This individual would undergo all of the cancer treatment, with associated morbidity, but with no possibility of benefit, because death occurs before the disease would even have become clinically evident. This is particularly a problem when screening for relatively slow-growing disease in older patients. Overdiagnosis must be considered as a harm of screening and remains at the center of much of the ongoing controversy, particularly for breast and prostate cancer screening. Unfortunately, pseudo-disease can never be directly quantified because pathology cannot accurately predict growth rate and because time of death is never known in advance.

UNDERSTANDING THE VALUE OF IMAGING

Critically evaluating the literature is only the first step in evidence-based imaging. To be useful, the existing evidence must be applied to determine if an imaging test will have value in a specific patient. However, understanding the value of imaging in patient care and clinical outcomes is complex and requires more than simply knowing the accuracy of a diagnostic test. Fryback and Thornbury in the 1990s developed a tiered effectiveness model to enable better understanding of the value of imaging in context. Based on this model (Table 10.2), imaging must obtain value at each successive level before achieving value at the highest levels, patient outcomes

TABLE 10.2   **Tiered Effectiveness Model for Understanding the Value of Imaging**

Level of Effectiveness	Definition	Measures
Technical effectiveness	Ability to generate an image	Signal to noise, freedom from artifacts
Accuracy	Ability for the image interpreter to distinguish between normal and abnormal	Sensitivity, specificity, receiver-operator characteristic curve
Diagnostic certainty	Ability of the test to change the perceived probability of disease in a given patient	Pre- and posttest probability of disease, level of diagnostic certainty
Therapeutic effectiveness	Ability of the test results to change choice of treatment in a given patient	Change in management
Patient outcomes	Effect of use of test on patient outcomes, mediated through change in management or provision of prognostic information	Morbidity, mortality, patient satisfaction, quality of life
Societal value	Opportunity cost of resources consumed to provide imaging when compared to other interventions in medicine	Cost-effectiveness analysis, cost-utility analysis, cost-benefit analysis

and societal value. At the most basic level, tests must have technical effectiveness. This means that an image must be obtainable, free from artifacts, and have sufficient signal-to-noise to generate meaningful information. It is at this level that core basic science radiology research occurs in trying to develop new or improved imaging tests. However, producing an image is not sufficient to provide value to the patient; the imaging study must be able to differentiate pathology from normal. This second level of effectiveness, accuracy, is dependent on the radiologist who interprets the imaging study and is generally measured as the sensitivity and specificity of the test. Sensitivity is the ability of a test to detect disease when it is present, and specificity is the ability of a test to identify subjects as normal when they do not have disease. There is a trade-off between these two because having a lower threshold to call a test abnormal will increase sensitivity at the expense of specificity and vice versa. This trade-off is captured in the receiver-operator characteristic (ROC) curve and can be summarized as the area under the curve. The diagnostic likelihood ratio is an alternate measure of the effectiveness of a diagnostic test that captures results in both diseased and nondiseased subjects as a single metric to compare tests.

Accuracy is core to our understanding of imaging and is foundational to radiology research. However, accuracy itself is not sufficient evidence to determine that an imaging study has overall value or indeed that it should be performed. Levels 3 and 4 of the Fryback and Thornbury hierarchy are diagnostic certainty and clinical decision making, which are related. In diagnostic certainty, the results of the diagnostic tests are not simply interpreted in a vacuum but are applied to an individual patient. Diagnostic certainty is the potential change in the likelihood of a particular disease(s) in a given patient. Sensitivity and specificity are useful metrics to compare diagnostic tests, but care is better driven by the probability of disease in a specific individual with a specific test result. This is known as the positive predictive value when the test is positive (the probability of disease in an individual with a positive test result) and the negative predictive value when the test is negative (the probability of an individual not having the disease when the test is negative). The positive and negative predictive values are based not only on the test result but also on the probability of

disease in the population. The trade-off between sensitivity/specificity and positive/negative predictive value can be brought home through the use of Bayes theorem. In simplest terms, Bayes theorem is the precept whereby the probability of disease in a particular patient is based on a test result but also on the probability of disease based on the clinical findings before the test was performed, known as the pretest probability. In effect, Bayes theorem tells us that we cannot interpret imaging studies in isolation but, rather, that the results of an imaging study must be considered in the clinical context. More formally, Bayes theorem mathematically combines pretest probability with sensitivity and specificity to determine the probability of disease after the test results, through the equation:

$$p\,[\text{posttest}] = \frac{(p\,[\text{pretest}])\,(\text{sensitivity})}{\{(p\,[\text{pretest}])\,(\text{sensitivity})\}\{1 - p\,[\text{pretest}])\,(1 - \text{specificity})\}}$$

where p[pretest] is the pretest probability and p[posttest] is the posttest probability of disease. Although it is not practical to calculate a posttest probability with every interpretation of an imaging test, it is useful to understand Bayes theorem when making decisions about the appropriateness of imaging.

The next level of the hierarchy, therapeutic efficacy or medical decision making, goes one step further and relates how imaging affects not only the perceived probability of disease in an individual but also how imaging might potentially drive changes in management. Bayes' theorem allows estimation of the probability of disease in a specific patient and can therefore directly drive treatment depending on the treatment threshold. The treatment threshold is the level of certainty required that the disease is present before treatment is initiated. The treatment threshold in turn is determined by the severity of the disease and the potential complications of the treatment being considered. For example, antibiotics for pediatric otitis media are a relatively benign treatment and therefore have historically been prescribed even though the certainty of bacterial otitis media is far less than 100% based on otologic examination of a squirming infant. Thus, the treatment threshold is low. Conversely, the aggressive chemotherapy, surgery, and radiation commonly prescribed for a glioblastoma is

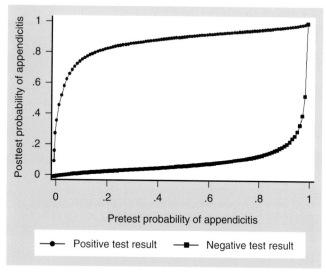

FIG. 10.1 The relationship between pretest and posttest probability of acute appendicitis after a positive or negative CT result. (From Blackmore CC, Terasawa T. Optimizing the interpretation of CT for appendicitis: modeling health utilities for clinical practice. *J Am Coll Radiol.* 2006;3:115–121.)

extremely toxic and would only be prescribed when the diagnosis is certain, requiring biopsy. Thus, although we might treat (appropriately or inappropriately) otitis media in a young child with only a 50% posttest probability of disease, we would require virtually 100% certainty before treating glioblastoma.

CT imaging for suspected appendicitis is a useful example for understanding Bayes theorem and therapeutic efficacy and one that is commonly used because much is known about the accuracy of CT, the pretest probability of disease, and the treatment threshold. The sensitivity and specificity of CT for appendicitis are available from published meta-analyses. The pretest and posttest probabilities can be calculated from Bayes theorem (Fig. 10.1). Finally, the treatment threshold for appendectomy can be understood from the historical rate of unnecessary appendectomy. Prior to the cross-sectional imaging era, surgeons would accept a 15% rate of incorrect diagnosis of appendicitis at laparotomy. Therefore, they would effectively operate when only 85% certain of the diagnosis, indicating a treatment threshold of 85%. To be useful, a result at CT must have the potential to change the probability of disease from below to above the treatment threshold (or vice versa). From Fig. 10.1, only when the pretest probability of disease is very low (<20%) will the treatment be the same regardless of the CT results. At all other disease probabilities, the positive and negative posttest probabilities will be on different sides of the treatment threshold at 85% and therefore indicate different treatments. Based on this model, we can conclude that if there is a reasonable probability of appendicitis, then CT has the potential to change management and is appropriate. Of course, this is an oversimplification because there may be more than one treatment threshold because patients at less than 85% probability of appendicitis might potentially still be treated with antibiotics or observation.

Level V in the tiered efficacy model involves clinical outcomes. Changing diagnostic certainty and changing

treatment may be desirable but only if, ultimately, patient outcome is improved. Regardless of the accuracy of an imaging study, if there is no effect on patient outcome, then the imaging should not be performed. This of course means that there must be effective treatment. Alternately, imaging may produce prognostic information. Though potentially not driving treatment itself, prognostic information may be of value to patients and family members. Thus, clinical outcomes encompass morbidity and mortality but also patient satisfaction and quality of life, which may be affected by knowledge of prognosis. Unfortunately, there is little research data on the value of prognostic information to patients and family members.

Regardless however, fundamentally, if imaging does not have the potential to change therapy and therefore affect clinical outcomes, or at least provide prognostic information that improves patient satisfaction and well-being, there is no reason to perform that imaging. From a research perspective, this makes understanding of the value of imaging challenging, because that value is directly linked to the availability of effective treatments. As an example, chest x-ray screening for lung cancer was popularized in the 1970s. Research at that time demonstrated that chest x-ray was more sensitive and specific than clinical exam for identification of early cancer. This led to changes in diagnostic certainty and changes in management, with patients undergoing lobectomy for pulmonary nodules. However, ultimately, there was no effect on clinical outcome, because by the time of diagnosis by chest x-ray, most such cancers had spread locally or metastasized, indicating that treatments available at the time were not effective. Thus, screening chest x-ray was not appropriate imaging. Current CT screening for lung cancer, because of the smaller size at detection, and because of improvements in therapy, does have effects on clinical outcome in smokers at appropriate age and thus may be appropriate.

The final step in determining the effectiveness of imaging is to understand the societal perspective. Implicitly or explicitly, only a finite amount of resources can be allocated to healthcare. Accordingly, use of such resources for one medical intervention will have an opportunity cost in not having those resources available for other interventions. As new expensive drugs come to market or advanced imaging modalities are used more, other interventions must be performed less, or cost must increase. Ideally, new imaging approaches would eliminate costly treatments through earlier detection, saving money for society. Unfortunately, this seldom seems to be the case. Historically, society has tolerated increasing cost, but it is clear that such increases are no longer sustainable, and efforts at cost containment have increased. Accordingly, one must not only look at whether imaging improves clinical outcome but whether the resources devoted to that imaging are providing value. Cost-effectiveness analysis is a former way of defining the amount of benefit per unit of cost for any intervention in medicine and is applicable to imaging. As an example, formal cost-effectiveness analysis of CT colonography compared to colonoscopy or sigmoid colonoscopy plus fecal occult blood testing revealed that CT colonography was more cost-effective than no screening but less cost-effective than screening with the other modalities. Such information can then be used for policy makers in determining whether an imaging study should be covered under government or private insurance plans.

Thus, understanding the value of imaging is complex. The tiered efficacy model provides a framework for using research evidence about imaging. The model also highlights where we have more abundant evidence (technical effectiveness and accuracy) and where the evidence driving imaging practice is sparse (diagnostic certainty, therapeutic effectiveness, patient outcomes, and societal value).

SHOULD IMAGING BE PERFORMED?

Evidence-based imaging in practice involves distilling what is known about the value of imaging from research at different levels of the tiered efficacy model into the clinical questions of whether imaging is appropriate to be performed at all and, if so, which imaging modality should be used. This balances the benefits of imaging in terms of diagnostic certainty and guiding therapy versus the costs of imaging in terms of dollars but more importantly in terms of patient outcomes, including complications from incorrect diagnosis, incidental findings, and radiation or other side effects of the imaging modality itself. Time may also be a cost of imaging, particularly in the emergency setting.

Appropriateness of imaging is an area of increasing interest. Some estimates are that up to 30% of medical imaging in the United States is not necessary, with cost estimations of $30 billion per year. National and international calls for improving the appropriateness of imaging have included the "Choosing Wisely" campaign, a large-scale Medicare Imaging Demonstration project using clinical decision support to improve appropriateness of imaging and recent federal legislation under the Protecting Access to Medicare Act of 2014. There are now multiple for-profit companies offering appropriate imaging criteria, as well as the American College of Radiology.

Identifying when imaging is appropriate is extremely challenging given the myriad imaging modalities and approaches available, as well as the incredible complexity of medical decision making. However, there are a number of common clinical scenarios where there is strong evidence that imaging is not necessary. This evidence usually takes the form of validated clinical prediction rules to identify clinical criteria for when imaging is not necessary. As discussed earlier, the probability that a patient actually has a disease after a positive test result is based not just on the accuracy of the test but also on the pretest probability that the disease was present. Thus, for a test to be useful, there must be at least some reasonable probability that an individual has the disease in question. In some circumstances, sets of clinical criteria, known as clinical prediction rules, can be used to identify individuals who have essentially zero pretest probability of a specific clinical condition. These clinical prediction rules can therefore be used to identify subjects who should not undergo imaging, because the condition has been effectively excluded on clinical grounds. To provide strong evidence that imaging is not appropriate, these clinical prediction rules must be validated, meaning that they

have been tested on actual patients in clinical practice and shown to be effective. Clinical prediction rules with strong evidence exist for appropriate use of imaging for topics including trauma to the head, cervical spine, ankle, foot, and knee and to rule out pulmonary embolism. There are other sets of clinical criteria to define when imaging is unnecessary, which are at least supported by the existing evidence and the basis for broad consensus, although they may not have undergone rigorous validation. This includes imaging for nontraumatic low back pain, imaging for headache, and imaging for sinus disease. The Choosing Wisely campaign emphasizes several of the clinical areas where evidence-based criteria can be defined to identify where imaging is unnecessary.

The areas where clinical criteria can define inappropriate imaging can also form the basis for clinical decision support systems. These systems provide point-of-order clinical information to clinicians to advise them of unnecessary imaging or potentially enforce whether imaging is or is not necessary. Clinical decision support systems can define a finite number of appropriate indications for specific imaging studies, blocking the ordering of imaging when these criteria are not met. When applied to areas of imaging with a strong evidence basis, such clinical decision support can help eliminate 20% to 30% of imaging that is not indicated. The challenge with clinical decision support is that it requires simple evidence-based criteria to define where imaging is appropriate. In the more nuanced clinical scenarios commonly driving performance of imaging, such criteria may be difficult or impossible to define. For example, there are well-supported criteria for when lumbar MRI should be performed, including presence of risk factors for more severe systemic conditions (infection, cancer, trauma), cauda equina syndrome, progressive motor weakness, or failure of conservative therapy. Absent these criteria, lumbar imaging for acute low back pain is not indicated. However, in contrast, a simple set of criteria for when abdominal CT for abdominal pain should or should not be performed cannot be defined. Features of the abdominal pain (duration, severity, location, etc.), other clinical features (nausea, vomiting, fever, etc.), or comorbidities (diabetes, hypertension) are insufficient to reliably define when imaging for abdominal pain is appropriate.

Although determination of whether imaging should or should not be performed ultimately requires an understanding of outcome and cost-effectiveness, the choice between imaging modalities may be a simpler decision, often based on accuracy. For a given clinical condition, simple comparison of the sensitivity and specificity of competing imaging modalities may provide the basis for choosing the optimal course. Of course there are other considerations, including cost, radiation dose, and potential for other diagnoses. In these circumstances, understanding of outcomes and cost-effectiveness through decision analysis modeling may be necessary. However, wide differences in accuracy will generally define the best imaging strategy even in the face of cost and radiation differences. For example, in adults, CT is a more accurate imaging study for the identification of acute appendicitis by a significant margin. Although there are risks associated with radiation, these risks are relatively small compared to the improvement in accuracy, decreased need for invasive laparotomy, or delayed diagnosis. In children however, the difference in accuracy between CT and ultrasound is decreased, due to the smaller body size in children allowing more accurate ultrasound imaging. In addition, the potential risk of radiation in children is greater. Accordingly, in children, it may be advisable to perform ultrasound first, with CT reserved for equivocal cases or those of high clinical suspicion in whom the ultrasound imaging is negative.

On a practical level, radiologists work with clinicians to understand whether an imaging study should be performed. For the radiologist, this should encompass an understanding of research that exists on appropriateness, including relevant clinical prediction rules. In addition, an understanding of the tiered efficacy model and Bayes theorem (described earlier) can help radiologists translate what is known about accuracy of an imaging study to the more valuable levels of diagnostic certainty and therapeutic effectiveness. In the simplest case, this is captured by the classic question, "How will this imaging study affect patient management?" However, the tiered efficacy model allows a deeper understanding and enables radiologists to provide guidance to clinical colleagues on how the test should influence clinical management.

CONCLUSION

In conclusion, evidence-based imaging requires application of the best available evidence to patient care. However, evidence is often biased and incomplete, and what is available tends to be limited to technical efficacy and accuracy. It is incumbent on radiologists to be able to translate measures of accuracy into the more clinically relevant therapeutic decision making and potentially even patient outcome levels of effectiveness. Further, imaging is not appropriate if there is no potential to change management based on the results of the study, with the important caveat that prognostic information can sometimes also provide value from the patient's perspective. As appropriate use of imaging becomes even more the focus of quality and cost-containment efforts in healthcare, radiologists should be uniquely positioned as experts on how to use the best evidence to maximize the value of imaging for patients and society.

SUGGESTED READINGS

Black WC, Welch HG. Screening for disease. *AJR Am J Roentgenol.* 1997;168:3–11.

Blackmore CC, Terasawa T. Optimizing the interpretation of CT for appendicitis: modeling health utilities for clinical practice. *J Am Coll Radiol.* 2006;3:115–121.

Blackmore CC. Clinical prediction rules in trauma imaging: who, how and why? *Radiology.* 2005;235:371–374.

Blackmore CC. Critically assessing the radiology literature. *Acad Radiol.* 2004;11:134–140.

Choosing Wisely. ABIM Foundation Website. <http://www.choosingwisely.org>; 2016 Accessed 29.03.2016.

Fryback DG, Thornbury JR. The efficacy of diagnostic imaging. *Med Decis Making.* 1991;11:88–94.

Medina LS, Blackmore CC, Applegate KE, eds. *Evidence Based Imaging: Improving the Quality of Imaging in Patient Care.* New York, NY: Springer Science + Business Media; 2011.

Sackett DL, Straus SE, Richardson WS, Rosenberg W, Haynes RB. *Evidence-Based Medicine-How to Practice and Teach EBM.* Edinburgh, Scotland: Churchill Livingstone; 2000.

Sox HC, Higgins MC, Owens DK. *Medical Decision Making.* New York, NY: Wiley-Blackwell; 2013.

Vanness DJ, Knudsen AB, Lansdorp-Vogelaar I. Comparative economic evaluation of data from the ACRIN national CT colonography trial with three cancer intervention and surveillance modeling network microsimulations. *Radiology.* 2011;261:487–498.

Welch HG, Black WC. Overdiagnosis in cancer. *J Natl Cancer Inst.* 2010;102:605–613.

Chapter 11
Patient-Centered Radiology

Jason N. Itri and David C. Mihal

INTRODUCTION

The Institute of Medicine highlighted the essential role of patient-centered care by including it as one of the committee's six specific aims for improving healthcare in *Crossing the Quality Chasm* (2001). In this report, patient-centered healthcare is defined as "providing care that is respectful of and responsive to individual patient preferences, needs, and values and ensuring that patient values guide all clinical decisions" and "encompasses qualities of compassion, empathy, and responsiveness to the needs, values, and expressed preferences of the individual patient." The committee's motivation for including patient-centered care as a specific aim is well-documented patient frustration with "their inability to participate in decision-making, to obtain information they need, to be heard, and to participate in systems of care that are responsive to their needs." Patients are highly variable in their preferences, want to obtain information about their diagnosis and treatment, and often make their own decisions with guidance from their physicians. In this paradigm, it is clear that physicians cannot make the best decisions for their patients without providing information and including patients and their families in the decision-making process.

PATIENT-CENTERED CARE IN RADIOLOGY

Redesigning processes to incorporate patient-centered principles in hospitals and outpatient imaging centers has received significant attention in the past several years, reflecting in part the growing need to improve patient satisfaction and demonstrate value in a healthcare system that is becoming more consumer and outcomes driven. Abujudeh's Quality Process Map for radiology provides a visual framework that concentrates on the patient first when it comes to radiology processes (Fig. 11.1). Providing a conceptual framework to help us understand the patient's experience of illness and healthcare is a prerequisite to redesigning radiology-specific processes that take into account patients' subjective experiences and measure satisfaction. In an effort to preserve the view that *patient-centered* radiology should be defined by *patients*, we will use the conceptual framework of patient-centered care provided by Gerteis et al. in which seven dimensions of patient-centered care are described based on extensive interviews and focus groups with patients, family members, physicians, and hospital staff.

1. Respect for patients' values, preferences, and expressed needs
2. Coordination and integration of care
3. Information, communication, and education
4. Physical comfort
5. Emotional support and alleviation of fear and anxiety
6. Involvement of family and friends
7. Transitions and continuity

This chapter provides an overview of the first six dimensions of patient-centered care adapted to radiology followed by a discussion of opportunities to improve patient centeredness in radiology. Review and discussion of the dimension *information, communication, and education* are focused on communication, given the critical role of communication in promoting patient centeredness. The final dimension of patient-centered care, *transitions and continuity*, is not reviewed because imaging is generally considered a clinical support service, and there is limited applicability of this dimension to radiology.

DIMENSIONS OF PATIENT-CENTERED RADIOLOGY AND OPPORTUNITIES FOR IMPROVEMENT

Respect for Patient Values, Preferences, and Expressed Needs

This dimension focuses on respecting patients as unique individuals. The patient's experience of illness encompasses not only the discomfort associated with being ill but all the social and psychological consequences as well. Physicians focused on the objective tasks of diagnosis and treatment fail to adequately address the patients' subjective experience of illness, and therein lies part of the cultural discord between patients and physicians. There are several components of this dimension: (1) involving patients in their care, which includes determining patient preferences for involvement in decision making, open discussion of alternative medical procedures, and providing information about the course of illness and prospect of recovery; (2) understanding and respecting patients' therapeutic goals; and (3) understanding and respecting cultural beliefs and practices. These components form the foundation of patient-centered care and are broadly applicable to patient care in radiology.

Involving patients in their care can be accomplished by having radiologists or knowledgeable staff members engage in dialogue with patients about what to expect during imaging procedures and the risks and benefits of specific procedures with alternative options. A survey of patients at a cancer center indicated that 71% of patients would like explanatory brochures, 82% would like explanations from a member of the radiology team concerning the examination procedure, and 85% would like explanations from a member of the radiology team concerning possible risks. While 88% did not meet with the radiologist before the examination, 36% expressed a desire to meet with the radiologist to understand the purpose of the examination,

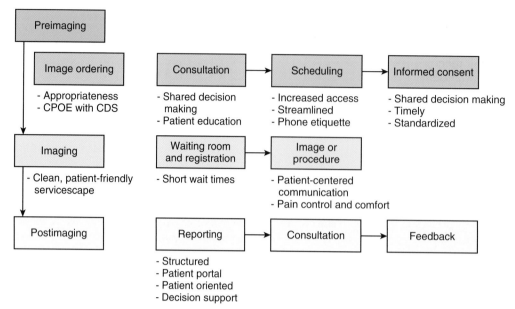

FIG. 11.1 PATIENT-CENTERED PROCESS MAP. *CDS,* Clinical decision support. *CPOE,* computerized physician order entry. (From Abujudeh HM, Danielson A, Bruno MA. A patient-centered radiology quality process map: opportunities and solutions. *AJR Am J Roentgenol.* 2016;207[5]:940–946.)

to be reassured, and to tell the radiologist about painful zones. That proportion increased to 77% when asked if they wanted to meet with the radiologist after the examination primarily to avoid waiting for the results.

Understanding and respecting patients' therapeutic goals is a concept that may not be considered by radiologists performing imaging studies. The critical role of patient preference in determining therapeutic goals is highlighted by a study of healthy volunteers asked to choose between radiation therapy and surgery to treat cancer of the larynx, revealing that 20% chose radiation to preserve speech even though it was associated with a significantly lower survival rate. Radiology departments may abdicate this important responsibility to referring physicians, routinely performing all imaging studies ordered with a "just do it" mentality. However, this mindset may not be consistent with patients' goals and invariably leads to inappropriate and costly overutilization. Patients' preferences and patient-defined outcomes can be incorporated into clinical practice guidelines, providing an opportunity for clinicians to place greater emphasis on patients' therapeutic goals when considering treatment options.

One way to promote patient-centered care is for clinicians to practice within a *shared decision-making* model: decision making involves at least the health provider and the patient but may also involve family members, relatives, friends, and multiple health providers; all parties take steps to participate in the process of decision making; information sharing is requisite; and an agreed-upon shared treatment decision is made. Shared decision making involves using guided-discussion tools such as flowcharts, videotapes, and interactive presentations that organize the disease information and treatment outcomes in language that is understandable by the patient. This model should improve patients' knowledge of options, perceptions of risks and benefits, and achieve clinical decisions that are consistent with patient values such as quality of life. This approach ensures that knowledge is shared and

information flows freely between patients and radiologists, who should also strive to provide the best available scientific knowledge. Shared decision making should be practiced in every patient encounter to accommodate differences in patient preference.

Understanding and respecting cultural beliefs and practices plays a significant role in access and utilization of radiologic services, particularly for screening exams. Interventions that incorporate cultural competency have been shown to improve the quality of healthcare in minority or underserved populations, such as patient tracking and reminder systems, healthcare provider education, and offering screening services directly to patients rather than through physicians. Similar improvements have been achieved by incorporating cultural competency into the use of medical imaging for screening. Disparate breast cancer–related mortality and survival outcomes between Caucasian women and ethnic minorities have been attributed to several factors, one of which is culturally grounded beliefs that act as a barrier to participation in conventional screening mammography programs. Improvements in the utilization of screening mammography among Korean American women were achieved by using a culturally relevant intervention consisting of interactive educational sessions focused on breast cancer, early screening guidelines, and Korean cultural beliefs.

Coordination and Integration of Care

Patient concerns with coordination of clinical care typically relate to the sense that members of the clinical team are not communicating critical information to one another based on the inconsistency of the message the patient is receiving from different members of the clinical care team. In contrast, coordination of clinical support services presents a different set of challenges for radiologists because the primary customer of clinical support services is typically the referring physician. These services are usually valued by how quickly, accurately, and completely information about confirming or excluding a diagnosis is conveyed to the clinician. As a result, patients too often describe diagnostic and therapeutic procedures as painful or dehumanizing experiences. This particular problem is aptly described by Gilda Radner in her book, *It's Always Something*, in which she describes her experience undergoing a barium enema during her struggle with cancer.

> *The technicians strapped me to a table and then put a tube in my rear end. As they poured a chalky liquid inside me and pumped gas into me so that my bowel would show up …, they were also turning me slowly around and around on the table. … I felt like I was trapped on an endless Ferris wheel with someone's fist up my butt. You can image how much I enjoyed the barium enema. I think the word that best captures the whole event is humiliating …*

A barium enema is considered a routine procedure by most radiologists, and this would have been the case with Gilda Radner as the study revealed nothing wrong. However, the factors that contribute to making the patient's experience painful and humiliating are the assembly-line style of technicians who have not developed a relationship with the patient, inadequate explanation of the procedure, being left alone and scantily clothed in a hospital gown in waiting areas and hallways, and being told that it will not hurt when it most likely will cause pain or discomfort. It is important for providers to be acutely aware of the pain and discomfort patients experience during *routine* procedures and to adequately address the patient's concerns prior to and during these procedures.

Fears that members of the clinical team are not passing along critical pieces of information to one another is another pervasive problem for radiologists. A lack of clinical history on radiology requisitions has been described as a universal problem for radiologists, and a systematic review evaluating the accuracy of diagnostic tests that are read with and without clinical information determined that clinical information improved test reading accuracy. When an important piece of information is lost or overlooked, patients see that the people taking care of them are uninformed, efforts are needlessly duplicated, procedures are delayed, and tasks are left undone. One of the greatest contributions an ordering provider can make to the radiologist's interpretation is to provide relevant clinical information with the order. Although computerized provider order entry offers opportunities to improve clinical histories, implementation is far from perfect. As a result, healthcare providers in radiology must be vigilant in obtaining the clinical information necessary to provide accurate, high-quality interpretations for imaging examinations, which can be accomplished by interviewing patients, reviewing the electronic medical record or patient's chart, and calling the referring physician's office.

Communication

Effective communication between patients and caregivers addresses both technical and nontechnical aspects of healthcare. Communication about the technical aspects of care is restricted to facts, diagnoses, recommended treatments, and likelihood of recovery; in this realm, patients are less knowledgeable, more passive, and more vulnerable than providers. The nontechnical aspects of care are emphasized in patient-centered communication, which places the patient and provider on equal ground by engaging both in the discussion of deep feelings and subjective experiences. An important area for radiologists to promote patient-centered care is in the communication of imaging results directly to patients. The traditional pattern of communication through referring physicians as intermediaries devalues the patient-radiologist relationship, has the potential for delay or miscommunication, and contributes to significant (and often unnecessary) patient anxiety.

A survey of patients' preferences in the *disclosure of imaging findings* shows a clear desire on the part of patients to hear the results of imaging examinations from the radiologist at the time of the procedure rather than hearing them later from the referring physician, regardless of the findings. Patients experience considerable anxiety waiting for the results of imaging procedures; half of the smokers undergoing lung cancer screening experienced discomfort waiting for results, whereas most patients undergoing imaging studies in a cancer center reported wanting to meet with the radiologist after the examination "to be reassured," "to avoid waiting for the results," "to have the preliminary results," for "rapid results before the visit with the doctor," and to know "if there is a problem." Patients are entitled to know the results of their examination, and radiologists should provide a mechanism whereby patients can choose if they want their results delivered immediately by radiologists or available through a patient portal, although disclosing the results directly to the patient requires that the referring physician be notified promptly as well.

According to Reynolds, "Health care practitioners in any specialty must possess soft skills to provide patient-centered care." Soft skills is a sociological term relating to an individual's personality traits, social graces, communication skills, language, personal habits, friendliness, and optimism, which characterize one's relationships with other people. The acronym AIDET (acknowledgment, introduce, duration, explanation, and thank you) represents a set of soft skills that can be used to improve communication between patients and healthcare providers in the radiology communication loop:

Acknowledgment: Greet and welcome the patient, apologize for delays, acknowledge concerns.

Introduce: Introduce yourself using your name and explain your role in the patient's care.

Duration: Describe the time the patient can expect to wait for a test or procedure.

Explanation: Describe what is going to happen to the patient and what he or she can expect.

Thank You: Thank the patient for his or her cooperation and participation.

Examples of patient-centered communication skills include encouraging patients to talk about psychosocial issues, using the patient's own words and language, using interruptions to reflect on the communication between physicians and patients, and providing information and counseling rather than asking questions and giving directions.

Language barriers contribute to health disparities in individuals with limited English proficiency and result in decreased patient satisfaction, decreased patient understanding of diagnosis and treatment, poorer adherence to treatment and follow-up for chronic illnesses, and increased medication complications. A systematic review by Karliner et al. indicates that the use of professional interpreters has positive benefits on communication with regard to errors and comprehension, use of clinical care, clinical outcomes, and satisfaction with care. According to Shams-Avari, "inexperienced interpreters have omitted questions about drug allergies; instructions for the dose, frequency and duration or antibiotics; and directions for rehydration fluids." It is important to note that although patients may prefer to use friends or family members for medical interpretation, this practice leads to a higher frequency of errors that are significantly more likely to have clinical consequences.

Hearing and vision impairment introduce significant barriers to effective communication within the healthcare setting and require specific approaches to minimize the impact of these barriers. In a study of patients with hearing impairment, six themes revolving around ineffective communication were described. Strategies proposed by the study participants included having physicians inquire about which method of communication patients prefer and having patients repeat critical health information to identify potentially dangerous miscommunication. A study using focus groups and interviews with individuals who were blind or had low vision, some of whom were healthcare experts, identified barriers to effective care and concluded that using common courtesy and individualized communication techniques could improve healthcare experiences of blind and low-vision patients.

Health literacy is the ability to understand health information and to use that information to make good decisions about your health and medical care. Low or limited health literacy can affect a patient's ability to fill out complex forms, locate providers and services, share personal information such as health history, manage chronic disease, and understand how to take medications. Low health literacy has been associated with higher rates of hospitalization, greater use of emergency care, lower receipt of mammography screening and influenza vaccines, poorer health status, higher mortality rates, and poorer use of healthcare services. In radiology, low health literacy could negatively impact a patient's ability to appropriately complete contrast or magnetic resonance imaging screening forms, follow preparatory instructions prior to procedures such as a barium enema, or seek medical assistance when experiencing pain after an interventional procedure. Several strategies have been proposed to address issues related to low health literacy (Box 11.1).

Cultural differences present unique challenges to healthcare providers, complicated by the complex interrelationships among culture, race, or ethnicity and the resulting healthcare disparities. Strategies incorporating cultural competency training have been shown to be effective in addressing cultural disparities by improving the attitudes and skills of healthcare workers. Engebretson et al. proposed a practice model integrating levels of cultural competency with components of evidence-based care in an effort to make cultural competence relevant

---

BOX 11.1 Strategies to Address Issues Related to Low Health Literacy

- Caregivers should focus on increasing patient recall and understanding.
- Information should be organized into logical blocks, and the main message should be simplified, made specific to the patient, repeated, and summarized.
- Patients' understanding should be checked by asking them to repeat information in their own words.
- Patient-centered interviewing skills should be employed.
- Medical concerns should be placed in a personal context by explaining the effect of treatment on the patient's daily activities.

---

to clinical practice. Educating healthcare providers to be more aware of their own cultural beliefs and more responsive to the cultural beliefs of their patients can lead to a higher level of self-awareness and new beliefs that will translate to better healthcare.

Communication of difficult results presents unique challenges that are best planned for in advance. A cancer diagnosis can involve imaging examinations in which the radiologist is primarily involved and delivers bad news to patients. It has been shown that women in the United States prefer that radiologists disclose findings from mammographic imaging immediately after the examination and that radiologists be prominent contributors in treatment and prognosis. Developing resources and making them available to guide radiologists in the position of delivering difficult news are a fundamental first step. Five stages of a difficult news delivery encounter have been described (Box 11.2). Potential barriers to communicating difficult news include the lack of a preexisting relationship with the patient, lack of education of physicians to deliver difficult news effectively, physician discomfort with stressful and/or emotional discussions, lack of a comfortable space to deliver the news, and variability in what actually constitutes difficult or bad news. With a bit of anticipatory preparation, all of these barriers can be mitigated to some degree.

Physical Comfort

The dimension of physical comfort encompasses two distinct tasks relevant to radiology, controlling acute pain and minimizing the stresses of the hospital's physical environment to provide a supportive atmosphere for healing and recovery.

Aggressive pain management is essential to patient-centered care, yet despite advances in the use of narcotics and other analgesics, pain control continues to be one of the most feared and debilitating aspects of illness and medical treatment. Studies assessing pain in various clinical settings indicate that a significant number of patients continue to experience moderate or severe pain despite treatment with analgesics, ranging from 20% to 75% of those questioned. For interventional procedures, radiologists should perform a baseline assessment by asking patients to rate their pain, make regular and ongoing assessments of pain, and monitor the effectiveness of pain control measures as well as side effects. A study measuring patient satisfaction during four diagnostic imaging

Discovery: At this stage, the imaging abnormality is identified. At this time, a point person should be assigned who is able to integrate and communicate information from both the staff and family in an effective manner while focusing on the patient's psychosocial needs. Providing a single person allows for one voice, which reduces the likelihood of conflicting information, personalizes the process and builds trust.

Evaluation: The patient is notified by the point person that there is a need to discuss the imaging findings. This provides a warning that something may be wrong and allows the patient a short period of time to prepare themselves for unexpected news. The point person should be updated with new information about the findings or impression and implications.

Alert: Escort the family to a private consult room and explain the following: "The radiologist is reviewing the images. As soon as we have more information, we want to share it with you. Let's go to a room where the doctor can easily find you." By now the patient has had time to mentally prepare himself or herself to receive information in a safe environment.

Communication: Have all contributing parties available who can participate in the conversation; the radiologist should be present no matter who has been assigned as the point person. The availability of the radiologist to answer questions or provide further detail is of tremendous value to the patient, even if unused. The disclosure should be initiated by evaluating what the patient already knows or suspects about his or her condition. This allows the point person to address the information as an extension of what the patient already knows and to clarify any points of confusion or misunderstanding.

Debriefing: The results are discussed with the patient and any caregivers or family. Because family members serve as an important source of emotional and social support, involving them when delivering difficult news may help the patient cope with his or her illness. When disclosing difficult news to patients, it is important to show compassion, acknowledge the patient's grief, and promote direct, honest communication.

procedures found that patients experienced the highest degree of pain during mammography and double-contrast barium enema examinations; the authors concluded that pain reduction strategies should be employed. General strategies that can improve pain management include educating patients about their right to pain relief, encouraging patients to take an active role in communicating and managing their pain, making pain assessment data more visible to caregivers, and educating staff about pain control protocols with a discussion of misconceptions about narcotics and their risks and benefits.

The *physical environment* can have a significant impact on a patient's experience, and a supportive environment may serve to help prevent illness and alleviate stress and depression. A key factor in determining customer satisfaction with radiology services concerns *tangibles*, which include the physical appearance of a department, its facilities, and the quality of the equipment. According to Alderson, tangible factors have a surprisingly large impact on the patient's opinion of a practice, because the patient's experience of service is much broader than the core skill brought by radiologists. Examples of physical features that support a patient-centered environment include general cleanliness, availability of parking in an area

that is easily accessible and well lighted, well-kept building and grounds, inviting waiting rooms, and comfortable exam rooms. The physical environment can be further individualized based on the patient population, with the Children's Hospital of Pittsburgh being an example of patient-centered design for pediatric patients and their families. The general trend in the design of healthcare facilities is toward more private, patient-friendly environments that are clean, reduce stress, and support patient well-being.

Emotional Support

A patient's experience of illness includes the emotional and psychological consequences of being ill, and healthcare providers must adequately address these subjective aspects of illness to provide the most effective care. Research has shown that addressing patients' emotional needs can influence their satisfaction with care, compliance with treatment regimens, side effects from drugs, recovery of function, need for pain medications, and length of hospital stay.

Anxiety and frustration are emotions experienced by patients as a result of waiting or not knowing what to expect, especially when a procedure has the potential to elicit discomfort or pain. Anxiety is often driven or magnified by the fact that critical clinical decisions may depend on the outcome of imaging procedures, and many diagnoses (e.g., cancer) have profound physical, emotional, and psychological implications for patients and their families. Survey results from a study of women undergoing percutaneous core biopsy of the breast indicate that being concerned about the results of the biopsy was a significant contributor to patient anxiety. Approximately 50% of patients surveyed in a cancer center reported that the radiology examination worried them during the days before the appointment, with 13% of respondents reporting being considerably worried. The reasons reported were fear of the results, waiting for the results, and fear of the risks and the examination procedure.

In a study of patients undergoing interventional radiologic procedures, subjective feelings of anxiety before procedures and patient pain during procedures were assessed on a visual analog scale to evaluate the effectiveness of conscious sedation. The authors found that all patients significantly overestimated their anticipated pain and concluded that interventionalists should spend more time assessing the patient's fear of pain and attempting to reduce that fear rather than dwelling on the technical aspects of procedures. High levels of anxiety experienced by women undergoing breast biopsy in a study evaluating correlates of anxiety led the authors to conclude that there is a need for future consideration and assessment of potential intervention strategies for anxiety. When discussing procedures with patients, it is important to give specific information with realistic expectations. Research has shown that giving patients information about the sensory aspect of procedural experiences helps reduce anxiety, whereas inaccurate expectations about the physical sensations (e.g., pain) can be a significant source of distress. Self-reporting instruments can be used to assess level of anxiety prior to procedures, and different types of educational material can be used to reduce anxiety depending on patient preference.

Radiologists who have relationships with patients beyond interpreting imaging examinations in the reading room should develop specific behaviors to provide

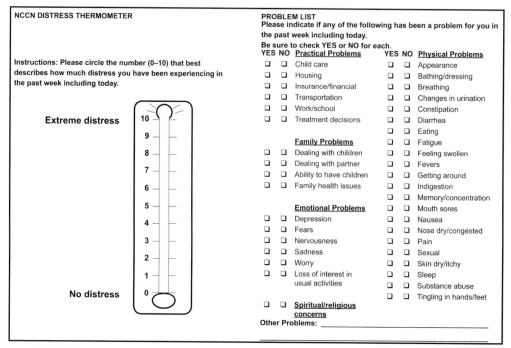

FIG. 11.2 **NATIONAL COMPREHENSIVE CANCER NETWORK (NCCN) DISTRESS THERMOMETER SCREEN-ING TOOL.** (From the NCCN Clinical Practice Guidelines in Oncology [NCCN Guidelines] for Distress Management V.2.2016. Copyright 2016 National Comprehensive Cancer Network, Inc. All rights reserved. The NCCN Guidelines and illustrations herein may not be reproduced in any form for any purpose without the express written permission of NCCN. To view the most recent and complete version of the NCCN Guidelines, go to NCCN.org. The NCCN Guidelines are a work in progress that may be refined as often as new significant data becomes available. NCCN makes no warranties of any kind regarding their content, use, or application and disclaims any responsibility for their application or use in any way.)

emotional support for their patients that convey a genuine sense of caring and concern. According to Walker, the most important category of support for patients is the expression of positive affect or bolstering of self-esteem, which includes such actions as expressing concern and empathy, showing special understanding of the nature of the problem, calm acceptance of the problem, and the expression of optimism or hope. Beyond these general behaviors, patients differ in their needs for support, and clinicians should ask patients about their fears and anxiety, as well as what kind of emotional support they find helpful. A variety of approaches have been described to reduce stress and relieve anxiety. Sims and Rilling have described a distress tool (Fig. 11.2) to evaluate and quantify patient psychosocial distress in interventional radiology patients with cancer, as well as psychosocial interventions that can be made within the interventional radiology clinic setting.

Involvement of Family and Friends

Families serve several functions in the setting of illness, including caregivers or care partners, long-term promoters of health and well-being, and providers of essential social and emotional support. Given these important roles, family involvement is an important component of patient-centered care and should be encouraged and supported. One of the most important functions of family members is to serve as proxy decision makers and patient advocates. This may put family members in an adversarial role with healthcare providers but ensures that someone is looking out for the patient's best interests. Family members monitor the patient's care both within the hospital setting and

at home and can participate meaningfully in healthcare decisions. Radiologists can support family involvement in a patient's care by including family members when providing information about imaging procedures or discussing abnormal findings. Including family members in the discussion of risks and benefits for imaging procedures facilitates shared decision making and is an opportunity for family members to provide information about the patient and ask questions. Family members caring for the patient at home can help ensure that patients follow postprocedural instructions, understand and identify warning signs to seek immediate care, and obtain necessary follow-up.

METHODS TO ASSESS PATIENT-CENTEREDNESS IN RADIOLOGY

Using experiences with focus groups and patient surveys, Lexa describes four groups or clusters of issues central to how patients perceive radiology services and evaluate them: time, safety, human interactions, and creature comforts. It is important to keep in mind, however, that there is considerable variability among patients related to several factors including age, gender, culture, type of illness, magnitude of illness, and regional variability in expectations. This variability leads to inhomogeneity in patient's definitions of subjective criteria and expectations for imaging services, emphasizing the need to assess satisfaction for patients undergoing imaging examinations at your particular facility. Box 11.3 provides a list of objective and subjective criteria that can be used to evaluate patient satisfaction with imaging service and quality using a rating scale ranging from very dissatisfied to very satisfied (e.g., Likert scale, 1 to 5).

TIME

1. Appointment availability for outpatient examinations
2. Appointment time for inpatient examinations
3. Wait time (time from the patient arriving at the imaging facility to examination completion)
4. Registration time (time to complete the registration process)
5. Study time (time from the beginning of the examination to completion)
6. Wait time (time from the patient arriving at the imaging facility to examination completion)
7. Report turnaround time (time from examination completion to final report available for the patient or referring physician to review)
8. Communication of critical results (time from examination completion to communication of critical results to the patient or referring physician)

SAFETY

1. Perceived safety of the imaging examination
2. Use of a screening tool for intravenous contrast
3. Use of a screening tool for magnetic resonance imaging
4. Verification of patient identity using two patient identifiers
5. Verification of imaging examination to be performed
6. Verification of the region or body part to be imaged

HUMAN INTERACTIONS

1. Courtesy and respectfulness of the scheduling and registration staff
2. Courtesy and respectfulness of the nurses or technologists
3. Courtesy and respectfulness of transport personnel
4. Explanation of preparation for an imaging examination
5. Explanation of what to expect during an imaging examination
6. Availability of educational material about an imaging examination
7. Explanation of the billing process and policies
8. Availability of staff members to answer questions

COMFORTS

1. Quality of the imaging equipment
2. Parking availability and cost
3. Cleanliness and accessibility of the imaging facilities
4. Overall appearance of the imaging facility

OVERALL

1. Overall satisfaction

Patient satisfaction surveys can be developed to gather qualitative feedback and suggestions from patients, obtain benchmarking and comparative data, determine baseline measurements to evaluate if progress is being made toward organizational goals, or provide continual measurements to evaluate the impact of service and quality initiatives.

NEXT GENERATION OF ASSESSING PATIENT-CENTEREDNESS IN RADIOLOGY

We have described a conceptual framework using dimensions of patient-centered care to help us understand the patient's experience of illness and healthcare adapted to radiology. The next step in using this information to redesign radiology-specific processes and measure progress toward goals is to convert the conceptual framework into a *conceptual map* describing the range of experiences during the delivery of imaging and image-guided services that matter to patients. A conceptual map helps answer questions about which aspects of care matter and why, how well these are reflected in survey instruments and other assessment tools, how they could and should be valued, and how information about them should inform service development. Various conceptual and theoretical frameworks have been described including the World Health Organization's responsiveness framework, the Institute of Medicine's domains of healthcare quality, and Nolan et al.'s SENSES framework. The conceptual map developed by Entwistle et al. is an example of a conceptual map providing a rich array of experiences that can be used to assess patient centeredness, including healthcare relationships and their implications for people's valued capabilities.

PATIENT-CENTERED AND PATIENT-DEFINED OUTCOMES IN IMAGING

Within radiology, patient-centered outcomes are much more complex to determine and measure than patient satisfaction. A recent systematic review of the use of patient-centered outcome measures in radiology revealed only 10 publications in which the primary aim of the study was to investigate patient-centered outcomes, and none of the outcome measures used were developed specifically for radiology. The authors indicated little patient engagement in outcome research in radiology, citing barriers such as radiology departments' research tradition, funding, and support for outcome research, coupled with the nature of the relationship between clinicians and radiology. The Patient-Centered Outcomes Research Institute is a nonprofit organization that funds comparative effectiveness research with the goal of determining which healthcare options will work best for patients in specific circumstances and then promoting policy change to promote those interests. A review of opportunities for patient-centered outcomes research in radiology was recently published.

PATIENT-CENTERED CARE COMPETENCIES AND TEACHING PATIENT-CENTERED SKILLS

The American College of Graduate Medical Education (ACGME) has transitioned to an outcomes-based milestones framework for determining resident and fellow performance within six core competencies including patient care and interpersonal skills and communication. This framework allows for the assessment of the development of resident and fellow physicians in key dimensions of the elements of physician competency in radiology. The milestone addressing interpersonal and communication skills tracks the development of effective communication with patients, families, and caregivers over five subcompetencies including communicating information about imaging results, obtaining informed consent, and communicating difficult news, performing each in a compassionate and sensitive manner that adapts to the wide range of cultural, language, impairment, and health literacy differences that exist among patients. The requirement for demonstration of "interpersonal and communication skills that result in the effective exchange of information and collaboration with patients, their families, and health professionals" requires a patient-centered approach that should be developed during residency.

Developing these interpersonal and communication skills during radiology residency is challenging because the opportunities may be relatively infrequent, particularly in circumstances where diagnostic errors, procedural complications, and bad news need to be communicated. To more effectively develop proficiency, manage the stress associated with these circumstances, and further develop this core competency, the Program to Enhance Relational and Communication Skills has developed an experiential workshop. Radiology residents and other healthcare professionals learn to address difficult situations by practicing each scenario with actors trained in improvisation. The result was a significant increase in comfort with discussing radiation risks, delivering difficult diagnostic news, and communicating about medical errors. There are various templates available in the literature to help promote patient-centered communication and assist radiology trainees and radiologists alike with the disclosure of emotional or distressing results.

CONCLUSION

Effective delivery of care in a modern healthcare environment requires that patients be the central focus of our efforts. Although we have discussed the core considerations of this approach, opportunities to expand on these principles in radiology are vast and only partially explored here. We noted that clear benefits in patient outcomes have been demonstrated when patient care is redesigned to accommodate patient differences, address socioeconomic and cultural barriers, engage patients in their care, and anticipate patient needs. Each dimension of patient-centered care discussed here (patient values, preferences, and needs, coordination of care, communication and education, physical comfort, emotional support, and involvement of family and friends) serves as a guide to help focus future improvement efforts. Moreover, the changing healthcare landscape requires that radiologists define and measure the value of services provided, in which patient centeredness is essential. To demonstrate value, current assessment tools for patient centeredness will require a new framework to help us understand the patient's experience of illness and healthcare. Using this framework, radiology practices can be redesigned to better align with patients' needs and values. This approach will allow us to overcome the challenges facing radiology today and play a meaningful role in shaping the future of the specialty.

SUGGESTED READINGS

ACGME Program Requirements for Graduate Medical Education in Diagnostic Radiology: ACGME. <https://www.acgme.org/Portals/0/PDFs/Milestones/DiagnosticRadiologyMilestones.pdf>.

Alderson PO. Customer service and satisfaction in radiology. *AJR Am J Roentgenol*. 2000;175(2):319-323.

Baile WF, Buckman R, Lenzi R, Glober G, Beale EA, Kudelka AP. SPIKES—a six-step protocol for delivering bad news: application to the patient with cancer. *Oncologist*. 2000;5(4):302-311.

Baker DW, Hayes R, Fortier JP. Interpreter use and satisfaction with interpersonal aspects of care for Spanish-speaking patients. *Med Care*. 1998;36(10):1461-1470.

Baker DW, Parker RM, Williams MV, Coates WC, Pitkin K. Use and effectiveness of interpreters in an emergency department. *J Am Med Assoc*. 1996;275(10):783-788.

Barry MJ, Fowler Jr FJ, Mulley Jr AG, Henderson Jr JV, Wennberg JE. Patient reactions to a program designed to facilitate patient participation in treatment decisions for benign prostatic hyperplasia. *Med Care*. 1995;33(8):771-782.

Bazzocchi M. Doctor-patient communication in radiology: a great opportunity for future radiology. *Radiol Med*. 2012;117(3):339-353.

Beach M, Cooper L, Robinson K, et al. Strategies for improving minority healthcare quality Baltimore: agency for healthcare research and quality. <https://archive.ahrq.gov/downloads/pub/evidence/pdf/minqual/minqual.pdf>.

Berkman ND, Sheridan SL, Donahue KE, Halpern DJ, Crotty K. Low health literacy and health outcomes: an updated systematic review. *Ann Intern Med*. 2011;155(2):97-107.

Berlin L. Communicating results of all outpatient radiologic examinations directly to patients: the time has come. *AJR Am J Roentgenol*. 2009;192(3):571-573.

Bohachick P. Progressive relaxation training in cardiac rehabilitation: effect on psychologic variables. *Nurs Res*. 1984;33(5):283-287.

Brock DW. The ideal of shared decision making between physicians and patients. *Kennedy Inst Ethics J*. 1991;1(1):28-47.

Brown SD, Callahan MJ, Browning DM, et al. Radiology trainees' comfort with difficult conversations and attitudes about error disclosure: effect of a communication skills workshop. *J Am Coll Radiol*. 2014;11(8):781-787.

Carey MP, Burish TG. Providing relaxation training to cancer chemotherapy patients: a comparison of three delivery techniques. *J Consult Clin Psychol*. 1987;55(5):732-737.

Carrasquillo O, Orav EJ, Brennan TA, Burstin HR. Impact of language barriers on patient satisfaction in an emergency department. *J Gen Intern Med*. 1999;14(2):82-87.

Charles C, Gafni A, Whelan T. Decision-making in the physician-patient encounter: revisiting the shared treatment decision-making model. *Soc Sci Med*. 1999;49(5):651-661.

Cincinnati Children's Hospital Medical Center. Communicating Difficult News to Patients and Families. <http://cchmcstream.cchmc.org/MediasiteEX/Play/352006b8b86c44378c1f0bb9dca868301d>.

Cobb SC. Teaching relaxation techniques to cancer patients. *Cancer Nurs*. 1984;7(2):157-161.

Cohen FL. Postsurgical pain relief: patients' status and nurses' medication choices. *Pain*. 1980;9(2):265-274.

Cohen MD, Alam K. Radiology clinical synopsis: a simple solution for obtaining an adequate clinical history for the accurate reporting of imaging studies on patients in intensive care units. *Pediatr Radiol*. 2005;35(9):918-922.

Cotanch PH, Strom S. Progressive muscle relaxation as antiemetic therapy for cancer patients. *Oncol Nurs Forum*. 1987;14(1):33-37.

Crane JA. Patient comprehension of doctor-patient communication on discharge from the emergency department. *J Emerg Med*. 1997;15(1):1-7.

Deber RB, Kraetschmer N, Irvine J. What role do patients wish to play in treatment decision making? *Arch Intern Med*. 1996;156(13):1414-1420.

Devine EC, Cook TD. A meta-analytic analysis of effects of psychoeducational interventions on length of postsurgical hospital stay. *Nurs Res*. 1983;32(5):267-274.

Emanuel EJ, Emanuel LL. Four models of the physician-patient relationship. *J Am Med Assoc*. 1992;267(16):2221-2226.

Engebretson J, Mahoney J, Carlson ED. Cultural competence in the era of evidence-based practice. *J Prof Nurs*. 2008;24(3):172-178.

Entwistle V, Firnigl D, Ryan M, Francis J, Kinghorn P. Which experiences of health care delivery matter to service users and why? A critical interpretive synthesis and conceptual map. *J Health Serv Res Policy*. 2012;17(2):70-78.

Fagan MJ, Diaz JA, Reinert SE, Sciamanna CN, Fagan DM. Impact of interpretation method on clinic visit length. *J Gen Intern Med*. 2003;18(8):634-638.

Fast Company. Patient Centered Design: children's Hospital of Pittsburgh. <https://www.fastcompany.com/1351198/patient-centered-design-childrens-hospital-pittsburgh>.

Flores G, Laws MB, Mayo SJ, et al. Errors in medical interpretation and their potential clinical consequences in pediatric encounters. *Pediatrics*. 2003;111(1):6-14.

Gandhi TK, Burstin HR, Cook EF, et al. Drug complications in outpatients. *J Gen Intern Med*. 2000;15(3):149-154.

Gerteis M. *Picker/Commonwealth Program for Patient-Centered Care. Through the Patient's Eyes: Understanding and Promoting Patient-Centered Care*. San Francisco: Jossey-Bass; 1993.

Gunderman RB, Brown BP. Teaching interpersonal and communication skills. *Acad Radiol*. 2012;19(12):1589-1590.

Hammond I, Franche RL, Black DM, Gaudette S. The radiologist and the patient: breaking bad news. *Can Assoc Radiol J*. 1999;50(4):233-234.

Hoe JW. Service delivery and service quality in radiology. *J Am Coll Radiol*. 2007;4(9):643-651.

Iezzoni LI, O'Day BL, Killeen M, Harker H. Communicating about health care: observations from persons who are deaf or hard of hearing. *Ann Intern Med*. 2004;140(5):356-362.

Institute of Medicine (US). *Committee on Quality of Health Care in America. Crossing the quality chasm: a new health system for the 21st century*. Washington, DC: National Academy Press; 2001:337p.

Itri JN. Patient-centered radiology. *Radiographics*. 2015;35(6):1835-1846.

Jacobs E, Agger-Gupta N, Chen A, Piotrowski A, Hardt E. *Language Barriers in Health Care Setting: an Annotated Bibliography of the Research Literature*. Woodland Hills, CA: The California Endowment; 2003.

Johnson JE, Christman NJ, Stitt C. Personal control interventions: short- and long-term effects on surgical patients. *Res Nurs Health*. 1985;8(2):131-145.

Johnson JE, Leventhal H. Effects of accurate expectations and behavioral instructions on reactions during a noxious medical examination. *J Pers Soc Psychol*. 1974;29(5):710-718.

Johnson JE, Rice VH, Fuller SS, Endress MP. Sensory information, instruction in a coping strategy, and recovery from surgery. *Res Nurs Health*. 1978;1(1):4-17.

Ka'opua LS, Park SH, Ward ME, Braun KL. Testing the feasibility of a culturally tailored breast cancer screening intervention with Native Hawaiian women in rural churches. *Health Soc Work*. 2011;36(1):55-65.

Karliner LS, Jacobs EA, Chen AH, Mutha S. Do professional interpreters improve clinical care for patients with limited English proficiency? A systematic review of the literature. *Health Serv Res*. 2007;42(2):727-754.

Karliner LS, Kerlikowske K. Ethnic disparities in breast cancer. *Womens Health (Lond Engl)*. 2007;3(6):679-688.

Keeri-Szanto M, Heaman S. Postoperative demand analgesia. *Surg Gynecol Obstet*. 1972;134(4):647-651.

Kim JH, Menon U, Wang E, Szalacha L. Assess the effects of culturally relevant intervention on breast cancer knowledge, beliefs, and mammography use among Korean American women. *J Immigr Minor Health*. 2010;12(4):586-597.

Lawlis GF, Selby D, Hinnant D, McCoy CE. Reduction of postoperative pain parameters by presurgical relaxation instructions for spinal pain patients. *Spine (Phila PA 1976)*. 1985;10(7):649-651.

Lexa FJ, Berlin JW. The architecture of smart surveys: core issues in why and how to collect patient and referring physician satisfaction data. *J Am Coll Radiol*. 2009;6(2):106-111.

Lexa FJ. 300,000,000 customers: patient perspectives on service and quality. *J Am Coll Radiol*. 2006;3(5):346-350.

Liu S, Bassett LW, Sayre J. Women's attitudes about receiving mammographic results directly from radiologists. *Radiology*. 1994;193(3):783-786.

Loy CT, Irwig L. Accuracy of diagnostic tests read with and without clinical information: a systematic review. *J Am Med Assoc*. 2004;292(13):1602-1609.

Mansell D, Poses RM, Kazis L, Duefield CA. Clinical factors that influence patients' desire for participation in decisions about illness. *Arch Intern Med*. 2000;160(19):2991-2996.

Manson A. Language concordance as a determinant of patient compliance and emergency room use in patients with asthma. *Med Care*. 1988;26(12):1119-1128.

Marks RM, Sachar EJ. Undertreatment of medical inpatients with narcotic analgesics. *Ann Intern Med*. 1973;78(2):173-181.

Mathers SA, Chesson RA, Proctor JM, McKenzie GA, Robertson E. The use of patient-centered outcome measures in radiology: a systematic review. *Acad Radiol*. 2006;13(11):1394-1404.

McNeil BJ, Weichselbaum R, Pauker SG. Speech and survival: tradeoffs between quality and quantity of life in laryngeal cancer. *N Engl J Med*. 1981;305(17):982-987.

Mueller PR, Biswal S, Halpern EF, Kaufman JA, Lee MJ. Interventional radiologic procedures: patient anxiety, perception of pain, understanding of procedure, and satisfaction with medication—a prospective study. *Radiology*. 2000;215(3):684-688.

Mumford E, Schlesinger HJ, Glass GV. The effect of psychological intervention on recovery from surgery and heart attacks: an analysis of the literature. *Am J Public Health*. 1982;72(2):141-151.

Niazkhani Z, Pirnejad H, Berg M, Aarts J. The impact of computerized provider order entry systems on inpatient clinical workflow: a literature review. *J Am Med Inform Assoc*. 2009;16(4):539-549.

Novy DM, Price M, Huynh PT, Schuetz A. Percutaneous core biopsy of the breast: correlates of anxiety. *Acad Radiol*. 2001;8(6):467-472.

Ollivier L, Apiou F, Leclere J, et al. Patient experiences and preferences: development of practice guidelines in a cancer imaging department. *Cancer Imaging*. 2009;9:S92-S97.

Ollivier L, Leclere J, Dolbeault S, Neuenschwander S. Doctor-patient relationship in oncologic radiology. *Cancer Imaging*. 2005;5:S83-S88.

Prabhakar AM, Harvey HB, Platt JT, Brink JA, Oklu R. Engaging our patients: shared decision making and interventional radiology. *Radiology*. 2014;272(1):9-11.

Puntillo KA. Pain experiences of intensive care unit patients. *Heart Lung*. 1990;19(5 Pt 1):526-533.

Radner G. *It's Always Something. 20th Anniversary Ed*. New York, NY: Simon & Schuster; 2009.

Revicki DA, Yabroff KR, Shikiar R. Outcomes research in radiologic imaging: identification of barriers and potential solutions. *Acad Radiol*. 1999;6(suppl 1):S20-S28.

Reynolds A. Patient-centered care. *Radiol Technol*. 2009;81(2):133-147.

Robinson JC. The end of managed care. *J Am Med Assoc*. 2001;285(20):2622-2628.

Roter DL, Rudd RE, Comings J. Patient literacy. A barrier to quality of care. *J Gen Intern Med*. 1998;13(12):850-851.

Schreiber MH, Leonard Jr M, Rieniets CY. Disclosure of imaging findings to patients directly by radiologists: survey of patients' preferences. *AJR Am J Roentgenol*. 1995;165(2):467-469.

Shams-Avari P. Linguistic and cultural competency. *Radiol Technol*. 2005;76(6):437-445.

Sims MJ, Rilling WS. Psychosocial management of distress in interventional radiology patients with cancer. *Tech Vasc Interv Radiol*. 2006;9(3):101-105.

Stacey D, Legare F, Col NF, et al. Decision aids for people facing health treatment or screening decisions. *Cochrane Database Syst Rev*. 2014;1. CD001431.

Strull WM, Lo B, Charles G. Do patients want to participate in medical decision making? *J Am Med Assoc*. 1984;252(21):2990-2994.

US Health and Human Services. What Is Cultural Competency? <https://www.cdc.gov/nchhstp/socialdeterminants/docs/what_is_cultural_competency.pdf>.

US National Library of Medicine, National Institutes of Health. Health Literacy. <http://www.nlm.nih.gov/medlineplus/healthliteracy.html>.

Van den Bergh KA, Essink-Bot ML, Bunge EM, et al. Impact of computed tomography screening for lung cancer on participants in a randomized controlled trial (NELSON trial). *Cancer*. 2008;113(2):396-404.

Vranceanu AM, Cooper C, Ring D. Integrating patient values into evidence-based practice: effective communication for shared decision-making. *Hand Clin*. 2009;25(1):83-96, vii.

Vydareny KH, Amis Jr ES, Becker GJ, et al. Diagnostic radiology milestones. *J Grad Med Educ*. 2013;5(1 suppl 1):74-78.

Waitzkin H. Information giving in medical care. *J Health Soc Behav*. 1985;26(2):81-101.

Weis OF, Sriwatanakul K, Alloza JL, Weintraub M, Lasagna L. Attitudes of patients, housestaff, and nurses toward postoperative analgesic care. *Anesth Analg*. 1983;62(1):70-74.

Wikipedia. Soft Skills. <http://en.wikipedia.org/wiki/Soft_skills>.

Winkel GH, Holahan CJ. The environmental psychology of the hospital: is the cure worse than the illness? *Prev Hum Serv*. 1985;(4 1-2):11-33.

Zygmont ME, Lam DL, Nowitzki KM, et al. Opportunities for patient-centered outcomes research in radiology. *Acad Radiol*. 2016;23(1):8-17.

Chapter 12
Professionalism and Ethics

Jared Meshekow and David M. Paushter

PRINCIPLES OF MEDICAL PROFESSIONALISM AND THE PHYSICIAN CHARTER

As societal norms have transformed and continued to evolve, physicians and other clinicians have faced significant legal, moral, and ethical quandaries that have influenced the practice of medicine. Although the development of professionalism stems from the core tenets of ethics and medicine, coined by Aristotle and Hippocrates respectively, it has been codified most famously by the Institute of Medicine in its white papers, *To Err Is Human: Building a Better Healthcare System,* and *Crossing the Quality Chasm: A New Healthcare System for the 21st Century.*

With the increasing emphasis of professionalism in radiology during the past decade, associated with shifting patient expectations, there has been a joint effort by the American Board of Radiology (ABR), the American College of Radiology (ACR), and the Radiological Society of North America (RSNA) to train and educate radiologists on professionalism and ethics. To support this endeavor, the RSNA Professionalism Committee adopted the Physician Charter and presented it at the opening session of their annual meeting in 2006. As adopted by the RSNA, professionalism is the basis of medicine's contract with society. It places the welfare of the patient above that of the physician, sets and maintains standards of competency and integrity, and provides expert advice to society on matters of health. The Physician Charter (Box 12.1) outlines three principles of medical professionalism and denotes 10 professional responsibilities.

PHYSICIAN-PHYSICIAN AND PHYSICIAN-PATIENT INTERACTIONS

As members of a profession, physicians must work collectively to enhance patient care, maintain a level of mutual respect, and participate in the processes of self-regulation. This involves remediation and discipline of members who do not adhere to strict predefined educational and professional standards. Physicians have both individual and collective duties to partake in these processes, including internal assessment and accepting third-party scrutiny of performance. Both the referring physician and the radiologist must demonstrate mutual respect for one another as well as take shared responsibility for the patient's welfare. Furthermore, it is the radiologist's obligation to review and interpret imaging studies in a timely manner and recommend additional studies when appropriate, while taking the patient's history and clinical symptoms into account.

In terms of the physician-patient relationship, physicians incur the responsibility of caring for patients when they are most vulnerable. Consequently, certain physician-patient interactions should be avoided because they promote impropriety within the profession. Physicians should never exploit patients' trust for personal financial gain, sexual advantage, or other private gain. Additionally, physicians must maintain a high level of discretion by maintaining patient confidentiality when interpreting and reporting studies. Treating the patient as a healthcare partner includes detailed but clear informed consent, patient-centered decision making, and disclosure of medical errors and diagnoses should they arise (Box 12.2).

DEALING WITH UNPROFESSIONAL BEHAVIOR

Disruptive behavior leads to medical errors, increased cost of care, patient dissatisfaction, attrition of personnel, and is common in high-pressure, high-stakes environments. Abusive, unethical, or intolerant behavior must be dealt with quickly and decisively, without consequence to the complainant. However, because disruptive behavior varies in its manifestations, intensity, and frequency, a variety of resources are required to approach potential solutions. Oversight can range from informal discussion between peers to legal action in the courts. Many institutions have developed formal, structured pathways to deal with troublesome behavior, as defined in the medical staff bylaws, with committees focusing on the disruptive physician and the impaired physician. There is training available for those dealing with unprofessional behavior as an avocation, as well as others who may be involved in the remediation process. Examples of professionalism programs include Brigham and Women's Hospital, the University of Pennsylvania Health System, and Vanderbilt University School of Medicine.

It is often useful to emphasize episodic behavior rather than values when working with disruptive physicians, because it is less threatening, focuses on the *what* rather than the *why*, and therefore may prove easier to accept and improve. An initial episode of disruptive behavior can often be handled by peer-to-peer mentoring, or the *cup of coffee* approach, focusing on the incident, listening to potential causative issues, and providing advice. This does require follow-up to verify that the behavior has ceased and that the physician has gained capability in dealing with precipitating issues. Typical concerns that increase the likelihood of unacceptable behavior include life stressors such as a demanding workload, job insecurity, financial difficulty, and marital discord. Discrimination against others based upon gender, ethnicity, or religion as a basis for the behavior necessitates adherence to workplace requirements based on a *no tolerance* policy. Many institutions now have a Committee on Professionalism to assist

Principles of Medical Professionalism

PRINCIPLE OF PRIMACY OF PATIENT WELFARE

This principle is based on a dedication to serving the interests of the patient. Altruism contributes to the trust that is central to the physician-patient relationship. Market forces, societal pressures, and administrative exigencies must not compromise this principle.

PRINCIPLE OF PATIENT AUTONOMY

Physicians must have respect for patient autonomy. Physicians must be honest with their patients and empower them to make informed decisions about their treatment. Patients' decisions about their care must be paramount, as long as those decisions are in keeping with ethical practice and do not lead to demands for inappropriate care.

PRINCIPLE OF SOCIAL JUSTICE

The medical profession must promote justice in the healthcare system, including the fair distribution of healthcare resources. Physicians should work actively to eliminate discrimination in healthcare, whether based on race, gender, socioeconomic status, ethnicity, religion, or any other social category.

BOX 12.2 **Commitments of Medical Professionalism Outlined by the Physician Charter and Endorsed by RSNA**

1. Professional competence
2. Honesty with patients
3. Patient confidentiality
4. Maintenance of appropriate relations with patients
5. Improvement of quality of care
6. Improvement of access to care
7. Just distribution of finite resources
8. Scientific knowledge
9. Maintenance of trust by managing conflicts of interest
10. Maintenance of appropriate relations with other physicians and healthcare professionals
11. Sensitivity to patients of diverse backgrounds*

RSNA, Radiological Society of North America.
*Additional tenet added by the RSNA.

in the process of dealing with unprofessional behavior, including trained professionals to assist with assessment and recommendations. It is incumbent on physicians to report impaired or incompetent peers, to assure safety of patients, protect other staff, and provide assistance for the professional in question.

Unfortunately, the disruptive physician may display repetitive, deep-seated behavior that requires alternate approaches for remediation. For personality disorders, compulsory counseling may be required. This situation is best handled by a specialized committee that can recommend resources and receive general professional feedback on success. The Committee on Professionalism or a sister committee may be charged with overseeing the evaluation and recommendation processes as well as gauging success of therapy. For some physicians, underlying psychiatric issues or substance abuse may lead to aberrant behavior, and evaluation and therapy should be handled by trained professionals. There is typically a mandatory requirement for counseling and/or addiction therapy coupled with a medical leave of absence. There is no return to work until professional therapists involved in care provide a

professional opinion that this is an appropriate course of action. In these instances, long-term follow-up is required, even with an apparent successful outcome, because the *relapse* rate remains high. External, professional academic programs allow the distressed physician to receive evaluation and treatment in a supportive and tailored environment with full confidentiality.

The issue of how to handle physicians who display continuing disruptive behavior despite intervention is complex, with ramifications that may involve suspension or loss of medical staff privileges, mandatory reporting to the state licensing bureau, involvement of the Equal Opportunities Commission, or legal action. The Joint Commission requires hospitals to provide procedures for identifying and referring impaired physicians for evaluation and treatment, in addition to educating physicians and staff about physician health and impairment. The bylaws of the medical staff typically specify the processes for evaluation, potential remediation, suspension or revocation of privileges, and reporting to the state licensing bureau or law enforcement. In addition, the bylaws also detail the rights of the accused caregiver and due process procedures. Reporting requirements to state licensing bodies vary from state to state but in general include ethical or competence breaches that put patients or others at risk. Unfortunately, many state licensing boards provide little guidance on the subject, with requirements for individual reported physicians at times shrouded in mystery. However, as the topic of physician behavior continues to expand in the public and professional domains, there is an increasing trend to recommend avenues for evaluation and treatment, in addition to punitive action.

PERSONAL BEHAVIOR AND RELATIONSHIP WITH THE EMPLOYERS

The ideals of professionalism include the physician's personal behavior. Physicians are expected to follow the rules and regulations of their governing bodies. This dictates that radiologists must not partake in substance abuse, fraudulent billing, deceptive clinical coverage, and/or disruptive personal behavior. Participation in such activities and behaviors can translate into suboptimal patient care, including medical errors, and result in a hostile work environment. Physicians should adhere to strict moral and ethical boundaries when negotiating and subsequently complying with contractual obligations set forth by their employer. As radiologists as healthcare system employees continues to escalate, this has new meaning for many.

CONFLICT OF INTEREST AND RELATIONSHIPS WITH VENDORS

Vendor-physician relationships, although an important part of medical practice, can lead to ethical conflicts, which have the effect of diminishing primacy of the patient and can erode the physician-patient relationship. These conflicts exist when physicians or practices have a fiscal relationship with or financial interests in a public or private company. In the past 20 years, a Pandora's box of relationships among industry, researchers, and academic institutions has emerged, leading to the development of potential conflicts and competing interests. Because these relationships have not always been well managed by physicians, the government instituted the Sunshine Act in 2013, which requires increased physician-vendor transparency, including public reporting.

In general, physician relationships with vendors and industry have not been shown to have a quantifiable influence on the decision-making process with regard to patient care. Nonetheless, ongoing debate has advocated that physicians should take a more active role in addressing conflicts of interest, which have the potential to compromise professionalism. In radiology, formal training on conflict of interest is rarely addressed, leaving trainees to formulate their own ethical standards and patients with no understanding of industry influence on their care. To deter any suspicions, radiologists should maintain transparency regarding potential conflicts, with full disclosure of any underlying affiliations with industry.

ETHICS OF RESEARCH AND PUBLICATIONS

When conducting research, physicians must take into account the core components of research, including study design, execution, reporting, and critical evaluation. Each of these elements is not without inherent ethical issues, which can impact study results and therefore interpretation by readers.

To further the field, radiologists must adhere to the legal and ethical bases for responsible research. A codified ethical foundation for research was conceived by the Department of Health, Education, and Welfare (now the Department of Health and Human Services [HHS]) in 1979. The resultant publication, *Ethical Principles and Guidelines for the Protection of Human Subjects of Research*, also known as the Belmont Report, serves as an ethical basis and a foundation for federal regulations governing research with human participants. Grounded in basic ethical principles, research involving human subjects must comply with the core tenets of respect of persons, beneficence, and justice. Not only must we *do no harm*, we are also expected to actively protect patients with diminished autonomy and maximize potential patient benefits. The HHS has established the Office for Human Research Protection, which has produced multiple regulations on research, including institutional review board (IRB) membership and function, study review, informed consent, and use of federal funds. Sunshine laws also apply to research, specifying the structure relationships between industry and academia.

Researchers must also conform to regulations set forth by IRBs at individual institutions. Additionally, researchers must protect patient privacy by complying with the Health Insurance Portability and Accountability Act.

Research misconduct is another potential threat to the integrity of radiology research, which endangers the reputations of the individual institutions, the specialty, and medicine as a whole, and reduces public confidence. Types of research misconduct include the following:
- Fabrication of data
- Falsification of results
- Plagiarism
- Templating
- Authorship, with inclusion of authors who did not provide a substantial contribution

- *Shotgunning*, defined as submission to multiple journals at the same time
- *Salami slicing*, defined as dividing research results among multiple publications
- Redundant publications

ETHICS IN GRADUATE AND RESIDENT EDUCATION

Graduate and medical education should be held to the same standard as all other core components of medical professionalism. Efforts should be made by medical educators, in conjunction with professional associations, and specialty boards, to educate trainees and practitioners on all aspects of professionalism. Exposure to formal content on professionalism in residency stresses and reinforces training experience as a means of learning professional values and behaviors in addition to interpretive and procedural competency. Didactic material does not suffice, underscoring the importance of mentoring and role models. However, the educational environment produces an inherently unequal relationship between the trainee and preceptor, which has the potential to interfere with the development of mutual respect and fair play. All parties involved within the residency educational program should promote and adhere to a set of principles that afford the optimal training environment, including the following:
- Mutual educator-trainee respect
- Intellectual and academic freedom
- Appropriate power, responsibility, and interpersonal relationships
- Confidentiality
- Fairness and equity, including nondiscrimination, nonfavoritism, and equal opportunity

Additionally, the Accreditation Council for Graduate Medical Education and therefore the specialty boards, including the ABR, have long focused attention on the critical importance of professionalism in graduate medical education by requiring curricula to support development of these six core competencies:
- Patient care
- Medical knowledge
- Practice-based learning and improvement
- System-based practice
- Interpersonal and communication skills
- Professionalism

By integrating these strategies into residency education, medical faculties are able to incorporate these competencies and serve as role models. This offers seamless integration and endorsement among physicians in training, to be used in the lifelong practice of medicine.

SUMMARY

Professionalism and ethics are an integral part of medical practice and have undergone a transformation in the past 15 years. As highly visible and publicized topics, physicians have an obligation to adhere to their basic principles and a tandem responsibility to monitor and report, if needed, the behavior of their peers. Improving treatment methodology assists healthcare professionals in dealing with unprofessional behavior in a logical and sympathetic manner, to maximize the likelihood of a positive outcome for the physician while protecting the patient and other employees. Principles of ethics and professionalism must be introduced early in the process of physician education and reinforced by role models by their behavior as well as didactic instruction.

SUGGESTED READINGS

2005 RSNA Professionalism Committee. Medical professionalism in the new millennium: a physicians' charter. *Radiology*. 2006;288:383-386.

ABIM Foundation. American Board of Internal Medicine, ACP-ASIM Foundation. American College of Physicians-American Society of Internal Medicine, European Federation of Internal Medicine. Medical professionalism in the new millennium: a physician charter. *Ann Intern Med*. 2002;136(3):243-246.

Accreditation Council for Graduate Medical Education. Common program requirements. <http://acgme.org/>.

Agrawal S, Brennan N, Budetti P. The sunshine act—effects on physician. *N Engl J Med*. 2013;368:2054-2057.

Barron BJ, Kim EE. Ethical dilemmas in today's nuclear medicine and radiology. *J Nucl Med*. 2003;44:1818-1823.

Behaviors that undermine a culture of safety. The Joint Commission. *Sentinel Event Alert*. 2008;40:1-3.

Bekelman JE, Li Y, Gross CP. Scope and impact of financial conflicts of interest: a systematic review. *J Am Med Assoc*. 2003;289(4):454-465.

Butler GJ. Keeping professionalism alive in radiology's new age: a choice—our future. *J Am Coll Radiol*. 2009;6:100-102.

Campbell EG, Weismann J, Ehringhaus S. Institutional academic industry relationships. *J Am Med Assoc*. 2007;298(15):1779-1786.

Cooper J. Responsible conduct of radiology research part I. Framework for human research. *Radiology*. 2005;236(2):379-381.

Cruess RL, Cruess SR. Expectations and obligations: professionalism and medicine's social contract with society. *Perspect Biol Med*. 2008;51:579-598.

Deitte L. The new residency curriculum: professionalism, patient safety, and more. *J Am Coll Radiol*. 2013;10(8):613-617.

Gilbert F, Denison A. Research misconduct. *Clin Radiol*. 2003;58:499-504.

Gunderman R. Fraud and abuse in radiology: perils and professionalism. <https://www.audioeducator.com/radiology/fraud-abuse-radiology-07-17-14.html>.

Halpern EJ, Spandorfer JM. Professionalism in radiology: ideals and challenges. *AJR Am J Roentgenol*. 2014;202(2):352-357.

Hendee W, Bosma JL, Bresolin LB, Berlin L, Bryan RN, Gunderman RB. Web modules on professionalism and ethics. *J Am Coll Radiol*. 2012;9:170-173.

Hickson GB, Pichert JW, Webb LE, Gabbe SG. A complementary approach to promoting professionalism: identifying, measuring, and addressing unprofessional behaviors. *Acad Med*. 2007;82(11):1040-1048.

Hryhorszuk A, Hanneman K, Eisenberg R, Meyer E, Brown S. Radiologic professionalism in modern health care. *Radiographics*. 2015;35:1779-1788.

Institute of Medicine (US) Committee on Quality of Health Care in America; Kohn LT, Corrigan JM, Donaldson MS, eds. *To Err Is Human: Building a Safer Health System*. Washington, (DC): Committee on Quality of Health Care in America, Institute of Medicine, National Academies Press (US); 2000.

Janower M. Ethics training for radiology residents. *AJR Am J Roentgenol*. 2005;184:701.

Office of the Secretary. *The Belmont report: ethical principles and guidelines for the protection of human subjects of research*. Department of Health and Human Services, Offices for Human Research Protections (OHRP); 1979.

Raymond J, Trop I. The practice of ethics in the era of evidence based radiology. *Radiology*. 2007;244(3):643-649.

Saxton R, Hines T, Enriquez M. The negative impact of nurse-physician disruptive behavior on patient safety: a review of the literature. *J Patient Saf*. 2009;5(3):180-183.

Shapiro J, Whittemore A, Tsen LC. Instituting a culture of professionalism: the establishment of a center for professionalism and peer support. *Jt Comm J Qual Patient Saf*. 2014;40(4):168-177.

Spandorfer J, Pohl CA, Rattner SL, Nasca TJ. *Professionalism in Medicine: A Case-Based Guide for Medical Students*. New York, NY: Cambridge University Press, 2010:7-21.

Speck RM, Foster JJ, Mulhern VA, Burke SV, Sullivan PG, Fleisher LA. Development of a professionalism committee approach to address unprofessional medical staff behavior at an academic medical center. *Jt Comm J Qual Patient Saf*. 2014;40(4):161-167.

Wynia MK. The role of professionalism and self-regulation in detecting impaired or incompetent physicians. *J Am Med Assoc*. 2010;304(2):210-212.

Chapter 13

Communication

James E. Kovacs

INTRODUCTION

Radiology reports are instrumental in decisions about patient management in most medical specialties. Clear communication requires written reports to be accurate, concise, and unambiguous. Constructing a quality report constitutes a critical, although often neglected, component of radiologists' training and practice. Four key areas of communications in radiology are reviewed in this chapter. The first section discusses communications between radiologists and both referring providers and patients. The second section presents various arguments for the best structure of the radiology report. The third section examines variation in reporting, and the final section provides an overview of systems for radiologist decision support.

REFERRING HEALTHCARE PROVIDERS AND PATIENTS

Direct Reporting to Patients and Patient Portals

The written radiology report has largely been a private communication between the radiologist and the referring physician. Although patients have never been legally denied access to their medical records, barriers to their access have been constructed, whether for fear of delivering records into the hands of a plaintiff's attorneys, over concerns that patients will find errors or admissions of uncertainty in reports and lose confidence in radiologists, or for fear it will start to shift the lopsided balance of the physician-patient relationship away from the physician. Until the passage of the Health Insurance Portability and Accountability Act (HIPAA) of 1996, which explicitly guarantees patients the right to their own health information, little consideration was given to increasing transparency in reporting. Since then, it has become progressively more common for radiologists to communicate results of diagnostic imaging examinations directly to patients. This trend has been fueled by a number of factors, including a national healthcare organization initiative (The Joint Commission National Safety Goals), various judicial rulings, professional society guidelines (American College of Radiology Practice Parameter for Communication of Diagnostic Imaging Findings [ACR PPCDIF]), the modish philosophy of patient-centered care, consumerism, and *entrepreneurial* radiology practice. Perhaps the most important driver of the trend toward direct reporting is the Mammography Quality Standards Act (MQSA), a federal mandate passed on October 27, 1992, as a result of efforts to encourage greater access to quality mammography. A provision therein mandates that "a summary of the written report shall be sent directly to the patient in terms easily understood by a lay person." Furthermore, "facilities must provide a summary of the results of the mammographic examination written in lay terms to all patients within 30 days." Although MQSA is perhaps the most significant legal mechanism enshrining the practice of greater transparency in radiology, the most significant practical tool has been patient use of online portals, which are electronic applications managed by healthcare providers that give patients access to their medical records through the Internet. The development and spread of online portals can be traced to advances in information technology and to initiatives such as patient-centered care, which encourage patients to more actively engage in their own healthcare decisions. The Joint Commission explicitly encourages patients to participate actively in their own healthcare through patient portals and has accordingly required hospitals to encourage patients to use them; to this end, in order to be in compliance with federal mandates for meaningful use of the electronic health records (EHRs), hospitals must prove that a minimum of 5% of their patients are using web-based access to their medical records. Although some critics of online patient portals have suggested that their use will prompt a greater number of phone calls directly to radiologists to discuss findings in their reports, early experience has not shown this to be the case.

Although advances in information technology, illustrated by the proliferation of web portals, is partly responsible for improvements in communications between radiologists and patients, a synergism of multiple external forces has driven radiology departments in recent years to improve the quality of their services. Although clinicians have long valued clarity, pertinence, and brevity in the written radiology report, new technologies in electronic data transmission have created an expectation of prompt reporting of findings. In this vein, ACR PPCDIF section I states that "quality patient care can only be achieved when study results are conveyed in a timely fashion to those responsible for treatment decisions." Especially at clinics at tertiary care centers to which many patients travel long distances for their appointments, it has become a common practice for patients to schedule their clinic appointments with their doctors within hours of their imaging examinations, thus placing greater pressure on the radiologist to communicate findings immediately.

Just as electronic data transmission has fueled tougher, if not qualitatively better, standards for timeliness of reporting, the quality of the radiology report has also come under greater scrutiny through increased patient access to reports via web-based portals. Studies show that patients are more critical than physicians of typographical errors, grammatical errors, sensitive topics, word selection, clarity, and overall organization. Inconsistencies such as right/left transposition and oversights such as failing to amend the default macro are common pitfalls, and while another physician who better understands the context of such errors might easily forgive them, these sorts of mistakes can be viewed by a patient as careless. A patient who sees an error-laden and disorganized report may lose confidence in the radiologist or even in the institution. The inevitable extrapolation that a sloppy report is the product of a harried, detached specialist understandably undermines confidence in the radiologist's work. Accordingly, serious medicolegal liability can result from patients' access to reports that contain such inaccuracies; plaintiff's attorneys may exploit a report with uncorrected errors and inconsistencies to portray the radiologist as inattentive and uncaring. The heightened expectations of quality incurred by greater transparency in reporting must be balanced against demands for greater productivity.

Although the legal implications of greater transparency deserve serious consideration, initial concerns that increased patient access to reports would increase the frequency of malpractice suits by effectively handing over a "blank check" to the trial lawyers has not translated into higher legal costs for most institutions. Acceptance of accountability, in fact, appears to mitigate patients' negative feelings. In 2001, the University of Michigan Health System (UMHS) adopted transparency and disclosure as its comprehensive claims management model, offering patients "the facts, a sincere apology, a commitment to prevent the error from recurring, and fair compensation" for harmful medical errors. The UMHS experience with error disclosure and transparency with patients and their families showed a decrease in the number of filed lawsuits, decreased time from claim to resolution, lower costs of compensation, and a reduction in legal costs. However, there is perhaps no stronger argument for reporting results of all radiologic examinations directly to patients than the byproduct of MQSA. Since the passage of the act, lawsuits alleging delay in communication of significant findings on mammography have been virtually eliminated.

The traditional method of communication of test results to the patient, which is for the referring physician to call or speak in person with the patient, is still preferred by most patients. In addition to understanding patients' preferences of how and which physicians relay examination results, it is important to consider how physicians might interact with patients and which physicians are most qualified to do so. To this end, the Radiological Society of North America (RSNA) campaign Radiology Cares promotes patient-centered culture within a radiology practice by assisting radiologists in becoming more comfortable with interacting with patients. However, even if radiologists were to receive training to minimize their discomfort in discussing results with patients, systems do not currently exist to accommodate this change in the workflow. Besides the overwhelming operational complexities of systematizing radiologist-patient interactions, any theoretical benefits could scarcely justify the expense incurred by loss of radiologist manpower. A radiologist's breadth of training would need to expand considerably to ensure he or she was qualified to answer any questions a patient might ask about the management of a problem uncovered by the radiologic exam. Furthermore, radiologists would, in addition to producing the written radiology report, also need to document what advice they rendered, which would incur both

a significant time drain and additional legal implications. Besides these logistical complications, serious underlying ethical questions arise when considering whether to more systematically integrate the radiologist into the patient experience. In other words, the gradual shift toward the practice of unrestricted and immediate patient access to radiology reports through portals raises the question of to whom the report is, and should be, directed: the patient, the referring physician, or the medicolegal record.

Although one might look to MQSA for guidance on this issue, the precedent of directly reporting results of screening mammography to patients is not analogous, because MQSA was a federal mandate and not a unilateral move by the radiology community to encroach upon the domain of the referring physician. A few progressive radiology practices have taken the step of giving patients preliminary results of their examinations on site before they leave the imaging center. A few groups who do provide this service give the patient the option to receive preliminary results. Referring physicians who request that the patient not be given preliminary results on site may do so for a variety of reasons. Many referring physicians maintain that it is their privilege and duty to relay results to their patients; a few do it for disingenuous financial purposes, but many do so because they believe their knowledge of the patient's problems, health history, and other ancillary studies best qualifies them to discuss the findings. Another criticism that referring physicians have of direct reporting by radiologists is that the patient may call the office to discuss the radiologic examination findings before the referring physician has even received the report. A simple solution to prevent the patient from viewing the results of his or her examination before the referring physician has had a chance to read the report is to impose an embargo of several days before the patient can gain access. The exception to this is mammography results (which the radiologist is legally bound to provide to the patient within a specific time frame). Furthermore, the complexity of the examination can tip the balance on the question of who is best qualified to explain the results to the patient. In either case, the medical professional must strike a balance between creating unneeded patient anxiety over observations that are likely to be incidental, benign, or of no clinical significance and alerting the patient of the need for follow-up on a finding that has a small risk of being a cancer. Adherence to guidelines published in the ACR white papers on incidental findings on computed tomography (CT) and following the guidance provided through clinical decision support (CDS) offer some degree of medicolegal protection on this front.

Although diagnostic imaging examinations are usually ordered by physicians or other healthcare providers with the expectation that the examination will answer a clinical question, issues with direct reporting also arise when patients are self-referred or referred by a third party, such as by a prospective employer or an insurer. In these cases, a direct communication between the radiologist and patient is necessary; on this point, the ACR PPCDIF states,

Interpreting physicians should recognize that performing imaging studies on self-referred patients establishes a doctor-patient relationship that includes responsibility for communicating the results of imaging studies directly to the patient and arranging for appropriate follow-up.

Although sometimes the pretest probability of a serious disorder is low, and the examination is ordered only with the intent to reassure the patient that a serious medical condition does not exist, the ACR PPCDIF says,

Regardless of the source of the referral, the interpreting physician has an ethical responsibility to ensure communication of unexpected or serious findings to the patient. Therefore, in certain situations the interpreting physician may feel it is appropriate to communicate the findings directly to the patient.

Nonroutine Communication

Although direct reporting and patient portals deal with more routine communications between radiologists and patients, there are circumstances in which the duty of the radiologist extends beyond interpretation, dictation, and signature of the final report. Findings on medical imaging examinations that demand immediate medical attention place moral and legal obligations on the radiologist to make direct contact with a patient. The ACR PPCDIF states that the following situations may warrant nonroutine communication:

1. *Findings that suggest a need for immediate or urgent intervention. Generally, these cases may occur in the emergency and surgical departments or critical care units and may include such findings as pneumothorax, pneumoperitoneum, or a significantly misplaced line or tube. Other urgent conditions typically included in "critical values" categories in most healthcare institutions would also be included in this group.*

2. *Findings that are discrepant with a preceding interpretation of the same examination and where failure to act may adversely affect patient health. These cases may occur when the final interpretation is discrepant with a preliminary report or when significant discrepancies are encountered upon subsequent review of a study after a final report has been submitted.*

3. *Findings that the interpreting physician reasonably believes may be seriously adverse to the patient's health and may not require immediate attention but, if not acted on, may worsen over time and possibly result in an adverse patient outcome. For example, acute infectious processes, possible malignant lesions, or other unexpected findings that may impact patient care if not treated in a timely fashion would fall into this category. This may be particularly applicable when there is a potential break in the continuity of care (such as can occur in emergency department encounters or the outpatient setting) that is unexpected by the treating or referring physician.*

In situations where nonroutine communication is necessary, logistical obstacles often arise. Berlin noted that contacting the referring physician concerning urgent or unexpected findings is not always possible; offices may be closed by the time the study is interpreted; phone calls are answered by an answering machine; the patient may receive medical care from more than one physician or at a clinic with rotating physicians or physician extenders; or the name of the ordering physician may not be listed. Although they demand greater

time and effort, in these instances it is appropriate for the radiologist to disclose the results of the examination directly to the patient. This duty to disclose has since been reiterated in revisions of the ACR Practice Parameter for Communication, and adherence to these guidelines reduces the chance of malpractice litigation and reinforces quality medical care. The ACR and judicial rulings clearly indicate that it is incumbent upon radiologists to relay significant findings to referring physicians, and this duty has been increasingly extended to include a duty to inform patients as well.

In addition to nonroutine and direct communication with patients, communications that are not part of the final report but are important for medical and legal purposes may be documented by way of digital "sticky notes." Examples include preliminary reports by residents; documentation of communication of emergent findings in emergency department, trauma, or critical care patients before the examination is viewed in its entirety and a final report submitted; two-way communication with technologists; flagging cases for performance improvement and quality measures; and posting memos to radiologist associates that supplemental information pertinent to the case is available.

Informal Communication

Radiologists' work does not just involve cases in which the radiologist is officially consulted. In fact, radiologists are commonly asked by their nonradiologist colleagues to render curbside consults, which often take the form of an outside examination that is rendered for unofficial review; in these cases, the examination technique and quality are not controlled by the consulted radiologist; the viewing conditions may be less than optimal; and the clinical information may be incomplete. Many practices do not have a mechanism for the radiologist to document the communication from these encounters, and consequently these situations are replete with (legal) traps for the radiologist. The ACR Practice Parameter II.C.3. states,

Informal communications carry inherent risk, and frequently the ordering physician's/health care provider's documentation of the informal consultation may be the only written record of the communication. Interpreting physicians who provide consultations of this nature in the spirit of improving patient care are encouraged to document those interpretations. A system for reporting outside studies is encouraged.

Commercial vendors have developed systems to archive data from varied sources and integrate these studies with the institution's picture archiving and communication system (PACS). With a system in place, reports can be generated, accurate and timely communication can be documented for optimal patient care and for legal protection, and codes can be applied for billing of second-read consultations.

Costs of Poor Communication

Lack of effective communication, whether formal or nonroutine, can have serious consequences in both human and financial terms. Data on the medical implications of poor communication has been collected by the Joint Commission, a not-for-profit organization founded in 1951 that evaluates, inspects, and accredits healthcare organizations in the United States. Since 2002, the organization has published an annual list of National Patient Safety Goals, and improvement in communication among caregivers has been on the list every year. Communication is the primary root cause of serious injury or death related to a delay in treatment; the second largest contributor to sentinel events arising from op/postop complications, transfer-related events, unintended retention of foreign objects, and wrong-site, wrong-patient, wrong-procedure incidents; and the third leading root cause overall. Aside from the material harm to the patient, the financial costs of poor communications can also be significant as a result of prolonged length of hospital stays, more expensive and/or prolonged care, lower reimbursement, lower patient satisfaction scores, and damaged institutional reputation. Inefficiencies in communication waste an estimated $12 billion a year, according to Agarwal, and increased length of stay accounted for more than 50% of that amount.

The Physicians Insurers Association of America, an association of physician- and dentist-owned or operated medical malpractice liability insurance companies, has also collected information on the legal implications of poor communications in radiology. In a survey of its 56 member companies in 1997, in which it collected data on more than 150,000 claims, communications errors were the fourth most frequent primary complaint against radiologists. In 10% of claims, the radiologist failed to send the report to the appropriate physician or patient, and in another 10% the delivery of the report was delayed and "directly affected the outcome of the case 75% of the time." However, the most significant breakdown in communication in almost 60% of the claims occurred when the radiologist did not notify the appropriate referring physician of "urgent or significant unexpected findings." The Healthcare Information and Management Systems Society (HIMSS) reported that in 2009, 75% of malpractice cases at Yale-New Haven Medical Center are communication related. These statistics underscore the serious moral, legal, and financial imperatives of efficient formal and informal communications.

Key Steps in Communication

A helpful framework for considering an effective communication process in radiology is critical to quality care. Thomas H. Berquist, editor-in-chief of the *American Journal of Radiology* in 2009, described four major steps in the process of communication:
1. The first step pertains to the appropriate imaging examination to answer the clinical question posed by the ordering physician. Appropriateness criteria based on evidence should be readily available to the referring physician when selecting the optimal imaging examination, but the choice of exam or technique of the examination may be modified by pertinent clinical information that may not have been provided to the radiologist.
2. Berquist's second step in good communication pertains to "a shared responsibility among the referring physician, patient, and radiologist to be certain the

patient understands the examination and any potential risks." Situations in which a patient refuses a scheduled examination because the risk of the examination was not explained in advance, or in which the patient could not undergo the examination because he or she was not adequately informed of the necessary preparation for the examination, can largely be avoided.
3. The third step involves effective communication between the radiologist and technologist to ensure that the correct views, imaging planes, or sequences are obtained to maximize the likelihood that the examination will be of good diagnostic quality.
4. Berquist's fourth step to good communication provides for alternatives to routine communication in cases where a delay can result in inappropriate, ineffective, or delayed treatment of significant findings. As telephone contact is not always successful, radiologists must use alternative methods to make contact and document confirmation that a responsible healthcare provider has received a report of the findings.

Critical Test Results Management

Critical test results management (CTRM) is an area in which closed-loop communication has become essential. Critical results include findings such as pneumoperitoneum, pneumothorax, and a significantly misplaced tube, which are findings from tests and diagnostic procedures that fall significantly outside the normal range and may indicate life-threatening situations. The radiologist's objective, therefore, is to provide the designated caregiver with the test results within a specific window of time so that the patient can begin treatment. Underscoring the particular importance of swift and accurate communication in relaying these findings to the appropriate individuals, The Joint Commission (an accreditation organization) and the American College of Radiology (ACR) have developed guidelines for communication of these time-sensitive findings. The Joint Commission requires hospitals to implement procedures for reporting critical results and evaluating the effectiveness of the procedures, although definitions of critical results and the acceptable length of time for a report to reach an actionable provider are left to each healthcare institution. There are no national standards for reporting time of critical results, and the definition of a *critical result* remains the discretion of each institution. One method adopted by some institutions to stratify abnormal findings is to color-code alerts, analogous to the Department of Homeland Security threat levels. Red alert signifies an immediate life-threatening condition, requiring notification of a caregiver within 60 minutes. Orange alert applies to conditions that, if not treated urgently, may increase morbidity and mortality, for example, acute diverticulitis. A yellow alert designation applies to conditions that do not require urgent attention or action but may lead to increased morbidity/mortality, such as a small pulmonary nodule. Recognizing the labor-intensive process of finding an actionable individual and its negative impact on radiologist productivity, vendors have developed automated solutions to CTRM. Current communication methods such as landline telephone, mobile telephone, fax, email, text messaging, and instant messaging have increased the options for communication, but none guarantee that the message has been received and understood by the intended individual.

The ACR's *IT Reference Guide for the Practicing Radiologist* states the following:

> *It is important for each participant in patient care to know that information sent has been successfully received and understood by the intended recipient. This is called "closed-loop communication" because the information is first sent out on one leg of a hypothetical loop to its intended recipient, and then a message returns back to the originator, confirming that the information was received.*
>
> *Confirmation of receipt and understanding is easy when communication is synchronous (i.e., both participants involved in the communication physically participate in the activity at the same time via telephone, online meeting, etc.), but when communication is asynchronous (e.g., e-mail) and separates participants in space and time, confirmation of successful communication may be more difficult. Additionally, permanent documentation of successful and timely communication is often critical for medicolegal and quality assurance activities, despite the challenges of asynchronous communication.*

CTRM solutions use advanced technologies to streamline communication between parties and document verification of receipt of critical test results (CTRs). Berlin strongly cautions that:

> *Once a radiologist decides that a finding needs a telephone report, he or she must continue efforts to reach the referring physician or an acceptable alternate to complete the communication. Terminating attempts at communication because the referring physician is not easily available…places the radiologist in greater medical and legal jeopardy than not having attempted to telephone in the first place.*

Escalation tools built into automated systems bypass the inefficient process of humans trying to contact the clinician by alternative methods or finding an alternate clinician responsible for the patient's care. Automating the process of closed-loop communication has many benefits: improved patient safety, savings of time and resources, and more precise documentation. Messages are tracked and stored in compliance with ACR PPCDIF II.C.2.c, which recommends that:

> *…non-routine communications be handled in a manner most likely to reach the attention of the treating or ordering physician/health care provider in time to provide the most benefit to the patient. …There are other forms of communication that provide documentation of receipt that may also suffice to demonstrate that the communication has been delivered and acknowledged.*

Automated closed-loop systems, which document confirmation that the message was received, ensure compliance with Joint Commission and ACR guidelines for communication of CTRs, thus lowering the risk of liability. Time stamps on communications facilitate monitoring of organizational compliance and quality performance.

American College of Radiology Practice Parameter for Communication

Guidelines for the components of the report and principles of reporting were first published by the ACR in 1991 in the publication ACR Standard for Communication: diagnostic radiology. The standard was revised in 1995, 1999, and 2001. The title was changed in 2005 when "Standard" was replaced by "Guideline." Additional revisions were made in 2010 and 2014. The guidelines are prefaced by the following paragraph cautioning its application as a standard of care, particularly in the context of legal defense:

> *This document is an educational tool designed to assist practitioners in providing appropriate radiologic care for patients. Practice Parameters and Technical Standards are not inflexible rules or requirements of practice and are not intended, nor should they be used, to establish a legal standard of care. For these reasons and those set forth below, the American College of Radiology and our collaborating medical specialty societies caution against the use of these documents in litigation in which the clinical decisions of a practitioner are called into question. The ultimate judgment regarding the propriety of any specific procedure or course of action must be made by the practitioner in light of all the circumstances presented. Thus, an approach that differs from the guidance in this document, standing alone, does not necessarily imply that the approach was below the standard of care. To the contrary, a conscientious practitioner may responsibly adopt a course of action different from that set forth in this document when, in the reasonable judgment of the practitioner, such course of action is indicated by the condition of the patient, limitations of available resources, or advances in knowledge or technology subsequent to publication of this document. However, a practitioner who employs an approach substantially different from the guidance in this document is advised to document in the patient record information sufficient to explain the approach taken.*

Irrespective of this cautionary language by the ACR, Berlin surmises that "the ACR standards are perceived by the legal community as a codification of the radiologic standard care as practiced throughout the United States." Conjecture on the impact of the ACR Standard for Communication: Diagnostic Radiology in a law review article in 2002 forewarned:

> *The purpose of the ACR Standards may be advisory, and may not include defining a legal standard of care; however, it would be naïve to believe that practice standards will not creep into medico-legal litigation as evidence of the applicable standard of care. It is difficult to predict an explosion of medical negligence actions against radiologists based on lack of urgent communication, but it is reasonable to suspect an increase in the incidence of this type of claim. The ACR Standards will likely be recognized as evidence of the standard of care, despite the disclaimer contained in the standard. …A jury might consider the ACR Standards tantamount to the standard of care. …This truly places radiologists in peril.*

STRUCTURED REPORTING

The main, and often the only, method of communication between the radiologist and the referring physician is the written report, which is the most tangible work product of radiologists' intellectual labor. Although prose has been the mainstay of reporting style since the beginning of radiology, great variation exists, with no rules or consensus on style or content. This form has been increasingly criticized for its lack of organization. This section reviews different formats of the radiology report.

Format of the Radiology Report

Radiology reports are formatted in one of two basic ways: prose (free text, narrative) or structured (tabular). Although prose is the predominant style, surveys of referring physicians report only a moderate level of satisfaction with this form of report. In a United Kingdom survey of general practitioners (COVER-GP) and hospital clinical specialists (COVER-SP), radiology reports were given scores of 7.8 (out of 10) for clarity by generalists and 6.7 for clarity by specialists. When asked whether they preferred free-text or itemized (structured) reports, clinicians strongly favored itemized reports (84%). These results have been mirrored by other surveys of referring providers and radiologists that indicate structured reports are favored over the prose (free-text) report format. The advantages of structured reports are numerous, including completeness, organization, fewer inconsistencies, and a tendency toward standardized lexicon. Organization into searchable fields facilitates data mining more easily than from prose reports, both by humans and by information systems, especially when standardized language is used. Information can be searched and retrieved by information systems for research, outcome, coding and billing, performance monitoring, quality improvement, and other operational purposes. Through additional data collection, individual and group practice parameters, including documentation of service for billing, throughput, and report turnaround time, can be monitored.

The European Society of Radiology (ESR) published its consensus opinion of what constitutes a *good* report in "Good practice for radiological reporting: guidelines from the European Society of Radiology." It expressed a clear preference for structured reports over free text in those guidelines:

> *Conventional radiology reports are stored as free text, so information is trapped in the language of the report, making it difficult to find specific details without reading the whole text. In structured reporting (SR), the information is standardised and presented in a clear, organised format, tracking the attributes of each finding (size, location, etc.) and prompting the radiologist to complete all required fields. It has been suggested that SR is more time-efficient than dictation, facilitates automated billing and order entry, and supports analysis for research and decision-support.*

The Royal Australian and New Zealand College of Radiology (RANZCR) drafted The Radiology Written Report Guideline Project in 2010. Although it did not endorse a particular report structure, it did recommend consistent ordering of the following broad categories: clinical referral, technique, findings, conclusions, and advice.

Several statements promoting the development and use of structured reporting have been issued the RSNA:

> *The Radiological Society of North America (RSNA) has sought to advance the concept of structured radiology reporting as a means of providing consistent, organized, and clear communication of radiologic results. The Reporting Subcommittee, which reports to the RSNA Radiology Informatics Committee, was created in 2008 to develop and promote the use of high-quality structured reporting throughout radiology.*
>
> *The clinical report is an essential part of the service that we provide to our patients. The report communicates information to referring physicians, records information for future use, and serves as the legal record that documents the episode of care. Ideally, the radiology report should be consistent, comprehensive, easily managed, and "readable" to humans and machines alike.*
>
> *The RSNA reporting initiative is improving radiology practice by creating a library of clear and consistent report templates. These templates make it possible to integrate evidence collected during the imaging procedure, including clinical data, coded terminology, technical parameters, measurements, annotations and key images.*
>
> *For researchers, these report templates capture information in a uniform, easily extracted format that facilitates clinical, translational and health services research. Educators find these templates can help trainees learn the important elements of reports in each subspecialty area and encourage the proper use of radiology terms, such as those found in RadLex.*

Examinations in which there is a high percentage of normal results, such as screening examinations, are most suited to structured reporting. A report is generated by simply accepting a template, which requires no amendments and no filling in of blank fields. A template, which can be defined as "a document with a preset structure, used as a starting point for a Report Creator, so that the structure does not have to be recreated each time it is used," can facilitate the capture of coded and/or quantitative information from imaging studies for transmission into patient registries. In trauma imaging or interventional radiology, for example, structured data from clinical radiology reports could support the development of local or national radiology results databases. Reporting templates can include features to help radiologists achieve quality benchmarks in their practices by making it easier for automated systems to summarize results.

Macros can be defined as any text or data stored and inserted by user command. The terms *macro* and *template* are often used interchangeably. Sometimes, template refers to a macro with blank spaces to be filled in by the user. A macro can consist of an entire report, a commonly used sentence or phrase, or even a problem word that is poorly recognized.

A white paper released by Integrating the Healthcare Enterprise (IHE) describes the modes typically used by radiologists in report creation:

> 1. *Text mode: In a purely text mode, the radiologist begins with a blank page, and creates the text of the report through automated speech recognition, or by typing and formatting the report narrative manually.*
>
> 2. *Fill in the blanks: Many radiologists start by applying a template that contains the overall structure of the entire report (e.g., by speaking "macro CT Abdomen*

normal"). Blanks within that template can be filled with customized text related to the study at hand. Because a template is used, the resulting report has a consistent ordering of report content.

3. *Serial assembly. Some radiologists use a large set of small templates, each containing only a small phrase or sentence related to the report (e.g., "macro atelectasis,""macro heart normal,""macro central line"). These small templates generally do not contain blanks that need to be filled in, and are assembled in series to create an entire report.*

4. *Nested or hybrid assembly. Radiologists who are "power users" of reporting systems often assemble their reports using a combination of fill-in-the-blanks and serial assembly. For example, they may begin with an overall template containing blanks and then fill in using serial assembly of smaller templates.*

An editorial by Winter responding to the article "Is structured reporting the answer?" by Gunderman urged caution in implementing structured reporting more broadly. He suggested that the benefits of structured reporting in disciplines of narrow domains such as mammography may not be achieved in other fields, such as in chest radiography, because "there is simply too much anatomy, and the range of pathologic processes is almost as wide as medicine itself. This situation is magnified even further in abdominal CT, which includes at least portions of most anatomic and physiologic systems."

Schwartz et al. posited that radiology may be slower in adopting structured reporting than other specialties because of the "limited nature of certain diseases" in certain specialties. Langlotz noted that structured reporting is "most widely accepted in breast imaging, cardiology and gastroenterology—disciplines that pertain to a limited anatomic area and a restricted set of diseases for which manageable template sets and straightforward user interfaces can be developed."

In general, the greater the degree of *structure* in a report, the less latitude afforded the individual radiologist with regard to their own personal writing style. Varied formats under the umbrella term *structured* may contain drop-down menus, require additional mouse clicks, include multiple blanks for free text, or entail other restrictions.

There are logistic and cognitive pitfalls in structured reporting. Productivity temporarily declines as radiologists acclimate to a new reporting system. The order of the report may also be discordant with the radiologist's search pattern; he or she may disagree with the format, order, style, or lexicon chosen by consensus of their department, leading to internal or external conflict. The radiologist may be distracted by menus, icons, text boxes, and so forth and spend less time viewing the medical images, missing opportunities to detect abnormalities. Use of standardized language and rigid formatting may depersonalize the process of reporting and promote professional dissatisfaction. Some veteran radiologists still regard the written radiology report as an art and argue that standardization constrains their creativity. On a cognitive level, Gunderman and McNeive express concern that:

Filling in blanks promotes a very fragmented approach to reporting, which may compromise a radiologist's ability to perceive connections between report elements and synthesize a truly coherent account of the case.

The use of checklists may undermine flexibility, making it difficult for radiologists to adapt their approach to the circumstances of the particular case at hand. It may undermine curiosity by shifting attention from "getting to the bottom of things" to filling out a form. It may poison imagination by focusing on the reciting of findings instead of the formulating and testing of hypotheses. It may get in the way of intuition, the somewhat mysterious process by which the elements of a case suddenly come together to produce a comprehensive and coherent account. ... It is quite possible that, in most cases, what referring physicians and radiologists really want from a radiologic report is not the ability to find and unambiguously interpret each component, but instead, a truly comprehensive and thoughtful assessment of the examination and its implications for further diagnostic workup and care. Here, the importance of conceptual synthesis may outweigh that of the clarity of each element.

Rosenkrantz et al. collaborated with a commercial vendor to "transform the report into an enhanced format complementing text with multimedia elements." Among the features of the enhanced report is a table populated with location and size of a lesion that tracks lesions across examinations. Such a table facilitates assessment of treatment response. Other groups have demonstrated added value in reports with attached images compared with text-only reports. The authors concluded that enhanced reports with select embedded images save time and increase physicians' confidence, suggesting that "[a]ttached images may circumvent the problem of not wording radiology reports in a manner most useful to clinicians."

Content of the Radiology Report

The following is a suggested format in the ACR PPCDIF for reporting:
1. Demographics
2. Relevant clinical information
3. Body of the report
   a. Procedure and materials
   b. Findings
   c. Potential limitations
   d. Clinical issues
   e. Comparison studies and reports
4. Impression (conclusion or diagnosis)

Many proponents of structured reporting regard listing the details of the procedure as superfluous. They argue that very few nonradiologists are interested in the technique, and many clinicians do not read radiology reports in their entirety. However, the radiology report serves several purposes, only one of which is transmitting meaningful information to the clinician. It is also an enduring medical record and a legal document through which the healthcare provider can prove that appropriate treatment was rendered and the standard of care was met. The ACR PPCDIF guidelines are explicit:

The report should include a description of the studies and/or procedures performed and any contrast media and/or radiopharmaceuticals (including specific administered activities, concentration, volume, and route of administration when applicable), medications, catheters, or devices used, if not recorded elsewhere. Any known significant patient reaction or complication should be recorded.

The following features should be addressed in the description of the findings: dimensions, shape, margins, location, attenuation/echogenicity/signal/activity/tracer avidity, enhancement, mass effect, and involvement of adjacent structures. When ambiguous terms, for example, *infiltrate* and *collection*, are substituted for description, accurate communication of the information is not assured, and so the radiologist is advised to qualify the *collection* as a hematoma/abscess/seroma/lymphocele/free fluid, etc. (also see ACR PPCDIF C.3). Conversely, lengthy discourse of a common familiar finding is clinically irrelevant and can distract the reader from a more significant finding hidden elsewhere in the report.

The recommended content of the impression or conclusion section is delineated in the ACR Practice Parameter:

"Impression" (conclusion or diagnosis)

a. *Unless the report is brief each report should contain an "impression" or "conclusion."*
b. *A specific diagnosis should be given when possible.*
c. *A differential diagnosis should be rendered when appropriate.*
d. *Follow-up or additional diagnostic studies to clarify or confirm the impression should be suggested when appropriate.*
e. *Any significant patient reaction should be reported.*

A variation of the report formatting is to place the conclusion at the beginning. Surveys found that this arrangement was more popular with general practitioners than with specialists. However, Friedman defends the standard order of placing the impression at the end of the report, where "the strength of my conviction depends on the logical development of the findings and commentary, and this determines how the diagnosis is expressed." Rothman has written that because radiologists are paid for using both "their eyes and their brains," a complete radiology report must include both sets of evaluations—not only a complete description of the abnormalities seen with the eyes of the radiologist but also a discussion of the findings that are important to the radiologist's brain. In 1923, Enfield, in the *Journal of the American Medical Association*, criticized radiologists who issued written radiology reports that "describe in detail all that the roentgenologist sees in the film but does not tell what he thinks about it, what conclusions he draws from it, and what it means to him." Enfield then exhorted radiologists to "give not only their opinion but also their method of arriving at that opinion."

Structured reporting continues to gather momentum, supported by commercial vendors and professional imaging societies. Referring physicians and the majority of radiologists favor structured reports over the narrative form. Advantages over prose reports are clear: structured reports are better organized, tend to be more complete, and contain fewer inconsistencies. They also foster a standardized lexicon and are more searchable, both by humans and by information systems; information can be stored, retrieved, searched, and parsed by radiology information systems for operational purposes, performance monitoring, quality improvement, coding and billing, and research. No single format for a structured report is universally accepted as being optimal, allowing flexibility for groups of radiologists to adapt them according to their practice needs.

DECREASED VARIATION IN REPORTING

Style and Quality

Transfer of meaningful information from the radiologist to the clinician is the objective of the written radiology report. For the communication to be effective, this written medium of transferring information must contain core content elements that are delineated in guidelines such as the ACR Practice Parameter for Communication of Diagnostic Imaging Findings (Revised 2014; Resolution 11), the RANZCR Written Report Guideline Project of 2010, and the Good Practice for Radiological Reporting Guidelines from the European Society of Radiology (ESR). However, the format, structure, and style of reports vary greatly between radiologists. Residents in radiology receive training in the content of the report, but few are given formal instruction in report style. Economic and institutional pressures to generate reports quickly foster a "continuous-flow mode" of rambling observations where there is little forethought as to what is being dictated. In this mode, insufficient time is typically allotted to contemplate the implications of the findings, to disregard the clinically irrelevant findings, and to integrate the observations with the clinical history to render a cohesive diagnosis or at least a limited differential diagnosis. A survey of physician faculty at a large Midwestern academic medical center asked what they considered to be most important in a high-quality radiology report. The characteristics listed in rank order were: *accurate*, *clear*, *complete*, and *timely*. Gunderman listed these qualities as *clear, concise*, and *complete*. Coakley et al. wrote, "A good report is not only accurate in content, but it is also concise, clear, and pertinent in style." Armas stated that a good radiology report comprises the "6C's": *clarity, correctness, confidence, concision, completeness*, and *consistency*. To those six, Reiner et al. added two more: *communication* and *consultation*.

Bruno et al. at the Penn State Milton S. Hershey Medical Center make several recommendations to improve the clarity and quality of the report: avoidance of medical jargon; regard for sensitivity when describing patient behavior; caution when discussing sensitive topics such as obesity, mental health, and substance abuse; and proofreading. The ACR Practice Parameter also recommends proofreading and discourages use of acronyms. Since 2009, Dr. Michael A. Bruno, vice chairman for quality and patient safety in the Department of Radiology at the Penn State University Milton S. Hershey Medical Center, has conducted a writer's workshop for radiology residents, in which he emphasizes careful word selection to avoid ambiguity. Determination of report quality is a mostly subjective assessment, influenced by numerous biases including educational, cultural, regional, institutional, subspecialty, and generational biases. To better understand assessments of quality, the Penn State group sought to measure quality by an objective method in collaboration with a psychometrician. As expected, they found higher quality in attending reports, but after training in reporting, residents showed statistically validated improvement in the quality of their reports.

Ambiguity and Vagueness

Ambiguity concerns terms that can be interpreted in more than one way. It can be broken into different classifications: syntactic, semantic, pragmatic, and semantic ambiguity. Syntactic ambiguity results from a problem in sentence structure where the placement of a punctuation mark or absence of punctuation leaves the intended meaning unclear. Pragmatic ambiguity pertains to a statement in which concepts within the statement are inconsistent or contradictory. Radiology reports are most prone to the third type, semantic ambiguity, which occurs when a statement can be interpreted in more than one way. A commonly encountered example of semantic ambiguity in radiology reports is the phrase "not seen on the prior study." This phrase leaves one wondering whether the finding was present on the prior exam but not noticed by the first radiologist or whether the abnormality developed since the prior exam.

Radiologists must convey important information to the clinician in a manner that is concise, and reports need to convey a message in unambiguous terms to elicit the correct response from the recipient. Different interpretation by the recipient than the one intended by the sender may lead to alteration in management of a condition and thus heighten the potential for medical error. Several medicolegal cases described by Berlin illustrate the importance of clarity in communicating significant findings to the referring physician. Applying a term such as *irregularity* and *density* or the archaic *shadow* to a finding that has moderate probability of malignancy exposes the radiologist to liability. The concept of a four-tiered hierarchy of radiology terminology was introduced by Friedman. He termed these levels shadows, anatomy, pathology, and diagnosis, reasoning that "It should be evident that the best radiologic report is one that interprets the findings to the highest level possible using all available information, but that uses the correct terms for the level of hierarchy that is being reported." He uses the chest radiograph findings of congestive heart failure as an example, wherein the radiographic findings in the clinical context indicate a pathologic process, so the pathologic terminology (level 3) *interstitial edema* should be applied, not the anatomic description *thickening of the interlobular septa* or the shadow description *Kerley B lines*.

Uncertainty is intrinsic to radiology. Castillo describes how we as radiologists make logical arguments about what we observe in the images and make deductive inferences. There are two main types of uncertainty relevant to the radiologist: (1) the degree of uncertainty as to whether there is an abnormality on the image and (2) the uncertainty as to what that finding represents in pathophysiologic terms. The first type is susceptible to errors of perception and is discussed in Chapter 14. The second type can describe the findings but arrive at an incorrect diagnosis, which is an example of a cognitive error. To communicate uncertainty in their reports, radiologists may invoke *hedge terms*, which may be perceived by the reader as vagueness rather than the intended message. For example, Baker recommended expunging the term *questionable* from radiology lexicon. First, it does not indicate which of the two types of uncertainty is involved;

and second, it does not convey to the reader the degree of uncertainty. The exception to this logical process is when we encounter something with a pathognomonic appearance.

Ambiguous terms for which there are several interpretations should perhaps always be avoided. The word *collapsed* in reference to the lung is problematic, because it means atelectasis to some and pneumothorax to others. Likewise, the word *clot* could be variably interpreted by the reader as a *sentinel clot, thrombus, embolus, hematoma,* or other. Nondescriptive phrases such as *nonobstructive bowel gas pattern* and *nonspecific bowel gas pattern* are widely denounced.

The pertinence of a negative depends on the recipient. In a survey of specialists and general practitioners in the United Kingdom, general practitioners were less interested than specialists were in reading a list of negatives in the body of the report. Without specific reference to the subject fields most relevant to the referring physician, the recipient of the report cannot know whether any particular attention was paid to those subjects if, in the finding section, the report merely states "normal." By stating a few pertinent negatives using the lexicon of the specialist, the radiologist has communicated to the clinician that the organs of particular interest were indeed scrutinized and found to be normal; that the radiologist was aware of the clinical question; and that the radiologist is up to date with the lexicon of the referring specialist's society.

Brevity is considered important by referring physicians, appearing as one of the top four characteristics that clinicians value most in a radiology report. There are circumstances where restating portions of two concomitant studies, such as transabdominal and transvaginal ultrasound of the pelvis, is required to comply with regulations for reimbursement. Some readers are annoyed to find a detailed description of the imaging planes and pulse sequences used for a magnetic resonance imaging (MRI) examination, but the ACR Practice Parameter defends this practice by stating:

> The report should include a description of the studies and/or procedures performed and any contrast media and/or radiopharmaceuticals (including specific administered activities, concentration, volume, and route of administration when applicable), medications, catheters, or devices used, if not recorded elsewhere.

The guideline does not specify to what level of detail the description should go. Although in private radiology practice this fine level of detail is of doubtful value, in teaching hospitals, a more detailed description serves several purposes: it provides a template for trainees in radiology, communicates to specialists what components have (and have not) been performed, and indicates what imaging protocol has been followed. The last point may be particularly important for patients who have ongoing serious health conditions such as malignancy, because these patients often undergo serial examinations.

The topic of substituting phrases for complete sentences is contentious, with Langlotz remarking that mixing sentence fragments with full sentences in the body of the report is "unacceptable," although he admits this practice may reflect a "generational divide." There are indeed numerous commonly used phrases that are nonessential, including those that are "content-free" such as "the examination is otherwise normal." Hall listed many of the common offenders:

This examination is provided, is obtained, is taken, or is submitted for interpretation; appearances are; a finding is seen, visualized or identified; as stated above, as noted, of note, or note is made of; is remarkable for; unremarkable; if clinically indicated; as well as; at this time; however; in addition to; in nature; otherwise normal; quite, unique, some and somewhat.

Langlotz labels these as "observational detachment hedges" and cautions that using such terms may unwittingly erode the confidence that a referring clinician has in the radiologist who is admitting his or her limitations. Excessively wordy reports also pose risks. Moreover, a "report's verbosity and lack of actionable information constitutes a medico-legal risk and serves primarily to distract from the most likely important diagnostic possibilities." Similarly, *tautology,* which is the needless repetition of an idea, statement, or word, should be avoided; common tautological phrases in radiology, according to Hall, include "oval in shape, close proximity, small in size, … direct comparison, interval change, time period, interval comparison, previous history, previous exam of (date), and completely asymptomatic." Langlotz applied the term *repetitive redundancy* to phrases like these. *Periphrasis,* another "stylistic device that can be defined as the use of excessive and longer words to convey a meaning which could have been conveyed with a shorter expression or in a few words," is indeed a common feature of radiology reporting, as are pleonasms, which occur when a writer uses many more words than are actually necessary for the expression of an idea. Common pleonasms include the following: "traverse across, perforate through,"…"total occlusion, very unique, somewhat unique, and … mm in diameter." A commonly misused word is *comprised,* which means the same as *contains.* The right upper lobe of the lung *comprises* three segments, rather than *is comprised of* three segments. Another common grammatical error is with use the phrases *compare to* and *compare with. Compare to* should be used to liken things, *compare with* to consider their similarities or differences.

Bruno et al. caution that abbreviations and jargon can unintentionally offend patients. A word several authors recommend avoiding is *gross,* which the radiologist may substitute for *obvious,* but the patient might interpret as an expression of disgust with the finding. The ACR Practice Parameter states: "Use of abbreviations or acronyms should be limited to avoid ambiguity." Sonographic prefixes and radiographic suffixes should not be combined to create neologisms such as *echodensity.* Coakley rebukes *no significant adenopathy* because -*pathy* (from Greek *pathos* meaning "suffering or disease") always denotes abnormality, so there cannot be insignificant adenopathy.

Describing a patient as *obese* may be medically correct, but in the era of patient portals, it is prudent to be tactful and use alternate terminology like *body habitus.* If the quality of an examination is lessened as a result of the patient's body habitus, it should be noted in the technique section (ACR Practice Parameter 3.c). Similarly, *poor inspiratory effort* is not only disparaging but is often wrong.

Many reasons for elevation of the diaphragm exist, including a large amount of intraabdominal fat, neuromuscular disorder, sedation, coma, mechanical ventilation, and language barrier/hearing loss preventing understanding of the radiologic technologist's breath-holding instructions. Stating the finding that the lungs are underinflated or that the diaphragm is elevated is correct and nonjudgmental. Rather than state that a patient *refused to* complete an examination, the prudent alternative would state the patient was *unable to* complete the exam. Similarly, instead of *noncooperative* or *uncooperative,* one could merely note the patient was *unable to tolerate* the procedure. Clinical history should not state the patient *complains of* a symptom, as this is also pejorative.

Quantification

Vagueness is akin to ambiguity and takes several forms in radiology reporting: underspecification, temporal vagueness, probabilistic terms, and quantitative vagueness. Underspecification is a form of vagueness that occurs when the amount or degree of detail provided is insufficient to render definitive interpretation. Temporal vagueness, probabilistic terms, and quantitative vagueness share the common feature that they may be represented on an ordinal scale. Terms at the extremes of scales, such as the temporal terms *always* and *never,* are not vague. Extremes of scales in probability are *definite* and *impossible.* At the extremes of the quantitative scale are *all* and *none.* In the middle of the scale are noncommittal hedge terms, such as *some,* an example of quantification vagueness. Radiologists in a large academic department and referring physicians were asked in one survey to rank the fifteen most common phrases used to express the level of diagnostic certainty on a scale of 1–15, with each number to be used only once. With the exception of "diagnostic of" at the extreme, there was little agreement among radiologists and nonradiologists. The study found that the phrases with the widest variability in conveying diagnostic certainty were *consistent with, worrisome for, suspicious for, may represent, probably,* and *possibly.*

Casford expanded the list of descriptors of diagnostic uncertainty to 100 and assigned a numerical rank to each word (Table 13.1).

A paper by Mosteller and Youtz reviewed multiple studies on opinions of probabilistic expressions. They reported what probability expressions meant to people, with the expectation that assigning numerical values to these verbal expressions would improve the precision of the language. Expressions with what they termed the highest modal acceptability are the ones that are *well anchored* at the extremes or in the middle: *always, certain, never, impossible,* and *even chance.* Surprisingly, the probabilistic term *possible* was used with the most variability between respondents, with likelihood percentages between 0 and 100. Some respondents "associate it with an event so rare that it can scarcely occur," and a few respondents interpreted *possible* as meaning a 50-50 chance. Mosteller and Youtz proposed that a codification of probability expressions, or assigning a numerical value to qualitative expressions, may improve communication, and terms with the lowest acceptability mode would not be codified.

TABLE 13.1   Complete List of Descriptors to Use in the Following Sentence: This Finding [UNK] Represents a Given Disease Process

Description	% Chance	Description	% Chance
Always	100[a]	As likely as not	50[a]
Definitely	99	Less likely than not	49
Virtually always	98[a]	Less often than not	48
Unceasingly	97	Does not normally	47
Invariably	96	Does not commonly	46
Universally	95	On occasion	45
Continually	94	Does not definitely	44
Constantly	93	Sometimes	43
Certainly	92	Does not usually	42
Classically	91	Does not uniformly	41
Consistently	90[a]	Occasionally	40[a]
Eternally	89	Irregularly	39
Habitually	88	Perhaps	38
Predictably	87	Not uncommonly	37
Uniformly	86	Now and then	36
Most typically	85	Does not always	35
Usually	84	Very occasionally	34
As a rule	83	Does not often	33
Is most likely to	82	Not ordinarily	32
Customarily	81	Is not likely to	31
Frequently	80[a]	Uncommonly	30[a]
Systematically	79	Very exceptionally	29
Likely	78	Does not repeatedly	28
Notably	77	Is unlikely to	27
Most often	76	Once in a while	26
Most frequently	75	Unusually	25
Persistently	74	Is very unlikely to	24
Very often	73	Very uncommonly	23
Not universally	72	Sporadically	22
Most commonly	71	Does not invariably	21
Commonly	70[a]	Infrequently	20[a]
Recurrently	69	Very infrequently	19
Normally	68	Does not frequently	18
Most generally	67	Hardly ever	17
Often	66	Only exceptionally	16
Not unusually	65	Scarcely ever	15
Ordinarily	64	Seldom	14
Is not unlikely to	63	Does not regularly	13
Perpetually	62	Very rarely	12
Habitually	61	Few and far between	11
Generally	60[a]	Rarely	10[a]
Typically	59	Once in a blue moon	9
More typically than not	58	Very seldom	8
Very regularly	57	Generally does not	7
Regularly	56	Does not typically	6
Repeatedly	55	At no time	5
Not rarely	54	Once in a great while	4
Not occasionally	53	Does not ever	3
More often than not	52	Virtually never	2[a]
More likely than not	51	Essentially never	1

0% = never.

[a]Descriptors used in abbreviated list.

From Casford B. Radiology lexicon. *Am J Roentgenol.* 2000;174(5):1463-1464.

Debate over the word *normal* has been rekindled by structured reporting. Some radiologists spurn its use, claiming that minor abnormalities such as degenerative disease or anatomic variations are encountered in the vast majority of cases and thereby exclude most patients from being entirely *normal*. Additionally, some believe, probably naively, that avoiding the word *normal* will absolve them of legal liability if a subtle or nonspecific finding is an early presentation of a developing serious condition. Taking the opposing position, Langlotz lauds the use of *normal* as:

> *...one of the most powerful words a radiologist can use. Normal makes a sweeping statement by indicating, in singular fashion, that all abnormalities have been considered and excluded. Using normal will enhance your reputation among referring clinicians, because it gives them the two things they want most: a definitive answer that halts the work-up and good news for their patient. Frequent use of normal also provides a counterpoint to the reputation of radiologists as wafflers who hedge against the risk of an incorrect conclusion.*

Langlotz also advises against using stand-ins for things larger than normal: *chunky, plump, generous*, or the frequent substitute, *prominent*. Adjectives used to quantify the number of things are variably interpreted and add to quantitative vagueness. More than one renal cyst may be variably reported as *a few, several, numerous, many*, and *multiple*. These semiquantitative terms are therefore ambiguous and should be avoided when possible. Findings that cannot be measured, such as things that are infiltrating rather than mass-forming, for example, periappendiceal stranding, can be semiquantitatively graded as mild, moderate, or severe. Things that can be precisely measured, such as fluid or a mass, can be semiquantitatively graded as small, moderate, or large.

The term *significant* is often misused in place of quantitative *largeness,* such as "a significant left pleural effusion," may merely mean a large one; in this way the true meaning can be rendered vague. It is also sometimes used to denote importance, for example, "Significantly, there is a new 3-cm mass in the pancreatic head." The word *significant* is best invoked for its statistical meaning, such as when a change in a dual-energy x-ray absorptiometry score reaches threshold significance. It can apply to statistical analysis of results of findings, particularly in research. It can be applied to quantify changes in tumor dimensions over time, a precept of Response Evaluation Criteria in Solid Tumors (RECIST) 1.1 or semiquantitatively applied, such as "no significant change in pleural effusion" between serial chest radiographs. It also has nonmathematical connotation in the field of medicine indicating something causing morbidity. It is a word that many believe ought to be used more judiciously and sparingly than it generally is.

Standardization of Terminology

Narrative (prose) radiology reports have been the object of criticism in medical literature for nearly 100 years. Studies show that prose reports are less likely to be complete. Prose or free-text reports often contain ambiguous terms, leading to uncertainty of their meaning by the referring clinician. Clear communication is hampered by the absence of shared common terminology by sender and recipient. Responding to contentions by the American Medical Association that recommendations in mammography reports were inconsistent and ambiguous, the ACR instituted the Breast Imaging Reporting and Data System (BI-RADS) initiative in 1995 to address these shortcomings. Collaboration between the American College of Surgeons, the College of American Pathologists, the American Medical Association, the Centers for Disease Control and Prevention, the National Cancer Institute, and the Food and Drug Administration ensured broad-based support for this initiative. Commonly understood terminology facilitates cooperation among radiologists, breast surgeons, pathologists, and radiation oncologists for optimal patient benefit. In addition to a lexicon of descriptors, the BI-RADS system also restricted the number of final assessment categories to standardize management. Through controlled vocabulary, the collection of data can be automated for purposes including storage and retrieval, performance tracking, and compliance requirements.

Other societies have followed the example of BI-RADS. A plethora of constrained terminologies from other disciplines have followed: BI-RADS US, BI-RADS MR, C-RADS, CAD-RADS, GI-RADS, Lung-RADS, PI-RADS, LI-RADS, and TI-RADS. The importance of standardization of terminology is illustrated in selection of patients for liver transplantation. In a retrospective analysis of data in 2006 of patients with hepatocellular carcinoma (HCC) who had undergone transplantation, the authors found that radiologic stage equaled pathologic stage in only 44% of patients. The organization realized that stricter diagnostic imaging criteria were needed for HCC diagnosis. A product of a consensus conference of the Organ Procurement and Transplantation Network (OPTN) United Network for Organ Sharing (UNOS) Liver Committee in November 2008 was a standard lexicon for imaging criteria for HCC. The reporting requirements state "A structured summary at the end of the clinician's report is strongly encouraged that lists the total number, location (liver segment), size (largest diameter), and OPTN class of all treated or untreated HCC."

Standardization is not as readily achieved without cooperative efforts by stakeholders. Kalra and Saini listed reasons for lack of standardization in CT scanning parameters and CT scanning protocols. At the level of oversight, there is no government body, professional organization, international committee of experts, or accrediting body tasked with regulating nomenclature for CT. Additionally, advances in multidetector CT technology outpace the assessment of these new technologies. Proprietary differences serve the need of the manufacturers to promote brand identity and create *brand inertia*, which is the difficulty users experience in moving from one manufacturer's platform to another.

Recommendations

Whether radiologists should make recommendations has been a long-standing debate without a foreseeable resolution. On the one hand, the radiologist is the most qualified specialist to recommend further imaging studies for a finding of indeterminate significance. On the other hand, the referring clinician knows the most about the patient, the patient's medical history, and the results of nonradiologic tests. A precarious balance exists between the professional duty to provide meaningful guidance to the recipient of the report and obligating the clinician to perform a procedure of dubious value or one that carries risks. Two related phrases of dubious merit that commonly appear at the end of a radiology report are "if clinically indicated" and "clinical correlation is recommended." Coakley decided that "[t]he terms 'if clinically indicated' or 'clinical correlation is suggested' should be used sparingly and should never be used as a substitute for offering a diagnostic opinion." Berlin concurred, stating that:

> Radiologists should minimize, if not eliminate altogether, the use of such phrases as "if clinically warranted," or "if clinically indicated may be of value," when assessing abnormal radiographic findings. Because radiologists are acknowledged to possess radiologic expertise derived from training and experience, they should not delegate to nonradiology physicians the responsibility of evaluating the potential significance of a purely radiographic finding that is unexpected or unusual.

The ACR PPCDIF makes a restrained statement that recommendations are within the purview of the radiologist in section IIA.4.d: "Follow-up or additional diagnostic studies to clarify or confirm the impression should be suggested when appropriate."

The ACR Practice Parameter Guideline recommends "a precise diagnosis when possible or a differential diagnosis when possible." A single-institution review of 5.9 million radiology reports from 1995 to 2008 found recommendations for additional imaging (RAI) in 10.5% of those reports. The authors noted an increase in the frequency of RAI over the study interval. Not surprisingly, breast imaging had the highest likelihood of RAI, followed by pelvis and chest. The likelihood of RAI decreased by about 15% for each decade of experience by the radiologist. The observed trend of lower frequency of RAI with increased experience of the radiologist is probably multifactorial. The case mix of the individual radiologist may change with experience and shift in the ratio of newly trained to experienced radiologists. Growing concerns of legal liability, quality improvement initiatives, and *information density* with better equipment, greater availability of high-cost imaging modalities, and increased use of higher-sensitivity modalities may all contribute to increased RAI. Counterintuitively, follow-up examinations may actually lower healthcare costs and promote patient safety by avoiding unnecessary procedures.

Despite the widening implementation of EHRs, radiologists continue to interpret many cases with sparse clinical information. Electronic ordering of imaging examinations remains flawed, and most studies can still be ordered with the barest of clinical information. The most elementary of clinical history such as pain, fever, or cough may be absent. Patients may be referred by a physician not affiliated with the radiologist's institution. Many EHR and hospital information systems are not fully integrated with PACS, requiring the radiologist to log on to a separate computer system and navigate multiple screens to access the medical record.

The absence of standard protocols for follow-up of incidental findings on medical imaging has led to wide variation between radiologists. Often these recommendations are not evidence based. These types of ad hoc recommendations are potential legal snares for radiologists and can also compromise patient safety in some cases. Recognizing the lack of guidance that radiologists have historically been afforded, professional organizations and societies have convened expert panels to promulgate consensus statements and guidelines for management, such as the Fleischner Society guidelines for solid pulmonary nodules. Several years later, the same society published guidelines for nonsolid and subsolid pulmonary nodules. The ACR has published several white papers, including management of incidental findings on abdominal CT. Once the findings are described by the radiologist in the report, the descriptions and parameters of the finding can be parsed by an ontology in the radiology decision support (RDS) system. Algorithms for management can be developed in-house by consensus of the radiologists in the department or can be adopted from professional societies. These guidelines can be embedded in RDS software so that recommendations are automatically generated, eliminating any variation and the chance that the radiologist might forget to recommend follow-up.

Ontology

For humans to communicate effectively, a standard lexicon is needed. None of the three existing medical lexicons in 2002 were specific for radiology, and none matched more than 50% of the radiologic terms. It was acknowledged that a lexicon specific to the needs of radiology needed to be created. This awareness of the limitations of the available lexicons and terminology guidelines led to the development by the RSNA of RadLex, replacing the ACR Index for Radiological Diagnosis. A lexicon specific to the needs of radiology, it facilitates indexing and retrieval of information through use of controlled terminology. The following statements on the RSNA website summarize the RadLex project:

> RadLex is a comprehensive lexicon—a unified language of radiology terms—for standardized indexing and retrieval of radiology information resources. With more than 68,000 terms, RadLex satisfies the needs of software developers, system vendors and radiology users by adopting the best features of existing terminology systems while producing new terms to fill critical gaps. RadLex also provides a comprehensive and technology-friendly replacement for the ACR Index for Radiological Diagnoses. It unifies and supplements other lexicons and standards, such as SNOMED-CT and DICOM.

No sooner after its development did Rubin recognize there were "significant obstacles" for RadLex to achieve its goals of:

> ...disseminating standardized terminology to researchers, radiologists, and developers to facilitate analysis of radiologic information, to permit uniform indexing of image libraries, and to enable new applications for structures capture of image information.

Data acquired and stored in the form of text files and spreadsheets were difficult to search and to modify, and flat file formats were difficult to analyze for errors of omissions and duplications. "[A]pplications that display

RadLex to users as well as programs that use RadLex terms for tasks such as structured reporting, teaching file coding, and indexing research data" needed a way to be updated that was not labor intensive and stayed abreast of advances in information technology. An ontology "describes a domain and comprises terms, attributes of those terms, and relationships among the terms." Representing RadLex as an ontology would make browsing easier for humans and computers, simplify analysis for errors, facilitate management of enlarging files, simplify modification, and enable integration into software and healthcare information suites. Its creators realized that, to maintain viability, RadLex must be robust to adapt to advances in information technology. RadLex was released in November 2006 in several forms, including a database file, a tabular format, and an ontology web language (OWL). Since its launch, it has grown to include over 68,000 terms. It is updated twice a year and is cross-linked with other medical vocabularies such as SNOMED-CT, International Classification of Diseases (ICD)-10, and Current Procedural Terminology (CPT).

RADIOLOGIST DECISION SUPPORT

Protecting Access to Medicare Act, Health and Human Services, and Centers for Medicare and Medicaid Services Legislation

The cost of performing inappropriate imaging studies is unsustainable. Durand et al. remarked on the inappropriate use of medical imaging and unnecessary exposure to ionizing radiation through low-utility studies: "Though often essential for diagnosis and management, medical imaging is known for low-value uses and as the single largest source of per-capita radiation exposure." Payer-led strategies to lower expenditures hinge on reducing fee-for-service reimbursement or by mandating preauthorization through radiology benefits managers (RBMs). Decisions by RBMs may not be evidence based, may delay needed patient care, and may actually increase healthcare costs by adding layers of healthcare administration. Denial of a high-cost medical imaging examination in the absence of evidence-based guidelines could be disingenuous and motivated by profit. The hidden cost of the inefficiency of requiring a physician to obtain preauthorization through an RBM is borne by the physician's practice.

Clinical Decision Support

CDS software ranks the appropriateness of diagnostic imaging examinations for a patient with certain symptoms and risk factors. Two federal programs enacted by congress and President Obama require healthcare organizations to adopt CDS. The Protecting Access to Medicare Act (PAMA), passed by Congress in April 2014, authorized the US Department of Health and Human Services (HHS) to implement CDS for medical imaging services rendered for Medicare beneficiaries. The act stipulated that appropriate use criteria (AUC) can only be "developed or endorsed by national professional medical specialty societies or other provider-led entities." In section 1834(q)(1)(B) of the Act, AUC are defined as evidence-based criteria (to the extent

feasible) that assist professionals who order and furnish applicable imaging services to make the most appropriate treatment decisions for a specific clinical condition. The US Government Accountability Office stated "CMS has proposed to qualify provider-led entities—such as national professional medical specialty societies—such that all AUC developed, endorsed, or modified by these entities would be eligible for use in the imaging program."

American College of Radiology Select

The ACR promotes stewardship of medical imaging to control healthcare costs and reduce the growing number of unnecessary tests. Its ACR Select program delivers up-to-date guidelines through EHR. The ACR has released the following statement on its implementation of appropriateness of use criteria through a newly created partnership:

> *The ACR has an exclusive agency agreement with the National Decision Support Company (NDSC) to provide the technical platform, support and licensing of its copyrighted appropriateness criteria under the name ACR Select. The College urges members, ordering physicians and administrative members to learn how ACR Select, a computer-based diagnostic imaging decision support system that uses ACR Appropriateness Criteria®, operates. NDSC provides electronic health record (EHR) vendors with a direct method for health care organizations to easily integrate and effortlessly use the ACR Appropriateness Criteria guidelines in daily practice. ACR Appropriateness Criteria are now available in a digitally consumable format to be incorporated into computerized ordering and EHR systems.*

The two major components of CDS systems are the computer software program and the clinical recommendations. Khorasami highlighted 10 attributes of effective medical imaging in "Ten Commandments for Effective Clinical Decision Support" (Box 13.1).

Appropriate-use guidelines change constantly, making it impossible for providers to keep up with the changes. CDS places the necessary resources to order the most appropriate examination at the physician's fingertips. Another benefit of decision support is instant access to practice guidelines, where the provider can show a difficult patient who makes a demand for a low-utility imaging study that the study is not recommended by a specialty society. It saves the physician or practice manager time that would otherwise have been spent on the phone with a radiology benefits manager seeking authorization for a study of dubious merit. CDS reduces the need for prior authorization by an RBM. Clinicians are required to consult CDS before making their selection of imaging exam but are not required to follow the recommendations of CDS. Consulting AUC is only required in physician offices, hospital outpatient practices, and emergency departments. Atypical clinical presentations and extenuating circumstances will prevent 100% compliance with CDS recommendations, and for those situations, most CDS systems require a free-text explanation before the order can continue. This data becomes part of the medical record, and ordering providers can be held accountable for choosing to ignore clinical evidence. CDS "has been shown to be effective in modifying physician behavior." Metrics can be applied to

BOX 13.1 Ten Commandments for Effective Imaging Clinical Decision Support

1. Effective imaging clinical decision support should be viewed as a multidisciplinary clinical program rather than an information technology initiative.
2. The strength of evidence supporting the clinical actions and recommendations embedded in imaging clinical decision support must be transparent to the user at the time of order entry.
3. Sources of evidence embedded in imaging clinical decision support must be diverse.
4. Evidence must be current.
5. Clinical recommendations and assessments embedded in imaging clinical decision support must be brief, unambiguous, and actionable.
6. Respect ordering provider workflow.
7. Establishing consequences for ignoring clinical decision support recommendations will enhance the impact of imaging clinical decision support as education alone.
8. Imaging clinical decision support initiatives that target well-defined clinical performance gaps are more likely to be effective.
9. Imaging clinical decision support must enable measurement of its impact.
10. Position imaging clinical decision support to improve workflow efficiencies for patients, providers, and payers.

From Khorasani R, Hentel K, Darer J, et al. Ten commandments for effective clinical decision support for imaging: enabling evidence-based practice to improve quality and reduce waste. *AJR Am J Roentgenol.* 2014;203(5):945-951.

a provider's pattern of use over time and compared with those of his or her peers. Benchmarks can be established, and the data can be used as an educational tool and part of a quality improvement process.

CONCLUSION

Vagueness and ambiguity in written radiology reports are barriers to clear communication. Many times, miscommunication can be prevented by simply avoiding a few commonly used terms that carry a high likelihood of misinterpretation. Adopting a standardized lexicon enables precision in communication where the sender and recipient share a common understanding of the terms. Terms can be retrieved manually or through ontologies from reports for various operational, performance monitoring, research, and other purposes. Appropriate utilization criteria can be embedded in CDS software and may lower the cost of healthcare by reducing the number of inappropriate or low-utility imaging examinations and other testing. As these systems evolve, it is expected that they will become more integrated from the time of the physician order entry process to the receipt of the finalized report. Radiologists will benefit from time saved (time which was previously lost) contacting a responsible individual to receive a critical test result and clinicians will benefit from receiving up-to-date, evidence-based recommendations from keywords electronically extracted from radiologists' reports. Legal liability exposure will also likely be diminished by widespread use of closed-loop communication methods and by adherence to guidelines developed by provider-led entities such as the ACR and other national professional societies.

SUGGESTED READINGS

American College of Radiology, Branstetter BF, Prevedello LM. IT Reference Guide for the Practicing Radiologist. Available at https://www.acr.org/~/media/ACR/Documents/PDF/Advocacy/IT%20Reference%20Guide/IT%20Ref%20Guide%20Reporting%20Communication.pdf.

American College of Radiology. *ACR Practice Parameter for Communication of Diagnostic Imaging Findings;* 2014 (Resolution 11). Available at https://www.acr.org/~/media/C5D1443C9EA4424AA12477D1AD1D927D.pdf.

Baker SR. The dictated report and the radiologist's ethos: an inextricable relationship: pitfalls to avoid. *Eur J Radiol.* 2014;83:236-238.

Berlin L. Pitfalls of the vague radiology report. *AJR Am J Roentgenol.* 2000;174:1511-1518.

Berlin L. Communicating findings of radiologic examinations: Whither goest the radiologist's duty? *AJR Am J Roentgenol.* 2002:809-814.

Berlin L. Communicating results of all radiologic examinations directly to patients: has the time come? *AJR Am J Roentgenol.* 2007;189(6):1275-1282.

Bruno MA, Petscavage-Thomas JM, Mohr MJ. The "open letter": radiologists' reports in the era of patient web portals. *J Am Coll Radiol.* 2014;11:863-867.

Burnside ES, Sickles EA, Bassett LW, et al. The ACR BI-RADS experience: learning from history. *J Am Coll Radiol.* 2009;6(12):851-860.

Good practice for radiological reporting. guidelines from the European Society of Radiology (ESR). *Insights Imaging.* 2011;2(2):93-96.

Hall F. Language of the radiology report: primer for residents and wayward radiologists. *AJR Am J Roentgenol.* 2000;175:1239-1242.

Khorasani R, Bates DW, Teeger S. Is terminology used effectively to convey diagnostic certainty in radiology reports? *Acad Radiol.* 2003;10:685-688.

Khorasani R, Hentel K, Darer J. Review. Ten commandments for effective clinical decision support for imaging: enabling evidence-based practice to improve quality and reduce waste. *AJR Am J Roentgenol.* 2014;203:945-951.

Morgan TA, Helibrun ME, Kahn CE. Reporting initiative of the Radiological Society of North America: progress and new directions. *Radiology.* 2014;273(3):642-645.

Radiological Society of North America. RadLex. Available at https://www.rsna.org/RadLex.aspx.

Chapter 14
Error in Radiology

Chandni Bhimani and Michael A. Bruno

INTRODUCTION

Errors are innate in every field of medicine and persist despite the best efforts of medical professionals to be (or become) flawless. In fact, the prevalence of errors by radiologists (i.e., the radiology error rate) has been remarkably constant in repeated studies dating to the 1930s. For radiologists, there are multiple contributing factors for this, including knowledge gaps and perceptual errors; flaws inherent in emerging technologies for image acquisition and reliance on the input of other professionals, especially technologists for image acquisition; and referring clinicians, who are relied upon for requesting the most suitable study and providing appropriate historical guidance. The underlying cause(s) of the most common radiologist error—simply failing to perceive a finding that sometime later seems obvious in retrospect—remains unknown. In the face of this harsh reality, it is crucial to create systems to attempt to reduce and prevent error but also to rapidly detect errors when they inevitably occur so that the appropriate remediation and prevention of harm can be accomplished. In approaching the subject of radiologist error, a classification of errors is needed.

EPIDEMIOLOGY OF ERROR

Leo Henry Garland was a radiologist in the mid-20th century. He was the pioneer in studying radiologic error and published an important article on diagnostic error in the *American Journal of Roentgenology* in 1939. Garland discovered a 30% miss rate when experienced radiologists interpreted positive chest radiographs and found that 2% of negative chest radiographs were overinterpreted. He also found that 20% of radiologists *disagreed with themselves* on a second reading! His work was not warmly embraced by his colleagues at the time, who were at best hesitant to acknowledge the significance of his results. Since Garland's time, more recent research on radiologist's error rates have repeatedly yielded results consistent with Dr. Garland's initial reporting of error frequency, without any appreciable improvement despite advances in radiologic technology and clinical knowledge. This suggests that the problem is a very basic one, not readily amenable to technological or educational intervention.

In multiple peer-reviewed publications (see Siegle et al.) the most realistic estimates for radiologist error rates are obtained when radiologist's performance is measured using case samples typical of actual practice, where the mix of studies interpreted includes a blend of normal and abnormal cases with a representative disease prevalence.

Studies of this type have generally revealed an error rate of 3.5% to 4%. If the case mix is enriched to include essentially 100% positive studies—a very artificial situation—the error rate rises to approximately 30%. Because most radiologists interpret a mix of studies with a low overall prevalence of positive findings, and because most radiologists interpret well in excess of 100 studies in a typical day, this translates to approximately three or four errors per day per radiologist, on average. Fortunately, only a small fraction of these errors result in patient harm, but it is worrisome that most go undetected; in most cases, radiologists are never made aware of the majority of their errors and receive useful, prompt feedback on an extremely small fraction of their actual errors.

In September of 2015, the Institute of Medicine (IOM) released a new report on the prevalence and range of diagnostic error, entitled *Improving Diagnosis in Healthcare*. This new IOM monograph, which is part of a series including *Crossing the Quality Chasm*, which was published in 2001, and *To Err Is Human: Building a Safer Health System*, published in 2000, once again called attention to the alarming magnitude of the problem, namely, the very large number of diagnostic errors in medicine. The report defined diagnostic error as "the failure to (a) establish an accurate and timely explanation of the patient's health problem(s) or (b) communicate that explanation to the patient." Based on that definition, the committee concluded that diagnostic error is so common that most people will experience at least one diagnostic error in their lifetime, sometimes with devastating consequences, and called for urgent change to address this challenge. Postmortem studies spanning many decades estimated that diagnostic errors contributed to approximately 10% of patient deaths, and review of malpractice claims data has shown that diagnostic errors are the most common cause of successful malpractice lawsuits.

Of course, radiologists' errors account for only a fraction of overall diagnostic error because imaging is only one of many factors that contribute to the diagnostic process. Other contributing factors include faulty information gathering by clinicians, insufficient consideration given to differential possibilities, inadequate performance of a physical examination or misinterpretation of physical exam findings and laboratory tests, lab and pathology errors, failure to act appropriately on the results of monitoring or testing once the results are reported, inadequate communication between caregivers, and so on. But because the specialty of diagnostic radiology exists primarily to reduce the uncertainty in establishing a diagnosis, the report carries significant implications for radiologists.

TYPES OF ERRORS

Various authors have attempted to provide classification systems for radiologist's diagnostic errors. The very comprehensive system proposed by Kim and Mansfield (discussed later in this chapter) includes 12 categories of error, although some error types were shown in their study to be much more prevalent than others. In this chapter we limit our discussion to *diagnostic errors* and do not consider the related issues of treatment, procedural, or medication errors, which are also common causes of patient harm. Often overlooked are errors related to *overdiagnosis*, in which radiologists contribute to placing a pathologic disease diagnosis on a normal, healthy patient, leading physicians to provide inappropriate (i.e., not indicated) care, such as when a normal appendix is removed because a radiologist misinterprets a normal structure for an inflamed appendix or laparoscopy is done for a presumed ectopic pregnancy due to misinterpretation of an ultrasound artifact. Other types of errors germane to radiologic practice (but not limited to radiology) include communication failures, equipment malfunction, or other system failures.

It is important to realize that, contrary to the prevailing culture within the medical profession, the vast majority of medical errors are not simply due to individuals being reckless, ignorant, incompetent, sloppy, or negligent. To the contrary, research has repeatedly demonstrated that nearly all medical errors are instead due to preventable failures in the systems, processes, and conditions in which caring, competent professionals practice.

DEFINITIONS AND CLASSIFICATIONS OF ERROR

In classifying errors, a few definitions are helpful.

An *active error* is one that can be attributed to specific human failures, equipment malfunction, or external failures. James Reason describes active errors as those that occur at the human interface with the larger healthcare system, often referred to as the "sharp end." They include procedural mistakes, diagnostic errors, and misinterpretations of test results. Active errors are more easily identifiable because they result from the consequences of the actions of an identifiable individual. In contrast, *latent errors* (or latent conditions) are usually not attributable to a single person but rather are the result of failures inherent in the system design, resulting in inadvertent (but often preventable) harm to a patient. These errors are said to occur at the "blunt end" of the system, and their causes are not as easily identified. The two often occur together; thus, an active error often occurs simultaneously with a latent error.

An *adverse event* is any injury caused by medical care and not by the patient's medical condition. Examples include pneumothorax post central venous catheter placement, anaphylaxis to penicillin, or development of deep vein thrombosis during hospital stay. Adverse events do not imply error or fault. The occurrence is defined as secondary to some aspect of diagnosis or therapy, not from an underlying disease process.

A *close call or near miss* refers to a mistake that did not lead to a negative outcome for a patient, but only by virtue of luck or chance.

The Joint Commission defines a *sentinel event* as "an unexpected occurrence involving death or serious physical or psychological injury, or the risk thereof." Serious injury in this context particularly refers to loss of limb or function. These events are called *sentinel* because they indicate that a serious systems issue may be present requiring immediate investigation and response.

Although not a specific error type, the presence of an *authority gradient* is a known risk factor for error in medicine. It was originally described in the setting of aviation when copilots had a difficult time communicating errors to pilots in time to prevent harm (such as an airplane crash), due to the copilot's feeling of hierarchical inferiority. Similarly, in medicine, there are many hierarchal levels in a medical team (e.g., doctor and nurse, attending and resident, and doctor and pharmacist) in which this authority gradient is applicable. This is a known significant cause of medical error and a well-documented cause of aviation errors that have led to significant loss of life in airline crashes.

RADIOLOGIC ERROR

Interpretation of imaging studies is performed by humans and thus involves all aspects of human error, especially error related to psychological and cognitive processes that are poorly understood. *Perceptual errors* involve both not seeing a finding and not becoming sufficiently aware of it to trigger an action or diagnosis on the part of a radiologist. Some of these are believed to actually represent errors in working memory, such as when a finding is annotated on an image but never mentioned in the final report and not taken into account when forming the differential diagnosis. Such findings are often readily apparent in retrospect to the person who made the perceptual error. *Cognitive error*, in contrast, arises when an abnormality is correctly identified visually, but the diagnostic implication or importance of the finding is not correctly understood and thus not relayed effectively in the report. The prevalence of perceptual errors is much larger than cognitive errors. Approximately 70% of radiologic errors are believed to be perceptual, and about 30% are believed to be some sort of cognitive error.

It is important to understand that a radiologist making such an error does not imply that the radiologist is being negligent and should be punished; careful research from the time of Garland onward has documented a *baseline* error rate (mostly perceptual errors), which represents errors that are not amenable to remediation by extra education or by having a solid work ethic. Knowing this basic fact, it is crucial to create a strong institutional infrastructure to identify radiologic errors as expeditiously as possible and to find ways to prevent errors and to detect them soon enough to avoid patient harm.

System errors are those to which individuals are predisposed due to flaws in the systems or processes in which they work. Most *communication errors* fall under this category, including lack of communication when it would have been needed or simple miscommunication, when the receiver does not *register* the intended message of the sender. In the teaching hospital setting, an example of a communication error may include an attending or resident radiologist not effectively communicating a change made to a preliminary radiology report to the appropriate clinician(s) in time for the new information to meaningfully change patient management.

COGNITIVE ERRORS IN RADIOLOGY: COGNITIVE BIAS

Cognitive bias is inevitable in every human-guided field, and many types of cognitive bias have been described. Although there is robust literature on the topic of cognitive *debiasing*, no technique for *debiasing* physicians has yet been shown to significantly reduce this type of error. Nonetheless, it is important for radiologists to be aware of the existence of these biases, be able to recognize them when they occur, and take steps to avoid being *caught* by latent bias in their daily work. The following are a few important categories of cognitive bias.

Anchoring bias is in effect when the interpreting radiologist fixates on a certain diagnosis early in the study and thus does not place emphasis on any further details that may otherwise point to the correct diagnosis. For example, knowing that the patient has an elevated brain natriuretic peptide on blood work, you have decided that the interstitial thickening in the lungs represents pulmonary edema, despite the presence of a lung mass and potential for lymphoproliferative spread of the cancer.

Availability bias occurs when someone allows easily recollected occurrences to exert undue influence on his or her diagnostic thinking, because frequent or recent events are easier to recall or imagine than infrequent ones. Thus, the same diagnosis may be considered for multiple patients because one has recently seen the diagnosis repeatedly, or if a disease has not been seen for a long time, it may tend to be underdiagnosed. For example, a radiologist who detected a renal cancer earlier in the week may tend to overdiagnose renal cysts as cancer later in that same week and encourage further tests or biopsy to prove the diagnosis. Availability bias is also at play when relying too much on a prior radiologist's imaging report. Availability bias can be mitigated if radiologists periodically remind themselves to treat each case individually and not to overdiagnose their recent missed cases or rare cases.

Confirmation bias comes into play when the interpreting radiologist looks for findings to support a suspected diagnosis and ignores other findings that may stray him/her from the originally sought-out diagnosis. For example, a study that is ordered for right lower quadrant pain with concern for appendicitis may see the finding of inflamed appendix with mild dilation but may overlook the edema and wall thickening of the cecum and ascending colon, which would lead the radiologist to consider the diagnosis of colitis with secondary reactive changes of the appendix.

Outcome bias involves opting for a diagnosis that will relay a better final outcome for the patient, such as when a radiologist is more prone to diagnose a tumor as benign despite features that suggest malignancy.

Hindsight bias is the inclination to attribute a correct diagnosis to one's own brilliant interpretive skills rather than realizing that the finding was much more easily recognized in hindsight, that is, after knowing the actual outcome. For example, once given the history of biopsy-proven malignancy, you are likely to find an abnormality that you feel is the location of cancer on a chest radiograph.

This is a very common problem with expert witness testimony, where the plaintiff's expert accuses the defendant radiologist of having missed something *obvious*, which may in fact be obvious only in hindsight.

Zebra retreat is a particular bias of knowledgeable radiologists, in which a rare *zebra* diagnosis is actually supported by the history and imaging findings, but the radiologist is reluctant to make the diagnosis of such a rare condition.

Framing bias or effect involves biasing your interpretation of a finding by the provided history. For example, when given the history of shortness of breath and cough with imaging findings of multifocal consolidation, the radiologist is likely to give the diagnosis of multifocal pneumonia. However, if given the full history of a patient with shortness of breath and cough status post cardiac arrest requiring chest compressions, the radiologist may interpret the consolidation as aspiration or hemorrhagic contusion from the trauma of performing chest compressions.

Satisfaction of search is the most-recognized bias in radiology. This occurs when a finding is interpreted as the cause for the patient's complaint, and so further search for another diagnosis is prematurely halted. For example, in a 6-month-old infant with a history of chronic lung disease presenting with cough and irritability, the radiologist may stop looking after finding the consolidation that would explain the patient's cough and fever. However, further review of the osseous structures is not given as much weight once the reason for the patient's symptoms is addressed. In glossing over the osseous structures, the radiologist could have missed multiple rib fractures indicative of nonaccidental trauma.

Premature closure is similar to satisfaction of search and involves deciding on a very specific final diagnosis before sufficient confirmation has been obtained. For example, in a patient with known myasthenia gravis, who has a thymic mass, one assumes thymoma without insisting on a tissue diagnosis. Although thymoma is classically associated with myasthenia gravis, this thymic mass could be thymic hyperplasia, lymphoma, or a germ cell tumor.

Commission/omission bias occurs when the radiologist fails to mention doubt or the possibility of a more fatal diagnosis due to self-doubt in the likelihood of an alternative diagnosis. For example, when reviewing a trauma case, linear high attenuation in the vicinity of the splenic artery may be assumed to represent calcification of the splenic artery. Another possibility would be a case involving active contrast extravasation, in which the radiologist's self-doubt, uncertainty, and the possibility of the patient facing further tests or surgery cause the radiologist not to include this in his or her report and not discuss the possibility with the ordering clinician. However, by bringing up this possibility, other noninvasive testing, such as a repeat noncontrast computed tomography of the abdomen, would help determine whether the finding is calcification or hemorrhage.

SYSTEM-RELATED ERRORS IN RADIOLOGY

System factors leading to diagnostic errors are typically related to policies and procedures, inefficiencies in the workflow, issues with teamwork and communication, inherent problems in electronic systems, or other

TABLE 14.1 **Just Culture Model of Manageable Behaviors and Appropriate Action**

Human Error	At-Risk Behavior	Reckless Behavior
Inadvertent slip, lapse, or mistake	A choice that is not believed to be a risk and is instead believed to be insignificant or justified	Consciously taking an unjustifiable risk
Manage by changing: • Choices • Processes • Procedures • Training • Design • Environment	Manage by: • Removing incentives for the behavior • Creating incentives for better choices • Increasing situational awareness	Manage by: • Remedial action • Punitive action
MANAGEMENT ACTION		
Console	Coach	Punish

infrastructural factors not directly under the control of the individual practitioner. For example, if staff shortages or mismanagement of staffing resources leads to radiologists working excessively long hours, simple fatigue and mental or visual fatigue (eyestrain or asthenopia) may ultimately lead to these radiologists making more errors of all types. In such a scenario, these additional errors over the baseline rate would be attributable to the work system rather than individual fault or normal human error.

ERROR CLASSIFICATION SYSTEMS

Kim-Mansfield Radiologic Error Classification System

Over the years, several error classification systems have been offered for radiology. The most recent and comprehensive of these is the Kim-Mansfield Radiologic Error Classification system, which uses a 12-category schema and expands on the previous error classification paradigm created by Renfrew. In their 2014 study, published in the *American Journal of Roentgenology*, Kim and Mansfield categorized over 1200 separate errors into 12 classifications based on the *cause* of the error: complacency (false-positive finding), faulty reasoning (true-positive finding misclassified), lack of knowledge, underreading (a missed finding), poor communication, technique, prior examination, history, location, satisfaction of search, complication, and satisfaction of report. Unique to their classification is the "lack of knowledge error," which is considered to have occurred when a finding is misinterpreted and attributed to the wrong cause simply because of a lack of knowledge that another cause exists to explain the findings. Such an error might be amenable to educational intervention.

Kim and Mansfield also point out that technical issues can lead to diagnostic error, such as when a potentially important finding is obscured due to limitations of the examination or subpar technique. An example of this would be if small foci of active bleeding/contrast extravasation following a motor vehicle accident are missed due to patient motion during the study, which degraded the image detail.

Kim and Mansfield also note that a finding can be missed because it is outside of the area of interest on an image, a phenomenon sometimes known as the *corner finding*. They also describe a new category of radiologist error, *satisfaction of report*, which occurs when a finding is missed due to overdependence on the previous examination's imaging report. An example would be if a highly respected colleague declared the liver to be normal, leading the second reader to overlook inhomogeneities that might actually reflect diffuse liver disease.

MANAGING ERROR: PUNITIVE, BLAMELESS, AND JUST CULTURE MODELS

Most experts agree that punishing people for making errors (i.e., a punitive culture) makes no sense and leads to errors being concealed or underdetected, ultimately undermining systemic learning from errors and finding meaningful solutions to systems-based problems. Initial efforts to change the punitive culture of medicine to a more blameless culture, where all persons involved in an error are held harmless, were resisted on the basis of concerns for fairness and self-policing of the profession. Social scientist David Marx proposed the *just culture* model, a system that blends the blameless culture with accountability for reckless behaviors on the part of individuals and focuses on the system in which workers are embedded. Under *just culture*, it is understood that human error is not to be punished, and people who unknowingly use potentially dangerous *workarounds* are to be coached not to do so in the future; however, if an individual's behavior is deemed reckless or careless under this system, punishment is indeed deemed to be appropriate.

Marx proposes three categories of manageable behaviors in the just culture model (Table 14.1): human error, at-risk behavior, and reckless behavior. Human error involves inadvertently doing something other than what was actually meant to be done. At-risk behavior occurs when shortcuts are taken to accomplish a task. Reckless behavior requires consciously taking a known inexcusable risk. In the just culture model, there is a proposed method for handling a specific error that is based on the classification discussed earlier, not on the severity of the event.

Another strategy to bring about system change in the hope of preventing future errors is known as the *forcing function*. A forcing function involves requiring that a specific action be completed prior to moving on to the next step. For example, medical records may not allow you to order a new drug without first acknowledging the patient's drug allergies.

It is generally agreed that creating *high-reliability systems*, ones that can be characterized as having very little process variation in how tasks are accomplished, is the most promising and effective strategy to reduce systems errors.

The topic of high-reliability systems in medicine and in manufacturing is a rich one and is the topic of Chapter 8; the interested reader is also directed to the following reading list.

SUGGESTED READINGS

Abujudeh HH, Boland GW, Kaewlai R, et al. Abdominal and pelvic computed tomography (CT) interpretation: discrepancy rates among experienced radiologists. *Eur Radiol*. 2010;20(8):1952-1957.

American Board of Radiology. *Noninterpretive Skills Resource Guide*. Available at: <http://theabr.org/sites/all/themes/abr-media/pdf/Noninterpretive_Skills_Domain_Specification_and_Resource_Guide.pdf>.

Berlin L. Accuracy of diagnostic procedures: has it improved over the past five decades? *Am J Roentgenol*. 2007;188:1173-1178.

Berlin L. Malpractice issues in radiology, hindsight bias. *Am J Roentgenol*. 2007;175:597-601.

Berlin L. Radiologic errors and malpractice: a blurry distinction. *Am J Roentgenol*. 2007;189(3):517-522.

Berlin L. Radiologic errors, past, present and future. *Diagnosis*. 2014;1(1).

Berner ES, Graber ML. Overconfidence as a cause of diagnostic error in medicine. *Am J Med*. 2008;121(5):S2-S23.

Brady A, O Laoide R, McCarthy P, McDermott R. Discrepancy and error in radiology: concepts, causes and consequences. *Ulster Med J*. 2012;81(1):3-9.

Brigham L, Mansouri M, Abujudeh H. Radiology report addenda: a self-report approach to error identification, quantification, and classification. *Am J Roentgenol*. 2015;205:1230-1239.

Brook O, O'Connell AM, Thornton E, Eisenberg R, Mendiratta-Lala M, Kruskal J. Anatomy and pathophysiology of errors in occurring in clinical radiology practice. *Radiographics*. 2010;30(5):1401-1410.

Bruno MA, Walker E, Abujudeh HH. Understanding and confronting our mistakes: the epidemiology of error in radiology and strategies for error reduction. *Radiographics*. 2015;35(6):1668-1676.

Cosby K, Croskerry P. Profiles in patient safety: authority gradients in medical error. *Acad Emerg Med*. 2004;11(12):1341-1345.

Croskerry P, Singhal G, Mamede S. Cognitive debiasing 2: impediments to and strategies for change. *BMJ Qual Saf*. 2013;22:ii65-ii72.

Garland LH. On the scientific evaluation of diagnostic procedures: presidential address thirty-fourth annual meeting of the Radiological Society of North America. *Radiology*. 1949;52:309-328.

Graber ML, Kissam S, Payne VL, et al. Cognitive interventions to reduce diagnostic error: a narrative review. *BMJ Qual Saf*. 2012;21(7):535-557.

Gunderman R. Biases in radiologic reasoning. *Am J Roentgenol*. 2013;192:561-564.

Institute of Medicine. *To Err Is Human*. Washington, DC: National Academies Press; 2000. Available at: <https://www.nap.edu/catalog/9728/to-err-is-human-building-a-safer-health-system>.

Kim YW, Mansfield LT. Fool me twice: delayed diagnoses in radiology with emphasis on perpetuated errors. *Am J Roentgenol*. 2014;202(3):465-470.

Kohn L, Corrigan J, Donaldson M, eds. *To Err Is Human: Building a Safer Health System*. Washington, DC: Committee on Quality of Health Care in America, Institute of Medicine, National Academies Press; 2000.

Krupinski EA, Berbaum KS, Caldwell RT, Schartz KM, Kim J. Long radiology workdays reduce detection and accommodation accuracy. *J Am Coll Radiol*. 2010;7:698-704.

Kundel HL. Perception errors in chest radiography. *Semin Respir Med*. 1989;19:203-210.

Larson D, Kruskal J, Krecke K, Donnelly L. Key concepts of patient safety in radiology. *Radiographics*. 2015;35:1677-1693.

Leape LL, Lawthers AG, Brennan TA, Johnson WG. Preventing medical injury. *Qual Rev Bull*. 1993;19(5):144-149.

Lee C, Nagy P, Weaver S, Newman-Toker D. Cognitive and system factors contributing to diagnostic errors in radiology. *Am J Roentgenol*. 2013;201:611-617.

Pinto A, Brunese L. Spectrum of diagnostic errors in radiology. *World J Radiol*. 2010;2(10):377-383.

Quekel LG, Kessels AG, Goei R, van Engelshoven JM. Miss rate of lung cancer on the chest radiograph in clinical practice. *Chest*. 1999;115(3):720-724.

Reason J. Human error: models and management. *BMJ*. 2000;320:768-770.

Siegle RL, Baram EM, Reuter SR, Clarke EA, Lancaster JL, McMahan CA. Rates of Disagreement in Imaging Interpretation in a Group of Community Hospitals. *Acad Radiol*. 1998;5:148-154.

Thammasitboon S, Thammasitboon S, Singhal G. Diagnosing diagnostic error. *Curr Probl Pediatr Adolesc Health Care*. 2013;43:227-231.

Tversky A, Kahneman D. Availability: a heuristic for judging frequency and probability. *Cognitive Psych*. 1973;5:207-232.

Wachter RM. Why diagnostic errors don't get any respect—and what can be done about them. *Health Aff*. 2010;29(9):1605-1610.

Chapter 15

Error Management and Reduction

Irina S. Filatova and Michael A. Bruno

INTRODUCTION

It is indeed human to err, yet unrealistic expectations for perfection persist throughout the practice of medicine. For radiology, the challenge has increased substantially in recent years due to rapidly advancing imaging technologies, increasing volumes of studies, each with massively increased volumes of images per study, as well as poor overall communication of needed clinical information from referring physicians, all of which contribute to an increased risk for radiologist error. If errors cannot be eliminated, then we must develop systems and procedures to reduce and manage them. If radiologists and their professional societies do not meet this challenge, governing bodies such as The Joint Commission (JC) will attempt to externally enforce the development of comprehensive error detection systems and procedures for active error prevention and remediation strategies.

In this chapter we discuss the various human factors involved in error occurrence in radiology, along with recommended strategies to address these factors with the aim of improving error detection, prevention, and finding the most effective ways to manage errors when they (inevitably) occur. We also focus on communication in radiology and strategies where improving the effectiveness of radiologic communication can lead to error reduction. The concept of a *sentinel event* response aimed at prevention of potential future harm is presented. We also wish to examine the types of occurrences that constitute an *error* in radiology and what methods exist that can be applied on a continuous basis to detect and prevent radiologic error in a rigorous fashion, including the role of (now mandated) peer review.

HUMAN FACTORS ENGINEERING

In a healthcare delivery system there are numerous daily interactions among workers, equipment, and environment, which ultimately lead to positive or negative outcomes in patient care. Human factors engineering is a relatively new but growing discipline in multiple fields, including healthcare. This discipline focuses on complex systems analysis and understanding of how a complex system, including people and machines, works in actual practice. The aim is to then design or optimize equipment and human-machine interfaces, with the human users' strengths and limitations in mind, to increase safety and minimize the risk of error in complex environments. This is done by *dissecting* complex activities or processes, breaking them down into smaller component tasks, and then assessing the individual demands of the operator at each stage, including things such as physical demands, skill demands, mental workload, team dynamics, and environmental adaptations (e.g., lighting, noise, distractors, ergonomics). This discipline attempts to pair human strengths and limitations in the performance of each task with the core design of the equipment and physical environment in which the task is performed.

Usability Testing

Usability testing refers to use of equipment and systems by trained *users* under *real-world* conditions to identify unintended flaws in these new technologies before they reach the user market. An example is a recent study that found an unexpected increase in patient mortality in a pediatric intensive care unit as a result of the use of a computerized order entry system (CPOE). Upon close evaluation, it was found that time demands resulting from a cumbersome order entry process were drawing clinicians away from the bedside, leading them to overlook signs of distress in their patients. Usability testing was later applied with simulated clinical scenarios and showed severe limitations of the installed CPOE.

Usability testing, as it applies to radiology, means testing the interaction between equipment and the user to find the best-suited equipment/technology or system to maximize ease and intuitive use to optimize radiologist performance. Usability in this sense is defined as the effectiveness, efficacy, and satisfaction with which a radiologist can interact with a system. In other words, *functionality* determines *usability*.

More simply put, usability testing answers the question: "How user-friendly is this system in achieving its desired purpose?"

Usability testing also impacts equipment design. Usability problems can arise not only when there is poor design of equipment but also when there are poor instructions for its use. One published example (see the Suggested Readings) is an implantable inferior vena cava (IVC) filter system that can be inserted by a femoral or brachial approach. Depending on the approach, the filter unit must be attached to the introducer sheath in a particular orientation for correct placement, and incorrect attachment of the filter (e.g., using the brachial attachment for a femoral approach procedure) can result in an incorrect orientation of the filter within the patient's IVC and thus lead to potential for harm by dislodgement or nonfunction. The authors point to the need for very clear documentation of how the system must be used and further suggest that usability problems in the future may be detected by use of a shared online database of users, as long as there is frequent database review by these users.

Workarounds

Workarounds are perhaps the most common class of methods in use to accomplish an activity when existing methods are cumbersome or are not working well. This involves both single instances and situations where practitioners consistently bypass established policies and safety procedures, increasing the risk of errors and patient harm. Although the goal is generally to get work done more efficiently, workarounds can be dangerous and illustrate the need for good system design. Flawed and poorly designed systems that force workers to spend an excessive amount of time or effort to complete a task when all safety steps are followed precisely lead workers to cut corners and find alternatives of varying effectiveness and safety. The identification of workarounds within a system can be a signal to leaders that a faulty process is in place.

Workarounds are often created spontaneously and used with good intentions by skilled staff to promote patient comfort or speed up medical interventions in an emergency situation. When cumbersome systems exist, healthcare workers may quickly determine that it is not always practical (or safe) in an emergency situation to follow all steps and comply with the prescribed process; these workers will generally find ways to circumvent the system to accomplish tasks more efficiently. There is substantial risk, however, of unintended downstream consequences: no matter how carefully done, and even with the best intentions, the use of workarounds promotes error and compromises patient safety, partly by overriding safety features that are built into systems. This is especially true in emergent situations with high tension when human attention to detail may be suboptimal.

In most instances, workarounds do not result in patient harm, and the increased efficiency of their use creates a type of *reward* for the creator of the workaround; there is the positive feedback of enhanced efficiency or ease, which reinforces the workaround's use, leading to complacency, which only serves to enhance their latent risks. An effective workaround can also serve to prevent the underlying system problems from being fully recognized and addressed.

Workarounds, however, can have positive effects. They can be viewed as a *trigger warning* for the existence of an underling system failure that requires attention and resolution. Analyzing a workaround process may lead to definitive solutions for more global issues within a poorly functioning or cumbersome system. It can identify problems with existing technologies or uncover unnecessarily complex processes. For example, it was discovered at a Veterans Affairs hospital that the staff was forced to use informal patient identification processes because barcodes on patient armbands were not water resistant and easily washed off. This example demonstrates how a significant patient identification error could easily occur as the result of working around an ineffective, unusable system. Addressing the underlying system failure, particularly by applying usability testing for the armbands, would resolve both the system failure and obviate the incentives for a potentially dangerous workaround.

In other words, a *workaround* process is most often an answer to the question, "How can I make this cumbersome, time consuming, or complicated system more user-friendly so that I can do my job more efficiently?" Usability testing can be employed in a scenario where the use of workarounds is identified. For example, when a new piece of equipment or a new system is introduced into the work environment, there perhaps ought to be a *beta testing* period where the new system is used by a limited number of staff to identify potential usability nuisances and provide feedback to the institution before the equipment or system is introduced to the larger group.

Forcing Functions

A forcing function is an aspect of system design that prevents an undesirable function from being performed or allows its performance only after another function is performed first, such as when a prefunction is needed to make the main intended function safe. A simple example of a forcing function in commonly used technology is how a microwave oven is designed not to function while the door is open. This forces the user to close the microwave door first. By applying principles of human factors engineering in error management and prevention, the design of forcing functions represents an attempt to anticipate the types of error that may occur and incorporate a function or failsafe directly into the design of products and processes that may prevent the occurrence of that error. (One must be careful not to create a function that only serves to force a workaround, however.)

Forcing functions are often embedded in medical equipment, from small syringes to complex magnetic resonance imaging (MRI) scanning machines. Although some make this equipment more cumbersome to use and require specialized training, this type of human factors engineering works to ensure patient safety as long as the forcing function mechanism is intact. One such example is the use of a Luer-Lok system for syringes and indwelling lines, which must be matched to catheters before an infusion is possible. Another common example is how the connectors for anesthetic and oxygen gas lines are incompatible with each other, so it is not possible to inadvertently misconnect them.

An example of a forcing function related to radiology equipment is the use of automatic exposure control (AEC) in both film screen and digital radiography. The purpose of AEC is to limit patient radiation dose and still generate the most optimal image by controlling exposure time. An AEC system uses radiation detectors in the form of ionization chambers (usually three to a system), which are calibrated based on phantoms and positioned in a specific orientation. AEC reduces radiation exposure by controlling the total milliampere second (mAs) output of the x-ray tube.

Another example of a forcing function, designed specifically for use in procedural environments, is the use of a preprocedural *time-out*. Instituting this practice forces performers to stop what they are doing and focus on the pertinent details of the case about to start, including having the correct patient, performing the requested procedure, and confirming optimized laboratory studies and presence of any possible limitations such as drug allergies. This also focuses the attention of multiple attendees present in the room for the case and enables someone to speak up if the presented information is incorrect to his or her knowledge before the case is started. This *universal protocol* is a requirement for all hospital procedures today.

Simply put, a forcing function is similar to a constraint because a constraint makes it more difficult to do the wrong thing; a forcing function at least theoretically makes it impossible to do the wrong thing. Employing the concept of the forcing function answers the following questions: How do I make this system impossible to mess up? What steps can I anticipate and pre-perform or take out of the hands of the operator? How can I make my system's safety more operator independent?

Standardization

Human factors engineering was responsible for bringing about many of the equipment and processes standards that we enjoy today in various medical domains. A key concept is that equipment and processes should be standardized whenever possible to increase reliability, improve information flow, minimize cross-training needs, and prevent operator confusion. Consistency with equipment function, for example, prevents potential for error due to alterations from the usual or expected workflow. It also allows staff to alternate between sites without learning how to use different equipment.

Although standardization of equipment is optimal, it may or may not be possible in a large institution, which may have equipment that differs by age and by manufacturer due to economic considerations such as contracting variability over time. It is, however, always possible to strive for standardization of processes. Constantly following the same steps over time minimizes variation and has been shown to improve both efficacy and safety. Standardizing processes ensures that the same processes are followed by different staff working in a rotation or in a changing environment. It builds resiliency into a system. More importantly, it allows for detection of variation from the norm more easily, which can trigger closer analysis and error prevention. The use of checklists and templates can help to promote standardization in radiology.

Checklists ensure consistency of procedural steps and communication. They allow for a concrete listing of required information so that all parties involved in a procedure are completely aware of the circumstances and can speak up if something seems off. They also allow for organized and readily available lists of proceedings in an emergency or high-risk situation. Some groups even advocate the printing of resuscitation or contrast reaction steps on cards with lanyards that are worn by primary staff, so this information is readily available when needed.

In surgery, institution of checklists prior to operative procedures has been shown to reduce mortality from 1.5% to 0.8% and complications from 11% to 7% (see Suggested Readings). Radiology checklists are useful in both diagnostic and procedural settings. In diagnostic radiology, TJC mandates the use of magnetic resonance (MR)

and computed tomography (CT) screening questionnaires. These questionnaires are designed to detect potential safety issues prior to scan administration so that they can be corrected or scanning prevented where potential harm may outweigh the benefits of the scan. Potential safety issues screened by these questionnaires include contrast material allergies, pregnancy and breast-feeding status, renal function, medication interactions and allergies, intravenous access, and presence of a cardiac pacemaker or aneurysm clips. In procedure-based radiology practices, such as interventional services, drainage services, aspiration, and injection services, checklists are used in the form of *time-outs* with an actual pause prior to the procedure and active participation in the *surgery safety checklist* by all team members, which is also mandated by TJC. This checklist includes a review of patients' identification, allergies, correct procedure, site of procedure, labs, collection of specimens, and medications that must be discontinued and those that must be administered.

The use of *report templates* is a form of standardization of the radiology report and has generated much controversy in recent years among radiologists but is gaining traction throughout the country. Although TJC recommends use of templates for reporting, it is not yet mandated, except in reporting of mammography results. Reports written using templates have been shown to have more clarity and consistency of content, leading to improved clinician understanding. For example, in one study evaluating the introduction of templated radiology reporting for presurgical staging of pancreatic cancer, surgeons reported an increase in presence of all information needed for surgical planning in radiology reports (an increase from 69% to 98% in structured reporting, compared to an increase from 25% to 43% in unstructured reporting, which was used as a comparison standard). Currently, several radiologic societies, including the Radiological Society of North America (RSNA) and the American College of Radiology (ACR), offer sample report templates in their Breast Imaging Reporting and Data System and Liver Imaging Reporting and Data System in an effort to standardize the reporting process across the nation. However, each radiology practice remains free to implement their own versions of templates as appropriate for their own specific practices.

Some authors in radiology have suggested that a checklist approach to imaging interpretation ought to decrease error rates in radiology. The use of a checklist function embedded in a template might well help to prevent error due to human perception where a finding is simply missed, by reminding the radiologist to look for it to fill in a blank in the template. A radiology checklist in this scenario might include common diagnoses and misdiagnoses typically seen on a specific body part or condition so that these are always checked prior to finalizing a radiology report.

Resiliency Efforts

Resiliency effort is an aspect of human factors engineering that focuses on risk management, anticipation of error, and recovery from error. Resilience, as the word might suggest, defines the adaptive capability of a system and its ability to modify itself and continue functioning, by modifying risk both *prior to* and *after* a safety event occurs.

In a standard model of risk management, an event occurs, is detected, is analyzed, and then corrective functions are implemented to prevent further such events. In a resilient system, an impending safety error is detected before patient harm occurs. Anticipation, early detection, and response to error are a dynamic process in this kind of system. Resilience, therefore, is an intrinsic ability of a system to adjust its functions prior to, during, and following disturbances, so it can sustain operation under both expected and unexpected conditions. According to Hollnagel et al., there are four essential capabilities of a resilient system:

Knowing what to *do*: being able to respond to regular and irregular variability and disturbances by either adjusting the way things are done or activating ready-made responses.

Knowing what to *look for*: being able to monitor what changes or what may change in the near future so much that it will require a response.

Knowing what to *expect*: being able to anticipate potential disruptions or changing conditions in the future.

Knowing what has *happened*: being able to learn from experience.

An example of a resilient system in radiology is the early detection of high radiation exposure from a CT scanner and either repairing the equipment or revising CT protocols to lower radiation exposure before any patient injury occurs.

To create resiliency in a system there must be consistent, open, and nonthreatening reporting of safety data. Barriers to reporting safety issues hinder the ability of an organization to achieve resilience. The following have been recognized as some of the common barriers to reporting: an individual's hesitance to admit failure, fear of punishment or retribution, failure to recognize the importance of reporting anomalies that do not result in actual patient harm, and existence of authority gradients. In addition, it is essential to create a safe culture of reporting where the person who identifies an error or a potential source of error feels comfortable and empowered to voice concerns without fear of retaliation. All high-reliability organizations feature such an open *safety culture*, and all display resiliency.

Ergonomics

With the ever-increasing volume of radiologic studies performed and read, the increasing demands for production of relative value units (RVUs) by radiologists, and pressure for rapid report turnaround times, physical stresses on radiologists become a significant factor. The science of ergonomics has therefore recently come to play a major role in the workplace and workflow design for radiologists.

One of the most obvious ergonomic features of a radiology practice is the use of low levels of ambient light in the reading room to optimize visual comfort and performance. The use of office-style lighting or complete lack of light, except for light from the monitor, has been shown to reduce diagnostic efficacy. Inappropriate balance between ambient room light and monitor lighting has been shown to contribute to radiologist fatigue and decreases both efficacy and accuracy. Kruskal et al. have

recommended that the reading room light is kept to low levels and that monitor light is kept at 25 foot-lamberts or more. In addition, to address fatigue and eye strain and for optimal visualization, a combination of indirect overhead lighting and local task lighting should ideally be used. Moveable partitions should be installed between workstations, and walls should be made dark to avoid reflection. In addition to screen resolution and lighting, effects of eye strain are also related to screen flicker and glare, working distance and angles, and decreased blink rate due to observing a monitor. Symptoms include irritation and eye pain, blurry or double vision and headache, and fatigue, burnout, increased perceptual error, and decreased reaction time. To help reduce eye strain, one should optimize the lighting in the work environment as discussed and sit at an appropriate distance and angle from the monitor, read for less than 7 hours a day, and take at least one break per hour.

In addition to eye strain, musculoskeletal ergonomics is considered for optimal reading performance. Musculoskeletal complaints include general fatigue, neck and back pain, carpal tunnel syndrome, and cubical tunnel syndrome. Carpal tunnel syndrome occurs more often among radiologists than among other nonradiology physicians and other computer-related fields such as office staff. Carpal tunnel syndrome is associated with dorsiflexion of the wrist and ulnar deviation of the hand. Even the constant spinning of the mouse wheel, commonly done in radiology reading rooms, has been shown to produce increased rates of carpal tunnel syndrome.

COMMUNICATION

Communication is an essential and integral part of the practice of radiology because interpretation of radiologic findings is incomplete without a structured way of presenting the findings to the requesting parties. An effective communication according to the ACR should strive to support the ordering clinician in providing optimal patient care, be timely, and minimize the risk of error. Communication in radiology takes on a variety of forms. Standard communication involves the creation and delivery of the written radiology report.

Report Clarity

The radiology report is the final product of the department of radiology and a primary method of communication with the requesting party and the patient. The analysis of many lawsuits filed against radiologists, some successful, led the ACR in 1991 to publish the first set of Standard Guidelines for Communication. There have since been multiple revisions (the most recent in 2014) that attempt to establish minimal standards for the content and structure of the radiology report. The ACR suggests that radiologists' written reports should include all of the following: demographics, including facility and location, patient identifiers, examination parameters (type of exam, date, time, and date and time of dictation), and the name of the requesting party; relevant clinical information; the procedures and materials used (contrast, other medications, radiation dose); findings; and potential limitations (such as sensitivity and specificity of the examination). The ACR also mandates that the report answer the clinical question and provide comparison to prior studies that are available. Finally, the radiology report should contain a final impression—a clinical interpretation of the findings and its potential implications, diagnosis or differential diagnosis, and suggestions for further management steps. This section should also report on any pertinent adverse reactions if they occurred.

Many methods have been suggested to improve the clarity of reporting. The most prominent has been the suggestion for institutionalizing the use of reporting templates. This practice promotes standardization of reports with respect to content, allows residents in training to know what content is important and not to be overlooked, helps practicing radiologists not to mistakenly omit important sections of the report, and allows clinicians who become familiar with the report structure to quickly identify the pertinent sections of the report to find the information they need.

As noted earlier, structured reporting is not yet the standard way of reporting even complex studies in most radiology departments and practices and remains a controversial topic among radiologists. Most clinicians and radiologists confirm their preference for structured reporting. One study, by Bosmans et al., found that 84.5% (592 of 701) of clinicians and 65.7% (88 of 134) of radiologists would opt for itemized reporting. Moreover, two-thirds of the radiologists and the referring clinicians would favor the use of a standardized lexicon for radiologic reporting. Since the report of the COVER and ROVER surveys in 2011, more and more movement toward some sort of standard reporting, at least within an institution, has been made, and residents are being trained in standardizing report organization and lexicon in each critical section.

The *American Journal of Roentgenology* (AJR) regularly addresses improvement in report clarity in their column on language at the end of every issue. For example, the March 2016 issue suggests clearly stating "no change" in the impression of the report if that is what the findings show. Other statements such as "no significant change, no interval change, stable" can mean different things to different specialty clinicians and can baffle some patients who increasingly read the radiology reports via patient online portals. The lexicon suggested by AJR is to report, "There is no change given differences in imaging technique" as a standard lexicon of reporting. Other authors have suggested putting a high premium on proofreading and editing every report before publishing for the reader so that such slips as "The liver is normal with metastatic disease," where the report author may have meant "without metastatic disease," do not take place! There also have been warnings regarding the errors typical of voice-recognition transcription, especially when using prefixes that can be misunderstood by such systems; for example, "aseptic" may be mistranscribed as "a septic." Such a simple, small error, if it leads to a clinical misunderstanding, can potentially cause severe consequences for patients.

Critical Results Reporting

Routine reporting of imaging findings is communicated through the usual channels established by the institution for such communication, such as a written radiology report published in a patient's chart, through the imaging interface, or printed and inserted in the medical record manually. However, in emergent or atypical situations, the radiologist should make an effort to deliver imaging findings in a more expedited manner. Several successful lawsuits have been won against radiologists when worrisome findings on an imaging report were not communicated to the clinician in such an atypical situation, and as a result, adverse patient events ensued. In such cases, radiologists were held responsible for patient harm caused by the resulting delay in treatment. Courts have consistently opined that the burden of delivery of critical results rests with the interpreting radiologist.

The ACR, therefore, has made recommendations for critical results reporting, noting that such results should be reported directly to the ordering party or to the patient if the ordering clinician cannot be reached. Such communication should take place by phone or in person. These methods guarantee the receipt of communication and that the message is understood. Such confirmation of receipt of the message is an essential element in critical results reporting.

According to the ACR guidelines, there are several situations that require this sort of *nonroutine* communication of critical results directly to the clinician in addition to the standard written radiology report. These situations include:

> *findings which require immediate intervention, findings that are discrepant with a preceding interpretation of the same examination and where failure to act may adversely affect patient health, and findings that the interpreting physician reasonably believes may be seriously adverse to the patient's health and may not require immediate attention but, if not acted on, may worsen over time and possibly result in an adverse patient outcome.*

Other authors further assign levels of importance based on urgency for communication of findings that require intervention. In one system, a level 1 finding is one that requires immediate, urgent intervention (e.g., tension pneumothorax, leaking aortic aneurysm, cerebral hemorrhage, pulmonary aneurysm). A level 2 finding is one that requires urgent intervention (i.e., within 2–3 days) to avert patient morbidity or mortality (e.g., intraabdominal abscess or impending pathologic fracture). A level 3 finding is something that is new or unexpected and that can lead to patient harm if not acted upon but is not immediately life threatening (e.g., new lung nodule or solid renal mass).

TJC first published their National Patient Safety Goals (NPSG) in 2002. These are renewed yearly, and compliance with them is now a requirement for hospitals to maintain TJC accreditation. One NPSG requires that communication of critical results be done in a timely manner with acknowledgment of the communication by the receiving party. However, TJC does not define any specific mandate or consensus for an appropriate method of communicating these results or any specific timeline for doing so. The implementation of these communications, therefore, is determined by the particular institution or practice, although telephone contact is currently the most commonly used method. Once the communication has occurred, proper documentation of the communication event is necessary. Usually this is inserted directly into the written radiology report. Four elements must generally be included: name, time, date, and write-down-read-back. For the name identifier, the use of first and last name is recommended, but first name and job description are also acceptable (e.g., Nurse Betty of the South ICU night team). The use of first name and general descriptor alone (Nurse Betty) is not sufficient. It is best if the receiving party writes down the communicated result, but many times this may be impractical. Read-back of the critical finding by the recipient party is perhaps the best way to determine whether the result was appropriately understood. Some even suggest the communicating party should then ask the receiver for a follow-up plan, particularly if speaking to the treating clinician. For example, one might state, "Findings are highly suspicious for ovarian torsion. Is there a plan to take this patient to the operating room?" The perceived response to this type of follow-up question may give the communicating party a better perspective on whether the implications of the communicated critical result were perceived and understood by the receiving party.

It is also recommended to perform a periodic check for compliance with critical results communications policies. One can initially settle for about a 90% compliance rate but should strive to slowly raise the rate to 100%. Data on critical results compliance should be collected, analyzed, and reported by departmental quality committees.

In addition to this, some radiology report communications, specifically those of mammography reports, are heavily regulated. For example, the US Food and Drug Administration requires communication of mammography findings to the referring provider and directly to the patient, through the Mammography Quality Standards Act (MQSA) of 1994. In addition to providing the report to the ordering clinician through the usual channels, a report in lay terms must be provided to the patient within 30 days of the examination, no matter what the findings are. In the case of critical mammography findings (Breast Imaging Reporting and Data System [BI-RADS] 4 and 5 lesions), an immediate and direct communication to the ordering clinician must be made. The patient will still receive a report summary within 30 days of the examination. In case the patient is self-referred, the breast imaging center must refer the patient with abnormal findings to a healthcare provider able and willing to provide further care to the patient.

Verbal Communication

Effective communication between patients and caregivers has been shown to decrease medical costs, increase patient satisfaction, and have a positive effect on health management outcomes, whereas at least 30% of patient dissatisfaction with their care is related to incomplete, abrasive, or ineffective communication. Although most radiology communication takes place in the form of a written radiology report, sometimes it is necessary to communicate urgent findings verbally, via phone or in person, as discussed earlier, with proper documentation of such communication then appearing in the radiology report. There is also a place for informal verbal communication in the form of a *curbside consult* or *wet read*, which may occur in clinical interdisciplinary conferences, when radiologists provide a preliminary verbal interpretation prior to publication of an official report, provide informal verbal interpretation of outside or prior studies, or provide on-the-spot interpretations at the time of imaging (such as in the trauma bay during level 1 trauma cases). These formal or informal verbal communications often occur without benefit of later written documentation. As such, informal communications of this type contain inherent risks that the information shared may be misunderstood or misremembered. It is encouraged that radiologists who provide these types of informal communications document what was discussed and recommended from their radiologists' perspective contemporaneously. A system for formal interpretation of outside studies as opposed to *curbside consults* is also encouraged to minimize misunderstandings, which may easily arise from informal, unscheduled interactions.

Informed Consent

Obtaining a patient's informed consent for a procedure is a specialized type of communication. Many physicians are familiar with the process of informed consent. In clinical practice and in research, this practice is widespread, providing documentation of patients' or subjects' understanding and agreement to the proposed intervention or study. In radiology, consent is typically obtained before administration of intravenous contrast, before interventional procedures, and before administration of sedation. However, there has been some ongoing discussion among radiologists in recent years that consent also needs to take place regarding medical radiation exposure in noninterventional imaging as well.

The concept of informed consent refers to the actual discussion between healthcare provider and patient. This process should provide complete information to allow the patient to understand the implications of the decision and to allow the patient to make the best, most well-informed decision. This is, however, not always feasible in practice due to study volumes and the time required to allow for such sufficient and comprehensive discussion regarding each examination. There was a joint proposal published by the RSNA and by members of the International Atomic Energy Agency and select European imaging specialists that an informed-consent discussion ought to be provided to patients for studies likely to expose patients to at least 1 mSv of ionizing radiation or more. Included in the discussion should be risks of radiation exposure, a risk-benefit analysis for performing the examination, and discussion of alternative means of imaging without the use of ionizing radiation, such as ultrasound or MRI. This proposal specified that only higher-dose studies be discussed at this time because the sheer volume of imaging studies with much less radiation exposure and much less overall risk would overwhelm the system if such discussion were mandated with every such minor study. The authors suggested that it would be ideal for radiologists to take an active role in initiating these discussions with patients, rather than await the imposition of governmental regulations to do so.

Penn State Radiology's "Failsafe" Program

In recent years, there has been a substantial increase in the use of imaging in the emergency department (ED) setting. This has resulted in radiologists detecting a large number of *incidental findings* that are unrelated to the patient's acute ED visit but that require follow-up and evaluation. Typically, such follow-up is *not* provided via the ED, and patients often fail to seek follow-up for these findings (if they become aware of them) after their discharge from the ED. Our radiology practice typically provides a written report detailing such findings only to the requesting physician, in this case an emergency physician, and not to the patient's primary care physician (PCP) of record, who often cannot be identified at the time of the ED visit.

This common scenario creates a unique type of communication challenge for radiologists and is a significant potential source of a communication error. Patients may be lulled into false complacency that no problem exists because they believe the ED would have taken care of whatever their workup revealed. At the Penn State Milton S. Hershey Medical Center, we have developed our own stopgap communication method in recognition of the problem, in which we notify patients directly by mail (and increasingly, by phone) that there were findings from their ED studies that require nonurgent follow-up (as urgent findings are directly communicated to the ED and handled during the patient's visit).

Our Failsafe Letter (Fig. 15.1) was developed in concert with a team of stakeholders from the Departments of Radiology, Emergency Medicine, Family and Community Medicine, the office of General Counsel for Penn State, and the Chief Quality and Safety Officer. Each letter is personally signed by a radiologist; it is identified as a communication from the radiology department and notifies the patient that a finding was made on a radiology study. It also states that the patient's own physician of record, and not the radiologist or the emergency physician, is the provider who can best decide with him or her what the appropriate follow-up for

---

PENNSTATE HERSHEY
Milton S. Hershey
Medical Center

[Date]

Dear [Patient name, *e.g.,* "Mr. Smith"],

I am writing to you today because you recently had an imaging study in the Dept. of Radiology here at Penn State Hershey Medical Center (PSHMC) as part of your visit to our Emergency Department. Your study was interpreted by a PSHMC radiology doctor, who felt there were findings that may require follow up.

The PSHMC radiologist who reviewed your study does not know the details of your health history, and therefore can only give general recommendations; it is up to your primary care doctor to customize those recommendations and make a follow-up plan that is right for you. Therefore, we are writing to ask you to please contact your primary doctor directly and inform them that they need to evaluate the findings related to your recent radiology test for follow-up.

If your primary care doctor is here at PSHMC, he or she can obtain the full Radiology report and decide what, if any, follow-up is right for you. If your doctor is not affiliated with PSHMC, you can obtain a copy of our report yourself by contacting our Health Information Services Department, at 717-531-8055. If you plan to make an appointment with your doctor to discuss the findings of the radiology study, you should request a copy of the report at least seven (7) days prior to your appointment, so that you will be sure to have it with you when you see your doctor.

If you do not have a primary care physician at this time, you may obtain a referral to a provider from our Department of Family and Community Medicine by calling the PSHMC Care Line at 717-531-6955 or if you are outside of our local calling area, you can use our toll-free Care Line number, which is 1-800-243-1455. The Care Line is available 24 hours a day, seven days a week.

Thank you for allowing us to participate in your care.

Sincerely,

[Committee Member], M.D.
[Academic title]
Department of Radiology, Hershey Medical Center

FIG. 15.1 **SAMPLE FAILSAFE LETTER.**

this finding ought to be. Each letter is addressed to a specific patient and mailed to his or her address of record, and the radiologists' signature is original for each letter; the letter content is not otherwise customized, and the letter does not inform the patient what the finding of concern is nor what should be done about it. The Failsafe Program has been very enthusiastically received by our clinical colleagues here in Hershey because it increases safety without compromising their autonomy. The impact of this relatively new program is currently being evaluated.

SENTINEL EVENTS

A sentinel event, according to TJC, is an "unexpected occurrence involving death or serious physical or psychological injury, or risk thereof." The term *serious injury* refers to loss of limb or function. The phrase *risk thereof* refers to any event where a recurrence, if it were to occur, would cause death or serious harm and therefore must be addressed immediately.

A sentinel event is not the same as a medical error. Not all sentinel events occur as a result of error, and not all errors result in sentinel events. An error is defined as "failure of a planned action to be completed as intended, or use of the wrong plan to achieve an aim." A sentinel event, on the other hand, is an adverse "unexpected occurrence," including simply the *risk* of such an event. A sentinel event may result from equipment failure or system failure where no misjudgment on the part of the operator occurred, but patient harm resulted or may have resulted. For example, a sentinel event might be extravasation of contrast in a patient's extremity (with or without causing tissue damage).

Many of the sentinel events in radiology are related to interventional and procedural radiology; however, events related to radiation dose, MRI safety, radiology reports, and notification of results are also considered. Examples of sentinel events include occurrences such as the following:

- Foreign body retention (e.g., a broken fragment of wire after catheter pull)
- Fall
- Burn (patient develops a thermal injury after radiofrequency ablation; patient develops a radiation burn in a malfunctioning or maladjusted CT scanner)
- Wrong interventional procedure performed, wrong site, or wrong patient
- Medication error
- Use of a device with function other than intended or use of a contaminated device

Radiology is a unique field for sentinel events because there is a possibility for occurrence of not only events that are immediately identifiable or identifiable within a reasonably short interval of time (such as performing a wrong intervention on a wrong patient) but also adverse events that may manifest much later. For example, TJC in 2006 added an item to the list of reviewable events under the Sentinel Event Policy. This item was "Prolonged fluoroscopy with cumulative dose >1500 rads to a single field or any delivery of radiotherapy to the wrong region or >25% above the planned dose." This type of event can be associated with death or major permanent loss, which may occur months or years after the event.

By definition, sentinel events are preventable, and when such an event occurs, or when its potential is identified, the overall organization is required to conduct a root cause analysis (discussed in other chapters of this textbook) to analyze, learn from, and develop strategies for prevention of patient harm, even before any outcomes of the event are evident. All such events are generally reportable, to state regulators, TJC, or both. TJC publishes the *Sentinel Event Alert Bulletin* and distributes it to all TJC-accredited institutions. Each *Alert Bulletin* identifies a specific event, describes its common underlying causes, and suggests steps to prevent such occurrences. These sentinel events are geared toward all of medical and surgical practice including radiology. Each published event addresses a potential problem that has occurred and may reoccur and therefore attempts to alert other institutions and providers before similar events have a chance to occur at those facilities.

FINDING ERRORS/TRIGGER FUNCTIONS

What Is Fair to Call an Error?

Diagnostic errors in radiology are as common as in any medical field and can occur in multiple phases of care provided within the radiology department. Mistakes have been made in patient identification, study protocol or protocol execution, radiation dose, image interpretation, communication of findings, and errors in radiologic interventions. Of these, arguably the most important is image interpretation because it has a strong connection with patient health outcomes.

However, it is not always clear what is *fair* to call an *error in interpretation*. Radiologic study interpretation is as much an art as it is a science, as is any other medical subspecialty where trained personnel are called on to make decisions based on the information they possess. There is wide variability in medical subspecialties. This variability is due in part to the high degree of natural variation in both normal anatomy and pathology. A *trigger function* is something that allows early detection of such errors, before patent harm ensues.

There are three possible sources of error in image interpretation: (1) differences in observation (detection), (2) differences in interpretation of a perceived finding (interpretation), and (3) different thresholds of concern about a perceived abnormality (level of confidence). Errors differ from normal variability because they imply an *incorrect* interpretation *when a correct one is possible* and *variability is low*. Thus, error is only possible in cases where the correct interpretation is without dispute and not subject to great variability.

Peer Review

One common method to improve quality of radiology performance and reduce error in medicine in general is to conduct peer review in a regular and nonthreatening, nonpunitive process. The practice of medicine has long relied on the peer-review process to uphold its professional standards and maintain a high quality of care. Peer review is now a requirement of TJC to ensure ongoing quality healthcare delivery; however, the methods employed by radiology practices are highly variable.

In addition to TJC quality requirements and other government and professional organizations (such as Medicare, the American Board of Medical Specialties, and the

American Board of Radiology maintenance of certification programs), reasons to perform periodic peer review include: (1) maintenance of professional standards (results of peer review can be an incentive for accuracy and consistency of individual physician performance) and (2) institutional medial staff obligations (it is an obligation of the medical staff as a whole to take mutual accountability for quality).

The peer-review process is just one way to measure and enhance quality and consistency among radiologists. Over the years, this process has evolved and has been refined to where current peer-review programs are generally conducted by committees of radiologists, and decisions about the significance of discrepant reviews are made by consensus. This makes the peer-review process more fair and credible. An ideal peer-review system should be nonpunitive, consistent, and fair to those being evaluated and the evaluator. There should also be timely feedback of the peer-review results. The process should steer away from putting all the effort on the department chair or any single individual having to discuss matters of error, which may have stigma of emotion attached. The steps in peer review should include case identification, case screening and assignment of a radiologist reviewer, the review of the case by the assigned reviewer and the review committee, input from the involved radiologist, committee decision, communication of findings, and plan for improvement or follow-up.

Peer review can also be achieved via outsourced mechanisms in the event a practice is too small to form a peer-review committee or when there is doubt of obtaining an unbiased or objective internal peer-review process. RADPEER is a web-based program created and implemented by the ACR to assist member practices in the process of conducting peer review. The program is based on interpretation of prior imaging (when available) by the reviewer engaged in current study interpretation. The reviewer scores the prior report based on a predetermined scoring system based on the reviewer's impression of the conspicuity of the findings and the accuracy of the report. The automated system provided by ACR (which is fee-based) collects the data and provides the practice with a summary of statistics from data collected from all member practices.

CONCLUSION

In summary, error management in radiology is a complex, multifactorial process involving careful examination of ongoing practices in the setting of continuous process improvement. Managing and preventing errors involve the continuous examination of human factors involved in error occurrence, as well as all system factors that increase the potential for error, from user-unfriendly computer systems to ergonomically uncomfortable chairs. By understanding and analyzing clues that problems exist, such as widespread use of workarounds, radiology practices can be proactive in managing risks, rather than reactive in dealing with failures and patient harm.

It is also essential to understand and appreciate the power of good, effective written and verbal communication in radiology, which carries its own great potential for error reduction through increasing report clarity and improving verbal communication between the interpreter and the clinician and documentation of such events. Appropriate response to sentinel events, a reliable peer-review system, and development of *trigger tools* to allow early detection of errors are also valuable in this effort.

By arming ourselves with detailed knowledge of the inner workings of our own systems, by being committed to pursuing our work with constant vigilance, and by eagerly implementing evidence-based best practices, we believe that it is possible for radiology practices to continuously reduce errors and enhance patient safety—which is, after all, our primary responsibility as physicians.

SUGGESTED READINGS

Boland GW. From herding cats toward best practices: standardizing the radiologic work process. *AJR Am J Roentgenol.* 2009;193:1593–1595.

Bosmans JM, Weyler JJ, De Schepper AM, Parizel PM. The radiology report as seen by radiologists and referring clinicians: results of the COVER and ROVER surveys. *Radiology.* 2011;259(1):184–195.

Brook OR, Brook A, Vollmer CM, Kent TS, Sanchez N, Pedrosa I. Structured reporting of multiphasic CT for pancreatic cancer: potential effect on staging and surgical planning. *Radiology.* 2015;274(2):464–472.

Cockton G, Lavery D, Woolrych A. Inspection-based evaluations. In: Jacko JA, Sears A, eds. *The Human-Computer Interaction Handbook.* Mahwah, NJ: Lawrence Erlbaum; 2003:1119–1138.

Donaldson MS. An overview of to err is human: re-emphasizing the message of patient safety. In: Hughes RG, ed. *Patient Safety and Quality: An Evidence-Based Handbook for Nurses.* Rockville, MD: Agency for Healthcare Research and Quality (US); 2008.

Ellenbogen PH. Standardization in radiology—protocols, procedures, and reports: best for patients and providers. *J Am Coll Radiol.* 2013;10(9):641.

Gawande A. *The Checklist Manifesto: How to Get Things Right.* New York, NY: Metropolitan Books/Henry Holt; 2009.

Goo JM, Choi JY, Im JG, et al. Effect of monitor luminance and ambient light on observer performance in soft-copy reading of digital chest radiographs. *Radiology.* 232(3):762–766.

Harisinghani MG, Blake MA, Saksena M, et al. Importance and effects of altered workplace ergonomics in modern radiology suites. *Radiographics.* 2004;24:615–627.

Haynes AB, Weiser TG, Berry WR, et al. A surgical safety checklist to reduce morbidity and mortality in a global population. *N Engl J Med.* 2009;360(5):491–499.

Herrmann TL, Fauber TL, Gill J, et al. *Best Practices in Digital Radiography.* Albuquerque, NM: American Society of Radiologic Technologists; 2012.

Hoang J. If there is no change, just say so. *J Am Coll Radiol.* 2016;13(3):236.

Hollnagel E, Pariès J, Woods DD, Wreathall J. Epilogue—RAG, the resilience analysis grid. In: Hollnagel E, Pariès J, Woods DD, Wreathall J, eds. *Resilience Engineering in Practice: A Guidebook.* Famham: Ashgate Publishing; 2011:277–280.

Hussain S. Communication of radiology results. In: Abujudeh H, Bruno M, eds. *Quality and Safety in Radiology.* New York, NY: Oxford University Press; 2012:59–67.

ISO 9241-11. *Ergonomic requirements for office work with visual display terminals (VDTs)—Part 11: guidance on usability.* Geneva: International Organization for Standardization; 1998.

Jorritsma W, Cnossen F, van Ooijen PMA. Merits of usability testing for PACS selection. In: Jorritsma W, ed. *Human-Computer Interaction in Radiology.* Groningen: Rijksuniversiteit Groningen; 2016:13–32. [Adapted from Jorritsma W, Cnossen F, Van Ooijen PMA. Merits of usability testing for PACS selection. *Int J Med Inform.* 2014;83:27–36.

Kim YW, Mansfield LT. Fool me twice: delayed diagnoses in radiology with emphasis on perpetuated errors. *AJR Am J Roentgenol.* 2014;202:465–470.

Kruskal JB, Siewert B, Anderson SW, Eisenberg RL, Sosna J. Quality initiatives managing an acute adverse event in a radiology department. *Radiographics.* 2008;28:1237–1250.

Kuzminski SJ. Sticks and stones can break your bones, words can also hurt you. *J Am Coll Radiol.* 2016;13(1):7.

Larson DB, Kruskal JB, Krecke KN, Donnelly LF. Key concepts if patient safety in radiology. *Radiographics.* 2015;35:1677–1693.

Launders JH, et al. The Joint Commission. *Sentinel Event Alert.* August 24, 2011; (Issue 47).

Pennsylvania Patient Safety Advisory. Let's stop this "epi"demic! Preventing errors with epinephrine. *PA PSRS Patient Saf Advis.* 2006;3(3):16–17.

Pennsylvania Patient Safety Authority. Workarounds: a sign of opportunity knocking. *PA-PSRS Patient Safety Advisory.* 2005;2(4).

Radiological Society of North America. *RSNA Informatics Reporting.* <http://www.radreport.org/>.

Robinson TJ, DuVall S, Wiggins 3rd R. Creation and usability testing of a web-based pre-scanning radiology patient safety and history questionnaire set. *J Digital Imaging.* 2009;22(6):641–647.

Ross JR. Standardization: an answer to three of radiology's vexing problems. *Radiol Bus.* Oct 15, 2014.

Schwartz LH, Panicek DM, Berk AR, Li Y, Hricak H. Improving communication of diagnostic radiology findings through structured reporting. *Radiology.* 2011;260(1):174–181.

Semelka RC, Armao DM, Elias Jr J, Picano E. The information imperative: is it time for an informed consent process explaining the risks of medical radiation? *Radiology*. 2012;262(1):15-18.

Siewert B, Hochman MG. Improving safety through human factors engineering. *Radiographics*. 2015;35:1694-1705.

Wiley G. Devising a blueprint for radiology: standardization. *Radiol Bus*. Jul 02, 2013.

Wood DL, Brennan MD, Chaudhry R, et al. Standardized care processes to improve quality and safety of patient care in a large academic practice: the Plummer Project of the Department of Medicine, Mayo Clinic. *Health Serv Manage Res*. 2008;21(4):276-280.

Chapter 16

Accounting in Radiology

Saurabh Jha

DOMINANT PAYERS IN AMERICAN HEALTHCARE

Most healthcare costs, roughly 72% by current estimates, are paid by third-party payers. Insured patients still have out-of-pocket expenses, for example, to meet copayments and deductibles, depending on the actuarial value of their plan. Approximately 12% of the US population is uninsured, or *self-pay* (Fig. 16.1).

Third-party payers include private insurance, Medicare, and Medicaid. The majority of the funds, roughly 45%, are contributed by several private insurers, followed by Medicare (28%) and Medicaid (21%). However, Medicare is the largest single payer, larger than any single private insurer. This is important because private insurers tend to follow Medicare regarding decisions about which services to cover and, in particular, how much to pay for technology.

MEDICARE REIMBURSEMENT FOR IMAGING

The government-administered Medicare and Medicaid programs were established in 1965 as part of the Social Security Act. These programs are administered by the Centers for Medicare and Medicaid Services (CMS) in the US Department of Health and Human Services.

Medicare reimburses healthcare providers for services deemed "reasonable and necessary for the diagnosis or treatment of illness or injury or to improve the functioning of malformed body member." The level at which Medicare reimburses providers for imaging services depends on where the imaging is performed. In CMS's view, there are essentially two settings where imaging services are rendered:
1. Outpatient physician practices/independent facilities
2. Hospitals

Medicare further divides hospital services into *inpatient* and *outpatient* services performed *in hospitals*.

Medicare may pay for imaging prospectively, via capitation, but in general, Medicare reimbursement is mostly rooted in fee-for-service (FFS) payments, which is a specified fee paid for a defined unit of work, such as interpreting a computed tomography (CT) scan. Under FFS, the more units of work that are completed, the greater the reimbursement. This is the basis of the Physician Fee Schedule (PFS), which is how imaging performed in outpatient physician practices/independent facilities is reimbursed.

EVOLUTION OF PAYMENT UNDER MEDICARE/ MEDICAID

When it was initially created, Medicare's FFS payment system set fees according to what was considered a *usual,* *customary and reasonable* (UCR) fee. Under the UCR system, physicians' charges were based on what the billing physician *usually* charged for a given service (usual), on what was *commonly* charged by their peers (customary), or anchored to what private insurance paid (reasonable). UCR had many limitations. Under UCR, the charges were arbitrary and varied widely. The prices set had no basis in the supply-demand schema seen in other markets because healthcare, for multiple reasons, is not a free market. For example, proceduralists, such as urologists, received disproportionately higher reimbursements than physicians such as internists, who did nonprocedural/cognitive work.

This all changed in 1992 when a team led by health economist William Hsiao devised a much more granular method for fair reimbursement known as the resource-based relative value scale (RBRVS).

RESOURCE-BASED RELATIVE VALUE SCALE

The Omnibus Reconciliation Act of 1989 mandated the use of the RBRVS by 1992, and this system is now the sole means of determining physician payments for all third-party payers. The RBRVS is a granular method of reimbursement used by Medicare, which attempts to compensate physicians fairly for the skill, risk, and unit cost of their work by a scale known as the relative value unit (RVU). The scale is relative—how one service is valued against another—making RBRVS a unified scale for all physician payments for all services across all medical specialties.

The RVU is divided into two components: technical and professional. The final reimbursement is calculated by using a single monetary conversion factor. The professional component, the component related to the physician's work, has three parts.
1. Physician work
2. Malpractice expense
3. Practice expense

Practice expenses may be direct or indirect. Direct practice expenses include salaries of support staff, cost of disposables, and costs related to durable equipment. Direct practice expenses are determined by both the Relative Value Scale Update Committee (RUC) and CMS. Indirect practice expenses, or overhead, are expenses not directly related to individual patient care. Indirect practice expenses vary from specialty to specialty. The indirect practice expenses are determined by surveys. There are several modifications, including the following:
1. Cost of living: geographic practice cost index
2. Malpractice expenses
   Factors that affect practice expense for imaging include:
1. Technology utilization assumption rate: duration of equipment usage
2. Equipment depreciation rate

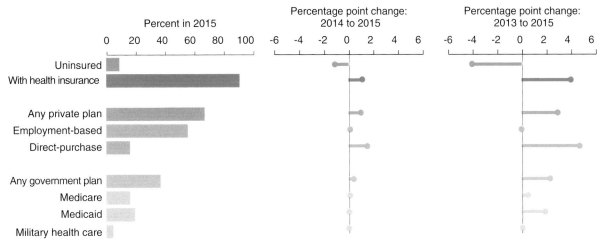

FIG. 16.1 Percentage of people by type of health insurance coverage and change from 2013 to 2015 (population as of March of the following year). Military healthcare includes TRICARE and Civilian Health and Medical Program of the Department of Veterans Affairs, as well as care provided by the Department of Veterans Affairs and the military. Note: Between 2014 and 2015, there was no statistically significant change in the percentage of people covered by employment-based health insurance, Medicaid, or military healthcare. Between 2013 and 2015, there was not a statistically significant change in the percentage of people covered by employment-based health insurance or military healthcare. For information on confidentiality protection, sampling error, nonsampling error, and definitions in the Current Population Survey, see http://www2.census.gov/programs-surveys/cps/techdocs/cpsmar16.pdf. (From US Census Bureau, Current Population Survey, 2014 to 2016 Annual Social and Economic Supplements.)

For example, echocardiography (Current Procedural Terminology [CPT] code 93306) has a technical component of 3.75 RVUs (which covers costs related to staff time, disposables, and depreciation costs), a professional component of 1.3 RVUs, and practice expense of 0.48 RVU. The technical component is paid to the physician, or physician group, if they own and operate the equipment, or to the hospital if the hospital owns and operates the equipment.

In the future, however, it has become clear that Medicare will increasingly move away from FFS and RVU-based reimbursements, preferring to shift physician payment into systems based on quality, value, and outcomes of care provided (i.e., value-based purchasing), rather than merely paying physicians a standard level of reimbursement for defined units of work (volume-based payment). Although some health economists and policymakers feel that the days of FFS payment are soon drawing to a close, many experts maintain that the ultimate result of current reforms will be a hybrid payment system blending elements of traditional FFS and value-based payment systems and that such a mixture of payment models will endure for the foreseeable future, such that FFS payment based on the RBRVS will never be entirely eliminated.

MEDICARE ACCESS AND CHIP REAUTHORIZATION ACT

The Medicare Access and CHIP Reauthorization Act of 2015 (MACRA) was a sweeping piece of bipartisan federal legislation signed into law on April 16, 2015. MACRA specifies a new schema for physician payments whereby a growing fraction of physician payments will be based on quality and effectiveness metrics rather than on the volume of services provided.

MACRA includes two new reimbursement structures: (1) the Merit-Based Incentive Payment System, which combines portions of the older physician quality reporting system with a *value-based payment modifier* and specified incentives for documenting meaningful use of electronic health record (EHR) technology to derive a composite performance score that can adjust physician payments up or down, or (2) alternative payment models, which are more comprehensive than the Merit-Based Incentive Payment System and involve prospective, risk-sharing financial arrangements such as the patient-centered medical home, accountable care organizations, and bundled payment models. These changes to physician reimbursement are scheduled to be phased in between 2019 and 2022 and are expected to have the effect of altering physician payments by ±9%. The basic concept behind MACRA is that physicians will increasingly bear risk for financial losses for healthcare inefficiencies and quality deficits and will increasingly be paid based on measured outcomes of their care, although the precise outcomes measures to be used under these schemes have yet to be selected and defined.

NEW PAYMENT MODELS VERSUS TRADITIONAL FEE-FOR-SERVICE PLANS

- Medicare will pay for quality, value, and outcomes.
- Medicare will pay for patient satisfaction.
- Under capitated payment systems, a primary care physician or an accountable care organization will be paid a fixed amount, per patient per month, for all care delivered to the patient. The rationale, or hope, is that the fixed payment will encourage efficiency, including better care coordination and a collaborative attempt to keep the patient healthy.

- In bundled payment systems, the physician or hospital will be paid a fixed amount to provide care related to a specific disease or presentation, such as acute stroke.

MEDICARE PAYMENT FOR IMAGING TECHNOLOGY, INTERNATIONAL CLASSIFICATION OF DISEASES-10, AND CURRENT PROCEDURAL TERMINOLOGY CODING

Medicare may issue a national coverage determination for a type of imaging study, such as magnetic resonance imaging (MRI). For technology that Medicare has not made a national coverage decision, it allows the local contractors (local administrators of Medicare) to decide if they wish to cover costs related to the use of that technology.

Medicare reimburses for services, imaging, or procedures if they are used for an *approved* medical indication. The medical indication is determined by a series of codes for symptoms and diseases, which are taken from the International Classification of Diseases (ICD), which is now in its 10th edition (ICD-10). ICD-10 only very recently supplanted ICD-9, the former version of the coding system. ICD-10 introduced a great deal of increased complexity to the coding system for symptoms and diseases, a change that had significant ramifications for radiology practices.

The ICD-10 codes define medical necessity, that is, why an imaging study was used. What was actually done for the patient is based on the CPT coding. New or revised CPT codes must be approved by the CPT Editorial Panel, selected by the American Medical Association's Board of Trustees, based on recommendations from diverse stakeholders such as specialty societies, industry, or the general public. CPT codes determine the medical service (cognitive, imaging, and procedural) actually performed.

There are three categories of CPT codes. Category 1 codes are for services that are common and backed by evidence. An example is CT of the chest with contrast to diagnose pulmonary embolus. Category 2 codes are supplementary tracking codes that help with performance measures and compliance. Category 3 codes are used for new and emerging technologies that are yet to be approved by the Food and Drug Administration or those for which more research is needed.

Once a CPT code has been approved, it is sent to the RUC, which decides on the relative value of the code under the RBRVS. The RUC determines the relative value of the physician work and sends its conclusions as a recommendation to CMS. Thus, the RUC acts as an unofficial advisor to CMS in determining the level of payment for particular imaging technologies and applications. CMS may choose to follow or ignore the recommendations of the RUC. By law, however, CMS must evaluate the relative value of each procedure every 5 years. In 2006, the CPT Editorial Panel and RUC formed the Relativity Assessment Workgroup to help CMS identify misvalued codes. In general, the *updated* relative values of medical imaging have resulted in lowering payments to physicians and hospitals.

MEDICARE REIMBURSEMENT FOR INPATIENT IMAGING

There are two components of Medicare payment for inpatient imaging, a professional and a technical component. The professional component follows the Medicare PFS.

Medicare pays prospectively for hospital in-patient services (which includes the technical component of imaging) using the Medicare Severity Diagnosis-Related Groups (DRGs). For a specific DRG, Medicare pays a fixed amount; this is a global payment that is the same regardless of how many imaging studies are done for that episode of care. Of note, the DRG does not include the professional component of physician services.

The cost estimates for each particular DRG have been based on historical data and self-reporting. Medicare plans, however, to use EHRs for more granular cost calculations for DRGs in the future.

The Hospital Outpatient Prospective Payment System (HOPPS) determines payment for hospital care lasting fewer than two midnights. HOPPS was introduced after the Balanced Budget Act of 1997. Before that act, hospitals rendering services like outpatient facilities were paid identically to outpatient facilities. HOPPS slightly modified that scenario by grouping similar services into the ambulatory payment classifications (APCs), so that services within any given APC are paid the same. The APCs are designated by the Healthcare Common Procedure Coding System (HCPCS). Under HOPPS, hospitals are paid on a fee-for-service basis based on HCPCS codes. The costs are determined by the charges recorded by the hospitals for the HCPCS code, which are then converted to costs using specific charge-to-cost ratios.

CHANGES IN MEDICARE REIMBURSEMENT FOR IMAGING

The Deficit Reduction Act of 2005 mandated that Medicare reimbursement for the technical component of imaging services rendered in the physician's office could not be greater than what is paid for the same service in the hospital outpatient setting. This affected cardiac CT very severely, for example, because the PFS payment ($350.59) was greater than the HOPPS payment ($261.75). Similar adjustments occurred throughout the practice of radiology.

CMS considers imaging services that are performed and billed together to contain duplicative work. This has led CMS to bundle multiple procedural codes into one solitary code, which carries a lower RVU value than the sum of the two previously independent codes that have been bundled. For example, 2-D Doppler and color Doppler were bundled into one code, 93306. Similarly, codes for nuclear myocardial perfusion imaging, wall motion, and ejection fraction (CPT codes 78465, 78478, 78480) were bundled into a single code (78452).

The rationale behind multiple procedure payment reduction is that when more than one imaging service is rendered on the same day for a patient, there are efficiencies because of duplication of services and resources, for example, when imaging is performed on two contiguous body parts such as the abdomen and pelvis, or brain and neck. The payment reductions from this bundling were quite substantial. In 2012, for example, the multiple procedure payment reduction was 50% for technical and 25% for professional fees paid.

CLINICAL DECISION SUPPORT

Clinical decision support (CDS) is a system that is integrated into the EHR, which acts at the point of physician order entry to guide physicians in selection of what diagnostic imaging, if any, to perform. The basic idea behind CDS is to provide an *appropriateness score* of some kind for a particular imaging modality for a particular indication for any given patient *just in time* to influence a physician's imaging test decision. There are many systems currently available or under construction, including a proprietary system endorsed by the American College of Radiology (ACR), known as ACR Select, which is based on the ACR Appropriateness Criteria, an evidence-based guideline for imaging utilization.

In the ACR system, the appropriateness score is on a nominal scale from one (least appropriate) to nine (most appropriate). CDS aims to ask the right clinical question so that the patient receives the best imaging test for the particular indication. If a clinician investigates a patient with long-standing headache, for example, the CDS will ask whether any new symptoms are present. If new symptoms are present, MRI receives a score of 8 and CT a score of 5, meaning MRI is the preferred modality to investigate the patient's symptoms. If the patient has no new symptoms, both CT and MRI receive a score of 4. CDS tries to increase the value of imaging by encouraging the use of tests with high appropriateness scores and discouraging the use of tests with low appropriateness scores. There is currently much enthusiasm for the use of CDS among private insurers as well as CMS.

BILLING PRIVATE HEALTH INSURERS

There are several steps in generating a bill to a private insurer (e.g., Aetna, Blue Cross/Blue Shield). First and foremost, the study used must be appropriate, that is, medically indicated. Particularly if advanced imaging is used, insurers often require preauthorization of the study to ensure that it is clinically appropriate prior to being performed. Preauthorization is often carried out by third-party radiology benefits managers. Once the study is preauthorized and carried out, a qualified radiologist interprets it, and a report is generated. The report must contain various elements to support billing. For example, the report must clearly state the medical indication in the patient history. For the purpose of billing and coding, a medical indication in a radiology report cannot be stated as merely the exclusion of a diagnosis such as *rule out pneumonia*. Medical indication must include the symptoms that prompted the search for the diagnosis, such as *fever and cough*.

The report must also include the minimum technical elements of the exam that justify the billing. For example, it should be stated whether contrast has been given

and, if so, how much. If an exam includes contiguous body parts such as head and neck, the report should specifically mention the findings within the organs in those body parts, such as posterior fossa and thyroid, so that it is clear that the radiologist interrogated the separate body parts.

Preauthorizations are increasingly code specific; that is, if a contrast-enhanced MRI of the brain is approved but the MRI exam is ultimately performed and billed without contrast, even though the charge for a noncontrast MRI is lower than was authorized, the payment will be denied. This phenomenon is known as *deauthorization*.

IMPORTANCE OF ACCURATE CODING

Accurate and complete coding are extremely important because improper, incorrect, or incomplete coding generally results in underpayment. But coding is also important because incorrect coding can be construed as abuse (incorrect billing) or fraud (intentionally incorrect billing) by CMS. Although it is always considered fraud when billing practice is willfully incorrect, fraud can even be construed when billing is merely systematically and continuously incorrect, albeit unintentionally so. Because the penalties for fraud and abuse can be quite severe, it is important for providers to be acutely aware of correct and proper coding and billing practices, a complex topic that is beyond the scope of this chapter.

RADIOLOGY ACCOUNTING 101: ACCOUNTS RECEIVABLE AND COLLECTIONS

Accounts Receivable

Radiology is essentially a credit-based service. Radiologists render a service with the expectation of being paid at some time in the future. Accounts receivable (AR) are payments yet to be received for services provided. AR, though not cash at the time of billing, is still considered to be an asset, equivalent to cash, inventory, property, and equipment. However, one's practice and other expenses cannot be paid with AR. It is therefore in the best interests of a practice to convert AR to cash as soon as possible because of the time value of money.

To initiate an AR, a study must be completed and an appropriate ICD code and CPT code should be attached. If the payment received is less than expected, an invoice might be sent to the patient. If payment received is the same as that billed, the payment can be recorded as cash. If payment cannot be received, it can be recorded as charity or bad debt.

Gross charges are the list price for the services. Insurers do not pay the gross charges but the adjusted charges, which typically involve a large discount. The adjusted charges are negotiated between the practice and the insurance for a particular service. In general, only the uninsured (self-pay) patients are assessed the gross charges, as all third-party payers receive a (typically large) discount. The difference between gross charges and adjusted charges is known as the adjustment. Adjustments are amounts that are never expected to be collected. A write-off is the amount that was expected to be legitimately collected for services rendered but was not, possibly because claims were denied, copays were left unpaid, or other bad debt was incurred.

Accounting Metrics to Measure Accounts Receivable Performance

A few commonly used accounting metrics are worth mentioning:

1. *Adjusted collection percentage.* This is the adjusted collection/adjusted charges ×100. This is a measure of how much the practice gets paid relative to what it expected. The benchmark for APC is high, over 95%.

2. *AR days outstanding.* This is a measure of how fast bills are paid, and AR is converted to cash. The formula is = Total AR balance/Average daily gross charges. Average daily gross charges are the average monthly gross charges per 30 days. The benchmark is less than 60 days; bills should generally be paid in less than 2 months.

3. *Collection expense percentage.* This is the amount a business spends to get paid relative to the cost of collections. The formula is = Collection expense/Adjusted collection ×100. The usual range is 4% to 10%.

4. *AR aging percentage over 120 days.* This is calculated as (AR ÷ 120 days)/Total AR balance ×100. This is an indicator of how well the group follows up on account activities; it is a quantitative measure of how many bills are unpaid after 4 months.

Chapter 17
Radiology Informatics

Ron Gefen and Paul Chang

Informatics is the science and practice of computer information systems. Imaging informatics encompasses the use of information technology to deliver efficient, accurate, and reliable medical imaging services within a healthcare network. Its imprint is felt in every step of the process of patient imaging, from order entry to results communication. Radiologists have key roles as leaders in imaging informatics and are the liaisons between the clinical needs of the healthcare enterprise and the applicability of an information technology team. Ultimately, radiologists can serve as innovators in a constantly evolving field to optimize the flow of medical information within a radiology department and throughout a healthcare institution.

This chapter is devoted to introducing the major components of imaging informatics. The workflow cycle begins with physician order entry, usually using the hospital information system (HIS) or electronic medical record (EMR). Data necessary to support imaging workflow are communicated to radiology departments via the radiology information system (RIS). The picture archiving and communication system (PACS) then organizes medical images for review by radiologists or other healthcare providers, as well as long-term storage (Fig. 17.1). The technical standards involving the organization and communication of these systems will be discussed.

The radiologist reading room environment will also be reviewed. The basic viewing requirements of modern reading room workstations will be introduced, as well as the ergonomics of desktop computer stations and related health concerns. Radiologists' workflow beyond image review and interpretation at the workstation involves multiple postprocessing applications, including advanced three-dimensional (3D) imaging and computer-aided detection. The software and hardware components of imaging reporting are varied and often vendor specific; however, there are physician-driven initiatives for report dictation that rely heavily on the standardized language and structure of reporting. Finally, postreporting computer applications will be introduced, including data mining, peer review, and critical results communication.

The breadth of imaging informatics covers practically all aspects of radiology. In one sense, every part of the radiologist's reporting workflow outside of image interpretation involves informatics. The depth of these topics reaches beyond the goals of this chapter. As an introduction, these outlined topics will create a foundation of nomenclature and technologic components that can be built upon throughout a career in radiology.

HEALTHCARE AND RADIOLOGIC INFORMATION SYSTEMS

Hospital Information System and Electronic Medical Record

A medical imaging study begins with a patient-physician encounter that generates an order or prescription. From within a healthcare enterprise, patient demographic and medical data are collected and distributed by a HIS, which may or may not be completely computerized and paperless. An EMR is such a data system that is completely paperless. In an EMR environment, the imaging study can be ordered by clinicians via computer. Such a computerized physician order entry carries the potential advantages of providing relevant patient history and providing point-of-need decision support, such as image exam appropriateness criteria.

Radiology Information Systems

Regardless of the method of study order, radiology study orders must be communicated to a RIS. A RIS is a computer application that manages patient demographic data and scheduling and tracks associated images and reporting results. Once an imaging study order is entered into a RIS, the study is associated with a unique identifier code such as an accession number. The accession number and medical record number allow unambiguous association of the image dataset with the correct patient demographics; this also allows coordination of the patient's scheduling and imaging encounter at the imaging modality. This system enables a patient study to be accessed at any site of a radiology department network for acquisition and communication of results and images back to the HIS/EMR. In addition, many of the business/operational analytics (scorecards, dashboards, and reports) necessary to monitor operational quality/efficiency are generated by the RIS or depend on RIS data.

Picture Archiving and Communication Systems

The RIS organizes patient data regarding a study but does not include the images themselves. The PACS is the information technology architecture that orchestrates the workflow of image acquisition, display, and storage across a network. Modern PACSs have largely replaced the need for hard copy film creation and transportation. The PACS also allows for quality improvement initiatives through additional software programs. PACSs have four main components:

1. The imaging modalities (radiography, computed tomography [CT], magnetic resonance imaging [MRI], ultrasound, etc.)

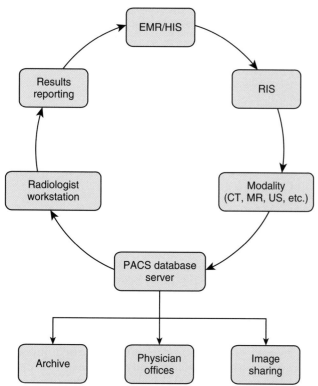

FIG. 17.1 **FLOW OF MEDICAL INFORMATION.** *CT*, Computed tomography; *EMR*, electronic medical record; *HIS*, health information system; *MR*, magnetic resonance; *PACS*, picture archiving and communication system; *RIS*, radiology information system; *US*, ultrasound.

2. A secure transmission network
3. Computer workstations for viewing and manipulating images
4. Digital archives for storing images and reports for later retrieval

Ideally, one PACS serves all of the imaging modalities across an institution's radiology services. Once imaging modalities acquire images scheduled by the RIS, image data is sent to the PACS database server. PACS servers typically communicate through a local area network (LAN) to various workstations, where images can be reviewed by radiologists, technologists, or caregivers throughout a health network. Networks, as well as digital archives, must maintain the security of patient data according to the regulations defined by the Health Insurance Portability and Accountability Act. A LAN maintains relatively high privacy as all computers on a network are physically wired to servers within a protective enterprise firewall. Large healthcare centers with multiple hospitals may have several LANs that intercommunicate and comprise a wide area network. In contrast, radiologists or caregivers may want to view images from outside a LAN, such as logging in through the Internet from home. In this case, a virtual private network (VPN) can be created. A VPN connects to the LAN with a comparable level of security to allow access to the PACS or EMR from outside the wired network.

PACS database servers send patient imaging studies to computer workstations for healthcare worker use and to archival storage. At larger institutions, storage servers can

be maintained off-site at dedicated data centers. Archival storage must be secure, scalable, and have redundancy or backup. The performance of storage servers is dependent on the media technology used; however, the decreasing cost of magnetic spinning disc drives has allowed for its use to become preferred and commonplace. Current and near future enterprise requirements have driven the need for a scalable enterprise image/multimedia archive and image consumption architecture. Examples include the vendor-neutral archive, archive-neutral PACS vendors, and PACS-neutral archives.

PACS software packages include the radiologist's tools for effectively and rapidly interpreting images. Preset window and level settings and hanging protocols are customizable for end users to fit individual personal preferences. Measurement tools, zoom, pan, and window adjustment are a few of the many assessment features needed. PACSs must also display patient information and prior studies, and their reports must be available. Modern offerings go beyond simple image study presentation and navigation and attempt to support more complex radiology workflow orchestration (e.g., real-time decision support, advanced visualization, advanced communication/collaboration, analytics, peer review).

Radiology Information Systems: Picture Archiving and Communication Systems Integration

There is clearly a need for RIS and PACS to communicate efficiently. Some vendors offer hybrid products comprising both RIS and PACS; however, that is not always the case. In scenarios where health networks work with different vendors, the radiologists' workflow is derived by either the RIS or the PACS as the primary *source of truth*. A RIS-driven workflow seems intuitive based on having patient and study information and being the primary tool for schedulers and technologists. However, a PACS-driven workflow would use the imaging studies themselves to drive a worklist and would be within the software workspace that radiologists mainly use, acquiring additional data from the RIS via the accession number or other identifier. Regardless of the method used, optimized and localized integration of RIS-PACS to offer efficient workflows for both radiologists and technologists is vital for a reliable and accurate department system.

TECHNICAL STANDARDS

For the various components of a healthcare system to communicate effectively, there are technical standards that enable the interoperability of different systems, both within radiology and throughout the enterprise. Standards are maintained and updated by corresponding associations and are continually evolving to improve efficient communication.

Health Level 7

Healthcare networks have many components in an information system, including the EMR, RIS, order entry systems, laboratory information systems, etc. Health Level 7 (HL7) is the computer standard governing the communication of these various information systems within and between healthcare networks. HL7 is responsible for communicating with a RIS and sharing information with an EMR. In imaging, this encompasses study ordering, registration, and results communication. HL7 characterizes each interaction as an event and can disseminate the associated message electronically to other systems.

Digital Imaging and Communications in Medicine

Although HL7 is the standard spanning the breadth of healthcare, Digital Imaging and Communications in Medicine (DICOM) is the technical standard for display, storage, and transmission of medical images. DICOM began as a collaborative effort by the American College of Radiology (ACR) and National Electrical Manufacturers Association in the early 1980s and was renamed DICOM in 1993. Now it has become the universal standard data format for images and communications among all medical imaging devices and software applications. A DICOM image also contains information regulated by the standard: media display, security profiles, data storage, and data encoding and exchange.

DICOM has been the critical enabler for interoperability of hardware and software spanning all aspects of radiology workflow (image acquisition modalities, PACS servers, workstations, networks). DICOM also allows image databases to be shared as PACSs develop and expand and maintain communication with other information systems.

DICOM does not have a centralized body to certify or enforce implementation of the standard. It is up to various vendors to conform to the standard. Although the standard can be followed, the mechanisms of use are not specified. Vendors almost universally provide DICOM conformance statements that explicitly state how a specific vendor's offering supports DICOM. Also, vendors may opt to carry additional proprietary technical parameters, which may impact interoperability.

Integrating the Healthcare Enterprise

Despite the presence of HL7 and DICOM standards, there are still variations in interconnectivity and efficiency. An initiative called Integrating the Healthcare Enterprise (IHE) began in 1998 with a goal to improve the communication of different standards. IHE does not create its own standard but instead promotes the coordinated and *best practice* use of established standards. IHE identifies common system integration challenges requiring HL7-DICOM or other communication and creates an *IHE profile* of an expected technical workflow that can consistently deliver expected results. IHE initiatives grow in parallel to updates from HL7 and DICOM, and compliance can further increase an accurate and efficient workflow.

Image Data Compression

Image data can be electronically compressed into smaller files by mathematical algorithms, with a goal of decreasing storage needs and image transfer time. Image compression can be lossless, which is reversible, or lossy, which is irreversible.

Lossless image data storage is used by many PACS systems and removes any doubt regarding potential loss in diagnostic quality of medical images. Lossless compression involves removing redundant data, and a commonly known example file is the Graphics Interchange Format. The degree of compression is limited, however, and is typically in the range of 1.5:1 to 3:1.

Lossy image compression methods remove potentially relevant pixel data from image files. The compression ratio improves to greater than 10:1. Joint Photographic Experts Group (JPEG) uses lossy image compression and is widely applied in digital photography, with minimal impact on image quality. JPEG is also supported by the DICOM standard. Studies have shown that some lossy image compression techniques can be used effectively in medical imaging without an impact on diagnostic relevance.

Lossy image compression that does not affect a particular diagnostic task is referred to as diagnostically acceptable irreversible compression. The ACR does not have a general advisory statement on the type or amount of irreversible compression to be used to achieve diagnostically acceptable irreversible compression, and only methods defined and supported by the DICOM standard should be used, such as JPEG, JPEG-2000, or Moving Picture Experts Group. In addition, the US Food and Drug Administration (FDA) requires that images with lossy compression are labeled, including the compression ratio and method used. The FDA prohibits the use of lossy compression of digital mammograms for interpretation, although lossy compression can be used for prior comparison studies.

IMAGE DISPLAY

To support numerous computer workstations throughout a department or institution, many PACS systems use thin client software or web-based platforms for viewing images to minimize the hardware memory requirements of individual computers. For interpreting radiologists, workstations must, in addition, meet minimum requirements for image display characteristics (Table 17.1). Liquid crystal display (LCD) monitors are ubiquitous, with high-resolution flat

TABLE 17.1 Image Display Components

Characteristic	ACR Requirement/ Recommendation
Color/grayscale depth	8 bit
Luminance	Lmax >350 cd/m^2 Lmin 1.0 cd/m^2 LR >250
Mammography	Lmax >420 cd/m^2 Lmin 1.2 cd/m^2
Pixel pitch	<0.21 mm; 0.20 mm recommended
Aspect ratio	3:4 or 4:5 ideal

ACR, American College of Radiology; *Lmax*, maximum grayscale luminance; *Lmin*, minimum grayscale luminance; *LR*, luminance ratio.

panels that can absorb ambient light and minimize glare and reflection.

Color and Grayscale Contrast

Color or grayscale contrast is characterized by bit depth to describe the number of colors or grayscale levels in an image pixel. An 8-bit system means that a pixel is comprised of an 8-bit byte. For example, a true-color 8-bit system assigns eight specific colors (three red, three green, two blue; red, green, blue [RGB] palette), which in combination form 2^8 colors, a 256-RGB color palette. In grayscale, all RGB values are equal for 256 shades of grayscale. Higher-bit-depth displays such as 30-bit systems are available and require support of the operating system and graphics card. No evidence has shown that radiologic interpretations are affected by the use of greater than 8-bit systems.

Color systems require pixels formed by color elements that are not precisely superimposed, resulting in pixels that may lose sharpness compared to grayscale monitors. The use of color displays has grown and is at times favored, such as in Doppler ultrasound and nuclear fused positron emission tomography and computed tomography images. The technology for comparable display brightness and sharpness has improved recently to be similar in quality to grayscale displays; however, color displays that also provide superior grayscale performance remain more expensive, and grayscale displays are still common and practical.

Luminance

The brightness and contrast of grayscale images are affected by the monitor luminance for a given grayscale value. Luminance is a measure of light intensity, and the standardized unit is the candela per square meter (cd/m^2), or nit. LCD monitors have luminance properties based on the light source and panel properties. LCD panels are lit by cathode fluorescent lamps or newer light-emitting diodes, which have lower power needs and potentially longer life. Regardless of source, monitor backlight luminance decays over time and requires periodic quality control. Monitors carry a maximum luminance dictated by the light source, Lmax, which is the luminance for the maximum gray value. Minimum luminance, Lmin, is the luminance of the darkest gray level and is dictated by the panel's ability to block the light source. The ACR has an established standard for Lmax of a white level of 350 cd/m^2 or greater for diagnostic viewing and 420 cd/m^2 for mammography and an Lmin baseline of at least 1.0 cd/m^2 or 1.2 cd/m^2 for mammography.

The luminance ratio (LR) is the ratio of Lmax to Lmin, and a high LR is required for good image contrast. LR should always be greater than 250, and an LR of 350 is considered effective. If the LR or Lmax is too high, however, the human eye will acclimate to the brightness, and subtle darker imaging findings can be missed. On the other hand, if the Lmin is too low, dark grayscale levels cannot be differentiated. The DICOM standard covers grayscale bit depth based on a nonlinear perception model. Because humans can better differentiate between lighter grayscale levels than darker levels, adjacent darker levels are assigned greater differences in luminance compared to lighter pixels.

Pixel Pitch and Resolution

Display monitors have a resolution typically characterized by the number of pixels (picture elements). Medical displays are often labeled as 2-, 3-, or 5-megapixel (MP) monitors based on the number of pixels in the display, with a pixel dimension such as 1600 × 1200 (pixels in the width of the monitor × height). However, it is more useful to characterize a monitor by its display size (diagonal length) and pixel pitch. Pixel pitch is the measure of one side of a pixel square. In addition, the perception of an image also depends on the viewing distance from the monitor.

The ACR standard recommends a pixel pitch of 0.20 mm for diagnostic interpretation and no larger than 0.21 mm. If the pixel pitch is too large, the image may appear *pixelated* with a fine grainy pattern of staircase artifacts. There is no advantage to using a smaller pixel pitch and doing so will result in smaller images when displayed at full resolution. Medical images are acquired with a resolution of varying detector element sizes that are different from a monitor's pixel pitch. In such instances, zoom and pan presentation tools should be used and may show subtle detail not detectable at initial image size.

For example, a CT image may have a resolution of 0.25 MP. When viewed at a diagnostic workstation with a 2-MP monitor, the image can be viewed at full resolution of one image pixel per display pixel. Zooming in and magnifying such an image will quickly make artifacts visible due to individual pixel identification. On the other hand, a chest radiograph image typically has an image resolution of 5 MP. When viewed on a 2-MP display, the image is minified to fill the size of the display. This can be routinely done without losing diagnostic information. However, if there is an area of abnormality, digitally zooming in on the area expands the region to its full pixel resolution, maintaining a smooth visual appearance and maximizing the image details. The routine minification of radiographs for monitor display is termed down-sampling.

Display Size

Radiologists interpreting images focus on the center of a display, but attention to the edges is also done using peripheral vision. The optimal visualization of a display is achieved when the display size is approximately 80% of the viewing distance. A workstation with a viewing distance of 25 to 35 inches (64–89 cm) corresponds to a monitor size of 21 inches (53 cm).

TELERADIOLOGY

Teleradiology is the electronic transmission of medical imaging to remote sites for consultation, review, or formal interpretation. The network technology may include the LAN or wide area network, as well as the Internet via VPN or *cloud computing*. Security and privacy standards must be maintained on par with typical data transmission and storage. In addition, the imaging data must be transmitted in a timely fashion using appropriate bandwidth, and the transmission must have no loss of clinically significant information.

The goals of teleradiology are varied. Hospitals or other facilities may require timely review of studies without having radiologists on site, such as providing emergency on-call study interpretations. Radiologist groups may use teleradiology among themselves or outsource their call to other practices. Sites can also be served in areas of need or areas that require subspecialty radiologic support. Finally, teleradiology can be used to send interpreted images to additional providers for quality improvement or educational opportunities. The use of teleradiology grew rapidly after the turn of the century, with a reported 50% of radiology practices outsourcing at least some call responsibility in 2010. More recently the trend has withdrawn from this peak as more practices have reverted to keeping calls in-house.

The methods and personnel can vary, and reports can be preliminary or final based on the desired contractual obligations. Ultimately, the services provided should be as similar as possible to direct on-site care. Ideally, the radiologist working remotely would have image and EMR access and report creation tools identical to those on site, including the ability to see prior imaging studies and their reports. There remain teleradiology practices with limited chart access, and separate lines of communication such as using email or fax machines. These considerations as well as lack of a face-to-face presence at a medical site have fueled the discussion on the potential negatives of teleradiology as compared to the positive impact of delivering timely patient care.

The ACR technical standard outlines the technologic and professional qualification needs for teleradiology. Practicing radiologists should meet the licensing needs of both the transmitting and receiving sites, which typically involves licensure in the transmitting state but not necessarily the receiving state. Radiologists should have medical privileges at the transmitting site. The teleradiologist or teleradiology company bears the responsibility of privacy and security protocols, monitor characteristics, and ergonomic conditions. Connectivity demands and infrastructure redundancy and reliability must also be met to serve patient interests.

WORK ENVIRONMENT AND HEALTH-RELATED ISSUES

Ergonomics in the workplace is the science of equipment design and use to maximize productivity by reducing user fatigue and discomfort. In the computerized era of radiology, the potential harmful health impact of computer desk workers is an important consideration in reading room and workstation design. Factors include the display monitors, ambient lighting, and position of the work chair, desktop, keyboard and mouse, and dictation microphone. Flexibility is also vital to accommodate variations in worker size and preference. Table 17.2 outlines basic methods to reduce health concerns at the workstation.

Ambient Lighting

The level of ambient lighting is an important consideration in the radiologist or caregiver environment. Ambient background light and glare degrade the observed display quality by increasing luminance of darker image regions, thereby

TABLE 17.2 Workstation Ergonomics

Potential Health Effect	Methods of Improvement
Eye strain	Hourly breaks Work shift 7 hours/day Artificial tears Increased blinking
Carpal tunnel syndrome	Wrist rest Wrist in neutral position Flat or ergonomically split keyboard
Cubital tunnel syndrome	Padded armrests Dictation headsets Elbow flexion >90 degrees
Other musculoskeletal/ postural strain	Neutral neck and shoulder position Eye gaze oriented 15–20 degrees down Hip flexion >90 degrees

decreasing contrast ratio. Therefore, ambient light can decrease the discrimination of low-contrast observations. Increased ambient light has been shown to decrease the detectability of lung nodules on digital chest radiographs. Such lighting situations occur with typical office lighting and can be frequently encountered in nonradiologist settings of image interpretation. In low ambient light settings and with appropriate monitor luminance, diagnostic accuracy is unlikely to be affected when applying adequate window width and level.

Too little or no ambient lighting can also have a negative impact on diagnostic accuracy, and study results have been similar to environments with excessive lighting. The impact of ambient lighting on reader fatigue is also a potential concern. Observers have reported greater levels of fatigue with a high level of ambient light and with higher levels of monitor luminance. The recommended ambient lighting level is 20 to 40 lux in the workspace environment. Lighting should be indirect and glare free, and fluorescent lighting should be avoided because it markedly increases ambient lighting.

EYE STRAIN

Computer worker eye strain is an established condition that can be ameliorated by the design of the working environment as well as work habits. Eye strain is a temporary condition encompassing a range of symptoms including eye irritation, blurry or double vision, tearing, and headache. For radiologists, eye strain is a potential component of fatigue and can increase perceptual errors and decrease reaction time. Display factors contributing to symptoms include screen resolution and contrast, image refresh rates, and screen flicker and glare. Decreased blink rate and working distances and angles are also factors.

Radiologists surveyed in a 2005 study by Vertinsky and Forster reported a 36% prevalence of eye strain. Symptoms were independently associated with longer work days, fewer breaks, screen flicker, female gender, and reading CT scans. Interestingly, there was no difference in eye strain rate between reading on computer displays or hard copy films, probably owing to the level of concentration with fixed gaze and decreased blinking related to interpretive activity.

Strategies for improving eye strain include reading cases for less than 7 hours per day and taking short breaks at least once per hour. Artificial tears and increased blinking may also help.

Monitor Positioning

The ideal display is situated about arm's length from the eyes, no closer than 25 inches. Placement further away has shown no deleterious effects. If characters are too small to read, it is preferable to increase the font size rather than to move closer to the monitor. The top of the monitor should be at or slightly below eye level, so that the worker's gaze is centered below the horizontal in the range of 15 to 20 degrees down. The monitor should be angled up slightly so that the top of the monitor is further away from the eyes than the bottom. A final consideration is the number of monitors at a workstation, which typically ranges from two to four. Although increasing the number of monitors allows for obviously desirable increased real estate, they also require more head and body movement, increasing the potential for visual fatigue or postural problems.

Posture and Musculoskeletal Concerns

Radiologists should be centered at their workstation with the keyboard directly in front of them. Adjustable chairs with appropriate lumbar support are essential to accommodate various heights and sizes. Chair height should be set so that the neck is in a neutral position while viewing monitors, with hips flexed at an angle of 90 degrees or greater. Footrests may be helpful to achieve such posture because a chair that is set too high causes the worker to slide forward with the back unsupported in an upright position. Keeping an upright posture with shoulders at rest is important to reduce back strain. Slouching increases pressure on intervertebral disks possibly leading to back pain. Adjustable workstations that allow work both in the seated and standing positions are also helpful.

Carpal tunnel syndrome is a well-known concern for computer desk workers. Carpal tunnel syndrome is caused by median nerve compression from inflammation and thickening of flexor tendons coursing between the flexor retinaculum and wrist bones. Signs and symptoms include pain and paresthesia in the wrist and radial side of the hand and muscle weakness. Potential causes of carpal tunnel syndrome are wrist dorsiflexion due to a high mouse position and wrist palmar flexion due to improper position of the keyboard. It is also associated with wrist ulnar deviation while typing. It is therefore important to have an adjustable-height tray table for the keyboard and mouse, set so that the wrist is in a neutral position while operating the mouse and typing. A wrist rest and negative-tilt tray table may also help or keeping the keyboard flat without the use of the small kickstands designed to make keys readable. An ergonomic split keyboard may improve ulnar deviation while typing.

Cubital tunnel syndrome is also associated with poor posture at the workstation. Cubital tunnel syndrome is the result of ulnar nerve compression between the humeral medial epicondyle, olecranon, and overlying cubital tunnel retinaculum. Signs and symptoms include pain in the medial elbow, paresthesia along the ulnar nerve distribution, and muscle weakness. At the workstation, it is related to prolonged elbow flexion. This is associated with the keyboard and mouse tray set too high, excessive use of handheld dictation microphones or telephones, and direct ulnar nerve trauma. Potential solutions involve maintaining the desk tray and chair heights so that the elbow is at or slightly greater than 90 degrees of flexion and using headsets for voice recognition dictation software and phones. Padded armrests diminish the impact of direct trauma on the nerve.

POSTPROCESSING IMAGING APPLICATIONS

Thus far the chapter discussion covered areas of informatics related to information systems, image and display standards, and workstation ergonomics. At the time of image interpretation, there are additional ancillary workstation tools that are used to improve accuracy and efficiency, such as computer-aided detection and 3D image rendering/advanced visualization.

COMPUTER-AIDED DETECTION

Computer-aided detection (CAD or CADe) is the technology of pattern recognition software that identifies suspicious features on an image and brings them to the attention of the radiologist. The goal is to decrease false negative rates of radiologists' interpretations alone by decreasing observational oversights. This is different from computer-aided diagnosis (also called CAD or CADx), which refers to software that is designed to classify lesions (i.e., benign or malignant) rather than just highlight them. For this discussion, CAD refers to CADe, with CADx programs not currently commercially available.

The FDA has approved the use of CAD in mammography, both film and digital, for screening and diagnostic imaging. The method of use is also outlined by the FDA: the radiologist first interprets the mammogram alone and then interprets an image with the CAD marks overlaid on it. This is in part designed to avoid satisfaction of search errors, overlooking areas of the image not marked by the CAD system. CAD algorithms are designed to highlight the same features that a radiologist looks for on images, in this case microcalcifications and masses. The CAD images may be integrated within the PACS or displayed on a separate monitor. Ultimately, CAD, like all decision support tools, is a supportive aid for the radiologist, who must accept or reject the CAD interpretation. The radiologist assumes final responsibility for the interpretation.

The benefits of CAD in improving the false negative rate for mammography have been well demonstrated. In prospective studies where mammograms are sequentially read without CAD and then with CAD, there has been a 7% to 20% increase in the cancer detection rate using CAD. Similarly, there is an increase in the overall recall rate of 9% to 18%. The ability to use software that can offer this benefit without requiring additional radiologist manpower (double reading) has led to its widespread use. CAD is not vulnerable to fatigue, emotion, or environmental distractions. The potential for reduced specificity can be partially offset by time and continuing education, because the radiologist learning curve for using CAD with reproducible results has been shown to take up to a year.

CAD has also been used to detect lung nodules on radiographs and chest CT scans and to detect colon polyps on CT colonography. Retrospective studies evaluating CAD algorithm detection rates of clinically missed lung cancers on chest x-ray range from 35% to 52%. Available CAD programs for lung nodule detection have not penetrated the market as well as they have for mammography. This may be because chest radiographs have not been shown to be effective in screening for lung cancer, and the time and reimbursement allotments for radiographic interpretations are less than for CT or mammography. Chest CT CAD programs as an adjunct for nodule detection may evolve quickly given the recent approval of the use of low-dose chest CT for lung cancer screening; however, its use remains more time consuming compared to the single image overlays of CAD for mammograms or chest x-rays.

Postprocessing and Two-Dimensional/Three-Dimensional Reconstruction Imaging

After image acquisition at the modality, image postprocessing techniques are applied to facilitate improved interpretive accuracy or efficiency. Some functions are performed by the modality itself and are ubiquitous, such as applying bone algorithms on CT images. Other techniques are used on a case-by-case basis, whether they are performed at the modality or at an independent workstation, such as bone removal algorithms for CT images. It is this type of human-driven manipulation of images requiring additional resources that are considered postprocessing tools for this discussion.

Postprocessing of cross-sectional imaging has become ubiquitous. Improvements in computer workstation central processing have allowed for software applications to run on standard out-of-the-box equipment, at a fraction of the hardware cost when these applications first appeared. Thin client software programs are also widely available. Server-side solutions are designed to require minimal hardware upgrades at the local workstation, while processing is performed centrally on a more powerful server.

The benefits of postprocessing vary based on the type of study but overall are designed to display a diagnosis with improved visibility. Most applications requiring additional time and human effort are for CT scans; however, there are programs across all types of advanced imaging including MRI and ultrasound. For CT, the use of postprocessing is often termed *3D reconstruction* regardless of whether actual volume-rendered 3D images are created. CT scanners have improved utility recently and are able to create preset image sequences, such as maximum intensity projection (MIP) series and basic 3D vascular or orthopedic series. Beyond this, radiologists or technologists must create other reconstructed images on their own, using image manipulation software that could be integrated within the PACS or standalone software connected to the network. Larger institutions have 3D labs that employ dedicated technologists who generate image sets for the interpreting radiologists, whereas images in other centers are generated by the technologists at the modality or the radiologist.

In 3D reconstruction imaging for CT, the postprocessing serves two main goals. Foremost, images are created to improve the detectability of abnormalities that may be subtle on standard image planes and slice thicknesses that are used for PACS storage and viewing. Examples include vessel mapping with curved planar reformation, MIP imaging for vessels or urographic images, and multiplanar reformation possibly in thinner sections or off-axis planes. Secondly, images can be created to depict abnormalities easily, such as for clinician viewing or education. Such images can use 3D volume rendering or thick slab MIP series to display disease states in one or a few images that are useful in communicating with referring physicians or even patients.

Postprocessing techniques apply mathematical algorithms to the volume of acquired imaging data. Each image voxel or cubic pixel in a 3D grid is set to be visible or not and to a specific degree of color/grayscale shading and translucency to create images. Individual images or series that are created independently can be saved and transmitted to the PACS as DICOM images attached to the patient's study.

Advanced visualization is also applicable to other modalities. Many MRI postprocessing applications are performed fully at the MRI console, with vendors packaging dedicated software for hardware components of the scanner. Examples include cardiac functional analysis and neuroradiologic applications of white matter tractography, MR perfusion, and MR spectroscopy. 3D ultrasound can be acquired and manipulated at the scanner and is most commonly used in obstetrical or gynecologic imaging. Regardless of the location or method by which images are acquired, it is important that all saved images are reviewed by the radiologist prior to finalizing a report.

REPORTING TOOLS

The process of creating a radiology report is another step in the radiologist's workflow that can be positively affected by informatics. Speech recognition dictation systems are very prevalent, have largely replaced other forms of reporting, and offer the benefit of immediate electronic availability of a report. Commercial vendors of speech-to-text dictation software have various add-on components that may integrate with the RIS or PACS or create cumulative data reports. There are also several unified efforts across the field of radiology to improve the radiology report.

Structured Reporting

A structured radiology report offers consistent organization of information in a structured format with headings and subsections. Basic components include patient demographic information, exam title, patient history, exam technique, comparison studies, findings, and impression. The findings section is typically subdivided into anatomic regions or organs. Taken a step further, structured reporting can also incorporate a standard lexicon of terms to represent imaging findings, impressions, and recommendations. Speech dictation software systems allow relative ease of use of structured reports via templates or macros that have dedicated text fields for each section of the report that are manipulated by the reporting radiologist.

Structured reporting improves clarity, consistency, and communication between radiologists and referring providers. The content of the report itself may also be improved through the guidance of a well-structured template. The Radiological Society of North America has developed a template library of reports that can be shared and adopted for organizational use. In addition, standard structure and language allow for information to be captured and used in quality improvement and safety initiatives. Standardized vocabulary systems, or lexicons, for reporting exist in various forms across different radiology subspecialty areas in an effort to promote high-quality reporting with reproducible results.

The most widely used and well-known lexicon is the ACR Breast Imaging Reporting and Data System (BI-RADS) Atlas. The BI-RADS lexicon was established in collaboration with the FDA, the American Medical Association, the American College of Surgeons, the College of American Pathologists, and the Centers for Disease Control and Prevention. The BI-RADS system's most significant benefit is forcing the classification of imaging findings into categories. In addition to the assessment categories for all mammography reports, BI-RADS also defines standard language to describe abnormal findings. Other, newer organ-specific lexicons have emerged more recently in efforts to standardize the reporting and management of specific imaging findings. The Liver Imaging Reporting and Data System lexicon defines assessment categories for liver lesions that indicate the likelihood of hepatocellular carcinoma. The Lung Imaging Reporting and Data System unifies lung cancer screening CT reporting and management recommendations. These lexicons serve to reduce confusion and variability in reporting and facilitate outcome monitoring.

RadLex

More broadly, a comprehensive standardization of reporting vocabulary and exam orders promotes clarity and plays a role in practice management such as billing and scheduling. The Radiological Society of North America has developed the RadLex project to create a single source for medical imaging terminology. The project began in 2005, and as of 2016, RadLex has more than 68,000 terms encompassing anatomy, pathology, imaging observations, and radiologic workflow. The RadLex project also comprises an index of exam titles to be standardized across health systems and improve billing coding, termed the RadLex Playbook. Perhaps most importantly for radiologists, RadLex lists names and description terms for imaging findings to be used in reporting. This is a further example of efforts to standardize reporting for improved direct patient care and data mining.

Radiology Decision Support

During interpretation and reporting of imaging studies, radiologists may use reference material to help the process. Internet-based searches and use of electronic books are typical methods of looking up information. In an effort to streamline the process during reporting, commercially available software bundles reference material with RIS systems or dictation programs. These tools also use the RadLex vocabulary for searching to give relevant search results. Semiautomated search engines can interface with radiology reports in real time, to quickly highlight associated reference terms. This type of technology applies natural language processing as a search method tool to evaluate dictated report text.

Future Reporting

Additional efforts are currently evolving to improve the radiology report by more closely interacting with the images themselves. Current standard reports are stand-alone text documents that accompany exam images. Through a process of annotation and image markup, future reports may include one or a few example images to better communicate findings and impressions. Image markups such as tumor measurements can be captured directly into table or chart format, displaying lesion sizes over time in a highly effective visual manner. These tasks can be integrated with DICOM and HL7 for widespread ease of use and report sharing.

Structured reporting has been defined here as a template of report fields to be used by the radiologist. In other instances, the term *structured reporting* has been used as a method of automatically filling required data fields of a report. The radiology report is typically a source of more information than just findings and impressions, and data such as contrast media and dose or radiation dose could potentially be populated directly in the report. If the modality interface enables it, image data such as ultrasound measurements performed by the technologist may also be prefilled in the report. These capabilities would improve efficiency and decrease potential error in reporting.

POSTREPORTING APPLICATIONS

Once a radiologist electronically signs a report, the exam closes and the radiologist moves on to the next exam. However, there is a trove of information in each report that may be important to track from the perspective of a department or institution. This includes critical results communication, peer review, or academic research pursuits. This section outlines areas where developing specialized computer programs improves the process of group data collection (Table 17.3).

Data Mining

Data mining is the process of analyzing pools of data and creating summaries of useful information. In radiology, data mining from within a RIS can involve a wide variety of topics, such as report turnaround times, scanner utilization, or preprocedure wait times. Text mining radiology reports for information retrieval is a more difficult process, because free text is unstructured, and language has a high degree of variability and complexity. Structured reporting can help in this regard somewhat. Nonetheless, dedicated programs are required to have algorithms to search reports and employ natural language processing.

Text data mining has multiple uses beyond the more straightforward reporting capabilities of a RIS. Critical results reporting can be tracked. The ACR Practice Guidelines for Communication of Diagnostic Imaging Findings stress timely reporting of critical results and the documentation of such communications into the radiology report. The Joint Commission's National Patient Safety Goals also require the prompt reporting of critical results. Although it is well engrained in radiologists to document critical results communications, tracking this activity is a challenge. An optimal program can search for key phrases or diagnoses and list and summarize these communications, without the need for additional activity by the radiologist.

Report mining can also broadly be used for academic research. Text mining allows for relatively accessible retrospective analyses of particular diagnoses. For example, comparative research of the effectiveness of different imaging modalities could be tracked with regard to their impact on patient care. This could also be tied into the associated clinical decision support software recommended exam types that were originally suggested at the time of order entry. The automated process of defining search terms, whether a particular diagnosis or tied to a particular modality, creates a highly efficient process for data collection.

Critical Results Reporting

Although critical results reporting can be documented by a dedicated software program using data mining, RIS platforms are increasingly creating additional pathways to track such communications. Software features may require that a report be electronically flagged so that critical results populate a specific spreadsheet report. In addition, although critical results are typically communicated directly by the radiologist to the ordering physician, other results that merit an additional level of results notification beyond the standard report may not require a phone call. Institutions may collectively organize other forms of communication to be used in certain settings.

For example, the reporting of solitary pulmonary nodules detected on chest x-ray, or other incidental findings, may significantly slow down a radiologist's workflow if he stops to make a phone call to notify the physician. Automated notification systems can significantly improve this work process efficiency. Software solutions can be embedded within a RIS, dictation system, or third-party add-ons and vary based on an institution's preference. The process of email or fax notification, or electronically highlighting a report, may still require some level of designation on the part of the radiologist at the time of reporting but will still decrease the time spent going through the notification process.

Quality and Safety Initiatives

Informatics software tools can use report or study information data mining in conjunction with additional data or applied work to track areas of patient safety and study quality. One of the most important areas of potential efficiency improvement is peer review. Peer review is the process of assessing radiologists' performance by having radiology reports rated for diagnostic accuracy by radiologist peers. The ACR requires peer review be performed as part of the facility accreditation process. The process of peer review can occur retrospectively without the use of specific software, but having a streamlined process that is

TABLE 17.3 Postreporting Informatics Tools

Category	Tool
Data mining	RIS reports
	Unstructured report mining
	Critical results communication tracking
	Academic research
Quality control	Peer review software
Image sharing	CDs; hard copy
	Shared PACS access
	Online sharing services

CDs, Compact discs; *PACS*, picture archiving and communication system; *RIS*, radiology information system.

incorporated into the RIS and PACS will increase usability and possibly make the process itself more accurate. Various applications of peer review can be embedded into the RIS, PACS, or speech recognition software with a goal of limiting the time spent on the activity.

Other radiology metrics can use data mining to automate the process of retrieving useful information from institutional activity. Software programs can be used to track radiation dose monitoring. In interventional or mammography procedures, complication rates could be followed, as well as biopsy yield. These data could be compiled for review by quality and safety committees as part of ongoing departmental analysis.

Image Sharing

One of the most recent frontiers of imaging informatics is the area of image sharing across healthcare institutions. Traditionally, a patient who seeks care at a new facility with its own imaging network would not bring along easy access to prior imaging exams or other medical record information. The realm of image sharing was limited to carrying compact discs or hard copy films from one facility to another. The benefits of having shared access to prior studies include increased quality of care, reduced costs of unnecessary repeat examinations or additional medical workup, and improved patient safety without having excess study radiation or risk of complication. Sharing access with individual PACS systems is one method of image sharing that is relatively straightforward, but it is limited by user variability, and the patient's imaging history may remain incomplete. Additional methods of image access are displayed in Table 17.3.

Online cloud-based image-sharing services can also be achieved with customized vendor solutions. Specifications are designed to fulfill the needs of an entire facility or physician group and include the capability to integrate with existing systems, image distribution and storage, and image viewing. Image viewers have recently been developed to include zero-footprint viewers that require no dedicated program download and can be used on any hardware device type or operating system. Facilities can make arrangements with vendors to make their studies available on online sharing services and subscribe to a sharing service. This can be particularly useful on a regional level. DICOM, HL7, and IHE are consistently adding to their programming platforms to improve the ability of computer systems to share medical information.

CONCLUSION

Imaging informatics is embedded in nearly every process of radiology workflow, from order entry to postreporting data collection. Some of the standards of informatics tools are well established. Others are quickly evolving or emerging as new areas of involvement. In particular, reporting tools, data mining, and image sharing are areas of rapid growth in terms of both quality of initiatives and use in the industry. Keeping track of all of the latest-and-greatest developments is a constantly changing task. A highly efficient radiology staff requires, at its core, an informatics foundation that can reliably keep up with the demands of a quickly changing landscape.

SUGGESTED READINGS

ACR-AAPM-SIIM Technical Standard for Electronic Practice of Medical Imaging. <http://www.acr.org/~/media/ACR/Documents/PGTS/standards/ElectronicPracticeMedImg.pdf>.

Birdwell RL. The preponderance of evidence supports computer-aided detection for screening mammography. *Radiology*. 2009;253:9–16.

Bolan C. Why CAD is here to stay. *Appl Radiol*. 2011;10:10–11.

Branstetter BF. Basics of imaging informatics: part 1. *Radiology*. 2007;243:656–667.

Branstetter BF. Basics of imaging informatics: part 2. *Radiology*. 2007;244:78–84.

Brennan PC, McEntee M, Evanoff M, Phillips P, O'Connor WT, Manning DJ. Ambient lighting: effect of illumination on soft-copy viewing of radiographs of the wrist. *AJR Am J Roentgenol*. 2007;188:W177–W180.

Calhoun PS, Kuszyk BS, Heath DG, Carley JC, Fishman EK. Three-dimensional volume rendering of spiral CT data: theory and method. *Radiographics*. 1999;19:745–764.

Castellino RA. Computer Aided Detection (CAD): an overview. *Cancer Imaging*. 2005;5:17–19.

D'Orsi CJ, Sickles EA, Mendelson EB, Morris EA. *ACR BI-RADS® Atlas, Breast Imaging Reporting and Data System*. Reston, VA: American College of Radiology; 2013.

Digital Imaging and Communications in Medicine (DICOM). <http://dicom.nema.org/standard.html>.

Dunnick LR, Langlotz CP. The radiology report of the future: a summary of the 2007 Intersociety Conference. *J Am Coll Radiol*. 2008;5:626–629.

Goldberg MA. Image data compression. *J Digit Imaging*. 1997;10:9–11.

Goo JM, Choi JY, Im JG, et al. Effect of monitor luminance and ambient light on observer performance in soft-copy reading of digital chest radiographs. *Radiology*. 2004;232:762–766.

Goyal N, Jain N, Rachapalli V. Ergonomics in radiology. *Clin Radiol*. 2009;64:119–126.

Harisinghani MG, Blake MA, Saksena M, et al. Importance and effects of altered workplace ergonomics in modern radiology suites. *Radiographics*. 2004;24:615–627.

Health Level 7 International. <http://www.hl7.org/index.cfm?ref=nav>.

Hirschorn DS, Krupinski EA, Flynn MJ. PACS displays: how to select the right display technology. *J Am Coll Radiol*. 2014;11(12B):1270–1276.

Huang HK. *PACS and Imaging Informatics: Basic Principles and Applications*. 2nd ed. Hoboken, NJ: Wiley Blackwell; 2010.

Huang HK. Short history of PACS. Part I: USA. *Eur J Radiol*. 2011;78:163–176.

Integrating the Healthcare Enterprise. <http://www.ihe.net/Technical_Frameworks/#radiology>.

Kansagra AP, Yu JJ, Chatterjee AR, et al. Big data and the future of radiology informatics. *Acad Radiol*. 2016;23:30–42.

Klein LW, Miller DL, Balter S, et al. Occupational health hazards in the interventional laboratory: time for a safer environment. *Radiology*. 2009;250:538–544.

Lakhani P, Kim W, Langlotz CP. Automated detection of critical results in radiology reports. *J Digit Imaging*. 2012;25:30–36.

Lakhani P, Kim W, Langlotz CP. Automated extraction of critical test values and communications from unstructured radiology reports. *Radiology*. 2012;265(3):809–818.

Langer SG, Ramthun S, Bender C. Introduction to digital medical image management: departmental concerns. *AJR Am J Roentgen*. 2012;198:746–753.

Liu BJ, Huang HK, Cao F, Zhou MZ, Zhang J, Mogel G. Informatics in radiology. A complete continuous-availability PACS archive server. *Radiographics*. 2004;24:1203–1209.

McEnery KW. Coordinating patient care within radiology and across the enterprise. *J Am Coll Radiol*. 2014;11:1217–1225.

McGinty GB, Allen Jr B, Geis JR, Wald C. IT infrastructure in the era of imaging 3.0. *J Am Coll Radiol*. 2014;11(12B):1197–1204.

Mendelson DS, Rubin DL. Imaging informatics: essential tools for the delivery of imaging services. *Acad Radiol*. 2013;20:1195–1212.

Mendelson DS, Erickson BJ, Choy G. Image sharing: evolving solutions in the age of interoperability. *J Am Coll Radiol*. 2014;11:1260–1269.

Nance JW, Meenan C, Nagy PG. The future of the radiology information system. *AJR Am J Roentgenol*. 2013;200:1064–1070.

Reiner BI. Strategies for radiology reporting and communication. Part I. Challenges and heightened expectations. *J Digit Imaging*. 2013;26:610–613.

Reiner BI. Uncovering and improving upon the inherent deficiencies of radiology reporting through data mining. *J Digit Imaging*. 2010;23(2):109–118.

RSNA RadLex. <http://radlex.org/>.

RSNA Reporting Initiative. <http://www.rsna.org/reporting_initiative.aspx>.

Ruess L, O'Connor SC, Cho KH, et al. Carpal tunnel syndrome and cubital tunnel syndrome: work-related musculoskeletal disorders in four symptomatic radiologists. *AJR Am J Roentgenol*. 2003;203(181):37–42.

Samei EJ, Seibert A, Andriole K, et al. AAPM/RSNA tutorial on equipment selection: PACS equipment overview. *Radiographics*. 2004;24:313–334.

Schwartz LH. Improving communication of diagnostic radiology findings through structured reporting. *Radiology*. 2011;260(1):174–181.

Silva III, Breslau J, Barr RM, et al. ACR white paper on teleradiology practice: a report from the task force on teleradiology practice. *J Am Coll Radiol*. 2013;10:575–585.

Sistrom CL, Langlotz CP. A framework for improving radiology reporting. *J Am Coll Radiol*. 2005;2:159–167.

Thrall JH. Teleradiology. Part I. History and clinical applications. *Radiology*. 2007;243:613–617.

Thrall JH. Teleradiology. Part II. Limitations, risks, and opportunities. *Radiology*. 2007;244:325–328.

Tran L, Wadhwa A, Mann E. Implementation of structured radiology reports. *J Am Coll Radiol*. 2016;13(3):296–299.

Vertinsky T, Forster B. Prevalence of eye strain among radiologists: influence of viewing variables on symptoms. *AJR Am J Roentgenol*. 2005;184:681–686.

Wang KC, Kohli M, Carrino JA. Technology standards in imaging: a practical overview. *J Am Coll Radiol*. 2014;11(12B):1251–1259.

Weiss DL. Structured reporting: patient care enhancement or productivity nightmare? *Radiology*. 2008;249(3):737–747.

Weiss DL, Kim W, Branstetter BF, Prevedello LM. Radiology reporting: a closed-loop cycle from order entry to results communication. *J Am Coll Radiol*. 2014;11(12B):1226–1237.

White CS, Flukinger T, Jeudy J, Chen JJ. Use of a computer-aided detection system to detect missed lung cancer at chest radiography. *Radiology*. 2009;252(1):273–281.

Chapter 18
Statistical Tools and Quantitative Reasoning

Michael A. Bruno and Christopher S. Hollenbeak

INTRODUCTION

The practice of medicine frequently requires that physicians make critical diagnostic and treatment decisions with incomplete information, working in a background of high uncertainty. The specialty of diagnostic radiology is not exempt from this reality. Although people in other walks of life might view such a high-uncertainty/high-stakes situation to be paralyzing, inaction is rarely an option in the practice of medicine. Many doctors consider this to be a fundamental part of the *art of medicine*, wherein a skilled physician must have the courage to commit to a presumptive diagnosis and initiate a treatment plan without the luxury of absolute certainty. Experience has proven, however, that achieving desired patient outcomes requires that physicians also understand the *science of medicine*, including the relative probabilities of the various disease entities they are considering for a patient's diagnosis, the limitations of available diagnostic tests to discriminate among them, and the strength of the evidence supporting the choices to be made among various available treatment options.

The nature of this evidence—and truly of all knowledge in medicine—is inherently stochastic; that is, it is subject to the laws of probability and statistics. It is therefore essential for physicians to understand the core mathematical concepts that underlie the data on which they rely, as well as how to use the tools of probabilistic, quantitative reasoning. Armed with a basic knowledge of statistical methods, physicians will be better able to interpret the relevant medical literature and draw the correct inferences from individual patient data, such as the results of a particular patient's various lab results and diagnostic imaging tests. This is arguably the most important of the noninterpretive skills.

Probability provides an approach to quantifying uncertainty in data that inform decisions. Without it, there is no modern scientific method. At the core of the scientific method is testing of hypotheses via experimentation. The answer to any hypothetical is almost never a simple "yes" or "no" but rather some probability that the outcome of any given experiment or test reflects reality, as opposed to reflecting random chance.

The diagnostic process similarly involves the formation and testing of hypotheses of what disease may be present, often relying on the findings of medical imaging studies. Diagnosis is thus a process analogous to that of testing a hypothesis by asking a scientific question (is disease XX hypothesis by asking a scientific question (is disease XX present) via an experiment (e.g., chest x-ray, computed tomography scan, complete blood count, or other lab test panel) that is sufficiently reproducible and reliable to allow actionable conclusions to be made. Quite often the *experiment* chosen is a modality of medical imaging. The answer to a diagnostic hypothesis being tested by imaging is rarely a simple "yes" or "no," because radiographic appearances are rarely (if ever) pathognomonic. Instead, radiologists frequently report the results of their tests in terms of a differential diagnosis—a rank-ordered list of the most likely underlying explanations for the observed findings. Most radiologists attempt to focus their differential diagnoses on their own professional assessment of the relative likelihood of the diagnostic possibilities under consideration and in doing so rely on Bayesian reasoning, updating their own personal understanding of the pretest probability of disease with diagnostic information provided by imaging and other tests. To inform this reasoning, radiologists depend on their training, their experience, and the medical literature. But to avoid being misled and drawing incorrect conclusions from the literature, radiologists also need to understand what constitutes statistical rigor in any research study being reported and thus be equipped to assess the reliability of the results. This chapter reviews the basic statistical tools and approaches to quantitative reasoning that underlie these tasks.

TAXONOMY OF DATA

A taxonomy of data is an important discussion because there are many different types of data, and the appropriate measure to summarize a variable and the appropriate statistical test that could be used to evaluate a particular experimental result depends first and foremost on the specific type of data under examination (Fig. 18.1).

The first and largest categories of data are *numerical* and *categorical*. As the name implies, numerical data are numbers. These data are actual measured values. There are two types of numerical data: discrete and continuous. Discrete numerical data are measured in integers. For example, the Glasgow coma scale is a discrete numerical variable and takes on only integer values between 3 and 15. Continuous numerical data are represented on some segment of the real line. The significance of occupying some segment of the real line is that numeric variables are sensibly divisible. We can divide them by, say, 2 and still have a sensible data point. For example, report turnaround time or hospital length of stay are examples of continuous

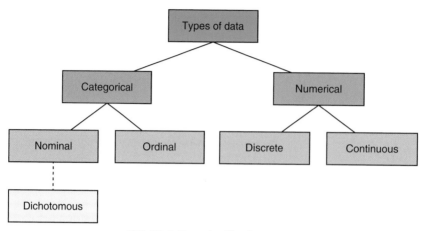

FIG. 18.1 Data classification types.

numerical variables; their values are on the real number line, and as such they can be divided by any real number and still have a sensible value.

Categorical data represent categories and not numbers, per se. Numbers may be used to represent the categories, but this is only for convenience. There are three types of categorical variables: *nominal, ordinal*, and *dichotomous*. Nominal data are variables that have categories with no particular order. Race/ethnicity and marital status are common examples. Numbers may be assigned to represent white non-Hispanic, black non-Hispanic, Hispanic, Asian, Native American, and others, but the number is for convenience, and the specific value and its implied order are irrelevant for nominal categorical variables. Ordinal categorical variables are also categories, but the order of the assigned number has significance. For example, in survey research, a Likert scale is commonly used to represent strength of response: 1, strongly disagree; 2, somewhat disagree; 3, neutral; 4, somewhat agree; 5, strongly agree. Thus, the fact that 3 is greater than 2 is meaningful because it indicates relatively more agreement. The third type of categorical data is dichotomous data. These data take on only two possible categories, for example, female or male, survived or died. It is conventional to use zeros and ones to represent these types of variables.

DATA SUMMARIES

Summarizing data appropriately depends on the type of data represented by the variables. We are usually interested in summarizing data by quantifying their central tendency (a number that represents a *middle* value) and its dispersion (how the data are distributed around the center). Continuous numerical data are best summarized using the average or *mean*, as well as the *median* or *mode* of a group of data. Variation of a variable is best summarized using the range of values, the *variance* or the *standard deviation*.

The most familiar measure of central tendency is the *mean*, or average, of a set of observed values, which is derived by taking the sum of all values divided by the number of observations. When the distribution of a variable is symmetric, the mean is a reasonable measure of central tendency. If the data are skewed or there are extreme values and outliers, then the median provides a more stable

measure of central tendency. The *median* is the value for which an equal number of other observations are found to lie above or below it, and the *mode* is defined as the most commonly occurring value of the variable in the dataset. *Variance* is a measure of dispersion of a variable and is calculated as the sum of the square of each value minus its mean, divided by 1 minus the number of observations:

$$\text{Variance} = \frac{1}{n-1} \sum_{i=1}^{n} (x_i - \overline{x})$$

Standard deviation is the square root of the variance. When a variable is normally distributed—symmetric and bell-shaped—the standard deviation provides a convenient summary of the dispersion of the data. When data are normally distributed, it can be shown that 68% of observations will fall within one standard deviation of the mean, 95% of observations will fall within two standard deviations of the mean, and 99.7% of observations will fall within three standard deviations of the mean.

Normally distributed data are very common in the physical sciences. The distribution of the timing of nuclear decays of any particular isotope around the mean half-life is an example of a normally distributed variable. Most variables in medicine, however, are not normally distributed, and in such cases the standard deviation does not provide the same rule of thumb for spread, and thus reliance on the standard deviation can be misleading. For one common example, the standard deviation is often misused by professors in evaluating test scores of their students (e.g., "the mean of the test was a 60 with a standard deviation of 20") or evaluating the teaching performance of radiology faculty (e.g., "the mean of Dr. Smith's teaching scores from radiology resident questionnaires this quarter was 3.46 with a standard deviation of 1.5"). Because there is no reason to suspect that these sorts of data are normally distributed, the usual interpretation of standard deviation is uninformative.

GRAPHICAL SUMMARIES

In addition to numerical summaries, data can be summarized using visual or graphical methods. Graphs can quickly convey a visual impression of the central tendency,

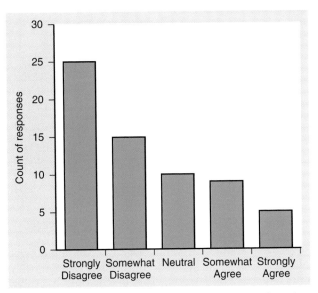

FIG. 18.2 Bar graph expressing counts of survey results using a Likert scale.

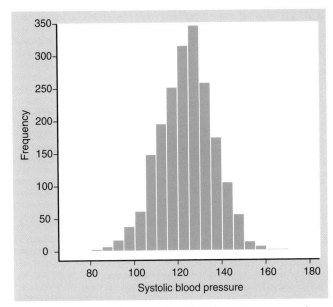

FIG. 18.4 Histogram showing the distribution of measures of systolic blood pressure in a sample of patients.

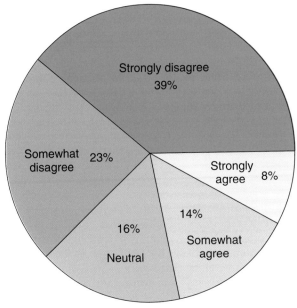

FIG. 18.3 Pie chart expressing proportions of survey results using a Likert scale.

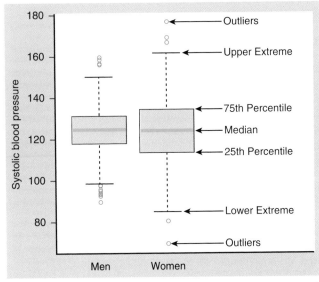

FIG. 18.5 Boxplot of systolic blood pressure measurements stratified by sex.

dispersion, and the distribution of data. Categorical data can be summarized using *bar charts*, which present counts (or percentages) of categories. The distribution of categorical data can also be displayed using *pie charts*, which present percentages of categories. Fig. 18.2 presents data from a survey question measured with a 5-point Likert scale. These data are ordinal categorical data. The bar graph presents counts of responses. Fig. 18.3 summarizes the same ordinal categorical data from survey responses in proportions using a pie chart. The graphical presentations of the data in Figs. 18.2 and 18.3 provide similar but complementary information about the responses to the survey question.

For continuous data, a *histogram* divides a variable into equally sized discrete units and then plots counts or percentages of observations that fall into each unit. An example is presented in Fig. 18.4, which shows the

distribution of systolic blood pressure in a sample of 2000 adults, including 1000 women and 1000 men.

When there is a need to summarize the distribution of more than one continuous variable at once, or to stratify a continuous variable by two or more groups, boxplots provide an excellent visual summary. A boxplot presents the quartiles of the data, extreme values (usually defined as 1.5 times the interquartile range, or the difference between the 25th and 75th percentile), and any outliers beyond the extreme values. An example of a boxplot of systolic blood pressure for men and women is presented in Fig. 18.5, with each summary indicated on the graph.

A visual summary of the correlation or relationship between two numerical variables can be made with a *scatterplot*. The scatterplot shown in Fig. 18.6 plots the relationship between body mass index and waist circumference. Note that by using separate colors we can

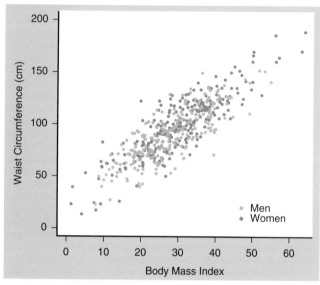

FIG. 18.6 Scatterplot of waist circumference and body mass index in men and women.

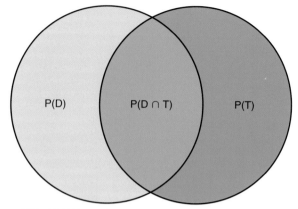

FIG. 18.7 Venn diagram of conditional probabilities.

distinguish the relationship between strata, in this case between men and women.

PROBABILITY

Probability is a measure of how likely it is that an event will occur. In other words, probability serves to quantify the level of uncertainty that is present in any given dataset. It is measured using a number between 0 and 1, where 0 represents absolute impossibility of the event and 1 represents absolute certainty of the event. Historically, there have been several definitions of probability. In most current scientific research, probability is interpreted according to the frequentist definition, which is that probability is the long-run relative frequency of the occurrence of an event. For example, we say that the probability of obtaining heads on a coin toss is 50%, not because heads is one of two possibilities, but rather because in a very large series of coin flips, heads occurs half of the time.

We call phenomena that have probabilities attached to them *random variables*. For example, a coin toss is a random variable; we know the set of possible outcomes of a coin toss (heads and tails), but we do not know which of these outcomes will be obtained before flipping the coin. Whether an individual has a disease is a random variable because we do not know whether the patient has a disease until we administer a diagnostic test. The *sample space* of a random variable is the set of all possible outcomes. The sample space for the random variable of whether an individual has a disease has two elements: yes and no. Probabilities describe the likelihood of each of the elements of the random variable. Sometimes probabilities are determined by two events. For example, assume we have two random variables: whether a patient has disease (*D*) and whether a diagnostic test result is positive (*T*). We use *P(D)* to denote the probability that a patient has disease, and we use *P(T)* to denote the probability that the patient tests positive for the disease. The probability that both events occur is the intersection of *D* and *T*, denoted *P(D∩B)*.

Fig. 18.7 contains a Venn diagram that demonstrates these relationships. The circle on the left contains all patients who have disease; the circle on the right contains all patients who test positive. The intersection of the circles is represented by the overlapping region and contains just patients who have disease and who test positive. Two random events are *independent* if the occurrence of one of the events does not affect the occurrence of the other. If, on the other hand, the occurrence of one event does impact the occurrence of another event, the probabilities are called *conditional*. Disease and diagnostic tests are conditional probabilities because if a diagnostic test is positive, the patient is more likely to have disease. We denote a conditional probability as *P(T | D)*, which is the probability of *T* (that a patient tests positive) given that *D* (the patient has disease) has occurred. We can compute *P(T | D)* in Fig. 18.7 as the area *P(T ∩ D)* divided by the area *P(D)*.

DIAGNOSTIC TEST PERFORMANCE

Conditional probability is the underlying concept of diagnostic test performance. The most common measures of the performance of a diagnostic test are sensitivity and specificity. Sensitivity is *P(T | D)*: the probability that a test result is positive given that a patient has disease. In a sample of patients, sensitivity is measured as the proportion of patients with disease who test positive. If a diagnostic test has high sensitivity, then it is informative about patients who have disease. Specificity is *P(T− | D−)*: the probability that a test result is negative given that a patient does not have disease. In a sample of patients, specificity is measured as the proportion of patients without disease who test negative. If a diagnostic test has high specificity, then it is informative about patients who do not have disease.

Fig. 18.8 illustrates how to compute these measures from a sample of patients. Suppose a diagnostic test with two possible outcomes (positive and negative) is administered to a group of patients who either do or do not have disease. In the diagnostic test matrix in Fig. 18.8, the number of patients who test positive and actually have disease (the true-positive results) is *a*, and the number of patients who test positive who do not have disease (the false-positive results) is *b*. Similarly, the number of patients who have disease who test negative (the false-negative results) is *c*, and the number of patients who do not have disease who test negative (the true-negative results) is *d*. Sensitivity measures the proportion of patients who actually have

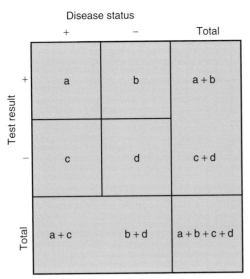

Disease status

FIG. 18.8 Contingency table for computing diagnostic performance characteristics.

disease among all patients who test positive: $a/(a + c)$. Diagnostic tests with a high specificity excel at ruling out disease, because negative test results suggest a low probability that disease is present. Specificity measures the proportion of patients who actually have no disease among all patients who test negative: $d/(b + d)$. Diagnostic tests with a high specificity excel at ruling in disease, because positive results suggest a high probability of the presence of disease. Overall test accuracy combines elements of sensitivity and specificity and measures the proportion of *true* results (i.e., true-positive plus true-negative) among all patients. Accuracy is defined as $(a + d)/(a + b + c + d)$.

Although sensitivity and specificity are important measures of diagnostic test accuracy, most clinicians are less interested in the probability that a patient who has disease tests positive and more interested in the probability that a patient has disease given that a test is positive. That is, rather than $P(T \mid D)$, clinicians need to know $P(D \mid T)$. This quantity can be computed using Bayes' theorem, which is a rule of conditional probability. Bayes' theorem is:

$$P(D \mid T) = \frac{P(T \mid D)\,P(D)}{P(T)}$$

Bayes' theorem allows us to compute one conditional probability from another: if we know $P(T \mid D)$, then we can compute $P(D \mid T)$. The first term in the numerator, $P(T \mid D)$ is the test sensitivity. The second term, $P(D)$, is the prevalence of disease in the population. The denominator, $P(T)$, is the probability that a patient will test positive. This term must be expanded into two parts, because there are two types of patients who test positive: those with disease and those without disease. Thus, $P(T) = P(T \mid D)P(D) + P(T \mid D-)P(D-)$. The second two terms can be identified as 1 − specificity, and 1 − prevalence. This means that if we know a diagnostic test's sensitivity and specificity, and the prevalence of disease in the population, then we can compute the probability that a patient has disease if he or she has a positive test. Assume a diagnostic test has a sensitivity of 76% and a specificity of 92%. In addition, the prevalence of disease in the population is

2%. If a patient received a positive result from a diagnostic test, then the probability she actually has disease is:

$$P(D \mid T) = \frac{0.76 \times 0.02}{0.76 \times 0.02 + 0.08 \times 0.98}$$

$$= \frac{0.0152}{0.0152 + 0.0784} = 16.24\%$$

This quantity is also called the *positive predictive value*. The *negative predictive value* is $P(D- \mid T-)$ and is the probability that a patient does not have disease given that she has received a negative result on the diagnostic test. If contingency table data are available as in Fig. 18.8, then the positive predictive value can be computed as $a/(a + b)$ and the *negative predictive value* can be computed as $d/(c + d)$.

SPECIAL TOPICS: SENSITIVITY, SPECIFICITY, ACCURACY, AND RECEIVER-OPERATING CHARACTERISTIC CURVES AND ANALYSIS

Many diagnostic test results are not dichotomous (positive/negative) but continuous, for example, the size of a mediastinal lymph node in a patient with lymphoma undergoing chemotherapy. In such cases we must dichotomize the result and choose a threshold value above which we declare the result positive. There are inevitable tradeoffs in this choice. At the lower end, a threshold of 0 would return a positive result for all patients, and give the test a sensitivity of 100%, but it would also give a specificity of 0%. As we increase the threshold value, the sensitivity falls and the specificity rises. Ultimately a threshold will be chosen that balances the tradeoff between sensitivity and specificity. The desired tradeoff may differ depending on the reason for obtaining the diagnostic test. For example, for a *screening test* such as screening mammography, which is performed on a large asymptomatic patient population, a very high level of sensitivity is desired, and one may be willing to sacrifice some degree of specificity to achieve that sensitivity.

The receiver-operating characteristic (ROC) curve provides a visual representation of the tradeoff between sensitivity and specificity of all possible thresholds for defining a positive diagnostic test. To construct an ROC curve, the test's sensitivity (true-positive rate) is graphed against 1 − specificity (false-negative rate) for each threshold value. The area under the curve (AUC) of the ROC curve also provides a measure of the performance of a diagnostic test. The AUC has a range of 0.5 to 1. Fig. 18.9 presents an ROC curve for a predictive model of low-birth-weight newborns. The AUC for this model is 0.65, which suggests only moderate performance. The worst possible diagnostic test, equivalent to flipping a coin, has an ROC curve that lies along the gray 45-degree line in Fig. 18.9 and has an AUC of 0.5. A perfect test that precisely predicts all positive and negative cases has an ROC with a right angle, covers the entire region, and has an AUC equal to 1.

PROBABILITY DISTRIBUTIONS

A probability distribution is a function that assigns a probability to all possible events in a sample space. Because events can be described according to our taxonomy of data, different probability distributions are required to

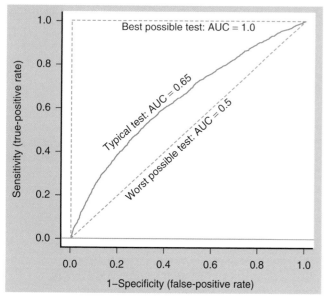

FIG. 18.9 Receiver-operating characteristic curve, with an area under the curve of 0.65.

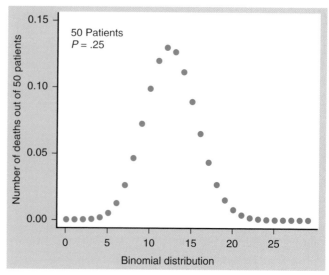

FIG. 18.11 Binomial distribution for a sample of 50 patients facing a probability of dying of 0.25.

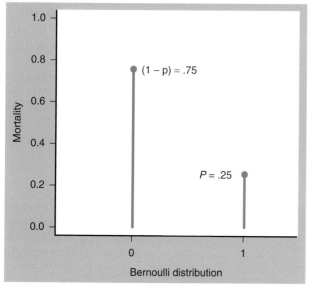

FIG. 18.10 Bernoulli distribution for a binary random variable.

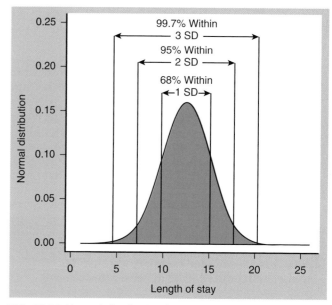

FIG. 18.12 Normal distribution for length of stay with a mean of 12 days and a standard deviation of 2.5 days.

describe different types of variables. For example, mortality (lived/died) is a dichotomous outcome, and a probability distribution for mortality would assign a probability value for each possible outcome: living and dying. This is the Bernoulli distribution, and an example is presented in Fig. 18.10, which shows a probability of dying of 0.25 and a probability of surviving of 0.75.

The Bernoulli distribution applies to the outcome of a single individual; in a sample, however, we may be interested in the number of deaths we might expect in N patients. This is modeled with a binomial distribution, which assigns a probability to the number of deaths that would occur in a sample of patients who each faced an identical probability of dying. Fig. 18.11 provides an example of the binomial distribution for a sample of 50 patients facing a probability of dying of 0.25. As seen in Fig. 18.7, the most likely number of patients who would die is 12, but there is some probability that it lies between 5 and 20.

Mortality and number of deaths are both discrete numerical variables, and the Bernoulli and binomial distributions are therefore discrete, with a point mass on each of the finite possible outcomes. However, for a continuous variable such as length of stay, a binomial distribution is inappropriate because length of stay can take on any number between 0 and infinity. A normal distribution, which is the classic bell-shaped curve, might be used to represent length of stay. Fig. 18.12 presents a normal distribution where length of stay has a mean of 12 days and a standard deviation of 2.5 days. It also shows how the standard deviation can be interpreted for normally distributed variables; 68% of events occur within 1 standard deviation of the mean, 95% of events occur within 2 standard deviations of the mean, and 99.7% of events occur within 3 standard deviations of the mean.

HYPOTHESIS TESTING

Although descriptive statistics are useful for describing and summarizing data, inferential statistics are useful for testing hypotheses. Probability distributions form the basis for testing hypotheses. Most inferential statistics assume that natural phenomena are driven by probability distributions. These probability distributions define the population, and the population parameters are unknown. However, because natural phenomena generate data, we can take samples of observations from the population, compute statistics, make inferences about the true population parameters, and test hypotheses about the true underlying population parameters.

When testing hypotheses, it is useful to think in terms of cause and effect and distinguish between variables that are causative and variables that are reactive. The variables that cause a result are called *independent* or *predictor* variables. The variables that are caused are called *dependent* or *outcome* variables. If we perform a randomized controlled trial of a lipid-lowering medication to test whether treatment reduces low-density lipoprotein (LDL) cholesterol, then drug treatment is considered to be the independent variable and LDL cholesterol is the dependent variable.

Hypotheses are statements about the location of population parameters. The most important hypothesis in radiology and biomedicine is the null hypothesis, which is a hypothesis of null effect. The null hypothesis always states that there is no effect of an independent variable on a dependent variable. So, for example, in our randomized controlled trial of lipid-lowering medication, the null hypothesis is that lipid-lowering medication does not impact the LDL cholesterol of treated patients relative to placebo controls.

POWER AND SAMPLE SIZE

Tests of hypotheses are not perfect. As we test hypotheses and either reject or fail to reject a null hypothesis, we will make mistakes. Sometimes we will reject a null hypothesis when it is true (i.e., we will conclude that there is a real effect of treatment when in reality there is none). This type of error is called a false-positive, or type I, error. Sometimes we will accept a null hypothesis when it is false (i.e., we will conclude that there is no real effect of treatment when in reality there is one). This type of error is called a false-negative, or type II, error.

We have some control over the likelihood of making type I and type II errors when we design studies and conduct experiments. The probability of making a type I error is noted as an α. We call it α *significance*, and we usually set it to .05. When we choose to reject a null hypothesis when a *P* value is .05 or less, or when the null value is outside of the 95% confidence interval, we are setting the α level to .05. This assures that there is only a 5% probability of rejecting the null hypothesis if in fact it were true. If we wanted to reduce the likelihood of a type I error to, say, 1%, then we would set the α level to .01 and only reject the null hypothesis if the *P* value were less than .01 or if the null value were outside the 99% confidence interval. We also have some control over type II errors. The probability of making a type II error is noted as β, and it is customary to set the level to .20. Thus, most experiments have a 20% probability of accepting the null hypothesis when in reality it is true.

Most of the time the type II error rate is quantified not using β but using $1 - β$. This is called quantity *power*. Thus, the power of a statistical test is the probability that you will *not* make a type II error. We can control the power of a study by adjusting its sample size. The larger the number of observations, all other things being equal, the more precisely a treatment effect is estimated and the less likely we are to make a type II error. In fact, there is a direct relationship between power and sample size. For a given treatment effect, it is possible to perform a sample size calculation to determine, a priori, how many patients must be enrolled to achieve a given level of power. In addition, if the sample size is fixed, it is possible to perform a power calculation that will tell you the power level that is achieved for a given sample size.

STATISTICAL TESTS

Statistical tests begin with an assumption about the probability distribution of the dependent variable under consideration. As such, the first consideration for any statistical test is the kind of data that are represented by the dependent variable: are they dichotomous, discrete, or continuous? We must, therefore, begin with an assumption about how the dependent variable is distributed that is consistent. For example, if we performed a clinical trial of a lipid-lowering medication on LDL cholesterol, the dependent variable is LDL cholesterol, which is continuous. The second consideration for any statistical test is what kind of data are represented by the independent variable. In the LDL-lowering trial, the independent variable is treatment, which is dichotomous. Once the type of data represented by the dependent and independent variables are identified, the statistical test follows. Table 18.1 presents the most common univariate statistical tests and the scenarios where they are used.

When the dependent variable and independent variable are both dichotomous, we are comparing two proportions, and the chi-squared test is appropriate. For example, if we wanted to compare mortality between a treated and a control group, this reduces to a comparison of two proportions, which could be done using a chi-squared test. When the dependent variable is dichotomous and the independent variable is discrete or categorical, we are comparing more than two proportions. This is also accomplished with a chi-squared test.

If the dependent variable is continuous, the independent is dichotomous, and patients serve as their own controls, then we are comparing two means in the same group of patients at two different time points. The appropriate univariate statistical test is a paired *t* test. If the dependent variable is continuous, the independent variable is dichotomous, and control patients differ from treated patients (the usual scenario for a placebo-controlled trial), then we are essentially comparing two means from two different groups of patients. The appropriate statistical test for such a comparison is the Student *t* test.

If the dependent variable is continuous and the independent variable is discrete or categorical, then the goal is to compare more than two means. Analysis of variance provides the appropriate statistical test.

The statistical tests contained in the first column of Table 18.1 are called *parametric* statistical tests. This is because they each begin with an assumption about the underlying

TABLE 18.1   Common Univariate Parametric and Nonparametric Statistical Tests

Statistical Test	Dependent Variable	Independent Variable	Description	Null Hypothesis	Nonparametric Alternative
Chi-squared test	Dichotomous	Dichotomous	Compare two proportions. Usually done with a 2 × 2 contingency table.	There is no difference in proportions between the two groups.	Chi-squared test
Chi-squared test	Discrete or categorical	Dichotomous, discrete, or categorical	Compare more than two proportions. Usually done with a N × K contingency table.	There is no difference in proportions across the groups.	Chi-squared test
Paired t test	Continuous	Dichotomous	Compare two means for the same group at two time points.	There is no difference in means between the two time points.	Wilcoxon signed rank test
Two-sample t test	Continuous	Dichotomous	Compare two means from different groups.	There is no difference in proportions between the two groups.	Mann-Whitney U test, Wilcoxon rank sum test
Analysis of variance	Continuous	Discrete or categorical	Compare more than two means.	There is no difference in means across the groups.	Kruskal-Wallis test

probability distribution and make inferences based on the parameters of that distribution. This works when the sample size is reasonably large. When the sample size is small, a *nonparametric* test is recommended. Nonparametric tests do not make assumptions about the underlying distributions of the data. Rather, they take advantage of ranks, orders, and sums that should be expected to follow under the null hypothesis. There is a nonparametric alternative to every statistical test; the most common nonparametric tests are presented in the last column of Table 18.1. Nonparametric tests are usually recommended when there are fewer than 20 observations in each group.

INFERENCE

Statistical tests are used to test hypotheses, specifically the null hypothesis. The P value from a statistical test is the usual object of inference. The P value does not provide a direct test of the null hypothesis. Rather, the P value assumes the null hypothesis is true and then asks the probability that one would observe a dataset with an effect as large, or larger, as was observed *if the null hypothesis was true*. Thus, if this probability is small, then the data are inconsistent with the null hypothesis (i.e., the effect is real), and we declare the result statistically significant; if this probability is large, the data are consistent with the null hypothesis (i.e., the effect is due to chance), and we declare the result not statistically significant.

The threshold for the determination of statistical significance is usually set at 0.05, but it should be noted that this is convention only, and there is nothing magic about 0.05 as a threshold for statistical significance. With a P value set at $P < .05$, there is still a 1 in 20 chance that the results were observed purely by chance. The choice of the $P < .05$ threshold often reflects the very high levels of uncertainty

that are inherent in biomedical research. In some studies the threshold may be set to $P < .01$ (a 1% probability that the null hypothesis is being rejected purely by random chance). This is in sharp contrast to the physical sciences, such as when physicists were determining the mass of the Higgs boson from millions of measurements conducted by two separate detector groups using very different methods at the Large Hadron Collider at CERN. In that example, the null hypothesis would not be rejected unless the P value was on the order of 5σ or 6σ, corresponding to $P < .00001$ or $P < .000001$, a threshold reflecting the much greater degree of accuracy in the measurements and the very large sample sizes available to the physical scientist, neither of which are generally achievable in medical research. So in a sense, the .05 threshold convention represents a compromise position for medical scientists. Our *signals* are so small and our *noise* is so large that we accept a level of significance in which we incorrectly reject a null hypothesis 1 time in 20 of our experiments.

PERILS OF $P < .05$: *REDUCTIO AD ABSURDUM*

The common practice of accepting a $P < .05$ threshold of significance to reject a null hypothesis has serious ramifications in biomedical research, which can serve to keep the individual clinician reasonably skeptical in relying on a particular test result as applied to a particular patient. First, statistical significance is designed to predict the likelihood of a particular test or treatment being accurate or effective when applied to a *population of patients*, but there is nothing in the statistical test that can inform you about your *individual* patient's results. Second, there is the very real (human) problem of cognitive bias on the part of the researchers themselves as well as their audience. These biases are not fully conscious modes of thought and can lead honest people to arrive at conclusions that grossly overreach the data, a natural human tendency that can be made even more problematic when combined with the sorts of perverse incentives that exist within the field of medical science today (e.g., the imperative to "publish or perish" to name just one). Many researchers joke about the practice of "torturing the data until it confesses," which is to say, finding creative and ostensibly valid ways of altering the parameters of the experiment, including exclusion of some unsupportive data points, until the $P < .05$ threshold is finally reached, rather than just accepting the null hypothesis and moving on. The underlying problem is that a P value that is set below any given threshold to reject the null hypothesis does not in itself prove causation but only establishes an acceptable level at which the results are considered *unlikely enough* to be due to pure, random chance.

Consider, for example, the following thought experiment, which was suggested by a very funny comic drawn by author Randall Munroe on his *xkcd* website (https://xkcd.com/882/) some years ago (Box 18.1). Sound far-fetched? It really isn't. We could cite a handful of examples of very similar scenarios unfolding in the past few decades. It is in reference to such silliness that people complain that there are three types of lies: lies, damned lies, and statistics. But it is not the math that is at fault but rather the realities of cognitive bias and our fallible human nature.

STUDY DESIGN AND OVERCOMING BIAS

Cognitive bias is a fundamental part of being human, and overcoming our own human cognitive biases is a challenge for everyone involved in performing research as well as those who must skeptically evaluate the results of published research as applied to clinical care. Unrecognized biases and hidden assumptions contaminating study data and skewing interpretation are a potential problem in all types of research. In evaluating a study reported in the radiology literature, one must be very careful not to simply accept the researchers' assumptions or take for granted that the journal reviewers have caught and corrected all of their reasoning or other errors. Instead, it falls to readers of a scientific paper to verify for themselves whether the expressed or hidden assumptions make sense with existing knowledge, whether the unique characteristics of the study population can truly be generalized to a population of patients, whether they have chosen an appropriate statistical method for their type of data, and so forth.

Dozens of cognitive biases have been described in the literature, a topic beyond the scope of this chapter. Suffice it to say that *all* experimental evidence presented in the scientific literature must be thoroughly questioned before one is certain that the results constitute strong enough evidence on which to base one's medical practice. One must also bear in mind the potentially perverse incentives that may be driving some of the research results encountered in the literature and, of course, the limitations that underlie of the concept of *statistical significance*.

When reading and evaluating a research paper, even one that is highly venerated and is felt to represent *settled science*, readers should ask themselves whether the data really justify the statistical test that was chosen; that is, has

---

BOX 18.1 Jelly Bean Thought Experiment

A researcher sets out to determine whether one or more of the 50 official flavors of Jelly Belly gourmet jelly bean candies might increase the survival time (measured in hours) of monkeys infected with Ebola virus. The makers of Jelly Bellies have never made any assertions that their product has any medicinal value, and so we can only speculate why a researcher would wish to carry out such a project; the candies may be his favorite, or he may have received a generous grant from a sugar-related foundation, or perhaps the scientist may have gotten the idea after a visit to the Reagan Presidential Library in Simi Valley, California. We can never know.

So, armed with some foundation money and with the significance threshold set to reject H_0 at $P < .05$, the scientist ought to know even before he begins that it is therefore possible that 1:20 of the flavors will show a significant effect purely by random chance. Indeed, after months of hard work running the experiment, he finds that *one* of the 50 flavors, *tutti-frutti*, did indeed appear to enhance survival in Ebola-infected monkeys by an average of 6.2 h. Of course, that is even lower than would be expected from the $P < .05$ threshold, and you as a prudent person would easily conclude that the null hypothesis is true, as expected.

But instead, our researcher somehow instead concludes that he has achieved a breakthrough! His research has proven that *tutti-frutti* Jelly Bellies have been shown to significantly increase survival in Ebola! The scientific paper is then eagerly written (he needs to publish his work in order to keep his job and get even more foundation funding, after all), and in his paper he somehow neglects to highlight the fact that actually all 50 flavors of the candies were tested and 49 of them had absolutely no effect. "*Who publishes negative results?*" he reasons. The paper is dutifully peer reviewed, and the three reviewers all note that the author has used rigorous statistical methods and achieved a $P < .05$, as is required by their journal. And so the paper is published in a prestigious medical journal with a picture of a *tutti-frutti* Jelly Belly on the cover of the issue.

You would think that the story would end there; skeptical readers would scoff at the paper. But wait! It is picked up by the press whose *talking head* scientific advisor, perhaps a distinguished retired medical school dean from an elite northeastern institution, opines on TV that perhaps the effect of the candies is because the Ebola virus is known to have polysaccharides in its envelope (see, e.g., a study by Ritchie et al. in 2010). The public needs no further convincing, and now every physician in the world comes to accept as *settled science* the unarguable fact that *tutti-frutti* Jelly Bellies should always be part of the standard treatment regimen for patients infected by the Ebola virus.

---

a linear regression method been used for data that should really not be expected to have a linear relationship? Consider also what potential cognitive biases might underlie the study design, the subject exclusion/inclusion criteria, or the data gathering. Finally, when interpreting the results of a research study involving thousands of patients or an individual patient's magnetic resonance imaging scan, it is imperative to bear in mind that every study (and every operator) has a unique ROC curve, that the underlying prevalence of disease within the study population matters a great deal, and that one must always apply an appropriate level of caution when considering the level of certainty that any result entails.

Medicine is a high-stakes environment with a very high level of uncertainty, yet inaction is rarely an option. Thus, we reliably err.

SUGGESTED READINGS

Ellenberg J. *How Not to Be Wrong: The Power of Mathematical Thinking*. New York: The Penguin Press; 2014.

Firestein S. *Failure: Why Science Is So Successful*. New York: Oxford University Press; 2016.

Hatch S. *Snowball in a Blizzard: A Physician's Notes on Uncertainty in Medicine*. New York: Basic Books; 2016.

Hough D. *Irrationality in Healthcare: What Behavioral Economics Reveals about What We Do and Why*. Stanford, CA: Stanford University Press; 2013.

Munro BH, Visintainer MA, Page EB. *Statistical Methods for Health Care Research*. Philadelphia, PA: J.B. Lippincott Co; 1986.

Ritchie G, Harvey DJ, Stroeher U, et al. Identification of *N*-glycans from Ebola virus glycoproteins by matrix-assisted laser desorption/ionization time-of-flight and negative ion electrospray tandem mass spectroscopy. *Rapid Commun Mass Spectrom*. 2010;24(5):571-585.

Savage SL. *The Flaw of Averages: Why We Underestimate Risk in the Face of Uncertainty*. Hoboken, NJ: Wiley & Sons; 2009.

Silver N. *The Signal and the Noise: Why So Many Predictions Fail—But Some Don't*. New York: Penguin Books; 2012.

Strogatz S. *The Joy of X: A Guided Tour of Math*. New York: Houghton Mifflin Harcourt; 2012.

Wasserstein RL, Lazar NA. The ASA's statement on *p*-values: context, process, and purpose. *Am Stat*. 2016;70(2):129-133.

SECTION III

Practice-Specific and Subspecialty Radiology Topics

Chapter 19

Imaging of Pregnant and Lactating Women

Manjiri Dighe and Jeff M. Moirano

INTRODUCTION

Radiation risks are of concern in pregnant patients due to the potential of harmful effects on the fetus. However, due to referring physician concerns about maternal health, some exams using ionizing radiation have to be performed in pregnant patients. A balance between appropriateness and overutilization of imaging techniques needs to be maintained to provide the best care to the patient. Any imaging technique performed should adhere to the "as low as reasonably achievable" (ALARA) principle. This chapter discusses the risks and safety issues related to imaging pregnant and lactating patients; reviews the evidence-based imaging recommendations, issues related to contrast administration, counseling, and informed consent and risk management; and discusses modality-specific considerations.

Radiation Dose Risk and Pregnancy

Almost any activity carries certain inherent risks, and the medical use of ionizing radiation is no exception. The mechanism of biological damage from x-ray interactions is well known. Although extensively studied, the risks from low doses of radiation in the ranges typically used in a clinical imaging setting remain highly controversial. Despite the controversy, it is important to recognize that the benefits of medical radiation are clear, and every effort should be made to ensure that these benefits continue to far outweigh any possible risk.

Maternal Risk

The detrimental effects of radiation are due to ionization within tissues, which occur directly with the genetic material itself, or more commonly through formation of free radicals in water molecules, which then react with DNA as shown in Fig. 19.1. This damage is typically repaired, but

unrepaired reactions fall into two categories of biological harm: cell death, which leads to deterministic or tissue effects, or alterations in the genetic code, which leads to stochastic effects.

Deterministic or tissue effects are rarely seen in adults at diagnostic exposure levels. These effects are associated with a threshold dose below which no effect is seen, and the severity of the effect increases with the dose. Although quite rare, the adult patient is at some risk of tissue effects due to complications or errors, particularly in interventional radiology cases or perfusion computed tomography (CT). Examples include erythema, epilation, or skin necrosis. Transient skin effects have an approximate threshold of 2 Gy single-site acute skin dose, while effects that may cause longer-term issues do not appear until 5 Gy.

At the low doses seen in diagnostic imaging, most of the risk to the adult is due to stochastic effects. Although highly debated, the scientific community generally assumes that stochastic effects have no dose threshold; therefore even the smallest radiation dose carries a nonzero risk. The stochastic effect of primary concern is cancer induction. Many factors significantly influence the risk of cancer development from exposure to radiation, including age, sex, the rate of exposure, and genetic considerations. As far as a risk estimate, the most widely used figure is a 5% risk of radiation-induced detriment per 1 Sievert (Sv) dose for the adult general population. It should be noted that the radiation-induced excess cancer risk associated with low levels of radiation as used in diagnostic imaging are orders of magnitude smaller than the spontaneous cancer risk.

Fetal Risk

Due to their high rate of cellular proliferation, developing organisms are much more sensitive to the effects of radiation, and thus the fetus is much more sensitive than adults

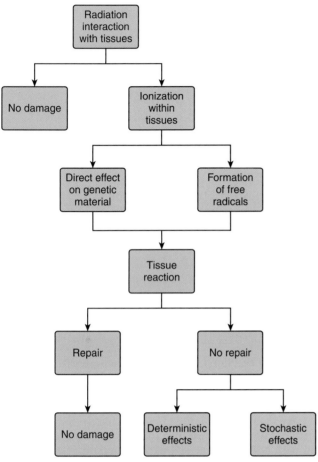

FIG. 19.1 Effects of radiation on tissues.

or children. The potential risks include deterministic effects such as microcephaly, mental retardation, organ malformation, fetal death, and stochastic effects such as carcinogenesis. The relative risk of effect depends primarily on gestational age and the total absorbed dose. Although the fetal risks at typical diagnostic imaging dose levels (as well as occupational levels) are minimal, careful consideration should be taken to maintain the fetal dose as low as possible while achieving the greatest diagnostic value from the exam.

In the preimplantation stage (0–2 weeks postconception), the developing embryo is very radiosensitive. The only potential risk is of fetal death, because the radiation-induced effects in this period are considered to have an *all-or-none* effect. Any nonlethal damage will be repaired to the extent that it will not manifest in any way after birth. The dose threshold for fetal death in this stage is 50 to 100 mGy. After the preimplantation stage, the threshold for fetal death rises to 250 mGy.

During organogenesis (2–8 weeks postconception), the main risk is for teratogenic effects such as microcephaly and organ malformations. The affected organ systems are at most risk during the period of their peak differentiation. The threshold for affects is 100 mGy. The organ group most at risk in humans is the central nervous system, which has a comparatively longer differentiation period.

The effects most likely during the fetal growth stage (weeks 8 to term) are neuropathologies such as mental retardation and lowering of IQ. Most of the risk is

negligible unless the doses are very high (>100–200 mGy). The most susceptible period is from weeks 8 to 16, after which the threshold dose for these effects is believed to be 500 mGy.

Carcinogenic risk is assumed to be constant post implantation, though some animal studies suggest a stronger sensitivity in the late fetal growth stage. The excess risk of childhood cancer incidence for exposures of 10 mGy is estimated to be 0.06%, compared to the background risk of 0.14%.

Fetal doses due to diagnostic imaging are rarely high enough to significantly increase risk to the fetus. If the fetus is not in the primary beam of the x-ray, the contribution from scatter radiation is insignificant. Typical fetal absorbed doses for abdominal exams range from 1 to 3 mGy for planar radiography to 16 to 31 mGy for a CT exam, depending on scan parameters and maternal size. Interventional cases can carry a greater radiation burden depending on the duration and complexity of the case, but it is rare for the total fetal dose to exceed 50 mGy.

The American College of Obstetrics and Gynecologists has stated, "Fetal risk of anomalies, growth restriction, or abortion have not been reported with radiation exposure of less than 50 mGy." The 50-mGy threshold under which prenatal effects of ionizing radiation are considered negligible or nonexistent is echoed in similar position statements issued by other regulatory and professional groups.

Fetal Dose Estimation

Estimation of the fetal dose is required for appropriate counseling and management of pregnant patients who undergo imaging exams. There are many factors that play a part in the estimation, including gestation age, depth and position of the fetus, entrance skin dose to the patient, radiation quality and quantity, geometry of the patient and beam, and others. Due to the complexity of the calculation, it is best to consult with an experienced medical or health physicist for detailed fetal dose estimates. However, a rule of thumb that may be used for gross estimation is that the fetus will receive one-third of the skin entrance dose for radiographic or fluoroscopic procedures. For CT exams or interventional procedures, or any set of exposures that approach 50 mGy, a more detailed estimate should be made to provide the most accurate information possible to the patient and physician.

In an ideal scenario, the pregnancy will be known in advance, and an estimate can be made using a direct measurement method such as placement of a thermoluminescent dosimeter on the abdomen before the exposure. This, in conjunction with other details, will allow an accurate estimation. In the more likely event of an unknown pregnancy that is revealed later, it is best to gather as much information about the case as soon as possible, interviewing anyone present about information they can recall that will aid in the calculation. Modern equipment should provide a detailed record of the exposure that is accessible. There are several methods that can be employed to estimate the fetal dose, depending on the amount of information that is available as shown in Table 19.1.

TABLE 19.1   Process for Prospective and Retrospective Fetal Dose Estimation

Prospective Dose Estimation	Retrospective Dose Estimation
Thermoluminescent dosimeter (TLD) placed on a patient at the uterus level	Physicist estimates the average dose to the uterus (fetus)
TLD is sent to a facility for readout	If fetal dose is <50 mGy (trigger level), dose info is entered in the dosimetry report
Physicists estimate fetal dose from TLD reading	If estimate is ≥50 mGy, physicists work up a detailed dosimetry report taking into account other variables (fetal depth and patient size)
If fetal dose is <50 mGy (trigger level), dose info is entered in the dosimetry report.	Detailed dosimetry report placed in patient's chart
If estimate is ≥50 mGy, the physicists work up a detailed dosimetry report taking into account other variables (fetal depth and patient size)	
Detailed dosimetry report placed in patient's chart	

From Wieseler KM, Bhargava P, Kanal KM, Vaidya S, Stewart BK, Dighe MK. Imaging in pregnant patients: examination appropriateness. *Radiographics.* 2010;30(5):1215–1229.

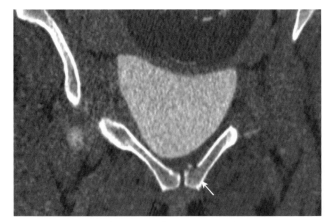

FIG. 19.2 Computed tomographic cystogram in a trauma patient showing a fracture in the left superior pubic ramus *(arrow)*.

MODALITY-SPECIFIC CONSIDERATIONS

Specific issues apply to modalities that use ionizing radiation (i.e., radiography, CT, nuclear medicine, and fluoroscopy) and those that do not use ionizing radiation (i.e., magnetic resonance imaging [MRI] and ultrasound).

Computed Tomography: Indication for Use

Currently, CT is mainly used in evaluating pregnant patients with trauma or suspected pulmonary embolism, which are the two main causes of maternal mortality.

Both major and minor trauma result in an increased risk of loss of pregnancy. The risk of pregnancy loss in trauma is reported to be between 1% and 34%; however, penetrating trauma has a higher rate of pregnancy loss, reaching almost 73%. Maternal death almost always results in fetal loss, although rare instances of emergency caesarean section despite lethal maternal injuries have been reported. The best chance of fetal survival is maternal survival. After maternal stabilization, imaging of the mother is performed with radiography, CT, or angiography as is necessary. Focused abdominal sonography for trauma is performed at the bedside for findings of free intraperitoneal or pericardial fluid. In cases of a positive focused abdominal sonography for trauma exam or if the suspicion is high, CT is the preferred modality for evaluation of hollow or solid organ trauma and vascular injury. In major trauma, risk of radiation exposure is small compared to the risk of maternal mortality or injury from missed or delayed diagnosis. Appropriate technique is used in imaging pregnant trauma patients, like nonextreme low-dose exams to ensure diagnostic quality of the exam, single-phase exams to decrease the radiation risk, and appropriate coverage of the anatomy. If delayed scans are required, they are focused on the

area of interest and are performed at a lower dose than the initial scan. CT cystography (Fig. 19.2) may be necessary in cases where bladder rupture is suspected and can be performed with low-dose techniques.

In cases with suspected pulmonary embolism, a positive diagnosis of deep venous thrombosis can obviate further workup, and therefore a chest radiograph with abdominal shield and vascular ultrasound are the first-line exams of choice. If the results of these exams are unavailable or equivocal, a CT pulmonary angiogram with abdominal shield is performed.

CT pulmonary angiogram has a dose similar to a ventilation-perfusion (V/Q) scan; however, CT is capable of providing an alternative diagnosis in cases of negative pulmonary embolism exams. The radiation dose in the first and early second trimesters is also low due to low scatter. If the patient is allergic to contrast, a V/Q scan (Fig. 19.3) can be performed. The American Congress of Obstetricians and Gynecologists and the Fleischner Society recommend CT pulmonary angiography for pregnant patients with suspected pulmonary embolism.

Another indication for using CT in pregnant patients is acute abdominal pain. In these cases, an attempt should be made to evaluate the pathology with ultrasound (e.g., appendicitis [Fig. 19.4]) and, if unsuccessful, a CT should be performed. Low-dose strategies should definitely be used when scanning the abdomen and pelvis in pregnant patients.

Dose Considerations and Dose Reduction Strategies

Even though the radiation exposure to the fetus is low when the fetus is not in the field of view, adhering to the principle of ALARA is important. Standard protocols should not be used in pregnant patients and should be replaced with low-dose protocols. To achieve this, the technologist should lower the tube potential (kilovolts) based on the patient's weight, decrease tube current-time product (milliampere second [mAs]), limit image length, increase pitch, and limit the number of acquisitions to one. Additional techniques like automated exposure control, automated tube potential selection, and iterative reconstructions should also be used. Techniques for reducing dose to the pregnant patient are listed in Box 19.1.

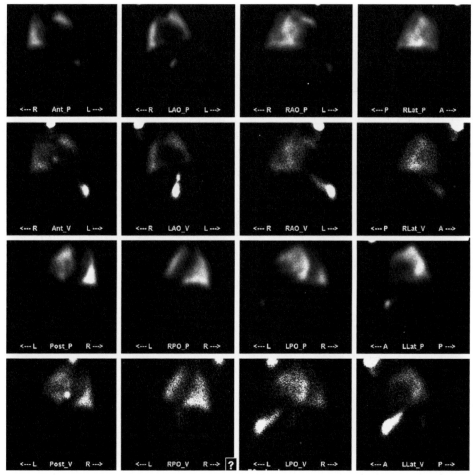

FIG. 19.3 Ventilation perfusion scan in a pregnant patient showing a very low probability of pulmonary embolism. Patient had a severe allergy to contrast and hence had to undergo an alternative exam.

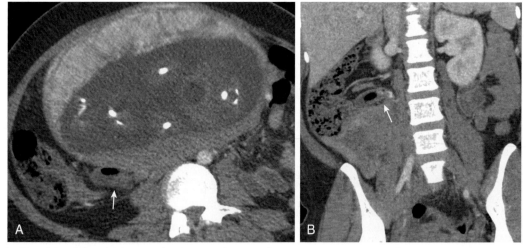

FIG. 19.4 (A) Axial and (B) coronal reformatted images from a postcontrast scan show a 30-year-old pregnant patient at 27 weeks of pregnancy with acute right lower quadrant pain. Note the dilated blind-ending tubular structure *(arrow)* in the right lower quadrant adjacent to the cecum with a small fecalith seen at the tip. This was suggestive of acute appendicitis.

Nuclear Medicine

The most commonly performed exam in pregnant patients is the V/Q scan for pulmonary embolism; however, this exam is performed only if CT cannot be performed for some reason or the CT is equivocal. The dose absorbed by the fetus from a V/Q scan is in the range of 0.1 to 0.37

mGy. Other exams are infrequently performed in pregnant patients. Studies using technetium-99m agents or positron emission tomography studies can be performed in patients with suspected peripartum cardiomyopathy because the fetal doses from these exams with a reduced radiotracer dose are less than 50 mGy. Treatment with iodide 131

BOX 19.1   Computed Tomography Dose Reduction Techniques

- One size does not fit all: DO NOT USE STANDARD PROTOCOLS.
- Decrease kilovolts for small patients.
- Decrease milliamperes and use automatic tube current modulation.
- Increase pitch >1.
- Perform a single scout view and avoid directly imaging the fetus for planning purposes.
- Limit the field of view.
- Avoid multiple phases.
- Use more recently available novel reconstruction algorithms to reduce noise in the image, thus allowing reduction of milliamperes or increase in noise level requirements during the scan.
- Lead shielding of the mother is most pronounced with circumferential shielding.
- Internal barium shielding with use of oral 30% barium sulfate solution
- Local QA program to monitor CT protocols and the resulting dose

From Wieseler KM, Bhargava P, Kanal KM, Vaidya S, Stewart BK, Dighe MK. Imaging in pregnant patients: examination appropriateness. *Radiographics.* 2010;30(5):1215–1229.

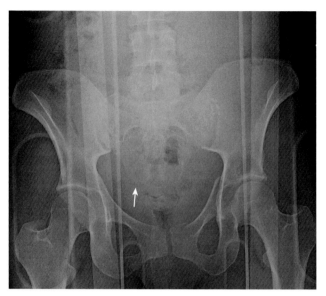

FIG. 19.5 Radiograph in a pregnant patient showing a fetus *(arrow)* at 24 weeks of gestational age and a fracture in the left pubic ramus.

(^{131}I-NaI) is contraindicated because it may lead to permanent hypothyroidism in the fetus. The American Congress of Obstetricians and Gynecologists recommends that therapy with ^{131}I-NaI be delayed until after delivery and that iodine 123 (123I) or technetium-99m be used for diagnostic thyroid examinations due to the lower radiation dose and shorter half-life.

Fluoroscopy, Interventional Radiology, and Radiography

Pregnancy status should be confirmed even with radiography (Fig. 19.5), even though there is negligible conceptus dose when the fetus is not undergoing direct exposure; however, the determination of pregnancy status should not alter the decision to proceed with the examination in these cases. In situations where an interventional procedure is needed, ultrasound guidance for the procedure should be used. When a nonionizing study cannot be avoided, exposure to the fetus should be reduced by minimizing the fluoroscopy time, decreasing the number of images acquired, using magnification only when necessary and employing the lowest possible frame rate, optimizing collimation, and using image hold instead of additional exposure.

Magnetic Resonance Imaging

The risks related to MRI are teratogenic and not carcinogenic. The primary concern with MRI is heating associated with the radiofrequency pulse B_0 strength, which may affect cell migration during the first trimester and acoustic noise produced during imaging, which may damage the fetal hearing. The American College of Radiology (ACR) Guidance document on magnetic resonance (MR) safe practices does state that MRI can be used at any gestational age when the information gathered is likely to alter

treatment, when it cannot be obtained by other nonionizing exams, and when the exam cannot be delayed until after delivery. Even though the risks of cell migration injury remain theoretical in humans and no detrimental effect has been reported, the International Commission on Nonionizing Radiation Protection recommends postponement of elective MRI until after the first trimester.

MRI is often performed to exclude appendicitis (Fig. 19.6), which is the most common cause of abdominal pain necessitating surgery in pregnant patients. MRI also allows evaluation of multiple additional structures in the abdomen and pelvis that may be the source of abdominal pain in the pregnant patient. Recently MRI has also been used to evaluate for pulmonary embolism in pregnant patients using noncontrast techniques (Fig. 19.7).

Ultrasound Examinations

Ultrasound is the first-line tool in imaging the mother and evaluating the fetus. Multiple societies agree that ultrasound is generally safe when performed for medical purposes. The only concerns with ultrasound include heating and cavitation effects; however, after 1992, the US Food and Drug Administration (FDA) mandated that ultrasound equipment adhere to the output display standard, which includes the thermal and mechanical indexes to guide users. These have been revised to suggested limits. Although no teratogenic effects have been demonstrated in humans, radiologists and sonographers should adhere to the ALARA principle by controlling output. Recommended mechanical and thermal indices should both be less than 1. Color, power, and spectral Doppler require higher-intensity acoustic output and hence should be replaced by M-mode when evaluating heart rate in the first trimester.

CONTRAST AGENT ADMINISTRATION IN PREGNANT PATIENTS

The maternal and fetal circulatory systems are interconnected systems with the dynamic barrier and interface

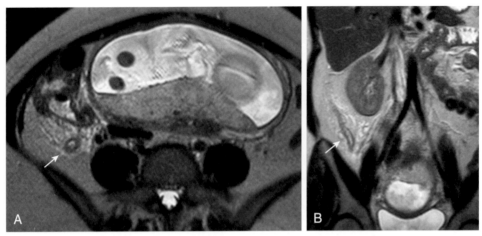

FIG. 19.6 Noncontrast magnetic resonance (A) axial and (B) coronal images in a 20-week pregnant patient showing a filling defect *(arrow)* in the right lower segmental branch suggesting a pulmonary embolism.

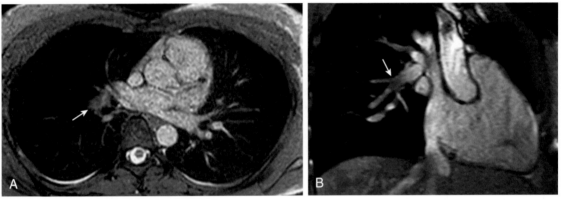

FIG. 19.7 A 34-year-old with acute right lower quadrant pain. (A) Axial T2-weighted and (B) coronal T2-weighted images show a dilated tubular structure in the right lower quadrant surrounded by fat stranding, suggesting a dilated appendix.

located in the placenta. Maternal blood passes into the intervillous spaces in the placenta, allowing nutrients and oxygen to pass into the fetal circulation with only a single layer of chorionic epithelium acting as the barrier. Drugs in maternal blood cross the placenta mainly by simple diffusion. Because the chorionic epithelium behaves like other lipid membranes in the body, lipid-soluble molecules and small nonionized water molecules cross readily as well, and larger water-soluble molecules cross less easily. Iodinated nonionic monomeric contrast agents and gadolinium contrast agents are water soluble and are hence expected to cross into the fetus; however, because they range in size from 500 to 850 Daltons (Da), they cross less readily than smaller water-soluble molecules. Gadolinium agents have been shown in the placenta following intravenous administration to the mother in animals and in human patients as well. No mutagenic effects were shown in vitro with ionic iodinated agents. No mutagenic or teratogenic effects have been described after administration of iodinated contrast media during pregnancy or after in vivo tests in animals. There is no evidence that gadolinium agents cause chromosomal damage or teratogenic effects.

IODINATED CONTRAST MEDIA ADMINISTRATION

When iodinated contrast media is given to the pregnant patient, it traverses the placenta and enters the fetal blood. It is then excreted by the kidneys into the bladder and reaches the amniotic fluid, which is then swallowed and enters the gut. It has also been suggested that iodinated contrast media enters the amniotic fluid directly from the maternal blood. Studies have demonstrated measureable amounts of iodinated contrast and gadolinium-based contrast agents in the fetus after intravenous administration to the mother. This is not of much concern because the contrast agent is eventually excreted by the maternal kidneys, but in patients with decreased renal function, the contrast agent may persist in the maternal circulation longer and lead to increased concentration of contrast agent in the fetus. The main deleterious effect of iodine-based compounds is their potential impact on the neonatal thyroid gland.

The fetal thyroid develops early in pregnancy at about 3 weeks of conception with thyrotropin hormone related between the 6th and 8th week of gestation. The hypothalamic-pituitary-thyroid axis begins to develop between the 8th and 10th weeks of gestation and is usually mature by 12 weeks, resulting in the release of thyroid-stimulating hormone. The fetal hypothalamic-pituitary axis is independent of the maternal hypothalamic-pituitary axis and continues to mature during the second and third trimesters. There is a normal increase of thyroid-stimulating hormone at delivery, with normalization of thyroid hormone levels by 2 weeks of age.

Depression of the thyroid function is the most important potential harmful effect of iodinated contrast media in the fetus because normal thyroid function is essential for normal development of the central nervous system. Congenital hypothyroidism is seen in one in every 4000 births and, if left untreated, can lead to failure to thrive and is the leading cause of treatable mental and developmental impairment.

Cases of hypothyroidism from administration of iodinated contrast medium in pregnant patients are rare, and most were seen decades ago when amniofetography was performed to detect congenital defects using lipid-soluble iodinated contrast agents. Bourjeily et al., from their study involving 343 newborns whose mothers had received a single dose of intravenous contrast medium during pregnancy for suspicion of pulmonary embolism, concluded that a single in utero exposure of high dose of water-soluble, low-osmolar, nonionic iodinated contrast medium is unlikely to have a clinically important effect on thyroid function at birth.

CURRENT RECOMMENDATIONS

The FDA considers iodinated contrast agents to be category B drugs; that is, reproductive studies in animals demonstrate no risk, but there have been no controlled studies in pregnant women. In their recent 2015 *Manual on Contrast Media*, the ACR does not recommend withholding the use of iodinated contrast agents in pregnant or potentially pregnant patients when it is needed for diagnostic purposes, given that there is no available data to suggest any potential harm to the fetus from exposure to iodinated contrast medium or intraarterial injection. However, the FDA recently announced that rare cases of underactive thyroid had been reported in infants following the use of contrast media containing iodine. They do believe that this effect is temporary and resolves without treatment or any long-lasting effects. The Contrast Media Safety Committee of the European Society of Urogenital Radiology, in their revised guidelines in May 2012, does recommend that iodinated contrast media be given to the mother only in exceptional circumstances and that when this occurs, neonatal thyroid function should be checked in the 1st week of life.

GADOLINIUM-BASED CONTRAST AGENTS

Even though there have been some reports of postimplantation fetal loss in rats, retarded development in rats and rabbits, and skeletal and visceral abnormalities in rabbits, to date there have been no known adverse effects in human fetuses when clinically recommended dosages of gadolinium-based contrast agents (GBCAs) have been given to pregnant women. However, no well-controlled studies

of teratogenic effects of these media in pregnant women have been performed.

Gadolinium chelate traverses the placenta and may accumulate in the amniotic cavity. The contrast medium cycles through the fetal gastrointestinal tract and genitourinary tract and can remain there for an indefinite period of time; however, recent studies show that only traces of contrast remain in the fetus after 24 hours. The free gadolinium ion is toxic to the fetus, and it is bound to a chelating agent to form a stable complex. When the gadolinium chelates accumulate in the amniotic fluid, there is the potential for dissociation of the toxic-free gadolinium ion, producing a potential risk for the development of nephrogenic systemic fibrosis in the child or mother.

CURRENT RECOMMENDATIONS

The FDA has classified gadolinium-based agents as category C drugs, meaning that animal studies have revealed adverse effects on the fetus and there have been no controlled studies in women. The ACR Committee on Drugs and Contrast Media published in 2015 recommends that "each case should be reviewed carefully by members of the clinical and radiology services and a GBCA should be administered only when there is a potential significant benefit to the patient or fetus that outweighs the possible but unknown risk of fetal exposure to free gadolinium ions." They also recommend that informed consent be obtained from the patient after discussion with the referring physician. In addition, the radiologist should document that the information requested from the MRI study cannot be acquired without the use of intravenous (IV) contrast or by using other imaging methods, it affects the care of the patient and/or fetus during the pregnancy, and that the referring physician does not think it is prudent to wait to obtain this information until the patient is no longer pregnant. The Contrast Media Safety Committee of the European Society of Urogenital Radiology, in their revised guidelines in May 2012, recommend using the smallest possible dose of one of the most stable GBCAs and only for a very strong indication for enhanced MRI. They do not recommend any monitoring of the neonate after the mother has been given GBCA during pregnancy.

CONTRAST AGENT ADMINISTRATION IN LACTATING PATIENTS

Iodinated Contrast Media

The plasma half-life of intravenously administered iodinated contrast medium is approximately 2 hours. Nearly 100% of the contrast is cleared from the bloodstream within 24 hours in patients with normal renal function. Due to its low lipid solubility, less than 1% of the administered maternal dose of iodinated contrast medium is excreted into the breast milk in the first 24 hours. With the small amount of contrast that may be excreted into the breast milk, less than 1% of the ingested contrast medium is absorbed from the infant's gastrointestinal tract. Hence the expected dose of iodinated contrast medium absorbed by the infant from breast milk is less than 0.01% of the IV dose given to the mother. The regular contrast dose for infants is 2 mL/kg and hence this dose represents less than 1% of the recommended dose.

Current Recommendations

The ACR recommends that based on the very small percentage of iodinated contrast medium that is excreted into the breast milk and absorbed by the infant's gut, it is safe for the mother and the infant to continue breast feeding after receiving iodinated contrast. The ACR also recommends that potential additional risks to the infant include direct toxicity from, and allergic sensitization or reaction to, contrast media, although these are theoretic concerns that have not been reported. The Contrast Media Safety Committee of the European Society of Urogenital Radiology, in their revised guidelines in May 2012, recommend that breast feeding should be continued normally when iodine-based agents are given to the mother, and in patients with impaired renal function, no additional precautions are necessary. The baby may notice a change in the taste of the milk due to excretion of contrast media in the milk.

Gadolinium

Less than 0.04% of the intravascular dose given to the mother is excreted into the breast milk in the first 24 hours, and less than 1% of the contrast medium ingested by the infant is absorbed from its gastrointestinal tract. Hence the expected dose absorbed by the infant from the breast milk is less than 0.0004% of the IV dose given to the mother.

Therefore the available data suggest that it is safe for the mother and infant to continue breast feeding after receiving contrast agents. If the mother desires, she may abstain from breast feeding for 24 hours with active expression and discarding of breast milk from both breasts during that period.

Current Recommendations

The ACR recommends that because of the very small percentage of gadolinium that is excreted into the breast milk and absorbed by the infant's gut, it is safe for the mother and the infant to continue breast feeding after receiving gadolinium. The Contrast Media Safety Committee of the European Society of Urogenital Radiology in their revised guidelines in May 2012 recommend that breast feeding should be avoided for 24 hours after contrast medium if high-risk agents are used, for example, gadodiamide, gadoversetamide, or gadopentetate dimeglumine. However, in patients with impaired renal function, they prefer not to administer gadolinium-based contrast agents.

As with iodinated contrast medium, the baby may notice a change in the taste of the milk due to excretion of contrast media in the milk.

SCREENING, INFORMED CONSENT, AND RISK MANAGEMENT

Pregnancy Screening

To reasonably minimize the number of unexpected exposures of pregnant patients to ionizing radiation, ACR recommends at least verbal screening before radiologic examinations are performed for women between 12 and 50 years of age. These age cutoffs are not absolute and depend on the menstrual status of the patient and relevant history like a previous hysterectomy or tubal ligation.

Screening could be tailored to the different types of imaging examinations, anticipated radiation to the fetus, and the urgency of the examination. Some examinations provide very low exposures to the pregnant uterus, if the beam is properly collimated and the patient is positioned to avoid direct irradiation to the pelvis. Such examinations include chest radiography during the first and second trimesters, extremity radiography or CT (excluding the hip), any diagnostic examination of the head and neck, and mammography. In these cases, screening documentation may not be required. In examinations that involve direct exposure of the female pelvis to ionizing radiation, screening should be an essential component. Screening can be in the form of a verbal question, as suggested by the ACR, or quantitative serum pregnancy tests. A screening questionnaire and/or direct questioning by the technologist should be used before the imaging examination. For exams involving high doses like multiphase CT or therapeutic doses of radiopharmaceuticals, the ACR and the Society of Nuclear Medicine and Molecular Imaging guidelines state that pregnancy status should be established with a β-human chorionic gonadotropin (BHCG) result obtained within 72 hours, a documented premenarche status, or history of hysterectomy. For high-risk interventional procedures, a quantitative test for pregnancy should be performed and patients should be counseled to abstain from sexual activity for 2 weeks before the procedure, or the examination should be scheduled within 10 days after the onset of the menstrual period.

Institutional policies should be adhered to because some of them have stricter policies for screening for pregnancy. In case of minors, state regulations on confidential pregnancy testing should be followed, although most states do allow minors to undergo pregnancy testing without parental consent when prenatal care is concerned.

In some situations, for example trauma, evaluation of pregnant status is not possible (such as with obtundation) or might lead to delay in patient care. In these situations, documentation by the referring physician in the medical record that pregnancy screening was waived due to the critical nature of the examination is essential.

Consent

It is imperative that the necessity of performing an exam with the potential to expose the fetus to radiation should be carefully evaluated with the patient and the referring team. After the necessity has been established and a decision has been made that the same or similar information cannot be obtained by using exams without ionizing radiation, consent must be obtained from the patient. This consent can be in the form of a verbal consent or written consent. Written consent should be retained in the medical record. The format of the consent can be detailed with a quantitative list of risks or a limited consent process with generalized benefits and risks explained. Regardless of the format, the information communicated should convey the benefits and risks posed by the procedure in an easily understandable format.

SUGGESTED READINGS

American College of Obstetricians and Gynecologists' Committee on Obstetric Practice. Committee opinion no. 656: guidelines for diagnostic imaging during pregnancy and lactation. *Obstet Gynecol.* 2016;127(2):e75-e80.

American College of Obstetricians and Gynecologists Committee on Patient Safety and Quality Improvement. ACOG Committee Opinion No. 447: patient safety in obstetrics and gynecology. *Obstet Gynecol.* 2009;114(6):1424-1427.

American College of Radiology. *ACR-SPR Practice Parameter for Imaging Pregnant or Potentially Pregnant Adolescents and Women With Ionizing Radiation. Resolution 39.* Reston, VA: American College of Radiology; 2014.

American Institute of Ultrasound in Medicine. AIUM practice guideline for the performance of obstetric ultrasound examinations. *J Ultrasound Med.* 2010;29(1):157-166.

American Institute of Ultrasound in Medicine. AIUM practice guideline for the performance of obstetric ultrasound examinations. *J Ultrasound Med.* 2013;32(6):1083-1101.

Angel E, Wellnitz C, Goodsitt M, et al. Radiation dose to the fetus for pregnant patients undergoing multidetector CT imaging: Monte Carlo simulations estimating fetal dose for a range of gestational age and patient size. *Radiology.* 2008;249(1):220-227.

Atwell TD, Lteif AN, Brown DL, McCann M, Townsend JE, Leroy AJ. Neonatal thyroid function after administration of IV iodinated contrast agent to 21 pregnant patients. *AJR Am J Roentgenol.* 2008;191(1):268-271.

Balter S, Hopewell JW, Miller DL, Wagner LK, Zelefsky MJ. Fluoroscopically guided interventional procedures: a review of radiation effects on patients' skin and hair. *Radiology.* 2010;254(2):326-341.

Bloomfield T, Hawkins D. The effects of drugs on the human fetus. In: Philipp E, Setchell M, eds. *Scientific Foundations of Obstetrics and Gynecology* 4th ed. Oxford: Butterworth-Heinemann; 1991:320.

Board on Radiation Effects Research Division on Earth and Life Studies National Research Council of the National Academies. *Health Risks from Exposure to Low Levels of Ionizing Radiation: BEIR VII Phase 2.* Washington, D.C: National Academic Press; 2006.

Bourjeily G, Chalhoub M, Phornphutkul C, Alleyne TC, Woodfield CA, Chen KK. Neonatal thyroid function: effect of a single exposure to iodinated contrast medium in utero. *Radiology.* 2010;256(3):744-750.

Bushberg J. *The Essential Physics of Medical Imaging.* 3rd ed. Philadelphia, PA: Lippincott Williams & Wilkins; 2011.

Centers for Disease Control and Prevention. Radiation and Pregnancy: A Fact Sheet for Clinicians. <http://emergency.cdc.gov/radiation/prenatalphysician.asp>.

Chen MM, Coakley FV, Kaimal A, Laros RK. Guidelines for computed tomography and magnetic resonance imaging use during pregnancy and lactation. *Obstet Gynecol.* 2008;112(2 Pt 1):333-340.

Colletti PM, Sylvestre PB. Magnetic resonance imaging in pregnancy. *Magn Reson Imaging Clin N Am.* 1994;2(2):291-307.

Colletti PM, Lee KH, Elkayam U. Cardiovascular imaging of the pregnant patient. *AJR Am J Roentgenol.* 2013;200(3):515-521.

De Santis M, Straface G, Cavaliere AF, Carducci B, Caruso A. Gadolinium periconceptional exposure: pregnancy and neonatal outcome. *Acta Obstet Gynecol Scand.* 2007;86(1):99-101.

Donandieu AM, Idee JM, Doucet D, et al. Toxicologic profile of iobitridol, a new nonionic low-osmolality contrast medium. *Acta Radiol suppl.* 1996;400:17-24.

Doshi SK, Negus IS, Oduko JM. Fetal radiation dose from CT pulmonary angiography in late pregnancy: a phantom study. *Br J Radiol.* 2008;81(968):653-658.

Fujikawa K, Sakaguchi Y, Harada S, Holtz E, Smith JA, Svendsen O. Reproductive toxicity of iodixanol, a new non-ionic, iso-tonic contrast medium in rats and rabbits. *J Toxicol Sci.* 1995;20(suppl 1):107-115.

Hall E. *Radiobiology for the Radiologist.* 7th ed. Philadelphia, PA: Lippincott Williams & Wilkins; 2011.

Hendee WR, O'Connor MK. Radiation risks of medical imaging: separating fact from fantasy. *Radiology.* 2012;264(2):312-321.

Horowitz NS, Dehdashti F, Herzog TJ, et al. Prospective evaluation of FDG-PET for detecting pelvic and para-aortic lymph node metastasis in uterine corpus cancer. *Gynecol Oncol.* 2004;95(3):546-551.

Hricak H, Brenner DJ, Adelstein SJ, et al. Managing radiation use in medical imaging: a multifaceted challenge. *Radiology.* 2011;258(3):889-905.

Huda W, Slone R. *Review of Radiologic Physics.* 3rd ed. Philadelphia, PA: Lippincott Williams & Wilkins; 2009.

Ilett KF, Paterson LP, Paterson JW, McCormick CC. Excretion of metrizamide in milk. *Br J Radiol.* 1981;54(642):537-538.

International Commission on Radiological Protection. The Recommendations of the International Commission on Radiological Protection. <http://www.icrp.org/publication.asp?id=ICRP%20Publication%20103>.

International Commission on Radiological Protection Report 84. Pregnancy and medical radiation. *ICRP publication 84. ICRP.* 2000;30(1).

International Commission on Radiation Protection. *Pregnancy and Medical Radiation.* Available at <http://www.icrp.org/publication.asp?id=ICRP%20Publication%2084>.

Johansen JG. Assessment of a non-ionic contrast medium (Amipaque) in the gastrointestinal tract. *Invest Radiol.* 1978;13(6):523-527.

Kanal E, Barkovich AJ, Bell C, et al. ACR guidance document on MR safe practices: 2013. *J Magn Reson Imaging.* 2013;37(3):501-530.

Krause W, Schöbel C, Press WR. Preclinical testing of iopromide. 2nd communication: toxicological evaluation. *Arzneimittelforschung.* 1994;44(11):1275-1279.

Kubik-Huch RA, Gottstein-Aalame NM, Frenzel T, et al. Gadopentetate dimeglumine excretion into human breast milk during lactation. *Radiology.* 2000;216(2):555-558.

Kuklina EV, Ayala C, Callaghan WM. Hypertensive disorders and severe obstetric morbidity in the United States. *Obstet Gynecol.* 2009;113(6):1299-1306.

Levine GN, Gomes AS, Arai AE, et al. Safety of magnetic resonance imaging in patients with cardiovascular devices: an American Heart Association scientific statement from the Committee on Diagnostic and Interventional Cardiac Catheterization, Council on Clinical Cardiology, and the Council on Cardiovascular Radiology and Intervention: endorsed by the American College of Cardiology Foundation, the North American Society for Cardiac Imaging, and the Society for Cardiovascular Magnetic Resonance. *Circulation.* 2007;116(24):2878-2891.

Little MP, Wakeford R, Tawn EJ, Bouffler SD, Berrington de Gonzalez A. Risks associated with low doses and low dose rates of ionizing radiation: why linearity may be (almost) the best we can do. *Radiology.* 2009;251(1):6-12.

Lowdermilk C, Gavant ML, Qaisi W, West OC, Goldman SM. Screening helical CT for evaluation of blunt traumatic injury in the pregnant patient. *Radiographics.* 1999:19. Spec No:S243-S255.

Marcos HB, Semelka RC, Worawattanakul S. Normal placenta: gadolinium-enhanced dynamic MR imaging. *Radiology.* 1997;205(2):493-496.

McCollough C, Schueler B, Atwell T, et al. Radiation exposure and pregnancy: when should we be concerned? *Radiographics.* 2007;27(4):909-917.

McCollough CH. CT dose: how to measure, how to reduce. *Health Phys.* 2008;95(5):508-517.

McJury M, Shellock FG. Auditory noise associated with MR procedures: a review. *J Magn Reson Imaging.* 2000;12(1):37-45.

Morisetti A, Tirone P, Luzzani F, de Haën C. Toxicological safety assessment of iomeprol, a new X-ray contrast agent. *Eur J Radiol.* 1994;18(suppl 1):S21-S31.

National Council on Radiation Protection and Measurements. *Medical Radiation Exposure of Pregnant and Potentially Pregnant Women. NCRP Report No. 54.* Bethesda, MD: National Council on Radiation Protection and Measurements; 1977.

National Council on Radiation Protection and Measurements. *Risk Estimates for Radiation Protection. NCRP Report No. 115.* Bethesda, MD: The Council; 1993.

Nelson JA, Livingston GK, Moon RG. Mutagenic evaluation of radiographic contrast media. *Invest Radiol.* 1982;17(2):183-185.

Nielsen ST, Matheson I, Rasmussen JN, Skinnemoen K, Andrew E, Hafsahl G. Excretion of iohexol and metrizoate in human breast milk. *Acta Radiol.* 1987;28(5):523-526.

Novak Z, Thurmond AS, Ross PL, Jones MK, Thornburg KL, Katzberg RW. Gadolinium-DTPA transplacental transfer and distribution in fetal tissue in rabbits. *Invest Radiol.* 1993;28(9):828-830.

Okazaki O, Murayama N, Masubuchi N, Nomura H, Hakusui H. Placental transfer and milk secretion of gadodiamide injection in rats. *Arzneimittelforschung.* 1996;46(1):83-86.

Pahade JK, Litmanovich D, Pedrosa I, Romero J, Bankier AA, Boiselle PM. Quality initiatives: imaging pregnant patients with suspected pulmonary embolism: what the radiologist needs to know. *Radiographics.* 2009;29(3):639-654.

Patel SJ, Reede DL, Katz DS, Subramaniam R, Amorosa JK. Imaging the pregnant patient for nonobstetric conditions: algorithms and radiation dose considerations. *Radiographics.* 2007;27(6):1705-1722.

Peck D, Samei E. How to understand and communicate radiation risk. <http://www.imagewisely.org/Imaging-Modalities/Computed-Tomography/Medical-Physicists/Articles/How-to-Understand-and-Communicate-Radiation-Risk>.

Petrone P, Talving P, Browder T, et al. Abdominal injuries in pregnancy: a 155-month study at two level 1 trauma centers. *Injury.* 2011;42(1):47-49.

Preston DL, Cullings H, Suyama A, et al. Solid cancer incidence in atomic bomb survivors exposed in utero or as young children. *J Natl Cancer Inst.* 2008;100(6):428-436.

Ralston WH, Robbins MS, Coveney J, Blair M. Acute and subacute toxicity studies of ioversol in experimental animals. *Invest Radiol.* 1989;24(suppl 1):S2-S9.

Raman SP, Johnson PT, Deshmukh S, Mahesh M, Grant KL, Fishman EK. CT dose reduction applications: available tools on the latest generation of CT scanners. *J Am Coll Radiol.* 2013;10(1):37-41.

Raptis CA, Mellnick VM, Raptis DA, et al. Imaging of trauma in the pregnant patient. *Radiographics.* 2014;34(3):748-763.

Remy-Jardin M, Pistolesi M, Goodman LR, et al. Management of suspected acute pulmonary embolism in the era of CT angiography: a statement from the Fleischner Society. *Radiology.* 2007;245(2):315-329.

Rofsky NM, Weinreb JC, Litt AW. Quantitative analysis of gadopentetate dimeglumine excreted in breast milk. *J Magn Reson Imaging.* 1993;3(1):131-132.

Sadro C, Bernstein MP, Kanal KM. Imaging of trauma: part 2, abdominal trauma and pregnancy—a radiologist's guide to doing what is best for the mother and baby. *AJR Am J Roentgenol.* 2012;199(6):1207-1219.

Schmiedl U, Maravilla KR, Gerlach R, Dowling CA. Excretion of gadopentetate dimeglumine in human breast milk. *AJR Am J Roentgenol.* 1990;154(6):1305-1306.

Shah KH, Simons RK, Holbrook T, Fortlage D, Winchell RJ, Hoyt DB. Trauma in pregnancy: maternal and fetal outcomes. *J Trauma.* 1998;45(1):83-86.

Siegel J. Nuclear Regulatory Commission Regulation of Nuclear Medicine. Guide for Diagnostic Nuclear Medicine. <http://www.nrc.gov/materials/miau/miau-reg-initiatives/guide_2002.pdf>.

Spalluto LB, Woodfield CA, DeBenedectis CM, Lazarus E. MR imaging evaluation of abdominal pain during pregnancy: appendicitis and other nonobstetric causes. *Radiographics.* 2012;32(2):317-334.

Thabet A, Kalva SP, Liu B, Mueller PR, Lee SI. Interventional radiology in pregnancy complications: indications, technique, and methods for minimizing radiation exposure. *Radiographics*. 2012;32(1):255-274.

Tirada N, Dreizin D, Khati NJ, Akin EA, Zeman RK. Imaging pregnant and lactating patients. *Radiographics*. 2015;35(6):1751-1765.

Torloni MR, Vedmedovska N, Merialdi M, et al. Safety of ultrasonography in pregnancy: WHO systematic review of the literature and meta-analysis. *Ultrasound Obstet Gynecol*. 2009;33(5):599-608.

Tremblay E, Thérasse E, Thomassin-Naggara I, Trop I. Quality initiatives: guidelines for use of medical imaging during pregnancy and lactation. *Radiographics*. 2012;32(3):897-911.

Tubiana M, Feinendegen LE, Yang C, Kaminski JM. The linear no-threshold relationship is inconsistent with radiation biologic and experimental data. *Radiology*. 2009;251(1):13-22.

US Food and Drug administration. <http://www.fda.gov/Drugs/DrugSafety/PostmarketDrugSafetyInformationforPatientsandProviders/ucm142882.htm>.

Wagner L. *Exposure of Pregnant Patient to Diagnostic Radiation*. Madison, WI: Medical Physics Publishing; 1997.

Wang PI, Chong ST, Kielar AZ, et al. Imaging of pregnant and lactating patients: part 1, evidence-based review and recommendations. *Am J Roentgenol*. 2012;198(4):778-784.

Webb JA, Thomsen HS, Morcos SK. (ESUR) MoCMSCoESoUR. The use of iodinated and gadolinium contrast media during pregnancy and lactation. *Eur Radiol*. 2005;15(6):1234-1240.

Weinmann HJ, Brasch RC, Press WR, Wesbey GE. Characteristics of gadolinium-DTPA complex: a potential NMR contrast agent. *AJR Am J Roentgenol*. 1984;142(3):619-624.

Wieseler KM, Bhargava P, Kanal KM, Vaidya S, Stewart BK, Dighe MK. Imaging in pregnant patients: examination appropriateness. *Radiographics*. 2010;30(5):1215-1229.

Zanzonico P, Stabin MG. Quantitative benefit-risk analysis of medical radiation exposures. *Semin Nucl Med*. 2014;44(3):210-214.

Chapter 20

Safe Use of Contrast Media

Khalid W. Shaqdan, Alexi Otrakji, and Dushyant Sahani

INTRODUCTION

Widespread use of medical imaging has led to a significant increase in the use of radiologic contrast media (CM). Half of the estimated 78 million computed tomography (CT) examinations and 37 million magnetic resonance imaging (MRI) examinations performed annually in the United States include the use of CM. Radiographic CM are used in imaging examinations to aid in the characterization, detection, and staging of disease. Although the CM currently in use have strong documented safety profiles, their use is not completely without risk. According to the World Health Organization, an adverse drug reaction is a harmful, unintentional, and often unavoidable response to normal therapeutic doses of a medicine. In general, most patients who receive a contrast agent have no adverse reactions (ARs), and when a reaction does occur it is usually mild and self-limiting. Therefore, establishing preventive measures against ARs from CM is essential for patient safety. Awareness of the various reactions that can occur and prompt management are critical in reducing the likelihood of an adverse outcome. Rapid evaluation and treatment of ARs requires adequate training, readily available equipment, and appropriate medications. This chapter discusses the important aspects of screening, recognizing, and managing the risks central to intravenously administered CM.

TYPES OF CONTRAST MEDIA, ADMINISTRATION OF CONTRAST MEDIA, AND GENERAL PRINCIPLES

Types of Contrast Media

Iodinated contrast media (ICM) can be classified according to their ionicity, relative osmolality, and chemical structure (Table 20.1). During the last 2 decades, the use of CM has transitioned from traditional ionic agents to safer nonionic agents, which are equally effective for imaging but cost much more. Traditional ionic agents, or high-osmolar CM, dissociate into charged particles when dissolved in water and, as a result, have an osmolality 5 to 8 times that of blood (normal blood osmolality is 285–295 mOsm/kg in adults). Charged particles are toxic irritants and can cause allergic reactions. Nonionic agents, or low-osmolar/isoosmolar CM, do not dissociate into charged particles when dissolved in water and have one-half the osmolality of ionic agents. As a result, nonionic agents are associated with a considerably lower incidence of ARs, particularly cardiovascular and allergic-like reactions. Due to the significant cost of nonionic CM, using new technologies, increasing the concentration, and decreasing the volume of CM are among the efforts to minimize the economic burden. Additionally, the cost of nonionic CM continues to decrease as manufacturers' patents expire and competing agents enter the market.

The majority of CM used for MRI are based on gadolinium (Gd) chelates and are extremely well tolerated by the vast majority of patients. Currently, there are nine gadolinium-based CM (GBCM) approved by the US Food and Drug Administration (FDA) that differ in a number of properties (Table 20.2). Generally, most GBCM present a distribution in the body similar to that of ICM. However, the mean dose of GBCM delivered is typically 5 to 15 times lower (ranges between 10 and 20 mL) than ICM. This is certainly one of the reasons why GBCM are considered safer to use, and their molecular structure and osmolality are less significant as far as safety is concerned in comparison with ICM. In terms of physical properties, stability and relaxivity are the most important criteria for patient safety optimization and diagnostic efficacy. Stability refers to the resistance of GBCM to break down into toxic components (Gd ions) in the blood circulation. GBCM with higher relaxivity provide greater contrast enhancement and increased signal intensity at lower doses, thereby achieving improved diagnostic efficacy while reducing the risk of an AR.

Administration of Contrast Media

CM administration depends on the clinical indication, vascular access, and type of examination. The method of CM delivery (hand injection vs. power injection) also varies depending on the requested procedure. Stable intravenous (IV) access is always necessary, and recognizing the importance of proper technique is critical to avoid potentially serious complications. Careful preparation of the power injection apparatus is crucial to minimize the risk of complications (Box 20.1). Power injection of IV CM should be through a flexible plastic cannula; metal needles must always be avoided. Vascular access guidelines for CM administration at our institution can be seen in Box 20.2. Power injection of CM through some central venous catheters can be performed safely, provided that certain precautions are followed (Box 20.3). Furthermore, obtaining the patient's full cooperation throughout the injection process is important to avoid or promptly identify a complication should one occur. The injection should always be discontinued if the patient reports pain or sensation of swelling at the injection site. Although not an adverse reaction of CM, a clinically significant venous air embolism can occur when IV CM is administered by hand injection. Venous air embolisms are potentially fatal but extremely rare complications commonly seen in the intrathoracic veins, main pulmonary artery, and right ventricle, and they appear as air-fluid levels or air bubbles on contrast-enhanced CT. Unintentional injection of large amounts of air into the venous system may result in dyspnea, expiratory wheezing,

TABLE 20.1 **Commonly Used Iodinated Contrast Media**

Name	Type	Iodine Content (mgI/mL)	Osmolality (osmol/kg)
NONIONIC			
Iodixanol (Visipaque 320)	Nonionic dimer	320	290, isoosmolar
Iohexol (Omnipaque 350)	Nonionic monomer	350	884, low osmolar
Iopamidol (Isovue 370)	Nonionic monomer	370	796, low osmolar
IONIC			
Ioxaglate (Hexabrix)	Ionic dimer	320	580, low osmolar
Metrizoate (Isopaque Coronar 370)	Ionic monomer	370	2100, high osmolar
Diatrizoate (Hypaque 50)	Ionic monomer	300	1550, high osmolar

TABLE 20.2 **Gadolinium-Based Contrast Media**

Brand Name	Chemical Name	Structure/Charge	Stability (log K_{eq})/T1 Relaxivity (L/mmol × s)	NSF Incidence (Based on EMA Classification)	Comments
Magnevist	Gadopentetate dimeglumine (Gd-DTPA)	Linear/ionic	22.5/4.1	High	Highest relaxivity of all extracellular GBCM
Omniscan	Gadodiamide (Gd-DTPA-BMA)	Linear/nonionic	16.9/4.3	High	Low thermodynamic stability
Optimark	Gadoversetamide (Gd-DTPA-BMEA)	Linear/nonionic	16.6/4.7	High	Low thermodynamic stability
MultiHance	Gadobenate dimeglumine (Gd-BOPTA)	Linear/ionic	22.6/6.3	Intermediate	Highest relaxivity of all extracellular GBCM
Eovist (US) Primovist	Gadoxetate disodium (Gd-EOB-DTPA)	Linear/ionic	23.5/6.9	Intermediate	Designed for liver imaging
Ablavar (US) Vasovist	Gadofosveset trisodium (Gd-DTPA-DCHP-MS-325)	Linear/ionic	22.1/16	Intermediate	Highest relaxivity of any agent due to reversible albumin binding
Gadavist (US) Gadovist	Gadobutrol (Gd-BT-DO3A)	Macrocyclic nonionic	21.8/5.2	Low	Highest viscosity; above-average relaxivity
Prohance	Gadoteridol (Gd-HP-DO3A)	Macrocyclic nonionic	23.8/4.1	Low	Lowest viscosity and osmolality of all agents; below-average relaxivity
Dotarem	Gadoterate meglumine (Gd-DOTA)	Macrocyclic ionic	25.8/3.6	Low	Designed for CNS-related MRI exams

CNS, Central nervous system; *EMA,* European Medicines Agency; *GBCM,* gadolinium-based contrast media; *MRI,* magnetic resonance imaging; *NSF,* nephrogenic systemic fibrosis.

BOX 20.1 Preparation of the Power Injection Apparatus

- Standard procedures should be used to clear the syringe and pressure tubing of air, after which the syringe should be reoriented with the tubing directed downward.
- Before initiating the injection, the position of the catheter tip should be checked for venous backflow.
- If backflow is not obtained, the catheter may need adjustment, and a saline test flush or special monitoring of the site during injection may be appropriate.
- If the venipuncture site is tender or infiltrated, an alternative site should be sought.
- If venous backflow is obtained, the power injector and tubing should be positioned to allow adequate table movement without tension on the intravenous line.

chest pain, cough, tachycardia, pulmonary edema, and hypotension. Stroke leading to neurologic deficits may also occur due to decreased cardiac output or paradoxical air embolism. Administering 100% oxygen and placing the patient in the left lateral decubitus position is the mainstay of treatment. To further reduce the size of air bubbles and help restore circulation and oxygenation, hyperbaric oxygen can be given. Closed-chest cardiopulmonary resuscitation should be started immediately if cardiopulmonary arrest occurs.

General Principles and Training

ARs can be prevented or minimized by applying certain principles for all patients. These include reassessing if CM is necessary, determining if a different IV CM can be used, and determining if 12–24 hours of premedication with corticosteroids and antihistamines can be started prior to CM administration. In some cases alternative imaging modalities can be diagnostic, thus avoiding the use of CM. If CM is necessary, the lowest possible dose to acquire the necessary clinical information should be administered. Because different types of CM have varying safety profiles, choosing the most suitable one for the patient may help avoid complications. In patients with a history of allergies or prior reaction to CM, premedication with corticosteroids and antihistamines can be attempted, although the efficacy

BOX 20.2 Vascular Access Guidelines for Contrast Media Administration at Massachusetts General Hospital

1. Mechanical injection of intravenous contrast media may be performed through the following power/pressure injectable devices:
   - Injection rates for 24 g catheters up to 2 mL/s
   - Injection rates for 22 g catheters up to 4 mL/s
   - Injection rates for 20 g catheters up to 5 mL/s
   - Injection rates for 18 g catheters up to 7 mL/s
2. Saf-T-Intima catheters, not to exceed injection rates of 2 mL/s regardless of the gauge size
3. Power/pressure injectable PICC lines:
   - PowerPICC: Manufacturer guidelines indicate injection rates up to 5 mL/s 300 psi. Product identification tags indicate maximum injection rates.
4. Power/pressure injectable chest port (must be accessed by a physician or registered nurse):
   - PowerPort implantable port, Xcela Power PICC: manufacturer guidelines state that the port must be identified prior to use and accessed with an identified power injectable PowerLoc safety infusion set. The product withstands 5 mL/s power injection at 300 psi pressure limit setting.
5. Central lines:
   - Pressure injectable ARROWg+ard Blue PLUS CVC Injection: manufacturer guidelines indicate rates up to 10 mL/s distal lumen 16 g 300 psi. Medial and proximal lumens 5 mL/s 18 g 300 psi. The injection rate is indicated on the identification tag of the lumen port access.
   - Central lines not indicated for power/pressure injections may be used for mechanical injections with the approval of the radiologist or requesting physician and must not exceed a rate of 2 mL/s.
6. The following devices are not approved for mechanical injections of iodinated contrast media. They are approved for manual injections via hand or gravity drip and must be approved by a radiologist for the examination value:
   - PICC lines not indicated for power/pressure injections
   - Chest ports not indicated for power/pressure injections
   - Midline catheters
   - Accessed femoral or lower extremity lines
   - Peripheral internal jugular accessed or external jugular accessed jugular lines
7. The following devices are not approved for any injection of iodinated contrast media:
   - Any catheter put in for the purpose of hemodialysis
   - Tunneled central venous catheters (e.g., Hickman, Broviac, NeoStar)
   - Any catheter placed intraarterially

CVC, Central venous catheter; *PICC,* peripherally inserted central catheter.

BOX 20.3 Power Injection of Contrast Media Through Some Central Venous Catheters

1. Check the computed tomography scout scan or a recent chest radiograph to confirm the proper location of the catheter tip.
2. Before connecting the catheter to the injector system tubing, test the catheter tip position for venous backflow.
3. Backflow will occasionally not be obtained because the catheter tip is positioned against the wall of the vein in which it is located.
4. If saline can be injected through the catheter without abnormal resistance, administer contrast media through the catheter.
5. If abnormal resistance or discomfort is encountered, seek an alternative venous access site. Injection with large-bore (9.5-F to 10-F) central venous catheters using flow rates of up to 2.5 mL/s has been shown to generate pressures below manufacturers' specified limits.

Contrast media should not be administered by power injector through small-bore, peripheral (e.g., arm) access central venous catheters (unless permitted by the manufacturer's specifications) because of the risk of catheter breakage. It cannot be assumed that all vascular catheters including a peripherally inserted central catheter can tolerate a mechanical injection. A number of manufacturers have produced power injector–compatible vascular catheters. The manufacturer's specifications should be followed.

contrast dose injection protocols on specific imaging scanners can be done to repeat studies without waiting.

Treating ARs requires adequate training with a proactive approach. Studies have shown that radiologists feel insufficiently prepared to manage acute incidents, particularly rare severe reactions. Didactic teaching, simulation courses, and virtual modules are great methods to help the radiologist maintain familiarity with methods for evaluation and treatment of reactions. A study by Tubbs et al. showed that radiology residents who underwent medical simulations showed considerable improvement in confidence and knowledge in management of ARs. Niell et al. demonstrated that didactic learning alone is inadequate because individuals in the study still felt that treating a reaction was difficult and distressing. Therefore, a combination of teaching methods with training repeated yearly or more often appears to be the most effective approach. All personnel who oversee CM injections are also encouraged to maintain current certification in basic life support.

RISK FACTORS AND PREMEDICATION

Risk Factors

For any imaging procedure, the referring physician and radiologist must weigh the risk-to-benefit profile of the requested CM-enhanced examination. Acquiring consent for the injection of CM is not customary because it is generally considered to be safe; however, most institutions collect information from patients to identify risk factors that may increase the likelihood of a reaction. Patients with a history of allergies, asthma, and those with features of atopy (e.g., urticaria) are 3 to 6 times more likely to develop a severe reaction to CM. Although there is no cross-reactivity, patients who have had allergic-like reactions to ICM are also at risk of AR to GBCM. It is important to note that seafood allergies have not been shown to predispose a patient to ARs, and patients with these allergies should be counseled appropriately. Patients with a previous AR

of premedication still remains controversial. If premedications will be administered, oral administration is preferable and should be given at least 6 hours prior to injection of CM whenever possible. Additionally, patients with prior reactions should be followed up more closely during CM administration and kept in observation for longer periods. If readministration of CM is required, it should be avoided for several days to a week after the first injection to allow the kidneys to recover. The American College of Radiology (ACR) recommends that the delay in CM readministration be balanced with the patients severity of renal disease and the medical urgency, whereas the European Society for Urological Radiology (ESUR) recommends the duration of delay be at least 7 days between two injections. If the patient did not reach the maximum daily CM dose, low

to CM are 5 to 6 times more likely to develop a subsequent reaction and are known as high-risk patients. For individuals with kidney diseases, the risk is proportional to the preexisting renal impairment. Other miscellaneous risk factors include patients on certain medications (e.g., metformin), history of multiple myeloma or sickle cell trait, poor cardiac status, anxiety, and history of thyroid cancer or pheochromocytoma.

Premedication

Corticosteroid premedication for high-risk patients is the standard of care in the United States. Corticosteroids produce antiinflammatory effects and cause decreased effectiveness of the innate immune system by impairing function of immune cells (e.g., neutrophils, mast cells). Prophylaxis with corticosteroids has been found to reduce the overall risk of a contrast reaction and is largely reserved for high-risk patients with previous anaphylactoid reactions to CM. However, its efficacy in the prevention of moderate and severe reactions is more controversial due to lack of evidence. Because steroids weaken the immune system, impaired immunity or active infection is seen as a relative contraindication. Additionally, steroids have their own side effects; therefore, the risks and benefits should be considered before administration. Typically, corticosteroids are well tolerated and cause no adverse effects when only a few doses are administered. When emergent contrast injection is required, higher doses of intravascular steroids may be considered. Elective and emergent premedication regimens with corticosteroids may also involve the use of antihistamines (Tables 20.3 and 20.4). All forms of antihistamines can cause drowsiness; however, second-generation antihistamines cause less drowsiness and may be beneficial for patients who

need to drive themselves home. Patients who are unable to take oral medications can have an IV dose of 200 mg hydrocortisone.

TYPES OF ADVERSE REACTIONS AND TREATMENT

Despite recognizing predisposing risk factors, ARs remain unpredictable and sporadic due to their multifactorial nature. ARs occur more commonly in ICM, and the incidence varies between studies (Table 20.5). Incidence of ARs ranges from 0.2% to 3% for ICM with severe reactions ranging from 0.005% to 0.01%. Incidence of ARs ranges from 0.03% to 0.5% for GBCM with severe reactions ranging from 0.002% to 0.01%. Most ARs occur in the first 5 minutes within the first hour of CM administration. ARs are typically classified into three categories of severity: mild (flushing, arm pain, nausea/vomiting, headache), moderate (bronchospasm, hypotension), and severe (cardiovascular collapse, laryngeal edema, convulsions, arrhythmias) (Fig. 20.1). The vast majority of ARs are mild, with the most common being transient injection site discomfort, headache, dizziness, nausea with or without vomiting, paresthesia, and itching. Mild reactions typically require no treatment because they are usually self-limiting and do not progress. However, if mild reactions become more severe, patients should be treated and monitored to ensure recovery. Moderate reactions with no or only mild hypoxia are usually not life threatening (e.g., bronchospasm); however, patients should be observed closely and managed until symptoms have resolved completely. Severe reactions should be identified and treated immediately to prevent permanent morbidity or mortality. For all ARs, practitioners should maintain IV access, measure vital signs, and assess the patient's well-being (e.g., appearance, voice quality, and symptoms). Facilities where injection of CM occurs must be equipped with the proper tools/supplies required to manage any form of reaction (Box 20.4). The management for different ARs as outlined by the ACR is shown in Table 20.6.

Anaphylactoid Reactions

The most clinically important ARs are anaphylactoid (allergic-like) reactions, which typically begin within several minutes of CM exposure. The incidence of allergic-like reactions to low-osmolar CM (LOCM) is relatively rare, with estimates in the range of 0.2% to 3.1%. Most of these reactions are mild to moderate in severity. The incidence of

TABLE 20.3 **Corticosteroid and Antihistamine Premedication Regimen for Adults: Elective Procedures**

	Dose
Steroids	Methylprednisolone, one 32-mg tablet, orally administered at 12 and 2 h before CM administration
	or
	Prednisone, one 50-mg tablet, orally administered 13 h, 7 h, and 1 h before CM administration
Antihistamine	Diphenhydramine 50 mg IV, IM, or orally administered 1 h before CM administration

TABLE 20.4 **Corticosteroid and Antihistamine Premedication Regimen for Adults: Emergent Procedures**

	Most Desirable in Emergency (First Choice)	Less Desirable Than First Choice	Least Desirable (Chosen When There Is Inadequate Time to Achieve Steroid Effect)
Steroid	IV methylprednisolone sodium succinate 40 mg	IV dexamethasone sodium sulfate 7.5 mg	Omit IV steroids; no effect when given less than 4–6 h before CM administration
	or	*or*	
	IV hydrocortisone sodium succinate 200 mg every 4 h until CM administration	IV betamethasone 6 mg every 4 h until CM administration	
Antihistamine	IV diphenhydramine 50 mg, 1 h before CM administration	IV diphenhydramine 50 mg, 1 h before CM administration	IV diphenhydramine 50 mg, 1 h before CM administration

CM, Contrast media; *IM,* intramuscular; *IV,* intravenous.

TABLE 20.5 Incidence Rates of Acute Adverse Effects for Contrast Media

Reference	Incidence
IODINATED CONTRAST MEDIA	
Cochran et al.	Overall rate 0.2% (LOCM)
Hunt et al.	Overall rate 0.15 (LOCM)
Mortelé et al.	Overall rate 0.7% (iopromide)
Wang et al.	Overall rate 0.6% (iohexol, iopromide, or iodixanole)
Dillman et al.	Overall rate 0.18% (pediatric)
Callahan et al.	Overall rate 0.46%
Caro et al. (meta-analysis)	Fatality rate of 0.9 per 100,000 injections of LOCM
GADOLINIUM-BASED CONTRAST MEDIA	
Hunt et al.	Overall rate 0.04%
Dillman et al.	Overall rate 0.07% (gadopentetate dimeglumine, gadobenate dimeglumine, gadodiamide)
Li et al.	Overall rate 0.48%
Murphy et al.	0.06% (gadopentetate dimeglumine) 0.03% (gadodiamide) 0.4% (gadoteriodol)

LOCM, Low-osmolar contrast media.

allergic-like reactions is higher in certain age and gender combinations (e.g., young females) compared to the general population. The increased incidence of ARs seen among younger patients may be due to psychological effects. Anaphylactoid reactions are mediated by type 1 hypersensitivity mechanisms, which involve the release of histamine and other mediators. Many patients have allergic-like reactions at initial exposure, unlike the classic allergic reaction that requires an initial sensitizing exposure. This is because mediators directly stimulate an allergic response through mast cell degranulation and other pathways, without involvement of immunoglobulin E (mediator of the classic allergic reaction). Because no previous exposure is required, patients do not usually have a more serious reaction with subsequent administration of IV CM. The small number of severe reactions that are mediated by immunoglobulin E can be identified by positive results at skin testing.

Dose-Dependent Reactions

Physiologic reactions that are chemotoxic in nature are believed to be caused by the dose and molecular toxicity of ICM as well as physical and chemical aspects such as viscosity or osmolality, among others. For example, high osmolality of ICM can lead to extracellular fluid shifts resulting in cellular dehydration and dysfunction. Physiologic effects of

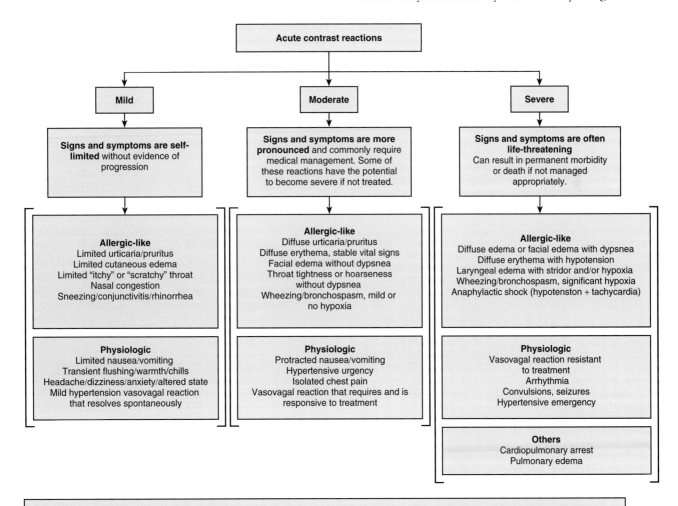

FIG. 20.1 Symptoms and signs of adverse reactions to contrast media based on severity. *ICM,* intravenous contrast media. (From American College of Radiology. ACR Manual on Contrast Media v10.1. <http://www.acr.org/quality-safety/resources/contrast-manual>.)

BOX 20.4   Equipment for Contrast Reaction Kits in Radiology

The following equipment must be readily available and within or nearby any room in which contrast media is to be injected (adult or pediatric sizes are optional for facilities that do not inject adult or pediatric patients, respectively):

- Oxygen cylinders or wall-mounted oxygen source, flow valve, tubing, oxygen masks[a] (adult and pediatric sizes)
- Suction: wall-mounted or portable; tubing and catheters
- Oral and/or nasal airways: rubber/plastic Ambu-type bag-valve-mask device; masks in adult and pediatric sizes; protective barriers for mouth-to-mouth respiration are optional if the bag-valve-mask device is stocked
- Stethoscope; sphygmomanometer
- Intravenous solutions (0.9% [normal] saline and/or Ringer lactate solution) and tubing
- Syringes and IV cannulas: various sizes; tourniquets
- Needles: various sizes
- Necessary medications:
  - Epinephrine 1:10,000, 10-mL preloaded syringe (for IV injection) *and/or*
  - Epinephrine 1:1000, 1 mL (for IM injection) *and/or*
  - Epinephrine IM auto-injector[b] (sizes for patients 15–30 kg and patients ≥30 kg)
  - Atropine, 1 mg in 10-mL preloaded syringe
  - Beta-agonist inhaler with or without spacer
  - Diphenhydramine for PO, IM, or IV administration
  - Nitroglycerin: 0.4-mg tabs, sublingual
  - Aspirin, 325 mg (for chest pain where myocardial ischemia is a consideration)
- Optional medications:
  - Lasix, 20–40 mg IV
  - Labetalol, 20 mg IV
  - Dextrose 50% 25 mg/50 mL syringe

The following items should be on the emergency/code cart[c] or within or near any room in which contrast media is injected:

- Defibrillator or automated external defibrillator
- Blood pressure/pulse monitor
- Pulse oximeter

The contact phone number of the cardiopulmonary arrest emergency response team should be clearly posted within or near any room in which contrast media is injected. For magnetic resonance imaging, to avoid any resuscitative equipment becoming a magnetic hazard, patients requiring treatment should be taken away from the imaging room immediately.

[a]Although oxygen can be administered in a variety of ways, use of nonrebreather masks is preferred because of their ability to deliver more oxygen to the patient.

[b]Examples: EpiPen Jr. or Auvi-Q 0.15 mg; injects 0.15 mg epinephrine (as 0.3 mL of 1:2000 or 0.15 mL of 1:1000 epinephrine, respectively) or EpiPen or Auvi-Q 0.3 mg; injects 0.3 mg epinephrine (as 0.3 mL of 1:1000 epinephrine).

[c]If in a hospital or clinic, the emergency/code cart should conform to hospital or departmental policies and procedures; it often includes these items.

CM can also affect several organ systems leading to various symptoms such as nausea, vasovagal reactions, bradycardia, and hypotension to name a few. It is important to distinguish allergic-like reactions from dose-dependent reactions due to the difference in management. For example, physiologic reactions do not require premedication in the future. On the other hand, patients who suffered an allergy-like reaction may likely need premedication with steroids for future CM-enhanced examinations.

Delayed Reactions

Delayed reactions (DRs) occur from 30 to 60 minutes up to 1 week after CM administration, with the majority occurring between 3 hours and 2 days. The incidence of delayed ARs is 5% to 6% for low-osmolar monomeric CM and 10.9% for isoosmolar dimeric CM. DRs are mostly seen in woman, young adults, and patients with a history of allergy. They are typically mild to moderate in severity and tend to be self-limiting cutaneous reactions (e.g., urticaria, maculopapular rash) that often require only symptomatic or no treatment. Cutaneous events in DRs have been seen significantly more often with dimeric nonionic CM than with monomeric nonionic CM (16.4% vs. 9.7%, respectively). Noncutaneous symptoms and signs include nausea, vomiting, fever, drowsiness, and headache. Symptoms such as salivary gland swelling (iodide *mumps*) and acute polyarthropathy are rare and more common in patients with renal disease. Premedication for future administration of CM is only warranted if the patient experienced a previous severe DR.

Breakthrough Reactions and Other Relevant Collateral Effects

Rarely, breakthrough reactions (BRs) can occur after injection of CM despite premedication with corticosteroids. Clinical appearance and severity of BRs often resemble those of the initial AR. Patients who suffer from BRs usually have a history of severe allergies to another substance or drug (including CM) have more than four allergies, or chronically use oral corticosteroids. After evaluation and treatment, patients should be counseled on the increased risk for future severe reactions if IV CM is administered. More recently, the FDA has been evaluating the risk of brain deposits with repeated use of GBCM and whether they lead to adverse health effects. Recent studies have

---

TABLE 20.6   Treatment of Adverse Reactions in Adults and Children

Type of Reaction	Adults	Children
Urticaria (Hives)		
Mild (scattered and/or transient)	• No treatment often needed • If symptomatic, consider diphenhydramine 25–50 mg PO* or fexofenadine 180 mg PO	• No treatment often needed • If symptomatic, consider diphenhydramine[a,*]
Moderate (more numerous/bothersome)	• Monitor vitals • Preserve IV access • Consider diphenhydramine 25–50 mg PO* or fexofenadine[†] 180 mg PO or diphenhydramine[b]	• Monitor vitals, preserve IV access, consider diphenhydramine[a,*]
Severe (widespread and/or progressive)	• Monitor vitals • Preserve IV access • Consider diphenhydramine[b,*]	• Monitor vitals • Preserve IV access • Consider diphenhydramine[a,*]

TABLE 20.6   Treatment of Adverse Reactions in Adults and Children—cont'd

Type of Reaction	Adults	Children
Diffuse Erythema		
All forms	• Preserve IV access • Monitor vitals • Pulse oximeter • O_2 by mask (6–10 L/min)	• Preserve IV access • Monitor vitals • O_2 by mask (6–10 L/min)
Normotensive	• No other treatment usually needed	• No other treatment usually needed

Hypotensive	• IV fluids: 0.9% NS or lactated Ringer solution (1000 mL rapidly)
	• If unresponsive to fluids or profound hypotension, consider:
	  • IV epinephrine[c] or IM epinephrine[d,‡] if no IV access available
	  • Consider calling emergency response team or 911
		• IV fluids: 0.9% NS or lactated Ringer solution (10–20 mL/kg; maximum 500–1000 mL)
		• If unresponsive to fluids or profound hypotension[‡]:
		  • IV epinephrine[e] or IM epinephrine[f]
		  • Consider calling emergency response team or 911

Bronchospasm		
All forms	• Preserve IV access • Monitor vitals • Pulse oximeter • O_2 by mask (6–10 L/min)	• Preserve IV access • Monitor vitals • O_2 by mask (6–10 L/min)
Mild	• Beta-agonist inhaler[g] • Consider sending patient to the emergency department or calling emergency response team or 911 based upon the completeness of the response	• Beta-agonist inhaler[g] • Consider calling emergency response team or 911, based upon the completeness of the response
Moderate	• Beta-agonist inhaler[g] • Consider adding IM epinephrine[d] or IV epinephrine[c] • Consider calling emergency response team or 911 based upon the completeness of the response	• Consider adding IM epinephrine[f] or IV epinephrine[e,‡] • Consider calling emergency response team or 911 based upon the completeness of the response
Severe	• IV epinephrine[c] or IM epinephrine[d,‡] and beta agonist inhaler[g] (may work synergistically) • Call emergency response team or 911	• Same treatment as moderate, with addition of beta-agonist inhaler[g] • Call emergency response team or 911
Laryngeal edema (all forms)	• Preserve IV access • Monitor vitals • Pulse oximeter • O_2 by mask (6–10 L/min) • Epinephrine IV[c] or IM[d,‡] • Consider calling emergency response team or 911 based upon the severity of the reaction and the completeness of the response	• Preserve IV access • Monitor vitals • O_2 by mask (6–10 L/min) • Epinephrine IV[e] or IM[f,‡] • Call emergency response team or 911
Hypotension (definition varies for children of different ages)		
All forms	• Preserve IV access • Monitor vitals • O_2 by mask (6–10 L/min) • Elevate legs at least 60 degrees • Consider IV fluids: 0.9% NS or lactated Ringer solution (1000 mL rapidly)	• Preserve IV access • Monitor vitals • O_2 by mask (6–10 L/min) • Elevate legs at least 60 degrees • Consider IV fluids: 0.9% NS or lactated Ringer solution (10–20 mL/kg [maximum 500–1000 mL])
With bradycardia (vasovagal reaction), pulse <60 beats/min	*If mild:* • In addition to above measures, no other treatment usually necessary *If severe* (patient remains symptomatic despite above measures): • Addition of atropine IV • 0.6–1.0 mg; administer into a running IV infusion of fluids; can repeat up to 3 mg total • Consider calling the emergency response team or 911	• Minimum normal pulse varies for children of different ages *If mild:* • In addition to above measures, no other treatment usually necessary *If severe* (patient remains symptomatic despite above measures): • Addition of atropine IV[h]
With tachycardia (anaphylactoid reaction), pulse >100 beats/min	*If hypotension persists:* • Give epinephrine IV[c] or IM[d,‡] • Consider calling emergency response team or 911 based upon the severity of the reaction and the completeness of the response	• Maximum normal pulse varies for children of different ages *If severe (symptoms persist):* • Give epinephrine IV[e] or IM[f,‡] • Call emergency response team or 911
Unresponsive and pulseless	• Activate emergency response team (call 911) • Start CPR • Get defibrillator or AED; apply as soon as available; shock as indicated • Epinephrine (between 2-min cycles) (0.1 mL/kg of 1:10,000 dilution [0.01 mg/kg]; administer quickly with flush or IV fluids; max dose of 10 mL [1 mg])[¶¶]	Same as for adults

Continued

TABLE 20.6   Treatment of Adverse Reactions in Adults and Children—cont'd

Type of Reaction	Adults	Children
Hypertensive crisis¶	• Preserve IV access • Monitor vitals • O$_2$ by mask (6–10 L/min) • Labetalol IV 20 mg; administer slowly over 2 min; can double the dose every 10 min (e.g., 40 mg 10 min later, then 80 mg 10 min after that) *or (if labetalol not available)* • Nitroglycerin tablet (SL) 0.4 mg tablet; can repeat every 5–10 min and furosemide (Lasix) 20–40 mg IV; administer slowly over 2 min • Call emergency response team or 911	
Pulmonary edema	• Preserve IV access • Monitor vitals • O$_2$ by mask (6–10 L/min) • Pulse oximeter • Elevate head of bed • Furosemide 20–40 mg IV; administer slowly over 2 min • Call emergency response team or 911	• Preserve IV access • Monitor vitals • O$_2$ by mask (6–10 L/min) • Elevate head of bed • Furosemide (IV 0.5–1.0 mg/kg over 2 min; max 40 mg) • Call emergency response team or 911
Seizures/convulsions	• Observe and protect the patient • Turn patient on side to avoid aspiration • Suction airway, as needed • Preserve IV access • Monitor vitals • Pulse oximeter • O$_2$ by mask (6–10 L/min) • *If unremitting,* call emergency response team or 911 and give lorazepam 2–4 mg IV; administer slowly to max of 4 mg	• Observe and protect the patient • Turn patient on side to avoid aspiration • Suction airway, as needed • Preserve IV access • Monitor vitals • O$_2$ by mask (6–10 L/min) • *If unremitting,* call emergency response team or 911
Hypoglycemia		
All patients	• Preserve IV access • O$_2$ by mask (6–10 L/min)	• Preserve IV access • O$_2$ by mask (6–10 L/min)
If patient is able to swallow safely	• Administer oral glucose[i]	• Observe • Administer oral glucose[i]
If patient is unable to swallow safely	IV access is available: • Dextrose 50% (IV D5W 1 ampule [25 g], administer over 2 min) *and* D5W or D5NS (IV) as adjunct therapy, administer at a rate of 100 mL/h If no IV access is available: • Glucagon IM 1 mg	IV access is available: • Dextrose 50% (IV D25 2 mL/kg; IV injection over 2 min) IV access is not available: • Glucagon (IM/SQ 0.5 mg if <20 kg or IM/SQ 1.0 mg if >20 kg)
Anxiety (panic attack)	• Diagnosis of exclusion • Assess patient for developing signs and symptoms that might indicate another type of reaction • Preserve IV access • Monitor vitals • Pulse oximeter • If no identifiable manifestations and normal oxygenation, consider this diagnosis	• Same as adult treatment
Reaction rebound prevention§	• Hydrocortisone[j] or methylprednisolone[k]	• Hydrocortisone[j] (max 200 mg) or methylprednisolone[k] (max 40 mg)

[a]1 mg/kg (max 50 mg) PO, IM, or IV; administer IV dose slowly over 1–2 min.

[b]25–50 mg IM or IV (administer IV dose slowly over 1–2 min).

[c]1 mL of 1:10,000 dilution (0.1 mg); administer slowly into a running IV infusion of fluids; can repeat every few minutes as needed up to 10 mL (1 mg) total.

[d]0.3 mL of 1:1000 dilution (0.3 mg); can repeat every 5–15 min up to 1 mL (1 mg) total or epinephrine autoinjector (EpiPen or equivalent), (0.3 mL of 1:1000 dilution, fixed [0.3 mg]); can repeat every 5–15 min up to 3 times.

[e]0.1 mL/kg of 1:10,000 dilution (0.01 mg/kg); administer slowly into a running IV infusion of fluids; can repeat every 5–15 min as needed; maximum single dose: 1.0 mL (0.1 mg); can repeat up to 1 mg total dose.

[f]0.01 mL/kg of 1:1000 dilution (0.01 mg/kg); max 0.30 mL (0.30 mg); can repeat every 5–15 min up to 1 mL (1 mg) total or epinephrine autoinjector (1:1000 dilution equivalent). If <30 kg, pediatric epinephrine autoinjector (EpiPen Jr or equivalent) 0.15 mL equivalent (0.15 mg); if ≥30 kg, adult epinephrine autoinjector (EpiPen or equivalent) 0.30 mL (0.30 mg).

[g]Two puffs (90 μg/puff) for a total of 180 μg; can repeat up to 3 times.

[h]IV 0.2 mL/kg of 0.1 mg/mL solution (0.02 mg/kg); minimum single dose of 0.1 mg and maximum single dose of 0.6–1.0 mg; maximum total dose of 1 mg for infants and children, 2 mg for adolescents; administer into a running IV infusion of fluids.

[i]Two sugar packets or 15 g of glucose tablet or gel or ½ cup (4 oz) fruit juice.

[j]IV 5 mg/kg; administer over 1–2 min.

[k]IV 1 mg/kg; administer over 1–2 min.

*All forms can cause drowsiness; IM/IV form may cause or worsen hypotension.

†Second-generation antihistamines cause less drowsiness and may be beneficial for patients who need to drive themselves home.

‡In hypotensive patients, the preferred route of epinephrine delivery is IV because the extremities may not be perfused sufficiently to allow for adequate absorption of IM-administered epinephrine. With respect to IM delivery of epinephrine, the EpiPen Jr package insert does not provide dosing recommendations for children <15 kg. Also, it can be difficult to dose medications accurately in neonates and infants.

§Although IV corticosteroids may help prevent a short-term recurrence of an allergic-like reaction, they are not useful in the acute treatment of any reaction. However, these may be considered for patients having severe allergic-like manifestations prior to transportation to an emergency department of an inpatient unit.

¶¶Also see BLS and ACLS booklets published by the American Heart Association.

¶Diastolic BP >120 mm Hg; systolic BP >200 mm Hg; symptoms of end organ compromise.

ACLS, Advanced Cardiac Life Support; *AED,* automated external defibrillator; *BLS,* basic life support; *BP,* blood pressure; *CPR,* cardiopulmonary resuscitation; *D5NS,* 5% dextrose in normal saline; *D25,* dextrose 25%; *D5W,* 5% dextrose in water; *IV,* intravenous; *IM,* intramuscular; *NS,* normal saline; *PO,* by mouth; *SQ,* subcutaneous.

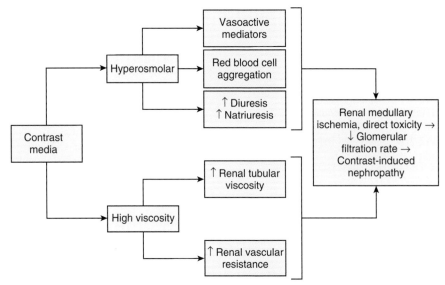

FIG. 20.2 Effects of high viscosity and hyperosmolarity of contrast media on the kidneys. (From McCullough PA. Contrast induced acute kidney injury. *J Am Coll Cardiol.* 2008;51[15]:1419–1428.)

demonstrated remaining deposits of GBCMs in the brain of some patients who underwent four or more MRI scans, long after the last administration. GBCMs are mostly eliminated from the body through the kidneys; however, trace amounts may stay in the body long term even in individuals with normal kidney function. Pseudohypocalcemia has also been reported with some GBCM, specifically with the use of less stable CM like Omniscan and OptiMARK. There is no actual reduction in serum calcium but merely falsely low serum calcium lab values as the CM interferes with the test. The importance of differentiating between pseudo- and real hypocalcemia is to avoid inappropriate management with calcium replacement, a therapy that has already been reported to cause death in at least one case. Other effects that may occur include a transitory increase in bilirubin (Magnevist, 3%–4% of patients) and iron serum levels (with Magnevist and Omniscan) that typically recede within 24–48 hours. Some GBCM agents (e.g., Eovist, Ablavar, MultiHance) may also cause QT prolongation, increasing the risk of arrhythmia.

CONTRAST-INDUCED NEPHROPATHY

Definition

Contrast-induced nephropathy (CIN) is the third most common cause of hospital-acquired acute renal failure (ARF). CIN is described as ARF occurring "within 48 hours of exposure to intravascular radiographic contrast material that is not attributable to other causes." Some have proposed that renal insufficiency (RI) up to 7 days post contrast administration can be considered CIN, as long as it is not attributable to any other identifiable cause of renal failure. The definition of ARF regardless of cause is defined as the increase in creatinine level of more than 0.3 mg/dL within 48 hours, an increase of more than 50% of the baseline creatinine level within 7 days, or oliguria lasting for more than 6 hours. The pathogenesis of CIN by CM is thought to be due to ischemic injury to tubular cells and due to direct toxicity by generation of reactive oxygen species (Fig. 20.2). Nevertheless, the clinical duration of

---

BOX 20.5   Risk Factors for Contrast-Induced Nephropathy

FIXED (NONMODIFIABLE)
- Preexisting renal dysfunction
- Chronic kidney disease
- Acute myocardial infarction
- Cardiogenic shock
- Diabetes mellitus
- Older age
- Intraaortic balloon pump
- Multiple myeloma
- Advanced congestive heart failure
- Left ventricular ejection fraction <40%

MODIFIABLE
- Dehydration
- Hypotension
- Anemia and blood loss
- Use of nephrotoxic agents
- Large volume dose iodinated contrast
- High-osmolar contrast
- Ionic contrast
- Short time interval between administration of 2 doses of contrast media

---

CIN depends on the patient's baseline renal function, coexisting risk factors, degree of hydration, and a few other factors. The major concern with respect to ARF is the high mortality rate (40%–90%) emphasizing the importance of understanding the clinical manifestations and subsequent management of CIN.

Risk Factors

There are several modifiable and nonmodifiable risk factors for CIN; however, preexisting impairment of renal function and diabetes appear to be the most important, particularly when coexisting (Box 20.5). The incidence of CIN is higher and may be as high as 20% to 50% in patients with underlying hypertension, cardiovascular

- Kidney:
  - Kidney disease/injury
  - Renal insufficiency/failure
  - Kidney surgery or kidney transplant
- Diabetes (treated with insulin or other medication)
- Cardiovascular disease:
  - History of congestive heart failure and hypertension requiring medication
  - Peripheral vascular disease: all computed tomography angiography runoff examinations
- Potentially nephrotoxic medications:
  - Chronic or high-dose nonsteroidal antiinflammatory drug therapy
  - Aminoglycoside antibiotics
- Inpatients and emergency department patients
- Age ≥70 years
- Certain diseases (e.g., multiple myeloma, systemic lupus erythematosa)

TABLE 20.7 Factors Affecting Serum Creatinine

Factors	Effect
Aging	Decreased
Female sex	Decreased
Race or ethnic group:	
Black	Increased
Hispanic	Decreased
Asian	Decreased
Body habitus:	
Muscular	Increased
Amputation	Decreased
Obesity	No change
Chronic illness: malnutrition, inflammation, deconditioning (e.g., cancer, severe cardiovascular disease, hospitalized patients), neuromuscular disease	Decreased
Diet:	
Vegetarian diet	Decreased
Ingestion of cooked meat	Increased

diseases, diabetes mellitus, or preexisting RI. Patients with stable renal function have a risk of CIN of less than 1%, especially in the absence of risk factors and serum creatinine (SCr) levels less than 1.8 mg/dL (159.12 μmol/L) at baseline. Patients with chronic kidney disease (CKD) have an increased risk of developing CIN that is more than 20 times that of a normal individual. For example, a study by Gussenhoven et al. reported that the incidence of CIN is elevated 5- to 10-fold in patients with RI (SCr >1.5 mg/dL [133 μmol/L]). Indications for obtaining a screening SCr are listed in Box 20.6 and Table 20.7, but changes in creatinine seen during ARF are delayed and not reliable for use in making treatment decisions. SCr is affected by many factors; thus, it is not the best way to determine renal function (see Box 20.6 and Table 20.7). The most important risk factor for the development of CIN in patients with preexisting

RI is an estimated glomerular filtration rate (GFR) equal to or less than 60. Guidelines to assess a patient's risk for CIN depending on his or her GFR are shown in Fig. 20.3. Additionally, a simple risk score for prediction of CIN can be done using the CIN risk stratification scoring system (Fig. 20.4). It is also important to remember that the choice of the CM agent to be used can affect the patient's risk of developing CIN. Randomized trials comparing CM with different osmolalities have demonstrated lower rates of CIN with LOCM compared to high-osmolar CM, and in high-risk patients the rate of CIN was significantly reduced when using isoosmolar contrast media (IOCM) rather than LOCM (Table 20.8). Ultimately, it is unusual for patients with CIN to develop permanent renal dysfunction.

Prophylactic Measures and Treatment

In addition to the general principles outlined earlier in the chapter, there are several strategies to prevent or minimize the occurrence of CIN (Fig. 20.5). The most important means of CIN prevention is fluid administration. Many studies have shown that hydration minimizes or decreases the incidence of renal injury induced by contrast material. In fact, the positive effect of adequate periprocedural hydration was first established by Solomon et al. in 1994. Although the exact mechanism is unclear, IV fluids seem to lead to expansion of intravascular space, weakening the vasoconstrictive effect of contrast in the medulla by inhibiting renin-angiotensin-aldosterone system (RAAS) vasopressin. Additionally, fluids blunt the direct toxic effect of contrast on tubules by reducing concentration and viscosity. Therefore, dehydrated patients are at increased risk for prolonged exposure of the tubules to CM unless they receive adequate hydration. Oral fluids are the easiest method of hydration, but efficacy is uncertain; therefore IV fluid is the mainstay of practice. Furthermore, IV fluid administration is the most reliable means to monitor and administer fluids. In addition to the route of hydration, factors such as fluid composition and fluid tonicity play a role. In a large prospective study, Mueller et al. showed that normal saline (NS; 0.9%) was superior to half-NS (0.45%) and that diabetic patients, female patients, patients undergoing emergent interventions, and patients receiving greater than 250 mL of contrast were the most likely to benefit from isotonic hydration. Isotonic fluids may be superior to hypotonic fluids, mostly because of their enhanced ability to expand intravascular volume. Sodium bicarbonate administration may provide added protection by alkalinizing renal tubular fluid and minimizing tubular damage. IV fluid loading regimens according to the Canadian Association of Radiologists can be seen in Table 20.9. In patients who are able to take oral fluids, moderate fluid intake up to 2 hours before CM administration and immediately after is also recommended. Salty foods may also be encouraged the day before the examination to promote volume expansion.

The use of N-acetylcysteine (NAC) is part of the standard of care but should not be considered as a substitute for hydration because efficacy in preventing CIN is still uncertain. NAC is a powerful antioxidant that reduces the depletion of glutathione and stimulates vasodilatory mediator release (e.g., nitric oxide). Tepel et al. first

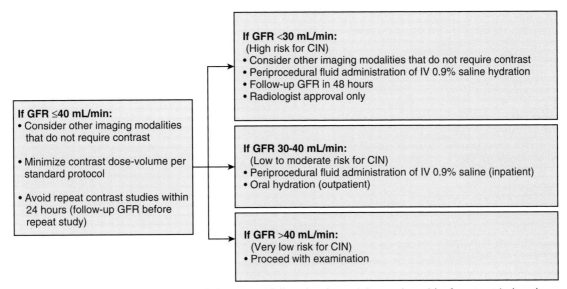

If GFR ≤40 mL/min:
- Consider other imaging modalities that do not require contrast
- Minimize contrast dose-volume per standard protocol
- Avoid repeat contrast studies within 24 hours (follow-up GFR before repeat study)

If GFR <30 mL/min:
(High risk for CIN)
- Consider other imaging modalities that do not require contrast
- Periprocedural fluid administration of IV 0.9% saline hydration
- Follow-up GFR in 48 hours
- Radiologist approval only

If GFR 30-40 mL/min:
(Low to moderate risk for CIN)
- Periprocedural fluid administration of IV 0.9% saline (inpatient)
- Oral hydration (outpatient)

If GFR >40 mL/min:
(Very low risk for CIN)
- Proceed with examination

FIG. 20.3 Canadian Association of Radiologists guidelines for determining patient risk of contrast-induced nephropathy (CIN) based on glomerular filtration rate (GFR). (From Owen RJ, Hiremath S, Myers A, Fraser-Hill M, Barrett BJ. Canadian Association of Radiologists Consensus Guidelines for the Prevention of Contrast-Induced Nephropathy: Update 2012. *Can Assoc Radiol J.* 2014;65[2]:96–105.)

CIN risk stratification scoring system	
Risk factor	**Points**
Chronic CHF	5
Hypotension	5
Intraaortic balloon pump	5
Age >75 years	4
Anemia (baseline hematocrit value <39% for men and <36% for women)	3
Diabetes	3
Contrast media volume (per 100 mL of contrast used)	1
Serum creatinine >1.5 mg/dL Or eGFR 40–59 mL/min Or eGFR 20–39 mL/min Or eGFR <20 mL/min	4 2 4 6

Risk score	Risk of CIN	Risk of dialysis
≤5	7.5%	0.04%
6–10	14%	0.12%
11–16	26.1%	1.09%
≥16	57.3%	12.6%

FIG. 20.4 Scoring system to assess a patient's risk of contrast-induced nephropathy. *CHF*, Congestive heart failure class III/IV by New York Heart Association classification and/or history of pulmonary edema; *CIN*, contrast-induced nephropathy; *eGFR*, estimated glomerular filtration rate. Hypotension defined as systolic blood pressure <80 mm Hg for at least 1 h requiring inotropic support with medications or intraaortic balloon pump within 24 h periprocedurally. (From Mehran R, Aymong ED, Nikolsky E, et al. A simple risk score for prediction of contrast-induced nephropathy after percutaneous coronary intervention. *J Am Coll Cardiol.* 2004;44[7]:1393–1399.)

described its efficacy in preventing CIN, but since then many trials have been published showing controversial results. However, NAC is still routinely administered due to the low cost and lack of major adverse effects (may cause anaphylactoid reaction but only if used at very large dose). Studies investigated doses ranging from 600 to 1200 mg by mouth twice daily before and after the procedure, with results showing that higher NAC doses may be more beneficial. To further minimize the likelihood of

CIN, medications such as aminoglycosides, nonsteroidal antiinflammatory drugs (NSAIDs), and diuretics should be withheld for at least 24 to 48 hours before and after exposure to CM. In patients receiving dialysis, there is no need for fluid hydration before CM administration. Furthermore, there is no obligation to coordinate the time of hemodialysis with CM administration. However, renal protective measures should always be considered for patients with residual kidney function.

TABLE 20.8 **Randomized Trials Comparing Contrast Media With Different Osmolalities**

Reference	Year	Patient Cohort	Procedure	Contrast Media Used	CIN, n/N (%)	RR	P Value
Barrett et al.	1992	249	Coronary angiography	LOCM (iohexol) HOCM (diatrizoate)	5/132 (3.8), 8/117 (6.8)	0.55	.39
Moore et al.	1992	929	Angiography + CT	LOCM (iohexol) HOCM (diatrizoate)	13/479 (2.7), 13/450 (2.9)	1.06	.87
Rudnick et al.	1995	1183	Coronary angiography	LOCM (iohexol) HOCM (diatrizoate)	19/591 (3.2), 42/592 (7.1)	0.45	.003
Schwab et al.	1989	443	Coronary angiography	LOCM (iopamidol) HOCM (diatrizoate)	24/235 (10.2), 17/208 (8.2)	1.25	.51
Taliercio et al.	1991	307	Coronary angiography	LOCM (iopamidol) HOCM (diatrizoate)	12/155 (7.7), 29/152 (19.1)	0.43	.008
Aspelin et al.	2003	129	Coronary angiography	IOCM (iodixanol) LOCM (iohexol)	2/64 (3.1), 17/65 (26.1)	0.12	.002
Chalmers et al.	1999	102	Angiography	IOCM (iodixanol) LOCM (iohexol)	2/54 (3.7), 5/48 (10.4)	0.35	.25
Hardiek et al.	2003	102	Coronary angiography	IOCM (iodixanol) LOCM (iopamidol)	7/54 (13.0), 10/48 (20.8)	0.62	.30
Jo et al.	2005	281	Coronary angiography	IOCM (iodixanol) LOCM (ioxaglate)	10/164 (6.1), 18/117 (15.4)	0.40	.01

AR, Adverse reaction; *CIN,* contrast-induced nephropathy; *HOCM,* high-osmolar contrast media; *IOCM,* isoosmolar contrast media; *LOCM,* low-osmolar contrast media; *RR,* relative risk.

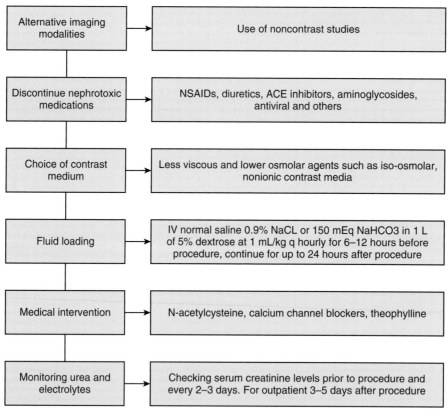

FIG. 20.5 Several strategies and recommendations to help minimize or prevent contrast-induced nephropathy. *ACE,* Angiotensin-converting enzyme; *NSAIDs,* nonsteroidal antiinflammatory drugs.

TABLE 20.9 **Intravenous Fluid Loading Regimens According to the Canadian Association of Radiologists**

Factor	Regimen
Inpatients	IV 0.9% saline at 100 mL/h 6-12 h before and continuing 4-12 h after CM
Outpatients	IV 0.9% saline at 100 mL/h 6 h prior to CM. Liberal oral fluids immediately following CM
Same-day procedures	NaHCO₃ or 0.9 NS at 3 mL/kg/h for 1-3 h before and 6 h after contrast media administration
	or
	NaHCO₃ 150 mEq in 850 mL D5W at 3 mL/kg/h for 1 h before and at 1 mL/kg/h for 6 h after CM administration

CM, Contrast media; *D5W,* 5% dextrose in water; *IV,* intravenous.

Other Medications

There has been much discussion regarding the benefit of other medications such as diuretics, vasodilators, and adenosine antagonists. However, the use of these medications has yielded varying results, some showing beneficial results, some showing no benefit, and in a few cases even causing harm. Larger trials are required to give a definitive answer and develop more concrete evidence as to their beneficial effects. Diuretics such as furosemide and mannitol are used in an attempt to increase or maintain the GFR and decrease the contact time of CM with tubular epithelium, thereby reducing epithelial damage to the kidney. A study by Marenzi et al. involving patients with chronic renal failure (eGFR <60 mL/minute/1.73 m²) showed significantly lower incidence of acute kidney injury (AKI) in patients who received a combination of hydration plus furosemide when compared to the patients treated with hydration only. In contrast, a study by Solomon et al. involving patients with SCr of 2.1 mg/dL concluded that hydration with 0.45% saline provides better protection against acute decreases in renal function when compared to saline plus mannitol or furosemide. Additionally, a study by Weinstein et al. even showed a decline in kidney function of patients treated with furosemide before IV CM administration. Calcium channel blockers have been hypothesized to have protective effects on the kidney by preventing vasoconstrictive response in intrarenal circulation due to intracellular calcium. However, the trials on calcium channel blockers do not detect clinically significant outcomes. Other vasodilators such as dopamine (e.g., fenoldopam) have controversial results; some are positive outcomes and others negative. The use of dopamine is controversial on the basis of its significant adverse effect profile and the difficulties associated with IV administration. Renal vasodilatory effects of certain prostaglandins have given some positive protective results on renal function in patients with preexisting renal impairment. There has been continued interest in the use of adenosine antagonists (theophylline, aminophylline) as a potential prophylaxis agent for contrast nephropathy, but their use has shown controversial results. Studies by Huber et al. and Erley et al. observed beneficial effects against AKI, while others such as Shammas et al. and Abizaid et al. denied any positive results. Larger clinical trials are needed on these medications, and currently no consensus has been reached regarding regimens involving these medications for the prevention of ARs to CM.

NEPHROGENIC SYSTEMIC FIBROSIS

Nephrogenic systemic fibrosis (NSF) is seen in patients with acute kidney failure or advanced CKD, most commonly following exposure to GBCMs. NSF is a progressive debilitating disease with no definite cure and may be fulminant in about 5% of cases, sometimes leading to patient death. NSF affects males and females in approximately equal numbers and most often affects middle-aged individuals. NSF typically occurs 16 days after GBCM administration and is a clinicopathologic diagnosis because there are no specific imaging findings. Clinical findings are classified into major and minor criteria (Box 20.7).

BOX 20.7 Clinical Criteria for Nephrogenic Systemic Fibrosis

MAJOR CRITERIA

- Patterned plaques: red to violaceous thin, fixed skin plaques showing polygonal, reticular, or amoeboid morphologies.
- Joint contractures.
- Cobblestoning of the skin.
- Marked induration/peau d'orange: unpinchable, firm, bound-down skin over the extremities. Peau d'orange refers to follicular dimpling. Must be present in the upper extremity or in the lower extremity above the knee.

MINOR CRITERIA

- Puckering/linear banding.
- Superficial plaque/patch: thin, irregularly bordered hypopigmented, pink, or flesh-colored macules coalescing into patches or thin plaques. Common on the upper extremities and unusual on the trunk.
- Dermal papules: slightly brawny papules without epidermal changes.
- Scleral plaques: new-onset white/yellow scleral plaques with dilated capillary loops in a patient <45 years.

As understood from literature, the incidence of NSF greatly depends on the residual renal function and the type and dose of the GBCM. The ACR and ESUR have released guidelines for identifying at-risk patients (Table 20.10). ACR risk assessment is based on whether the patient is an inpatient or outpatient, whereas ESUR risk assessment is based on the type of GBCM used. Both guidelines focus on the group of GBCMs with the highest risk of causing NSF, the use of which the FDA has contraindicated for patients with AKI or severe CKD. GBCMs with the highest risk of causing NSF include gadopentetate dimeglumine, gadodiamide, and gadoversetamide. Most reported NSF cases have been associated with GBCMs from this group, with gadodiamide being the most common. In patients with reduced renal function, the prevalence of NSF after use of gadodiamide is significantly higher than any other GBCM (3%–7% vs. 0%–1% per injection). For all other GBCMs, the ESUR recommends using them with caution in patients with stage 4 or stage 5 CKD. Despite some differences between the ACR and ESUR, these guidelines agree that all patients at risk for acute respiratory distress (ARD) or chronic renal disease (CRD) should be identified and that evaluation of renal function be required before the administration of a GBCM.

Once at-risk patients are identified, the principles for minimizing ARs that were discussed at the beginning of this chapter can be implemented to prevent or minimize occurrence. This includes considering alternative imaging modalities, selecting the most suitable CM, and using the lowest possible CM dose to obtain diagnostic information. There is no definite cure for NSF, despite sparse studies demonstrating partial response to several therapies such as thalidomide, plasmapheresis, and extracorporeal photopheresis. The most effective strategy observed from literature is the restoration of renal function, which appears to halt or slow the progression of NSF. Symptom reductions or cures have also been reported after successful renal transplantation. In general, the incidence of NSF has decreased following adherence and implementation of the guidelines on restrictive use of GBCMs. Thus, increasing clinician awareness and encouraging adherence to the updated guidelines are important to minimize or prevent the occurrence of new cases.

CONTRAST EXTRAVASATION

Contrast extravasation (CE) occurs when CM infiltrates the interstitial tissue during injection; it is usually reported with an incidence of less than 1%. For CT scans, the reported extravasation rates range from 0.14% to 0.9% and average 0.43%. Incidence rates of extravasation for MRI have been reported to range from 0.06% to 0.9% and are considered less common than CT due to the lower volumes of CM given and the higher frequency of manual injections. GBCMs are also less toxic to the skin and surrounding tissues than are equal volumes of ICM, and the small volumes typically injected for MR studies limit the chances for serious complications (e.g., compartment syndrome). Patients who develop CE are usually asymptomatic and heal spontaneously within 2 to 4 days. However, some may report a variety of inflammatory signs and symptoms at the injection site. The clinical presentation of CE ranges from minor swelling and redness to tissue death associated with progressive edema and skin ulceration. A number of clinical findings such as paresthesia, skin blistering, and persistent or increasing pain after 4 hours suggest severe injury, and a surgeon's opinion is warranted. Rarely, a few cases result in serious complications that can lead to tissue damage or pressure effects, such as compartment syndrome, which may require emergency fasciotomy to prevent neurovascular compromise. Damage due to direct toxicity from CM can continue for months and involve nerves, tendons, and joints. This can lead to longer hospital stays and increased morbidity and costs, with risk of surgical procedures needed to treat some complications.

Certain factors should be considered to assess the risk for CE, and in the case of extravasation, proper treatment and follow-up communication are necessary to avoid unfortunate consequences. Patient history should focus on risk factors that may indicate a contraindication to CM use or an increased likelihood of CM extravasation. For example, patients with altered circulations (e.g., insufficient venous drainage) increase their risk of extravasation and are less able to tolerate the complications. One study published by Shaqdan et al. found that the elderly (>60 years), females, and inpatients are at the highest risk of extravasation after contrast-enhanced studies in both CT and MRI. For MRI, power injections also increase patient risk for developing extravasation. The risk of CE also depends on various mechanical and pharmacologic factors (Box 20.8). For example, hypertonic GBCM such as gadopentetate dimeglumine are more likely to cause symptomatic extravasation than nonionic GBCM. Also, injections in the lower limb and small distal veins are more likely to result in an extravasation and are less ideal than the antecubital fossa. When more peripheral (e.g., hand or wrist) venipuncture sites are used, a flow rate of no greater than 1.5 mL/second may be more appropriate.

Communication with the patient before, during, and after the CM injection is essential to monitor for an extravasation. Directly palpating the catheter venipuncture site during the initial seconds of injection and asking the patient to report any unusual sensations at the injection site are effective methods of identifying CE. If no problem

TABLE 20.10 Guidelines for the Use of Gadolinium-Based Contrast Media in At-Risk Patients Regarding Nephrogenic Systemic Fibrosis

	ESUR	ACR
ADULTS		
Patients with end-stage renal disease on chronic dialysis	Contraindicated	Contraindicated
Patients with CKD 4 or 5 (eGFR <30 mL/min/1.73 m²) not on chronic dialysis	Contraindicated	Contraindicated
Patients with CKD 3 (eGFR 30-59 mL/min/1.73 m²)	Should be used with caution	eGFR 30-39: contraindicated eGFR 40-59: no special precautions required
Patients with CKD 1 or 2 (eGFR 60-119 mL/min/1.73 m²)	Not at risk of NSF: any GBCM can be administered	Not at risk of NSF: any GBCM can be administered
Patients with acute kidney injury	Contraindicated	Contraindicated
Hepatic insufficiency/hepatorenal syndrome	No special recommendation	No special recommendation
Pregnant women	Contraindicated	No special recommendation; however, gadolinium chelates should not be routinely used in pregnant patients
CHILDREN		
Neonates <4 wk	Contraindicated	Term neonates: same as adult
		Preterm neonates and infants with potential GFR <30 mL/min/1.73 m² due to immature renal function (not due to pathologic renal impairment): use with caution
Children 1 mo to 1 y	Should be used with caution	Same as adult
Lactating women	Stop breastfeeding for 24 h and discard the milk	Safe for the mother and infant to continue breastfeeding after receiving such an agent

ACR, American College of Radiology; *CKD*, chronic kidney disease; *ESUR*, European Society for Urological Radiology; *GFR*, glomerular filtration rate; *NSF*, nephrogenic systemic fibrosis.

is encountered during the first 15 seconds, the person monitoring the injection exits the room before the scanning begins. If an extravasation is detected, the injection is stopped immediately. The recommended management for CE involves three steps: initial therapy, surgical consult, and postextravasation management. The most common initial treatment of CE involves elevating the affected extremity above the level of the heart to reduce the swelling and applying cold compresses. Topical application of heat may also promote resorption of CM by causing vasodilation, while topical application of cold packs will suppress inflammation by way of vasoconstriction. Local injections of hyaluronidase have been administered to break down connective tissue and promote absorption of extravasated drugs into the lymphatic and vascular systems. Administration of sulfur sulfadiazine is recommended to prevent

secondary infection whenever blistering is evident. All patients with extravasation should be monitored for a period as long as the responsible physician considers sufficient. Few patients require surgical intervention, but such intervention is indicated if the patient's pain gradually increases over 2 to 4 hours, if skin blistering or ulceration develops, or if the circulation or sensation changes at or distal to the level of the extravasation.

Postextravasation management includes reassuring and providing an explanation to the patient/family. At discharge, the patient should be given home care instructions for the extravasation and should be contacted 24 to 28 hours following the incident by a physician or nurse to check on the status of the extravasation (Fig. 20.6). Home care instructions should include how and when to apply warm and cold compresses to help alleviate symptoms of pain or swelling. The instructions should also remind the patient to seek immediate medical care if symptoms become worse, a skin ulceration appears, or there are any circulatory or neurologic symptoms.

MISCELLANEOUS CONSIDERATIONS

Pregnancy

In general, intravascular CM should be avoided in pregnancy to prevent or minimize possible hazard to the fetus. In vitro experiments have demonstrated the mutagenic effects of ICM on human cells, but reassuringly, in vivo teratogenic effects were not seen in animal studies. Studies on the occurrence of neonatal hypothyroidism due to the iodine content of CM have shown conflicting results. Some studies have shown that intravascular ICM may induce hypothyroidism in the fetus in utero (placental passage) and in neonates, particularly preterm babies. On the other hand, studies performed by Rajaram et al. and Bourjeily et al. showed no adverse effects on the neonatal thyroid function in mothers who received ICM. In terms of intravascular nonionic CM, there have been no reports of adverse effects on neonatal thyroid function. Nevertheless,

---

BOX 20.8 Risk Factors for Contrast Extravasation

MECHANICAL FACTORS

- Small size and poor condition of veins
- Larger catheter size relative to vein size
- Choice of site (e.g., dominant hand)
- Unstable catheter
- Poor securing of implanted port access needle
- Patient activity
- Multiple venipuncture sites
- Use of an infusion pump or power injection
- Catheter port separation or catheter fracture

PHYSIOLOGIC FACTORS

- Clot formation above the cannulation site
- Thrombus or fibrin sheath at the catheter tip
- Lymphedema

PHARMACOLOGIC FACTORS

- pH
- Osmolality
- Vasoconstrictive potential
- Cytotoxicity

HOME CARE INSTRUCTIONS FOR EXTRAVASATION OF IV CONTRAST

Today on_____(date) during your radiology exam, some of the intravenous contrast that was injected into the vein in your arm leaked into the tissues surrounding the vein instead of staying in the vein. This is called an extravasation. Sometimes the extravasation of IV contrast produces swelling and bruising of the skin, accompanied by minor discomfort.

Warm compresses were applied immediately following the extravasation. When you get home you should apply cold compresses on the extravastion site, on and off for the next four hours. This will decrease the swelling and minimize any pain that you are experiencing.

On occasion, the extravasation is in an area where it may put pressure on the veins and or nerves in your arm or hand. If this happens, swelling of your hand and or numbness of your fingers may occur. Blistering of the skin or increasing pain after the initial 4 hours may sometimes occur. These are symptoms which should be evaluated by a doctor. Therefore, if you experience swelling, skin blistering or increasing pain, please contact your referring physician and follow his or her instructions. If you are unable to reach your physician, please call the Massachusetts General Hospital, Department of Emergency Radiology at 617 -726 -3050 and ask to speak with the radiologist on duty or go to the nearest emergency room and bring this information sheet with you.

We will contact you 24-48 hours following this incident to check on the status of your extravasation. If you prefer to contact us, please call us at the number below:

(xxx)- _____ and ask for _____ between the hours of 8:00am and 5:00pm.

Patient's Name _____

Medical Record Number _____

Date_____

FIG. 20.6 Sample document used at Massachusetts General Hospital to provide home care instructions for patients in whom contrast extravasation occurred. *IV*, Intravenous.

screening for hypothyroidism in neonates is part of standard practice and is particularly important in the infants of mothers who received ICM during pregnancy. Therefore, CT contrast should be administered as usual to avoid the risk of repeating a study if the initial exam was nondiagnostic due to lack of IV contrast.

In contrast with ICM, IV GBCM has shown to be teratogenic in animal studies (albeit at high and repeated doses). Even though teratogenic effects in pregnant patients were not observed in a small number of human studies, the recommendation is to avoid GBCM in pregnancy (particularly during organogenesis) unless there is an absolutely essential clinical indication. Gd is classified as a category C drug by the FDA and can be used "if the potential benefit justifies the potential risk to the fetus." Additionally, the prevalence of NSF and Gd brain deposits raises theoretical concerns of toxicity related to disassociation and persistence of free Gd. Such concerns emphasize the regulatory advice on Gd use in pregnancy. If GBCM will be administered, the risks and benefits must be discussed with the patient and referring physician.

Lactating Patients

Imaging studies requiring ICM or GBCM are occasionally required in patients who are breast feeding. Both the patient and referring physician may have concerns regarding potential toxicity to the infant from CM that is excreted into the breast milk. Actually, studies have shown that less than 0.01% of the CM administered to the mother is absorbed from the gastrointestinal tract of the breastfed infant. Based on a comprehensive literature review, the ACR and ESUR conclude that the very small risk associated with absorption of CM is not enough to necessitate cessation of breast feeding 24 hours following ICM or GBCM. Therefore, interruption of breast feeding after administration of ICM or GBCM is not warranted or recommended.

Metformin

Metformin is an oral hypoglycemic agent for patients with non–insulin-dependent diabetes mellitus and is typically excreted in the kidneys by glomerular filtration and excretion. The most significant side effect is the potential of metformin-associated lactic acidosis in certain patients. Frequently, lactic acidosis occurs because of other existing comorbidities such as renal or cardiovascular disease. Conditions that decrease metformin excretion or affect the metabolism of lactate acid or increase production of lactic acid blood lactate levels are also important risk factors. Therefore, patients on metformin who are at great risk of CIN have an increased tendency to develop lactic acidosis. Steps that can be taken to reduce the risk of CIN include discontinuing metformin approximately 48 hours before any contrast study, adequate hydration before the procedure, and limiting the amount of CM used. Patients with an estimated GFR less than 45 mL/minute should stop their metformin at the time of contrast injection and should not restart for at least 48 hours. Metformin should only be restarted if the patient's renal function remains stable (<25% increase compared with baseline creatinine).

TABLE 20.11 Iodine Load in Radiographic Studies Using Iodinated Contrast Media

Radiographic Study	Usual Volume of Contrast Agent	Total Iodine Load (g)
PCI	200 mL of 300–350 mgI/mL	60.0–70.0
Coronary angiography	100 mL of 300–350 mgI/mL	30.0–35.0
Coronary angiography + PCI	250 mL of 300–350 mgI/mL	75.0–87.5
CT: brain parenchyma	80 mL of 300 mgI/mL	24.0
Brain perfusion	50 mL of 350 mgI/mL	17.5
Neck and brain	100 mL of 350 mgI/mL	35.0
Liver/routine abdomen	100 mL of 350 mgI/mL	35.0
Routine chest	70 mL of 300–350 mgI/mL	21.0–35.0
CTA: peripheral runoff	125–140 mL of 350 mgI/mL	43.8–49.0
ERCP	25–50 mL of 300 mgI/mL	7.5–15.0

CT, Computed tomography; *CTA,* CT angiography; *ERCP,* endoscopic retrograde cholangiopancreatogram; *PCI,* percutaneous coronary intervention.

TABLE 20.12 Tolerable Upper Limits of Iodine (µG/Day)

Age Group	US Institute of Medicine	Scientific Committee on Food (European Commission)
1–3 y	200	200
4–6 y	300	250
7–10 y	300	300
11–14 y	300	450
15–17 y	900	500
Adults	1100	600
Pregnancy	1100	600

Thyroid Disease

Sudden exposure to high levels of iodide in patients receiving ICM can cause thyroid dysfunction (hyperthyroidism and/or hypothyroidism), particularly in susceptible patients. The link between exposure to ICM and new thyroid dysfunction is more common than was previously anticipated, with a prevalence of 0.05%–5%. If unrecognized and untreated, contrast-induced thyroid dysfunction (CITD) may result in life-threatening consequences. The usual iodine load in contrast-enhanced studies along with tolerable levels of iodine exposure can be seen in Tables 20.11 and 20.12. Determining who will be susceptible to thyroid dysfunction following ICM administration depends on the patient history and physical examination. CITD is more commonly seen in patients with preexisting thyroid disease. Risk factors include a patient or family history of thyroid dysfunction and nontoxic diffuse or multinodular goiters with thyroid autonomy, particularly among the elderly (≥65 years old) and inhabitants of iodine-deficient areas. Individuals with a history of partial thyroidectomy are particularly at risk of developing iodine-induced hypothyroidism. A study has also demonstrated the possibility of transient subclinical hypothyroidism in euthyroid patients receiving CM for coronary angiography or CT (iodine dose range of 300–1221 mg of iodine per kilogram). Clinically, CITD may be subclinical

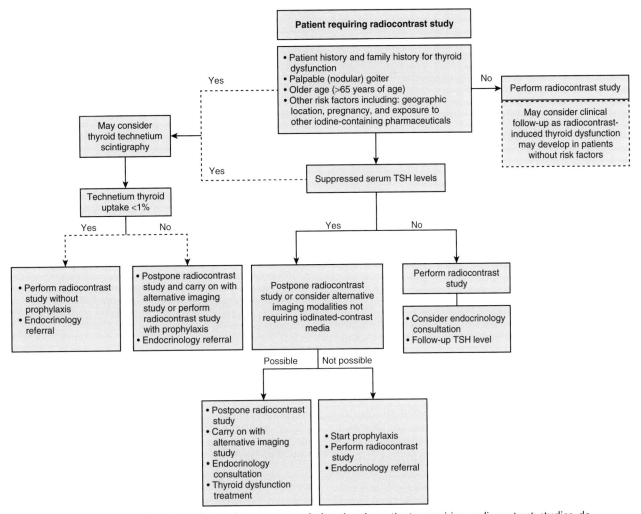

FIG. 20.7 Process for determining the recommended action in patients requiring radiocontrast studies depending on their thyroid status. *TSH*, Thyroid-stimulating hormone. (From Hudzik B, Zubelewicz-Szkodzinska B. Radiocontrast-induced thyroid dysfunction: is it common and what should we do about it? *Clin Endocrinol.* 2014;80:322–327.)

or overt and can occur up to 12 weeks after ICM administration. The decision to undergo radiocontrast studies depends on the patient's health status (Fig. 20.7). At-risk patients and individuals who are unable to endure thyroid dysfunction, notably those with cardiovascular disease, should be monitored closely by endocrinologists after ICM administration. Regimens that have been suggested to prevent iodine-induced hyperthyroidism include pretreatment with short-term thiamazole and/or perchlorate to decrease the risk of incident thyrotoxicosis (Box 20.9). Prophylaxis is not required in patients without any underlying thyroid disease and is only recommended in high-risk patients. Special consideration should be given for the use of IV contrast in patients who are anticipating treatment with radioactive iodine (I-131). Such patients should not receive ICM 4–6 weeks before radioiodine treatment, because the iodine load in the contrast bolus may render the treatment ineffective.

Children

Estimating the incidence of ARs to IV CM in children is difficult. This is due to the lack of controlled prospective studies and consensus regarding what represents a

---

BOX 20.9 Prophylaxis Regimen for Contrast-Induced Hyperthyroidism

ELECTIVE CONTRAST MEDIA ADMINISTRATION

Sodium perchlorate[a]: 300 mg 3 times daily
Begin the day prior to exam and continue for 8–14 days *and/or*
Thiamazole[b]: 30 mg once daily
Begin the day prior to exam and continue for 14 days

EMERGENT CONTRAST MEDIA ADMINISTRATION

Sodium perchlorate[a]: 800 mg directly prior to exam and continue with 300 mg 3 times daily for 8–14 days *and/or*
Thiamazole[b]: 30 mg once daily
Directly prior to exam and continue for 14 days

---

[a]Because perchlorate is not widely available, using a single antithyroid agent (e.g., thiamazole) remains a viable option, although combination therapy offers a higher level of efficacy.
[b]Pretreatment with short-term administration of thiamazole (inhibition of thyroid hormone synthesis) and/or perchlorate (inhibition of iodine uptake) has been proposed to decrease the risk of incident thyrotoxicosis.

true allergic reaction. A study by Dillman et al. showed a frequency of acute allergic-like reactions of 0.18% after administration of ICM in children. Another study by Callahan et al. showed an overall acute AR rate of

0.46% (physiologic and allergic-like). Guidelines for prevention and treatment of ARs in children are similar to those for adults (see Table 20.6). There has been no large prospective investigation of the possible nephrotoxic effects of CM in children. CIN may occur in children, but if so, it is rare. Few cases of NSF have been reported in children with severe renal dysfunction. Due to the renal immaturity and lower GFRs in pediatric patients, it is recommended that GBCM be used only when necessary.

Enteric Contrast Media

Barium sulfate is the ideal CM for opacification of the gastrointestinal tract and rarely results in ARs. When adverse allergic-like and physiologic reactions do occur, almost all are mild in severity and usually require no treatment. Moderate-to-severe allergic-like reactions occur more in patients with prior reactions to IV CM and in those with active inflammatory bowel disease because of impaired mucosal protection against CM absorption. Approximately 1% to 2% of ingested CM is normally absorbed, but the absorption is increased in patients with mucosal infection or inflammation. Theoretically, the small volumes of absorbed CM can cause dose-independent anaphylactoid reactions. One of the most worrisome complications is the leaking of CM into the mediastinal or peritoneal cavity. Leakage of CM into these cavities can cause mediastinitis or peritonitis; therefore, barium CM are contraindicated when bowel perforation is suspected. Instead, iodinated water-soluble CM (WSCM) can be given in patients suspected of having bowel perforation. WSCM can also be used before expected surgical or endoscopic procedures and to confirm the position of percutaneous feeding tubes. Aspiration of CM can lead to serious complications such as acute respiratory distress from high volumes of barium and severe pulmonary edema from high-osmolar WSCM. Therefore, IOCM or LOCM should be used in patients at risk of aspiration.

GUIDELINES FOR CONTRAST WARMING

Although studies have shown warming of CM alters the bolus kinetics and injection pressure of ICM, evidence that it affects AR rates in a meaningful way is not substantial. A study by Vergara and Seguel that included both adult and pediatric patients showed fewer ARs following injection of warmed CM when compared to CM administered at room temperature. In another study including both children and adults, both iopamidol-300 and iopamidol-370 were warmed to body temperature before being administered. The study by Davenport et al. showed that warming of iopamidol-300 had no effect, but warming of iopamidol-370 reduced the extravasation rate. This may suggest that lower-viscosity agents benefit less from warming than higher-viscosity agents. Because CM are designated as medications, the warming of CM is under regulation of the Joint Commission. The Joint Commission mandates that if CM are to be extrinsically warmed, there must be daily temperature recording for each warmer and proof of routine maintenance for the warming device(s). Recommended storage temperatures are included in the package inserts that come with the ICM product. According to the ACR, extrinsic warming of ICM to human body

---

BOX 20.10 Guidelines for Contrast Media Warming

Extrinsic warming of iodinated contrast material to human body temperature (37°C) may be helpful in the following circumstances:
- For high-rate (>5 mL/s) IV LOCM power injections
- For injections of viscous iodinated contrast (e.g., iopamidol 370 and presumably other contrast media with a similar or higher viscosity)
- For direct arterial injections through small-caliber catheters (≤5 Fr)
- For intravenously injected arterial studies in which timing and peak enhancement are critical features

Extrinsic warming of iodinated contrast material may not be needed or beneficial in the following circumstances:
- Low-rate (≤5 mL/s) IV LOCM power or hand injections
- Injections of iodinated contrast media with a relatively low viscosity (e.g., iopamidol 300 and presumably other contrast media with a similar or lower viscosity)
- Direct arterial injections through large-bore catheters (≥6 Fr)
- IV injections in which peak opacification and timing are not critical (e.g., routine portal venous phase chest/abdomen/pelvis computed tomography imaging)

IV, Intravenous; *LOCM*, low-osmolar contrast media.

---

temperature (37°C) may help improve vascular opacification and reduce complications in specific circumstances. Guidelines for contrast warming as outlined by the ACR are shown in Box 20.10. According to package inserts for GBCM, no external warming for clinical applications is indicated, and they should be administered at room temperature (15–30°C [59–86°F]).

CONCLUSION

Although CM is considered to be safe in medical imaging, their use may occasionally result in ARs and other complications. Knowledge of, familiarity with, and adequate training in ARs to CM are vital for an appropriate and effective response. Sufficient patient screening and adequate prophylactic measures are important to minimize or avoid such reactions from occurring in the first place. A basic understanding of ICM and GBCM, the risks of their administration, and premedication regimens for high-risk patients are useful in preparing patients for their contrast-enhanced imaging examinations. Additionally, immediate recognition and adherence to treatment guidelines are essential for adequate management of patients. Radiologists and their staff members are strongly recommended to review all the treatment algorithms frequently so they may carry out their roles efficiently and properly and seek clinical assistance when needed. We hope that this chapter has given the reader an understanding of the important aspects of screening, recognizing, and managing the risks central to IV-administered CM.

SUGGESTED READINGS

Abizaid AS, Clark CE, Mintz GS, et al. Effects of dopamine and aminophylline on contrast-induced acute renal failure after coronary angioplasty in patients with preexisting renal insufficiency. *Am J Cardiol*. 1999;83(2):260–263.

Abujudeh HH, Rolls H, Kaewlai R, et al. Retrospective assessment of prevalence of nephrogenic systemic fibrosis (NSF) after implementation of a new guideline for the use of gadobenate dimeglumine as a sole contrast agent for magnetic resonance examination in renally impaired patients. *J Magn Reson Imaging*. 2009;30:1335–1340.

Almén T. The etiology of contrast medium reactions. *Invest Radiol.* 1994;29(suppl 1): S37–S45.

American College of Radiology. ACR Manual on Contrast Media v10.1. <http://www.acr.org/quality-safety/resources/contrast-manual>.

American College of Radiology. ACR Manual on Contrast Media v10.1. <http://www.acr.org/quality-safety/resources/contrast-manual>.

Andreucci M, Solomon R, Tasanarong A. Side effects of radiographic contrast media: pathogenesis, risk factors, and prevention. *Biomed Res Int.* 2014;2014:741018.

Aspelin P, Aubry P, Fransson S-G, et al. Nephrotoxic effects in high-risk patients undergoing angiography. *N Engl J Med.* 2003;348:491–499.

Atwell TD, Lteif AN, Brown DL, McCann M, Townsend JE, Leroy AJ. Neonatal thyroid function after administration of IV iodinated contrast agent to 21 pregnant patients. *AJR Am J Roentgenol.* 2008;191(1):268–271.

Bae KT. Intravenous contrast medium administration and scan timing at CT: considerations and approaches. *Radiology.* 2010;256(1):32–61.

Baker ME, Beam C, Leder R, Gulliver D, Paine SS, Dunnick NR. Contrast material for combined abdominal and pelvic CT: can cost be reduced by increasing the concentration and decreasing the volume? *AJR Am J Roentgenol.* 1993;160(3): 637–641.

Barrett BJ, Parfrey PS, Vavasour HM, et al. A comparison of nonionic, low-osmolality radiocontrast agents with ionic, high-osmolality agents during cardiac catheterization. *N Engl J Med.* 1992;326(7):431–436.

Bartlett MJ, Bynevelt M. Acute contrast reaction management by radiologists: a local audit study. *Australas Radiol.* 2003;47(4):363–367.

Bellin MF, Stacul F, Webb JA, et al. Late adverse reactions to intravascular iodine based contrast media: an update. *Eur Radiol.* 2011;21(11):2305–2310.

Bona G, Zaffaroni M, Defilippi C, Gallina MR, Mostert M. Effects of iopamidol on neonatal thyroid function. *Eur J Radiol.* 1992;12:22–25.

Bottinor W, Polkampally P, Jovin I. Adverse reactions to iodinated contrast media. *Int J Angiol.* 2013;22:149–154.

Bourjeily G, Chalhoub M, Phornphutkul C, Alleyne T, Woodfield C, Chen K. Neonatal thyroid function: effect of a single exposure to iodinated contrast medium in utero. *Radiology.* 2010;256:744–750.

Brockow K, Christiansen C, Kanny G, et al. Management of hypersensitivity reactions to iodinated contrast media. *Allergy.* 2005;60(2):150–158.

Brown JJ, Hynes MR, Wible Jr JH. Measurement of serum calcium concentration after administration of four gadolinium-based contrast agents to human volunteers. *AJR Am J Roentgenol.* 2007;189:1539–1544.

Bruce RJ, Djamali A, Shinki K, Michel SJ, Fine JP, Pozniak MA. Background fluctuation of kidney function versus contrast-induced nephrotoxicity. *AJR Am J Roentgenol.* 2009;192(3):711–718.

Callahan MJ, Poznauskis L, Zurakowski D, Taylor GA. Nonionic iodinated intravenous contrast material-related reactions: incidence in large urban children's hospital—retrospective analysis of data in 12,494 patients. *Radiology.* 2009;250(3):674–681.

Caro JJ, Trindade E, McGregor M. The risks of death and of severe nonfatal reactions with high- vs low-osmolality contrast media: a meta-analysis. *AJR Am J Roentgenol.* 1991;156:825–832.

Chalmers N, Jackson RW. Comparison of iodixanol and iohexol in renal impairment. *Br J Radiol.* 1999;72:701–703.

Chamsuddin AA, Kowalik KJ, Bjarnason H, et al. Using a dopamine type 1A receptor agonist in high-risk patients to ameliorate contrast-associated nephropathy. *Am J Roentgenol.* 2002;179(3):591–596.

Chatham WW. Glucocorticoid effects on the immune system. <http://www.uptodate.com/contents/glucocorticoid-effects-on-the-immune-system>.

Christiansen C. Hypersensitivity reactions to iodinated contrast media: an update. In: Pichler WJ, ed. *Drug Hypersensitivity.* Basel, Switzerland: Karger; 2007:233–241.

Cochran ST, Bomyea K, Sayre JW. Trends in adverse events after IV administration of contrast media. *AJR Am J Roentgenol.* 2001;176:1385–1388.

Cohan RH, Ellis JH. Iodinated contrast material in uroradiology. Choice of agent and management of complications. *Urol Clin North Am.* 1997;24:471–491.

Cowper SE. Nephrogenic systemic fibrosis: an overview. *J Am Coll Radiol.* 2008;5:23–28.

CT Market Outlook Report. <http://www.imvinfo.com/index.aspx?sec=ct&sub=def>.

Daftari besheli LD, Aran S, Shaqdan K, Kay J, Abujudeh H. Current status of nephrogenic systemic fibrosis. *Clin Radiol.* 2014;69:661–668.

Davenport MS, Cohan RH, Caoili EM, Ellis JH. Repeat contrast medium reactions in premedicated patients: frequency and severity. *Radiology.* 2009;253(2):372–379.

Davenport MS, Wang CL, Bashir MR, Neville AM, Paulson EK. Rate of contrast media extravasations and allergic-like reactions: effect of extrinsic warming of low-osmolality iodinated CT contrast media to 37°C. *Radiology.* 2012;262: 475–484.

Dillman JR, Ellis JH, Cohan RH, Strouse PJ, Jan SC. Frequency and severity of acute allergic-like reactions to gadolinium-containing I.V. contrast media in children and adults. *Am J Roentgenol.* 2007;189:1533–1538.

Dillman JR, Strouse PJ, Ellis JH, Cohan RH, Jan SC. Incidence and severity of acute allergic-like reactions to I.V. nonionic iodinated contrast material in children. *AJR Am J Roentgenol.* 2007;188:1643–1647.

Eisenberg RL, Hedgcock MW, Shanser JD, Brenner RJ, Gedgaudas RK, Marks WM. Iodine absorption from the gastrointestinal tract during hypaque-enema examination. *Radiology.* 1979;133(3 Pt 1):597–599.

Erley CM, Duda SH, Rehfuss D, et al. Prevention of radiocontrast-media-induced nephropathy in patients with pre-existing renal insufficiency by hydration in combination with the adenosine antagonist theophylline. *Nephrol Dialysis Transplant.* 1999;14(5):1146–1149.

European Medicines Agency. Assessment report for gadolinium-containing contrast agents. In: Proced. No. EMEA/H/A-31/1097. <http://www.ema.europa.eu/docs/en_GB/document_library/Referrals_document/gadolinium_31/WC500099538.pdf>.

European Society of Urogenital Radiology. ESUR Guidelines on Contrast Media. <http://www.esur.org/guidelines>.

European Society of Urogenital Radiology. ESUR Guidelines on Contrast Media. European Society of Urogenital Radiology. <http://www.esur.org/guidelines/>.

Finn WF. The clinical and renal consequences of contrast-induced nephropathy. *Nephrol Dial Transplant.* 2006;21(6):i2–i10.

Gare M, Haviv YS, Ben-Yehuda A, et al. The renal effect of low-dose dopamine in high-risk patients undergoing coronary angiography. *J Am Coll Cardiol.* 1999;34(6):1682–1688.

Gartner W, Weissel M. Do iodine-containing contrast media induce clinically relevant changes in thyroid function parameters of euthyroid patients within the first week? *Thyroid.* 2004;14(7):521–524.

Gelfand DW, Sowers JC, DePonte KA, Sumner TE, Ott DJ. Anaphylactic and allergic reactions during double-contrast studies: is glucagon or barium suspension the allergen? *AJR Am J Roentgenol.* 1985;144(2):405–406.

Gilgen-Anner Y, Heim M, Ledermann H-P, Bircher AJ. Iodide mumps after contrast media imaging: a rare adverse effect to iodine. *Ann Allergy Asthma Immunol.* 2007;99:93–98.

Gomi T, Nagamoto M, Hasegawa M, et al. Are there any differences in acute adverse reactions among five low-osmolar non-ionic iodinated contrast media? *Eur Radiol.* 2010;20(7):1631–1635.

Gonzales DA, Norsworthy KJ, Kern SJ, et al. A meta-analysis of N-acetylcysteine in contrast-induced nephrotoxicity: unsupervised clustering to resolve heterogeneity. *BMC Med.* 2007;5:32.

Greenberger P, Patterson R, Kelly J, Stevenson DD, Simon D, Lieberman P. Administration of radiographic contrast media in high-risk patients. *Invest Radiol.* 1980;15(suppl 6):S40–S43.

Gupta RK, Bang TJ. Prevention of contrast-induced nephropathy (CIN) in interventional radiology practice. *Semin Intervent Radiol.* 2010;27:348–359.

Gussenhoven MJ, Ravensbergen J, van Bockel JH, Feuth JD, Aarts JC. Renal dysfunction after angiography: a risk factor analysis in patients with peripheral vascular disease. *J Cardiovasc Surg.* 1991;32:81–86.

Hans SS, Hans BA, Dhillon R, Dmuchowski C, Glover J. Effect of dopamine on renal function after arteriography in patients with pre-existing renal insufficiency. *Am Surg.* 1998;64(5):432–436.

Hardiek K, Katholi RE, Ogden C, Pianfetti L. Double blind, randomized, comparison of iopamidol 370 and iodixanol 320: renal response in diabetic subjects. In: *Radiological Society of North America Scientific Assembly and Annual Meeting Program.* Oak Brook, IL: Radiological Society of North America; 2003:541.

Huber W, Ilgmann K, Page M, et al. Effect of theophylline on contrast material-induced nephropathy in patients with chronic renal insufficiency: controlled, randomized, double-blinded study. *Radiology.* 223(3):772–779.

Hudzik B, Zubelewicz-Szkodzinska B. Radiocontrast-induced thyroid dysfunction: is it common and what should we do about it? *Clin Endocrinol.* 2014;80:322–327.

Hunt CH, Hartman RP, Hesley GK. Frequency and severity of adverse effects of iodinated and gadolinium contrast materials: retrospective review of 456,930 doses. *AJR Am J Roentgenol.* 2009;193:1124–1127.

Idée JM, Pinès E, Prigent P, Corot C. Allergy-like reactions to iodinated contrast agents: a critical analysis. *Fundam Clin Pharmacol.* 2005;19(3):263–281.

Jo SH, Youn TJ, Park JS, et al. Iodixanol is less nephrotoxic than ioxaglate in patients with renal insufficiency after coronary angiography. *J Am Coll Cardiol.* 2005;45(suppl A):32A.

Jung JW, Kang HR, Kim MH, et al. Immediate hypersensitivity reaction to gadolinium-based MR contrast media. *Radiology.* 2012;264:414–422.

Junior JE, Santos AC, Santos M, Barbosa MH, Muglia VF. Complications from the use of intravenous gadolinium-based contrast agents for magnetic resonance imaging. *Radiol Bras.* 2008;41(4):263–267.

Kanal E, Barkovich AJ, Bell C, et al. ACR guidance document for safe MR practices: 2007. *AJR Am J Roentgenol.* 2007;188:1447–1474.

Kanal E, Tweedle MF. Residual or retained gadolinium: practical implications for radiologists and our patients. *Radiology.* 2015;275:630–634.

Kanda T, Fukusato T, Matsuda M, et al. Gadolinium-based contrast agent accumulates in the brain even in subjects without severe renal dysfunction: evaluation of autopsy brain specimens with inductively coupled plasma mass spectroscopy. *Radiology.* 2015;276(1):228–232.

Katayama H, Yamaguchi K, Kozuka T, Takashima T, Seez P, Matsuura K. Adverse reactions to ionic and nonionic contrast media: a report from the Japanese Committee on the Safety of Contrast Media. *Radiology.* 1990;175(3):621–628.

Kelly AM, Dwamena B, Cronin P, Bernstein SJ, Carlos RC. Meta-analysis: effectiveness of drugs for preventing contrast-induced nephropathy. *Ann Intern Med.* 2008;148:284–294.

Koch J, Plum J, Grabensee B, Mödder U. Prostaglandin E1: a new agent for the prevention of renal dysfunction in high risk patients caused by radiocontrast media? *Nephrol Dial Transplant.* 2000;15(1):43–49.

Kopp AF, Mortele KJ, Cho YD, Palkowitsch P, Bettmann MA, Claussen CD. Prevalence of acute reactions to iopromide: postmarketing surveillance study of 74,717 patients. *Acta Radiol.* 2008;49:902–911.

Kwok CS, Pang CL, Yeong JK, Loke YK. Measures used to treat contrast-induced nephropathy: overview of reviews. *Br J Radiol.* 2013;86(1021):20120272.

l'Allemand D, Grüters A, Beyer P, Weber B. Iodine in contrast agents and skin disinfectants is the major cause for hypothyroidism in premature infants during intensive care. *Horm Res.* 1987;28:42–49.

Lameire N, Biesen WV, Hoste E, Vanholder R. The prevention of acute kidney injury: an in-depth narrative review Part 1: volume resuscitation and avoidance of drug-and nephrotoxin-induced AKI. *NDT Plus.* 2008;1:392–402.

Lasser EC, Berry CC, Mishkin MM, Williamson B, Zheutlin N, Silverman JM. Pretreatment with corticosteroids to prevent adverse reactions to nonionic contrast media. *AJR Am J Roentgenol.* 1994;162(3):523–526.

Ledneva E, Karie S, Launay-Vacher V, Janus N, Deray G. Renal safety of gadolinium-based contrast media in patients with chronic renal insufficiency. *Radiology.* 2009;250:618-628.

Li A, Wong CS, Wong MK, Lee CM, Au Yeung MC. Acute adverse reactions to magnetic resonance contrast media: gadolinium chelates. *Br J Radiol.* 2006;79:368-371.

Lightfoot CB, Abraham RJ, Mammen T, Abdolell M, Kapur S, Abraham RJ. Survey of radiologists' knowledge regarding the management of severe contrast material-induced allergic reactions. *Radiology.* 2009;251(3):691-696.

Marcos HB, Semelka RC, Worawattanakul S. Normal placenta: gadolinium-enhanced dynamic MR imaging. *Radiology.* 1997;205:493-496.

Marenzi G, Ferrari C, Marana I, et al. Prevention of contrast nephropathy by furosemide with matched hydration: the MYTHOS (induced diuresis with matched hydration compared to standard hydration for contrast induced nephropathy prevention) trial. *JACC: Cardiovasc Intervent.* 2012;5(1):90-97.

Marenzi G, Assanelli E, Marana I. N-acetylcysteine and contrast-induced nephropathy in primary angioplasty. *N Engl J Med.* 2006;354:2773-2782.

McClennan BL. Ionic and nonionic iodinated contrast media: evolution and strategies for use. *AJR Am J Roentgenol.* 1990;155(2):225-233.

McCullough PA. Contrast induced acute kidney injury. *J Am Coll Cardiol.* 2008;51(15):1419-1428.

Mehran R, Aymong ED, Nikolsky E, et al. A simple risk score for prediction of contrast-induced nephropathy after percutaneous coronary intervention. *J Am Coll Cardiol.* 2004;44(7):1393-1399.

Miller SH. Anaphylactoid reaction after oral administration of diatrizoate meglumine and diatrizoate sodium solution. *AJR Am J Roentgenol.* 1997;168(4):959-961.

Moore RD, Steinberg EP, Powe NR, et al. Nephrotoxicity of high-osmolality versus low-osmolality contrast media: randomized clinical trial. *Radiology.* 1992;182:649-655.

Morcos SK. Review article: acute serious and fatal reactions to contrast media—our current understanding. *Br J Radiol.* 2005;78(932):686-693.

Morcos SK. Review article: effects of radiographic contrast media on the lung. *Br J Radiol.* 2003;76(905):290-295.

Morisetti A, Tirone P, Luzzani F, de Haen C. Toxicologic safety assessment of iomeprol, a new x-ray contrast agent. *Eur J Radiol.* 1994;18(suppl 1):21-31.

Morélé KJ, Oliva MR, Ondategui S, Ros PR, Silverman SG. Universal use of nonionic iodinated contrast medium for CT: evaluation of safety in a large urban teaching hospital. *AJR Am J Roentgenol.* 2005;184:31-34.

MR Market Outlook Report. <http://www.imvinfo.com/index.aspx?sec=mri&sub=def>.

Mueller C, Buerkle G, Buettner HJ, et al. Prevention of contrast media-associated nephropathy: randomized comparison of 2 hydration regimens in 1620 patients undergoing coronary angioplasty. *Arch Intern Med.* 2002;162(3):329-336.

Murphy KPJ, Szopinski KT, Cohan RH, Mermillod B, Ellis JH. Occurrence of adverse reactions to gadolinium-based contrast material and management of patients at increased risk: a survey of the American Society of Neuroradiology Fellowship Directors. *Acad Radiol.* 1999;6(11):656-664.

Namasivayam S, Kalra MK, Torres WE, Small WC. Adverse reactions to intravenous iodinated contrast media: a primer for radiologists. *Emerg Radiol.* 2006;12(5):210-215.

Nelson JA, Livingston JC, Moon RG. Mutagenic evaluation of radiographic contrast media. *Invest Radiol.* 1982;17:183-185.

Nicola R, Shaqdan KW, Aran S, Mansouri M, Abujudeh HH. Contrast-induced nephropathy: identifying the risks, choosing the right agent, and reviewing effective prevention and management methods. *Curr Probl Diagn Radiol.* 2015;44(6):501-504.

Niell BL, Vartanians VM, Halpern EP. Improving education for the management of contrast reactions: an online didactic model. *J Am Coll Radiol.* 2014;11(2):185-192.

Okuda Y, Sagami F, Tirone P, Morisetti A, Bussi S, Masters RE. Reproductive and developmental toxicity study of gadobenate dimeglumine formulation (E7155)—study of embryo-fetal toxicity in rabbits by intravenous administration. *J Toxicol Sci.* 1999;24(suppl 1):79-87.

Owen RJ, Hiremath S, Myers A, Fraser-Hill M, Barrett BJ. Canadian Association of Radiologists consensus guidelines for the prevention of contrast-induced nephropathy: update 2012. *Can Assoc Radiol J.* 2014;65:96-105.

Panesar M, Yacoub R. What is the role of renal transplantation in a patient with nephrogenic systemic fibrosis? *Semin Dial.* 2011;24:373-374.

Parfrey P. The clinical epidemiology of contrast-induced nephropathy. *Cardiovasc Intervent Radiol.* 2005;28(suppl 2):S3-S11.

Pasternak J, Williamson E. Clinical pharmacology, uses, and adverse reactions of iodinated contrast agents: a primer for the non-radiologist. *Mayo Clin Proc.* 2012;87:390-402.

Pearce EN. Iodine-induced thyroid dysfunction: comment on "association between iodinated contrast media exposure and incident hyperthyroidism and hypothyroidism". *Arch Int Med.* 2012;172:159-161.

Perez-Rodriguez J, Lai S, Ehst BD, Fine DM, Bluemke DA. Nephrogenic systemic fibrosis: incidence, associations, and effect of risk factor assessment—report of 33 cases. *Radiology.* 2009;250(2):371-377.

Prince MR, Erel HE, Lent RW, et al. Gadodiamide administration causes spurious hypocalcemia. *Radiology.* 2003;227:639-646.

Prince MR, Zhang H, Morris M. Incidence of nephrogenic systemic fibrosis at two large medical centers. *Radiology.* 2008;248:807-816.

Rajaram S, Exley C, Fairlie F, Matthews S. Effect of antenatal iodinated contrast agent on neonatal thyroid function. *Br J Radiol.* 2012;85(1015):e238-e242.

Ralston WH, Robbins MS, James P. Reproductive, developmental, and genetic toxicity of ioversol. *Invest Radiol.* 1989;24(suppl 1):16-22.

Rhee CM, Bhan I, Alexander EK, Brunelli SM. Association between iodinated contrast media exposure and incident hyperthyroidism and hypothyroidism. *Arch Int Med.* 2012;172:153-159.

Rodesch F, Camus M, Ermans AM, Dodion J, Delange F. Adverse effects of amniofetography on fetal thyroid function. *Am J Obstet Gynecol.* 1976;126:723-726.

Rudnick MR, Goldfarb S, Wexler L, et al. Nephrotoxicity of ionic and nonionic contrast media in 1196 patients: a randomized trial. The Iohexol Cooperative Study. *Kidney Int.* 1995;47(1):254-261.

Runge VM, Dickey KM, Williams NM, Peng X. Local tissue toxicity in response to extravascular extravasation of magentic resonance contrast media. *Invest Radiol.* 2002;37:393-398.

Rydahl C, Thomsen HS, Marckmann P. High prevalence of nephrogenic systemic fibrosis in chronic renal failure patients exposed to gadodiamide, a gadolinium-containing magnetic resonance contrast agent. *Invest Radiol.* 2008;43:141-144.

Sanyal S, Marckmann P, Scherer S, Abraham JL. Multiorgan gadolinium (Gd) deposition and fibrosis in a patient with nephrogenic systemic fibrosis—an autopsy-based review. *Nephrol Dial Transplant.* 2011;26:3616-3626.

Schild HH, Kuhl CK, Hübner-Steiner U, Böhm I, Speck U. Adverse events after unenhanced and monomeric and dimeric contrast-enhanced CT: a prospective randomized controlled trial. *Radiology.* 2006;240(1):56-64.

Schopp JG, Iyer RS, Wang CL, et al. Allergic reactions to iodinated contrast media: premedication considerations for patients at risk. *Emerg Radiol.* 2013;20(4):299-306.

Schwab SJ, Hlatry Maipieper KS, Davidson CJ, et al. Contrast nephrotoxicity: a randomized controlled trial of a nonionic and an ionic radiographic contrast agent. *N Engl J Med.* 1989;320:149-153.

Shammas NW, Kapalis MJ, Harris M, McKinney D, Coyne EP. Aminophylline does not protect against radiocontrast nephropathy in patients undergoing percutaneous angiographic procedures. *J Invasive Cardiol.* 2001;13(11):738-740.

Shaqdan K, Aran S, Thrall J, Abujudeh H. Incidence of contrast medium extravasation for CT and MRI in a large academic medical centre: a report on 502,391 injections. *Clin Radiol.* 2014;69(12):1264-1272.

Solomon R, Werner C, Mann D, D'Elia J, Silva P. Effects of saline, mannitol, and furosemide to prevent acute decreases in renal function induced by radiocontrast agents. *N Engl J Med.* 1994;331:1416-1420.

Spargias K, Adreanides E, Demerouti E, et al. Iloprost prevents contrast-induced nephropathy in patients with renal dysfunction undergoing coronary angiography or intervention. *Circulation.* 2009;120:1793-1799.

Stone GW, McCullough PA, Tumlin JA, et al. Fenoldopam mesylate for the prevention of contrast-induced nephropathy: a randomized controlled trial. *J Am Med Assoc.* 2003;290(17):2284-2291.

Sun Z, Fu Q, Cao L, Jin W, Cheng L, Li Z. Intravenous N-acetylcysteine for prevention of contrast induced nephropathy: a meta-analysis of randomized, controlled trials. *PLoS One.* 2013;8:e55124.

Taliercio CP, Vlietstra RE, Ilstrup DM, et al. A randomized comparison of the nephrotoxicity of iopamidol and diatrizoate in high risk patients undergoing cardiac angiography. *J Am Coll Cardiol.* 1991;17:384-390.

Tapping CR, Culverwell AD. Are radiologists able to manage serious anaphylactic reactions and cardiopulmonary arrest? *Br J Radiol.* 2009;82(982):793-799.

Tavernaraki A, Skoula A, Benakis S, Exarhos D. Side effects and complications of magnetic resonance contrast media. *Hosp Chron.* 2012;7(4):208-214.

Telischak NA, Yeh BM, Joe BN, Westphalen AC, Poder L, Coakley FV. MRI of adnexal masses in pregnancy. *AJR Am J Roentgenol.* 2008;191(2):364-370.

Tepel M, Aspelin P, Lameire N. Contrast-induced nephropathy: a clinical and evidence-based approach. *Circulation.* 2006;113:1799-1806.

Tepel M, van der Giet M, Schwarzfeld C, Laufer U, Liermann D, Zidek W. Prevention of radiographic-contrast-agent-induced reductions in renal function by acetylcysteine. *N Engl J Med.* 2000;343:180-184.

Thompson JR, Henrich WL. Nephrotoxic agents and their effects. In: Jacobson HR, Striker GE, Klahr S, eds. *The Principles and Practice of Nephrology.* St. Louis, MO: Mosby; 1995:788-796.

Thomsen HS, Bush Jr WH. Adverse effects of contrast media: incidence, prevention and management. *Drug Saf.* 1998;19(4):313-324.

Tubbs RJ, Murphy B, Mainiero MB, et al. High-fidelity medical simulation as an assessment tool for radiology residents' acute contrast reaction management skills. *J Am Coll Radiol.* 2009;6(8):582-587.

Tweedle MF, Kanal E, Muller R. Considerations in the selection of a new gadolinium-based contrast agent. *Appl Radiol.* 2014;43(5 suppl):1-11.

Vergara M, Seguel S. Adverse reactions to contrast media in CT: effects of temperature and ionic property. *Radiology.* 1996;199:363-366.

Wang CL, Cohan RH, Ellis JH, Caoili EM, Wang G, Francis IR. Frequency, outcome, and appropriateness of treatment of nonionic iodinated contrast media reactions. *AJR Am J Roentgenol.* 2008;191(2):409-415.

Warakaulle DR, Anslow P. Differential diagnosis of intracranial lesions with high signal on T1 or low signal on T2-weighted MRI. *Clin Radiol.* 2003;58:922-933.

Webb JA, Thomsen HS, Morcos SK. Members of Contrast Media Safety Committee of European Society of Urogenital Radiology (ESUR). The use of iodinated and gadolinium contrast media during pregnancy and lactation. *Eur Radiol.* 2005;15:1234-1240.

Weinstein JM, Heyman S, Brezis M. Potential deleterious effect of furosemide in radiocontrast nephropathy. *Nephron.* 1992;62:413-415.

Weisbord SD, Palevsky PM. Prevention of contrast-induced nephropathy with volume expansion. *Clin J Am Soc Nephrol.* 2008;3:273-280.

Wertman R, Altun E, Martin DR, et al. Risk of nephrogenic systemic fibrosis: evaluation of gadolinium chelate contrast agents at four American universities. *Radiology.* 2008;248:799-806.

WHO. A guide to detecting and reporting adverse drug reactions. <http://apps.who.int/iris/bitstream/10665/67378/1/WHO_EDM_QSM_2002.2.pdf>.

Widmark JM. Imaging-related medications: a class overview. *Proc (Bayl Univ Med Cent).* 2007;20:408-417.

Chapter 21

Noninterpretive Skills in Ultrasound

Steven Tandberg and Michael R. Williamson

BIOEFFECTS OF ULTRASOUND

The benefit of diagnostic ultrasound as an imaging modality in clinical practice cannot be overstated. Avoiding the radiation of radiography and computed tomography and the restrictive nature of magnetic resonance imaging coupled with the portability of ultrasound machines make ultrasound an attractive diagnostic tool. Although there are no known deleterious effects in humans when used within normal ranges, knowledge of potential bioeffects of ultrasound is important to avoid improper use, especially with newer techniques and equipment. Imaging professionals should have adequate knowledge of the potential bioeffects and methods to reduce risk to the patient, especially fetal and neonatal patients. This chapter reviews the known and theorized bioeffects of ultrasound and presents current guidelines for safe practice.

Ultrasonic waves deposit energy in the tissues with transmission. Tissues also undergo compression and rarefaction under the mechanical force of ultrasound (Fig. 21.1). Whether or not the energy or waves cause deleterious outcomes to the cells depends on the characteristics of the ultrasound beam and time involved. Data have shown increased caspase levels in cells exposed to ultrasound, intimating an activation of an apoptotic pathway, although this has not been confirmed in the human model in the normal diagnostic range of output. The specific bioeffects of diagnostic ultrasound in the animal model have been examined for many years, through direct evaluation as well as applying results from other modalities.

DOSE

Ionizing radiation dosage can be measured and/or inferred and is related to time of exposure, whereas ultrasound dosage is related to indices of pressure and intensity but not associated with time of exposure.

BIOEFFECTS

There are two main bioeffects of ultrasound: thermal effects, resulting in localized tissue heating, and mechanical effects, resulting in tissue distortion and disruption. Another theoretical bioeffect is radiation force, although this is believed to be a minor effect in the output range of diagnostic ultrasound.

Thermal Bioeffects

Sound waves should be viewed as waves with energy. These waves lose amplitude as they pass through tissue by absorption and scatter, which leads to localized tissue heating. This localized increase in heat, if great enough, is presumed to create hydrogen peroxide, a free radical, which can create DNA strand breaks leading to cell death. Mild temperature increases have been shown to accelerate cellular processes without cellular detriment, but moderate increases in temperature can arrest or retard cellular division.

Tissue characteristics play a large role in temperature modulation. In regions of high blood flow, the blood acts as a heat sink and thus temperature increase is attenuated. In regions of poor blood flow, temperature increase is greatest. Due to low perfusion, the globe is particularly sensitive to ultrasound and thus output in ophthalmic ultrasound is limited to 50 mW/cm². Although ophthalmic ultrasound is routinely performed on pediatric and adult patients, ophthalmic ultrasound on a fetus should not be performed unless absolutely necessary.

There are many other modifying factors, including body habitus, perfusion, distance to the transducer, bone, and fluid presence. The first 5 mm of tissue experiences the greatest temperature increase as the sound wave loses energy. This effect is amplified with high-frequency ultrasound, which is common for superficial evaluations.

Different tissues absorb energy at different rates. Soft tissues such as adipose and muscle absorb less heat than bone and cartilage. Bone quickly absorbs energy resulting in heat.

There are many documented effects of temperature increase in fetal animal model studies, including neural tube defects, microphthalmia, cataracts, microcephaly, and functional and behavioral problems. Hyperthermia is also a proven teratogen in animals and is considered teratogenic in humans. None of these congenital abnormalities have been shown to be caused by diagnostic ultrasound.

In the animal model, significant temperature increases of more than 4°C for more than 5 minutes have been shown to cause developmental and congenital abnormalities. This temperature increase is much greater than expected in human diagnostic ultrasound.

There has been no documented adverse effect on an embryo or fetus of an increase of less than 1.5°C in maternal temperature. An increase of 2.5–5.0°C can occur with 1 hour of ultrasound exposure. Effects in nonfetal ultrasound likely require an increase of 18°C for at least 0.1 seconds.

Data from a study on effects of maternal fever on fetal development demonstrate an association of maternal fever exceeding 38.3°C with increased fetal abdominal wall defects. Although maternal fever is a systemic

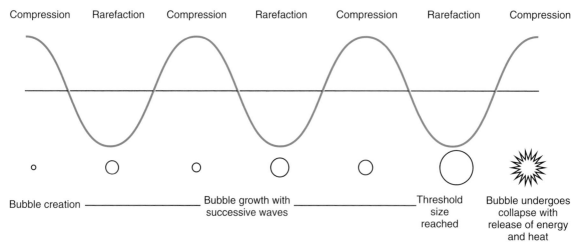

FIG. 21.1 Compression and rarefaction of tissue by ultrasonic waves. (Courtesy Steve Tandberg, MD.)

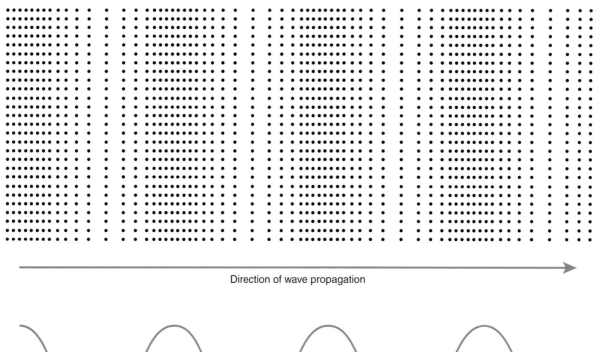

FIG. 21.2 Process of cavitation from bubble formation to collapse due to alternating compression and rarefaction. (Courtesy Steve Tandberg, MD.)

process affecting the entire fetus, it is postulated that an increase in temperature via ultrasound could result in similar effects.

Mechanical

The main mechanical bioeffect of ultrasound is cavitation. This occurs when gas bubbles or voids are trapped in tissue and, under the effects of alternating compression and rarefaction of the acoustic waves of ultrasound, increase in size until the energy reaches a threshold during compression, and the bubble violently collapses resulting in localized release of energy with associated potential for injury (Fig. 21.2). This process can occur where there are preexisting gas bubbles, such as within the lung and bowel. Lung hemorrhage has been observed in the animal model following ultrasound exposure. Cavitation is also the process of creating gas bubbles within tissue, which can then go on to cavitate. Although this is the desired outcome in new ultrasonic fat removal techniques, it is to be avoided in diagnostic ultrasound.

There are two types of mechanical cavitary effects, inertial/transient and noninertial. Inertial/transient effects result in cavitation, whereas noninertial effects result in only oscillation of the formed or preexisting gas bubbles. Noninertial mechanical effects are less likely to produce adverse bioeffects.

Ultrasound waves should be considered as high-pressure shock waves; when these waves produce cavitation, they release energy and heat as the gas bubble collapses. This localized release in energy and heat is believed to result in tissue damage.

Cavitation due to diagnostic ultrasound has not been documented in mammalian fetuses, presumably due to the lack of a gas-fluid interface, although theoretically, sustained high-powered ultrasound in a localized area could create gas bubbles that could subsequently cavitate. It should be noted that current epidemiologic data do not link fetal ultrasound with nonthermal adverse bioeffects. All of the adverse bioeffects in mammalian fetuses have been related to temperature effects.

The other ultrasound-induced mechanical bioeffects are radiation force and acoustic streaming. Radiation force is produced as the acoustic energy of the ultrasonic wave is absorbed along the path of the beam. As the ultrasound transducer produces pulses of ultrasonic waves, a pulsatile force is created. The result of the force can be seen in streaming debris within cysts.

ACOUSTIC OUTPUT AND INDICES

The acoustic output limit from diagnostic ultrasound equipment from 1976 to 1992 was restricted to 720 mW/cm^2 for peripheral vascular, 430 mW/cm^2 for cardiac, 94 mW/cm^2 for fetal and other, and 17 mW/cm^2 for ophthalmic applications. In 1992, the US Food and Drug Administration (FDA), under pressure from manufacturers and clinicians, raised the limit to 720 mW/cm^2 for all applications except ophthalmic (50 mW/cm^2). With the increased limit came a need for imaging professionals to know, in real time, the potential for bioeffects. The FDA developed a regulation known as the Standard for Real-Time Display of Thermal and Mechanical Acoustic Output Indices on Diagnostic Ultrasound Equipment, also known as the output display standard. This standard mandated that the thermal and mechanical indices be displayed on ultrasound equipment capable of outputs up to the FDA limit.

Thermal Index

Currently, the thermal index (TI) is used to measure the potential thermal bioeffects of ultrasound. The thermal index is the ratio of emitted acoustic power to the power required to raise tissue temperature by 1°C. A larger TI indicates a higher heating potential. This index was intended to estimate the magnitude of temperature increase after an exposure to ultrasound. Unfortunately, this is a general index and does not take into account the duration of exam.

There are three display options for the TI:
1. *TIS, soft tissue:* This option assumes that the beam impinges only on soft tissue; consider first trimester ultrasound examinations up to 10 weeks. After 10 weeks, the sonographer should change the machine settings.
2. *TIB, bone:* This option assumes that the beam impinges on bone at or near its focus; consider second and third trimester ultrasound examinations.
3. *TIC, cranial bone:* This option assumes that the beam impinges on bone of the cranium in the neonate, pediatric, or adult patient in transcranial ultrasound.

Mechanical Index

The mechanical index (MI) is meant to be an indicator of the potential for nonthermal bioeffects. The index is calculated as the maximum value of peak negative pressure divided by the square root of the acoustic center frequency. A larger MI indicates a higher potential for nonthermal bioeffects. There is a higher potential for damage above an MI of 0.4, particularly in organs such as the lung or intestines, which have surface gas bubbles.

BIOEFFECTS OF ULTRASOUND MODES

To understand the differing levels of potential bioeffects of the various ultrasound modes, an understanding of the physics of the specific mode is necessary.

B-mode, or brightness modulation or two-dimensional mode, produces a two-dimensional image using a linear array of transducers scanning simultaneously. This is the most commonly used ultrasound noted.

M-mode (motion mode) is not a Doppler-based ultrasound; instead, it is a real-time grayscale mode that uses high-frequency pulses in succession to evaluate movement of focal structures over time, predominantly for fetal cardiac imaging.

Doppler mode ultrasound uses the Doppler effect to visualize and measure flow away from and toward the transducer. Color Doppler overlays color-coded Doppler data on B-mode images. Continuous Doppler displays flow along a single line using a segmented transducer to allow continuous transmission and receipt of the Doppler signal. Pulsed-wave Doppler acquires the Doppler signal from a small volume designated by the sonographer. To localize the Doppler signal, there is a small delay between transmission and receipt of the Doppler signal.

Bioeffects are greatest with pulsed Doppler, followed by power and color Doppler, and finally B-mode and M-mode. Effects are additionally amplified with pulsed-wave Doppler because of sustained scanning in a relatively small focal area.

POWER OUTPUT

An increase in output, leading to higher TI and MI values, does not necessarily produce higher-quality images. Thus, it is prudent to begin exams with lower power output and adjust as needed. As in all of clinical imaging, as low as reasonably achievable (ALARA) techniques should be maintained.

CONTRAST AGENTS

There is now an FDA-approved ultrasound contrast agent, Lumason, for the evaluation of liver lesions. This contrast agent, and the other agents that are not FDA approved, contain gas microbubbles that produce nonlinear echoes in high-perfusion tissues. It is recommended that the MI be maintained under 0.4 if microbubbles are present due to the possible rupture of the gas-containing lipid molecule. If this occurs, energy may potentially be released, resulting in tissue damage.

LITERATURE ON BIOEFFECTS

Many of the prospective studies on ultrasound bioeffects analyzed the effects on animal models, including mice and other small animals. Although these studies revealed certain effects discussed in the following paragraphs, the doses tended to be whole-body doses due to the physical size of the model. In the human model, doses are more focal and superficial, although the fetal/neonatal doses can approach whole-body doses.

In 1989, Tarantal and Hendrickx evaluated the effect of ultrasound on *Macaca fascicularis* fetuses and found that fetuses exposed to ultrasound (5 times per week) demonstrated higher Apgar (appearance, pulse, grimace, activity, and respiration) scores, lower birth weights, and lower white blood cell counts. They found no effect on the rate of abortions, gross malformations, or stillbirths. At 3-month follow-up, there were no differences in weight or white blood cell count between the exposed and nonexposed fetuses.

Moore et al. evaluated 2444 neonates, 1500 of whom were exposed to prenatal ultrasound. They found that those exposed had a statistically significant reduction in birth weight compared to the nonexposed neonates. Further analysis revealed that many of those receiving multiple ultrasound evaluations had preexisting conditions that confounded results.

Lyons et al. compared siblings of the same sex and found no difference in height and weight at delivery or at 6 years between exposed and nonexposed siblings.

Newnham et al. randomized 2834 fetuses into two groups, an *intensive group*, which received five ultrasound exams with continuous-wave Doppler flow studies, and a *regular group*, which received a single ultrasound evaluation. They found a significantly higher rate of intrauterine growth restriction in the *intensive group*.

In a follow-up study, they found no significant differences in physical size, speech, behavior, or neurologic development between the cohorts at 1 or 8 years after the study. The actual acoustic exposure from these studies is not known.

Grether et al. used data from children born in the Kaiser Permanente health care system. Children with autism spectrum disorders were compared to controls based on the number of ultrasound exposures and trimester of exposure. They found no increased risk for autism spectrum disorders in patients exposed to antenatal ultrasound.

Schneider-Kolsky et al. evaluated ultrasound exposure of the fetal chick brain and the effects on learning and memory. They found that significant memory impairment occurred with greater than 3 minutes pulsed Doppler exposure during incubation. They also found no increase in memory impairment with B-mode ultrasound exposure.

CURRENT RECOMMENDATIONS

To reduce the risk of potential bioeffects of diagnostic ultrasound, we advise the following simple recommendations:
- For first trimester ultrasound, the TI should be maintained below 1.0 for no more than 30 minutes. It should be unusual that more than 30 minutes of imaging is required in nearly any clinical setting.
- Due to the theoretical increased risk of mechanical bioeffects, the MI should be maintained below 0.4 when using intravenous contrast agents.

Nelson et al. made the following more detailed recommendations:
- Maintain TI <0.5, especially in the first trimester, unless otherwise required.
- TI between 0.5 and 1.0: limit to under 30 minutes.
- TI >2.5: limit to less than 1 minute.
- Limit MI <0.4 if gas bodies are present (lung, intestines, etc.).
- Use TIS <8 weeks, TIB >8 weeks.
- TI = 0.7: Up to 60 minutes likely safe.
- TI = 1.0: Up to 30 minutes likely safe.
- TI = 1.5: Up to 15 minutes likely safe.
- TI = 2.0: Up to 4 minutes likely safe.
- TI = 3.0: Up to 2.5 minutes likely safe.

Nelson's recommendations for postnatal ultrasound are as follows:
- TI <2.0: no current time limit.
- TI = 2.0–6.0: limit to 15 minutes.
- TI >5: limit to 5 seconds.
- Limit MI <0.4 if gas bodies are present (lung, intestines, etc.).
- If no gas bodies are present: MI ≤1.9, which is the current FDA limit.

The American Institute of Ultrasound Medicine (AIUM) has an official statement on the safe use of Doppler ultrasound during scans between weeks 11 and 14 (or earlier in pregnancy):
1. Pulsed Doppler (spectral, power, and color flow imaging) ultrasound should not be used routinely.
2. Pulsed Doppler ultrasound may be used for clinical indications such as to refine risks for trisomies.
3. When performing Doppler ultrasound, the displayed TI should be 1.0 or less, and exposure time should be kept as short as possible (usually no longer than 5–10 minutes) and should not exceed 60 minutes.
4. When using Doppler ultrasound for research, teaching, and training purposes, the displayed TI should be 1.0 or less and exposure time should be kept as short as possible (usually no longer than 5–10 minutes) and should not exceed 60 minutes. Informed consent should be obtained.
5. In educational settings, discussion of first trimester pulsed or color Doppler should be accompanied by information on safety and bioeffects (e.g., TI, exposure times, and how to reduce the output power).
6. When scanning maternal uterine arteries in the first trimester, there are unlikely to be any fetal safety implications as long as the embryo/fetus lies outside the Doppler ultrasound beam.

INFECTION AND ULTRASOUND EQUIPMENT

For the first 30 years of clinical ultrasound, little attention was paid to the possible role of the transducer as a vector for infection. For perspective, this was also the era of physical exams without emphasis on handwashing between patients and neckties contaminated with bacteria. Many ultrasound transducers were difficult or impossible to clean thoroughly.

In the 1990s, the epidemic of methicillin-resistant *Staphylococcus aureus* as well as concern over hepatitis B, hepatitis C, and human immunodeficiency virus transmission raised awareness of medical instruments as a method of transmission of infection. Papers by Mullaney and Frazee documented colonization of ultrasound transducers by significant pathogens including methicillin-resistant *S. aureus*. In addition, other parts of the machine including keyboards and controls were vulnerable to contamination.

Endocavity transducers have been shown to be possible sources of human papillomavirus, herpes simplex virus, cytomegalovirus, and pathogenic bacteria. There are numerous other organisms that have not been thoroughly studied for contamination and transmission.

The Centers for Disease Control and Prevention (CDC) has issued recommendations for sterilization or disinfection of medical devices. The CDC recommendations are based on the Spaulding Classification, which categorizes infection risk and level of disinfection required.

Critical devices contact the bloodstream and must be sterilized. These may include intraoperative, endovascular, and endobronchial transducers. Critical items confer high risk if they are contaminated with any microorganism.

Semicritical devices may come in contact with nonintact skin or mucous membranes. Other examples are fluids, blood, and other infectious material. Examples of semicritical devices are endovaginal and endorectal transducers. Semicritical devices should be free of all microorganisms, but small numbers of bacterial spores are permissible. High-level disinfection is required.

Noncritical devices may come in contact with intact skin. Most exams on the body surface are in this category. Noncritical devices are disinfected with low-level disinfection. Any cover is removed, the gel is wiped clean or washed with running water, and a damp cloth with mild nonabrasive soap is used to cleanse the probe. A small brush should be used for crevices, and the probe should be rinsed thoroughly. Alternative means of cleaning include wiping with an appropriate chemical agent for low-level disinfection.

The AIUM guidelines for the cleaning, disinfection, and sterilization of ultrasound probes include the following:

All cleaning, disinfection, and sterilization represent a statistical reduction in the number of microbes present on a surface rather than their complete elimination. Meticulous cleaning of the instrument is the key to an initial reduction of the microbial/organic load by at least 99%. This cleaning is followed by a disinfecting procedure to ensure a high degree of protection from infectious disease transmission, even if a disposable barrier covers the instrument during use.

According to the CDC *Guideline for Disinfection and Sterilization in Healthcare Facilities* (2008):

Cleaning is the removal of visible soil (e.g., organic and inorganic material) from objects and surfaces and normally is accomplished manually or mechanically using water with detergents or enzymatic products. Thorough cleaning is essential before high-level disinfection and sterilization because inorganic and organic material that remains on the surfaces of instruments interfere with the effectiveness of these processes. Disinfection describes a process that eliminates many or all pathogenic microorganisms, except bacterial spores.

Low-level disinfection: destruction of most bacteria, some viruses, and some fungi. Low-level disinfection will not necessarily inactivate *Mycobacterium tuberculosis* or bacterial spores.

Mid-level disinfection: inactivation of *M. tuberculosis*, bacteria, most viruses, most fungi, and some bacterial spores.

High-level disinfection: destruction/removal of all microorganisms except bacterial spores.

Sterilization describes a process that destroys or eliminates all forms of microbial life and is carried out in healthcare facilities by physical or chemical methods. Steam under pressure, dry heat, ethylene oxide (EtO) gas, hydrogen peroxide gas plasma, and liquid chemicals are the principal sterilizing agents used in health-care facilities. …When chemicals are used to destroy all forms of microbiologic life, they can be called chemical sterilants. These same germicides used for shorter exposure periods also can be part of the disinfection process (i.e., high-level disinfection).

The following specific recommendations are made for the cleaning and preparation of all ultrasound probes. Users should also review the CDC document on sterilization and disinfection of medical devices to be certain that their procedures conform to the CDC principles for disinfection of patient care equipment.

1. *Cleaning:* Transducers should be cleaned after each examination with soap and water or quaternary ammonium (a low-level disinfectant) sprays or wipes. The probes must be disconnected from the ultrasound scanner for anything more than wiping or spray cleaning. After removal of the probe cover (when applicable), use running water to remove any residual gel or debris from the probe. Use a damp gauze pad or other soft cloth and a small amount of mild nonabrasive liquid soap (household dishwashing liquid is ideal) to thoroughly cleanse the probe. Consider the use of a small brush, especially for crevices and areas of angulation, depending on the design of the particular probe. Rinse the probe thoroughly with running water, and then dry the probe with a soft cloth or paper towel.

2. *Disinfection:* As noted previously, all internal probes (e.g., vaginal, rectal, and transesophageal probes) as well as intraoperative probes require high-level disinfection before they can be used on another patient.

For the protection of the patient and the healthcare worker, all internal examinations should be performed with the operator properly gloved throughout the procedure. As the probe cover is removed, care should be taken not to contaminate the probe with secretions from the patient. At the completion of the procedure, hands should be thoroughly washed with soap and water. Gloves should be used to remove the probe cover and to clean the probe as described above.

Note: An obvious disruption in condom integrity does not require modification of this protocol. Because of the potential disruption of the barrier sheath, high-level disinfection with chemical agents is necessary. The following guidelines take into account possible probe contamination due to a disruption in the barrier sheath.

After removal of the probe cover, clean the transducer as described previously. Cleaning with a detergent/water solution as described earlier is important as the first step in proper disinfection, because chemical disinfectants act more rapidly on clean and dry surfaces. Wet surfaces dilute the disinfectant.

High-level liquid disinfection is required to ensure further statistical reduction in the microbial load. Examples of such high-level disinfectants are listed in Table 21.1. A complete list of FDA-cleared liquid sterilants and high-level disinfectants is available at http://www.fda.gov/MedicalDevices/Safety/AlertsandNotices/ucm194429.htm, and other agents are under investigation.

To achieve high-level disinfection, the practice must meet or exceed the listed "high-level disinfectant contact conditions" specified for each product. Users should be aware that not all approved disinfectants on this list are safe for all ultrasound probes.

The CDC recommends environmental infection control in the case of *Clostridium difficile*, consisting of "meticulous cleaning followed by disinfection using hypochlorite-based germicides as appropriate" (2008). The current introduction and initial marketing of a hydrogen peroxide nanodroplet emulsion might provide an effective high-level disinfectant without toxicity.

The Occupational Safety and Health Administration and the Joint Commission (Environment of Care Standard IC 02.02.01 EP 9) have issued guidelines for exposure to chemical agents, which might be used for ultrasound probe cleaning. Before selecting a high-level disinfectant, users should request the Material Safety Data Sheet for the product and make sure that their facility is able to meet the necessary conditions to minimize exposure (via inhalation, ingestion, or contact through skin/eyes) to potentially dangerous substances. Proper ventilation, a positive-pressure local environment, and the use of personal protective devices (e.g., gloves and face/eye protection) may be required.

Immersion of probes in fluids requires attention to the individual device's ability to be submerged. Although some scan heads and large portions of the cable may be safely immersed up to the connector to the ultrasound scanner, only the scan heads of others may be submerged. Some manufacturers also note that the crystals of the array may be damaged if, instead of suspending the probe in the disinfectant, it rests on the bottom of the container. Before selecting a method of disinfection, consult the instrument manufacturer regarding the compatibility of the proposed agent with the probes. Relevant information is available online and in device manuals. Additionally, not all probes can be cleaned with the same cleaning agents. Although some agents are compatible with all probes of a given manufacturer, others must be limited to a subset of probes.

After soaking the probe in an approved disinfectant for the specified time, the probe should be thoroughly rinsed (especially to remove traces of toxic disinfectants in the case of orthophthalaldehyde) and dried.

In summary, transducers should be cleaned of visible soil. Endovascular transducers must be sterilized. Endocavity transducers and transducers used on nonintact skin must undergo high-level disinfection, where all microorganisms are killed with only a few bacterial spores permissible. Transducer condoms, either commercial or drugstore type, have a significant incidence of leaks. It must be assumed that these condoms are not intact and high-level disinfection must be performed. Transducers used in the setting of intact skin should undergo low-level disinfection as described previously. Cords and keyboards should be cleaned following manufacturer instructions.

TABLE 21.1 **Sterilants and High-Level Disinfectants Listed by the US Food and Drug Administration**

Name	Composition/Action
Glutaraldehyde	Organic compound ($CH_2(CH_2CHO)_2$) Induces cell death by cross-linking cellular proteins; usually used alone or mixed with formaldehyde
Hydrogen peroxide	Inorganic compound (H_2O_2) Antiseptic and antibacterial; a very strong oxidizer with oxidation potential of 1.8 V
Peracetic acid	Organic compound (CH_3CO_3H) Antimicrobial agent (high oxidization potential)
Orthophthalaldehyde	Organic compound ($C_6H_4(CHO)_2$) Strong binding to outer cell wall of contaminant organisms
Hypochlorite/ hypochlorous acid	Inorganic compound (HClO) Myeloperoxidase-mediated peroxidation of chloride ions
Phenol/phenolate	Organic compound (C_6H_5OH) Antiseptic
Hibidil	Chlorhexidine gluconate ($C_{22}H_{30}Cl_2N_{10}$) Chemical antiseptic

American Institute of Ultrasound in Medicine. AIUM official statement: guidelines for cleaning and preparing external- and internal-use ultrasound probes between patients. <http://www.aium.org/officialstatements/57>.

SUGGESTED READINGS

Abramowicz JS. Fetal Doppler: how to keep it safe? *Clin Obstet Gynecol.* 2010;53(4):842–850.

American Institute of Ultrasound in Medicine. AIUM official statement: guidelines for cleaning and preparing external- and internal-use ultrasound probes between patients. <http://www.aium.org/officialstatements/57>.

American Institute of Ultrasound in Medicine. AIUM Official statement: statement on the safe use of doppler ultrasound during 11–14 week scans (or earlier in pregnancy). <http://www.aium.org/officialStatements/42/>.

Bolyard E, Tablan O, Williams W, Pearson ML, Craig NS, Deitchman SD. Guideline for infection control in health care personnel, 1998. *Am J Infect Control.* 1998;26(3):289–327.

Frazee BW, et al. Bacterial growth on ED ultrasound machines. *Ann Emerg Med.* 2011;58(1):56–63.

Grether J, Li S, Yoshida C, Croen L. Antenatal ultrasound and risk of autism spectrum disorders. *J Autism Dev Disord.* 2009;40(2):238–245.

ter Haar G, Wells PNT. Ultrasound bioeffects and safety. *Proc Inst Mech Eng H.* 2009;224(2):363–373.

Lyons E, Dyke C, Toms M, Cheang M. In utero exposure to diagnostic ultrasound: a 6-year follow-up. *Radiology.* 1988;166(3):687–690.

Moore R, Diamond E, Cavalieri R. The relationship of birth weight and intrauterine diagnostic ultrasound exposure. *Obstet Gynecol.* 1988;71(4):513–517.

Mullaney PJ, et al. How clean is your probe? Microbiological assessment of ultrasound tranducers in routine clinical use and cost effective ways to reduce contamination. *Clin Radiol.* 2007;62(7):694-698.

Nelson T, Fowlkes J, Abramowicz J, Church C. Ultrasound biosafety considerations for the practicing sonographer and sonologist. *J Ultrasound Med.* 2009;28(2):139-150.

Newnham J, Doherty D, Kendall G, Zubrick S, Landau L, Stanley F. Effects of repeated prenatal ultrasound examinations on childhood outcome up to 8 years of age: follow-up of a randomised controlled trial. *Lancet.* 2004;364(9450):2038-2044.

Newnham J, Evans S, Michael C, Stanley F, Landau L. Effects of frequent ultrasound during pregnancy: a randomised controlled trial. *Lancet.* 1993;342(8876):887-891.

Rutala WA, Weber DJ, Healthcare Infection Control Practices Advisory Committee. Guideline for disinfection and sterilization in healthcare facilities. <http://www.cdc.gov/hicpac/pdf/guidelines/disinfection_nov_2008.pdf>.

Schneider-Kolsky M, Ayobi Z, Lombardo P, Brown D, Kedang B, Gibbs M. Ultrasound exposure of the foetal chick brain: effects on learning and memory. *Int J Dev Neurosci.* 2009;27(7):677-683.

Sheiner E, Abramowicz JS. A symposium on obstetrical ultrasound: is all this safe for the fetus? *Clin Obstet Gynecol.* 2012;55(1):188-198.

Tarantal A, Hendrickx A. Evaluation of the bioeffects of prenatal ultrasound exposure in the cynomolgus macaque (Macaca fascicularis): I. neonatal/infant observations. *Teratology.* 1989;39(2):137-147.

Chapter 22

Noninterpretive Skills in Magnetic Resonance Imaging

Jonathan Larson, Lindsey Berkowitz, and Neel Madan

INTRODUCTION

Magnetic resonance imaging (MRI) is used in the diagnosis of patients with many conditions, and while the interpretive skills necessary to appropriately interpret the MRI images are complex, so too are the noninterpretive skills. Many of these issues come to the radiologist's attention on a daily basis—for example, issues concerning magnetic resonance (MR) safety, whether a patient will be safe in the MRI environment, and issues regarding artifacts seen on an MRI. Intravenous gadolinium contrast (discussed in Chapter 20) adds another layer of complexity in the daily performance of MRI, especially in light of ongoing developments with regard to nephrogenic systemic fibrosis and gadolinium deposition in the brain. The two main practice domains that are important to understand are those pertaining to patient safety and those needed for quality improvement, for example, identification and improvement of image quality as well as establishing the best workflow environment.

MAGNETIC RESONANCE IMAGING SAFETY

MR scanners are classified as "nonsignificant risk devices" by the US Food and Drug Administration (FDA), as long as specified parameters and best practices are followed. In contrast to imaging modalities that rely on ionizing radiation, which is associated with carcinogenesis, cataract formation, and other complications, MRI uses static magnetic fields, time-varying gradient magnetic fields, and time-varying radiofrequency (RF) magnetic fields, which tend to be more benign. Nevertheless, each of these fundamental components of the MR system presents its own unique set of safety issues: the static magnetic field can result in projectile injury as well as the displacement of, interference with, and/or permanent damage to implanted medical devices; the time-varying RF magnetic field can result in tissue heating and/or burns; and the time-varying gradient magnetic field can result in peripheral nerve stimulation and/or acoustic injury. All of these risks, however, are generally the result of failure to appropriately follow safety guidelines. Therefore, MR safety risks are particularly important to recognize because they are largely preventable and potentially catastrophic.

A turning point in the history of MR safety occurred in 2001, when a 6-year-old boy died as the result of projectile injury during an MR exam. Many systematic issues were identified that played a role in allowing this tragedy to occur, such as deficiencies involving the safety policies and physical design of the MR facility and insufficient training of MR personnel. In response to this incident and others, the American College of Radiology (ACR) published the first edition of their guidance document on MR safe practices in 2002, which addressed many of the systematic issues identified in the 2001 tragedy, and offered MR facilities across the country a template to follow to develop and strengthen their own set of MR safety policies. Multiple organizations are currently involved in establishing and maintaining guidelines, regulations, and best practices related to MR safety. For example, the FDA establishes regulations for the safe operation of an MR scanner, such as setting exposure limits for RF power deposition, and also regulates MR contrast agents. The American Society for Testing and Materials (ASTM) develops standard test methods for determining the MR safety of medical devices, and several additional organizations, such as the ACR and Joint Commission, serve as accrediting bodies. Specific guidelines are in continuous evolution as technology advances and MR scanners are able to generate stronger static magnetic fields, faster gradient magnetic fields, and more powerful RF magnetic fields. Up-to-date MR safety information is available from many sources such as the ACR's website and MRIsafety.com.

Static Magnetic Field–Related Safety Issues

MRI was introduced as a clinical imaging modality in the early 1980s, thereby exposing large populations to powerful magnetic fields for the first time. Although the first MR scanners generated field strengths in the range of 0.05 to 0.35 T, modern MR scanners are able to produce field strengths greater than 10 T. For reference, the magnetic field strength of the Earth is approximately 0.05 millitesla (mT), or 0.5 gauss (G) (1 T = 1000 G). A large body of literature has characterized the interactions between magnetic fields and various biological processes, including cell growth and reproduction, DNA structure and gene expression, nerve conduction, cognition, vision, cardiovascular physiology, and immune function, among many other processes. Although more research must be done at field strengths greater than 3 T, there is currently no conclusive evidence of adverse biological effects resulting from exposure to field strengths used in clinical practice. The FDA has set an upper limit for static magnetic field exposure of 8 T for adults, children, and infants greater than 1 month of age and 4 T for infants less than 1 month of age, given the lack of data at very high field strengths (although field strengths greater than 4 T require Institutional Review Board approval and an investigational device exemption).

There are multiple safety issues associated with the static magnetic field including projectile injury and the displacement of, interference with, and/or permanent damage to, implanted medical devices. To understand the safety risks associated with the static magnetic field, it is first necessary to be familiar with the hardware of the main magnet and basic principles of electromagnetism, which will briefly be reviewed.

The main magnet fundamentally consists of a coil of wire wrapped around the bore through which electric current is applied. The flow of current induces a magnetic field, with its polarity depending on the direction of current flow, and its strength depending on several factors including the magnitude of the current. Because conductors inherently resist and dissipate current at temperatures significantly greater than absolute zero, a constant source of electricity would be necessary to maintain a given field strength under these circumstances, which is not practical at high field strengths due to cost. Therefore, modern MR scanners use superconducting coils, which are immersed in cryogens and cooled to a temperature approaching absolute zero. Current is applied to the superconducting coil over the course of several hours until the desired field strength is reached, and the coil is then able to maintain a given field strength without a constant supply of electricity, as long as its temperature is maintained. Modern MR scanners typically have an additional set of superconducting coils external to the main set, which generate a magnetic field that cancels out a portion of the fringe field, or the static magnetic field that extends beyond the confines of the MR scanner. The static magnetic field is strongest and most homogeneous at the center of the bore, or the isocenter. The rate at which the static magnetic field strength changes with distance is referred to as the spatial gradient.

It is also important to be familiar with physical principles that determine the interaction between magnetic fields and various types of matter with differing magnetic properties. All matter, including human tissue, is associated with some degree of magnetism, depending on its electron configuration. The degree to which a substance becomes magnetized in the presence of an external magnetic field is referred to as its magnetic volume susceptibility, or simply susceptibility. Substances are categorized as diamagnetic, paramagnetic, or ferromagnetic based on their susceptibility.

Diamagnetic substances have a negligible, negative susceptibility to magnetic fields and are minimally repelled by magnetic fields. These substances have paired valence electrons and therefore no net intrinsic magnetic moment. Examples of diamagnetic substances include water and most human tissues.

Paramagnetic substances have a weak, positive susceptibility to magnetic fields and are slightly attracted to magnetic fields. Paramagnetic properties are due to the presence of unpaired valence electrons, resulting in a small net intrinsic magnetic moment. Examples of paramagnetic substances include ions of certain metals such as iron and gadolinium. Although human tissues contain paramagnetic materials such as iron ions, they are distributed in various molecules such as hemoglobin and hemosiderin, which are only weakly paramagnetic and not sufficiently concentrated to routinely interact with an external magnetic field.

Ferromagnetic substances have a large, positive susceptibility and are strongly attracted to magnetic fields. Like paramagnetic substances, ferromagnetic substances have unpaired valence electrons. However, the much larger susceptibility of ferromagnetic substances is related to magnetic domains, within which large numbers of magnetic moments become aligned in the presence of an external magnetic field. Ferromagnetic materials are not naturally present in human tissues but may be present as foreign bodies or implanted medical devices. Examples of ferromagnetic materials include elemental iron, nickel, and cobalt. Metals or alloys that do not contain elemental iron, nickel, or cobalt are not ferromagnetic and therefore are not associated with a risk of projectile injury, although they are associated with a risk of burns, as all metals are efficient conductors of heat (see the next section for further detail).

The static magnetic field exerts translational and torque forces on ferromagnetic objects, which are related to a number of factors including the susceptibility, mass, and shape of the object; the distance and orientation of the object with respect to the magnet; and the strength and spatial gradient of the magnetic field. As an example, a 1.5-T magnet can lift and transport a car in a junkyard but exerts no significant force on a human body in an MR scanner due to differences in their magnetic properties. The translational force exerted by a static magnetic field may attract and accelerate ferromagnetic objects toward the magnet, resulting in the *projectile effect*. Given the presence of a ferromagnetic object in a strong static magnetic field, this force is largely dependent on the spatial gradient. Because the static magnetic field is very homogeneous near the isocenter, the spatial gradient within the central bore is small, and the translational force is weak. As a result of shielding techniques used in modern MR scanners, the fringe field is highly concentrated around the bore, resulting in very high spatial gradients at the periphery of the bore and the potential for overwhelming, abrupt, and unexpected translational force on a ferromagnetic object that is brought too close to the magnet (Fig. 22.1).

All ferromagnetic objects, regardless of mass, pose a safety risk in the fringe field. For example, even a paperclip can accelerate up to speeds of 40 MPH in a 1.5-T magnetic field and cause significant injury. The projectile effect is most likely to occur at field strengths greater than 30 G. However, translational attraction of a medical device can be more specifically characterized by the deflection angle test, which was devised by the ASTM. In this test, a device is suspended by a thin string at various static magnetic field strengths, and the angle at which the device is displaced from its vertical axis is measured. If the device deflects less than 45 degrees, then the magnetically induced force is less than the force exerted on the device by gravity, and it is assumed to be safe at that field strength.

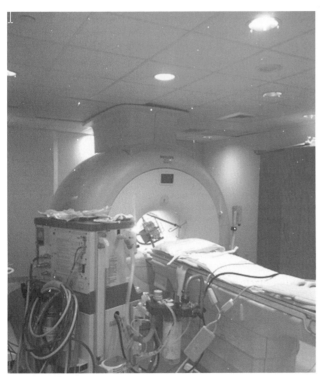

FIG. 22.1 The static magnetic field has the potential to attract and accelerate ferromagnetic objects toward the magnet with overwhelming, abrupt, and unexpected force, a phenomenon known as the projectile effect. The IV pole in this image was not magnetic resonance safe, became a projectile, and lodged inside the magnetic resonance imaging scanner. Thankfully this occurred as anesthesia was setting up for a magnetic resonance imaging study, and no patient was harmed.

The torque force exerted by a static magnetic field causes ferromagnetic objects to rotate and align parallel to the direction of the magnetic field. Given the presence of a ferromagnetic object in a strong static magnetic field, this force is largely dependent on the field strength and is strongest at the isocenter. Therefore, the torque force presents the greatest safety risk for patients with implanted medical devices with ferromagnetic components such as certain aneurysm clips, cochlear implants, and cardiac pacemakers. The ASTM has also devised a standard test to evaluate the torque force exerted on a medical device in a static magnetic field. In this test, a device is secured by a spring and placed on a holder at the isocenter, and the angular deflection of the holder is measured. If the maximal torque is less than the product of the longest dimension of the device and its weight, then the magnetically induced force is less than the force exerted on the device due to gravity, and it is assumed to be safe at that field strength with respect to torque forces.

The static magnetic field may also temporarily interfere with and/or permanently damage implanted electronic medical devices. For this reason, the *5-G line* must always be clearly demarcated in the MR environment; this line defines the perimeter within which the static magnetic field exceeds 5 G and poses a risk to the general public, particularly individuals with cardiac pacemakers and other implanted electronic medical devices (Fig. 22.2). Moreover, some medical equipment

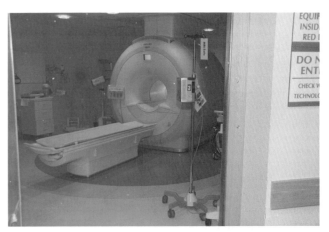

FIG. 22.2 A magnetic resonance (MR) imaging scanner demonstrating the 5-G line, which is represented by the periphery of the colored circle on the floor surrounding the scanner. This defines the area in which the static magnetic field poses a risk to the general public, particularly individuals with cardiac pacemakers and other implanted electronic medical devices. Some MR conditionally safe devices, such as a respirator, must also stay outside the 5-G line. Note the IV pole is labeled as MR safe.

(e.g., respirators) may be approved in the MR environment outside the 5-G line but can act as a projectile when brought within the 5-G line. More specific information with regard to various types of medical devices is separately discussed.

Although implanted medical devices are increasingly being composed of nonferromagnetic materials, there are many devices and metallic foreign bodies that may represent a contraindication to MRI. A metallic foreign body in the eye or in close proximity to large blood vessels or vital organs may represent an absolute contraindication (unless the composition of the foreign body can be determined or it can be removed). Implants that have not been rated as MR safe or MR conditionally safe also may be a contraindication to MRI, including cardiac pacemakers and implantable cardioverter-defibrillators, nerve stimulators, cochlear implants, ferromagnetic aneurysm clips, hemodynamic monitoring and temporary pacing devices, pulmonary artery monitoring catheters, retained transvenous pacemaker and defibrillator leads, and transdermal patches. However, many manufacturers are now making such devices that are MR conditionally safe (e.g., cochlear implants and cardiac pacemakers). Moreover, a handful of centers nationwide have instituted safeguards that allow them to successfully image patients with devices that are not MR safe or MR conditionally safe, such as cardiac pacemakers or implantable cardioverter-defibrillators. The MR safety of specific devices can be determined from published written or electronic resources, product manufacturers, and/or peer-reviewed publications.

An additional safety concern related to the static magnetic field is potential biological effects, particularly those due to the magnetohydrodynamic effect, or the induction of a voltage in a conductive fluid that flows through a magnetic field. Examples of such fluids in the human body include blood and endolymphatic fluid. For example, ions present in blood flowing through the aorta generate a voltage across the vessel that results in artificial T-wave elevation on ECG. Although this effect is far too weak to cause arrhythmias even at high field strengths, it may result in faulty triggering on gated cardiac MR exams. Additionally, magnetohydrodynamic forces on the semicircular canals, retina, and surface of the tongue are thought to be a source of nausea, vertigo, flashes of light (magnetophosphenes), and metallic taste, which have been reported, especially at high field strengths.

The use of cryogens presents an additional safety issue in MRI. Modern MR scanners contain over 1000 L of cryogens to maintain the superconductive properties of the magnet. Liquid helium is the most commonly used cryogen, which is not inherently toxic but is associated with dangerous physical properties, including a boiling point of approximately −450°F and a thermal expansion ratio of greater than 750:1. In the event of a magnet quench, or sudden loss of superconductive properties of the magnet, the cryostat temperature rises above the boiling point of liquid helium, which rapidly vaporizes. If the MR system functions properly, the cryogen gas enters an escape valve and is discharged into the atmosphere. However, if the ventilation system fails, there is the potential for hundreds of liters of cryogens to vaporize into the MR environment. Because of its high thermal expansion ratio, 1000 L of liquid helium may explosively expand into over 750,000 L of gas during a full quench, posing several safety risks including cold exposure and frostbite, asphyxiation from oxygen depletion, physical injury from ejected material, and increased atmospheric pressure. Therefore, an intentional magnet quench is rarely indicated other than in extraordinary circumstances, such as a projectile restraining a patient in the magnet.

Radiofrequency Magnetic Field–Related Safety Issues

The main safety risks associated with RF electromagnetic fields include tissue heating and burns. RF pulses are short bursts of nonionizing, electromagnetic radiation that are used to excite protons within a given slice thickness of the patient and generate a measurable signal. The excited protons emit RF radiation as they relax back into their resting state, some of which is received by a coil and used to generate an image. However, only a small portion of the emitted RF radiation reaches the receiver coil, with the majority of energy absorption occurring within the patient according to Faraday's law of induction. Because human tissues have some degree of conductivity, the RF field induces small electrical voltages within the patient, leading to induced currents and resistive heating, with the potential for tissue heating if the energy absorbed exceeds the patient's capacity to dissipate heat. Current may also be induced in metallic objects within the RF field, such as components of the MR scanner or medical devices or wires on or within the patient, resulting in the potential for severe burns. The specific absorption rate (SAR) is used to quantify RF radiation exposure during an MR exam and is one of the safety parameters regulated by the FDA. In general, SAR refers to absorbed power per unit mass, typically expressed in watts per kilogram. The FDA has set SAR limits for the whole body, whole head, and local tissue in the head, torso, and extremities. Varying limits are in place for different modes of operation of the MR scanner as defined by the International Electrotechnical Commission, which represent varying levels of risk to the patient. Imaging parameters in the normal operating mode do not result in physiologic stress to the patient, whereas those in the first-level controlled operating mode have the potential for physiologic stress to the patient, warranting a risk-benefit analysis and medical supervision; those in the second-level controlled operating mode pose significant risk to the patient and warrant Institutional Review Board approval.

The whole-body SAR refers to the SAR averaged over the whole body over a 15-minute time interval and is limited to 1.5 W/kg in the normal operating mode and 4 W/kg in the first-level controlled operating mode, with SARs greater than 4 W/kg in the second-level controlled operating mode. The whole-body temperature should not increase more than 1°C during an exam. The head SAR refers to the SAR averaged over the head over a 10-minute time interval and is limited to 3 W/kg in the normal operating mode, with SARs greater than 3 W/kg in the second-level controlled operating mode. The local tissue SAR refers to the SAR averaged over any 1 g of tissue over a 5-minute time interval and is limited to 8 W/kg in the head or torso for the normal operating mode, with SARs greater than 8 W/kg in the second-level controlled operating mode. The local tissue SAR in the extremities is limited to 12 W/kg in the normal operating mode, with SARs greater than 12 W/kg in the second-level controlled operating mode. Multiple prior studies have confirmed the safety of imaging at a whole-body SAR of 4, with only mild increases in body temperature of less than 0.6°C and physiologically insignificant increases in skin temperature.

The SAR is determined by many factors including the static magnetic field strength, RF power (i.e., repetition time, flip angle, and duty cycle), tissue density and conductivity, and patient size, among other factors. In general, the SAR increases with the square of the static magnetic field strength and flip angle. It also increases with patient size, tissue conductivity, and duty cycle. For example, doubling the static magnetic field strength from 1.5 to 3 T or the flip angle from 90 to 180 degrees results in a fourfold increase in the SAR. For this reason, fast-spin echo sequences with long trains of 180-degree RF pulses generally have a larger SAR compared to gradient echo sequences, which do not use 180-degree refocusing RF pulses. At the same time, parallel imaging techniques may help reduce the SAR by decreasing the scan length. Patient parameters may also affect the SAR. For example, medical conditions including hypertension, diabetes, obesity, cardiovascular disease, fever, and/or advanced age may affect the SAR, and medications including beta-blockers, diuretics, amphetamines, and sedatives may interfere with the capacity to dissipate heat. Of note, certain human tissues with relatively poor vascularization, such as the eye and testis, are at increased risk of thermal injury, because blood flow acts as a heat sink. Moreover, these organs are also at increased risk due to their superficial location; the majority of RF energy absorption occurs superficially, because the incident RF wavelength is relatively long compared to the wavelength of human tissues.

The SAR can be estimated by adding the total energy of RF pulses in a given period of time, dividing by the duty cycle to determine the power, and dividing by the patient's mass. MR scanners calculate the estimated SAR and do not permit imaging parameters outside of the normal operating mode without special authorization by MR personnel. There are multiple methods to reduce the SAR, such as increasing the time to repetition (TR), reducing the number of slices, reducing the echo train length, and reducing the refocusing pulse flip angle. Controlling the room temperature, humidity, and airflow also facilitates heat dissipation.

Metallic objects within the RF field may undergo significant heating because of their high conductive capacity, resulting in the potential for severe burns. Similar to the heating that occurs in human tissues, induced currents and resistive heating of metallic objects will occur if the time-varying RF or gradient field intercepts an electrically conductive loop. Metallic objects with an elongated or looped configuration, such as wires, leads, certain types of catheters, jewelry, and piercings, are therefore most likely to result in burns. Metallic substances such as tattoos, permanent makeup, and certain clothing microfibers may also pose a risk for burns. Of note, because the amplitude and duration of the gradient magnetic field are much smaller than the RF field, it does not pose a significant risk of thermal loading.

Although burns are one of the more common safety issues in the MR environment, they can be avoided if appropriate safety precautions are taken. The patient should change into a gown and remove any metallic objects such as piercings, MR-unsafe monitoring equipment, and drug-delivery patches. Care should be made to ensure that no metallic materials are in contact with the patient. If the patient has tattoos, permanent makeup, or other unremovable metallic objects, a cold towel should be placed over them to facilitate heat dissipation. The patient should be aware of the potential for thermal loading and burns and should always be able to communicate with MR personnel in the event of perceived heating. Additionally, leads, cables, and other potentially conductive objects should never be looped. Insulating material should be placed between the patient's skin and RF coil and between the patient and any electrically conductive material that must remain in the MR system.

In addition to the safety issues, some patients, especially larger patients, will report significant sweating during the MR examination as their bodies attempt to dissipate the heat deposition in their bodies. This impacts patient comfort during the examination, and some patients may be unwilling to continue with the study because of these effects.

Gradient Magnetic Field–Related Safety Issues

MR scanners contain three orthogonal pairs of gradient coils, which generate linear variation along the static magnetic field to spatially encode the RF signal and allow spatial localization of the signal. Gradient magnetic fields are characterized by a maximum amplitude, measured in millitesla per meter, and a rise time, or the time interval necessary for the gradient to reach its maximum amplitude, measured in microseconds. The slew rate, which reflects the speed and strength of the gradient, can be calculated by dividing the maximum gradient amplitude by the rise time and is measured in millitesla per meter per second. Modern MR scanners are capable of slew rates greater than 200 mT/m/s. However, because higher slew rates are associated with a greater change in magnetic field strength over time, or dB/dt, pulse sequences with high slew rates, such as echo planar imaging sequences, are more likely to cause inductive currents according to Faraday's law of induction. Although the RF and gradient magnetic fields vary rapidly with time, gradient magnetic fields are characterized by a greater dB/dt and a lesser maximum amplitude and are consequently more likely to result in induced currents and less likely to result in significant thermal loading.

Therefore, the primary safety issues related to gradient magnetic fields are caused by induced currents in the body or implanted medical devices, which can result in peripheral nerve stimulation, interference with the device, or burns. Stimulation of cells in the diaphragm, myocardium, or central nervous system are theoretical risks that could occur at much greater rates of change in magnetic field strength than those used in clinical practice. Additionally, because of the rapid time-varying nature of the gradient magnetic fields, vibration of gradient coils generates significant acoustic noise with the potential for temporary or permanent hearing impairment.

The potential for gradient magnetic field–induced physiologic effects at a given location in the body is determined by numerous factors, including the local dB/dt, average and maximum gradient magnetic field strength, and electrical properties of the tissue, among other variables. At the level of the cell membrane, the stimulation threshold varies with the amplitude and the duration of the applied pulse for a particular type of cell with a given excitability. The rheobase and chronaxie are measures of the excitability of cell membranes and refer to the minimum current amplitude that can depolarize the cell membrane and the minimum time required for an electric current of twice the rheobase strength to depolarize the cell membrane, respectively. For a peripheral nerve, the rheobase ranges from 6 to 20 T/s and the chronaxie ranges from 200 to 350 µs. Given these considerations, the FDA previously set an upper limit of 20 T/s for a pulse duration of 120 µs or more. However, following the introduction of echo planar imaging and other similar fast imaging techniques, which provide unique and valuable diagnostic information but rely on faster and stronger gradient magnetic fields, the FDA changed this recommendation and eliminated an absolute upper limit for dB/dt. Instead, the current FDA recommendation is to avoid severe discomfort or painful peripheral nerve stimulation, which effectively protects patients from more serious safety risks such as respiratory and cardiac stimulation, which occur at a much greater dB/dt. More specifically, the threshold for peripheral nerve stimulation is roughly 60 mT/s, at which point mild paresthesias may be perceived, with uncomfortable or painful peripheral nerve stimulation occurring at roughly 90 mT/s. Given this narrow margin between painless and painful peripheral nerve stimulation, it is important for the patient to alert the technologist of any perceived paresthesia so that corrective measures can be taken.

If painful peripheral nerve stimulation is avoided, there is a negligible risk of respiratory or cardiac stimulation, which occurs at roughly 900 and 3600 mT/s, respectively. Gradient magnetic fields may also induce currents in implanted medical devices or other metallic objects, particularly those with looped or linear metallic components, such as pacemakers, cables, or retained wires, and result in malfunction of the device or burns. There are several reported cases of death as a result of pacemaker malfunction during MR exams.

An additional safety concern regarding gradient magnetic fields is acoustic noise, which results from the vibration of gradient coils (and to a lesser extent RF coils) due to the Lorenz force. The acoustic noise generated by vibrating coils may interfere with communication between the patient and technologist and also has the potential for temporary, or in extreme cases, permanent hearing impairment. The FDA has set an upper limit of 140 dB for allowable acoustic noise, which is the level at which hearing damage may occur. Additionally, manufacturers must place warnings for pulse sequences exceeding 99 dB in acoustic noise. Although most pulse sequences generate acoustic noise ranging from approximately 80 to 90 dB, echo planar imaging sequences can generate up to approximately 130 dB. It is therefore important to provide ear protection such as ear plugs and/or headphones, which can reduce effective noise levels by roughly 30 dB.

Magnetic Resonance Imaging Environment

Zoning

An important means of preventing MRI-related accidents is the division of the MR environment into four distinct zones, with increasingly restricted access from zone I to zone IV.

Zone I represents the areas outside of the MRI environment, which may include reading rooms and the entrance into the MR environment. It is the only zone that is freely accessible to the general public.

Zone II represents the interface between the unrestricted zone 1 and highly restricted zone III and may contain the reception and waiting areas, as well as the screening area where potential safety issues are identified. Patients are under the direct supervision of MR personnel in zone II. Zone III represents the portion of the MR environment in which the magnetic field poses safety risks. It contains the MR control room and scanner room. Zone III is physically restricted from general public access with locked doors, for example, passkey locking systems, and is only accessible to patients under the direct supervision of MR personnel. Patients in zone III have been cleared for the MR exam and are prepared for entry into the scanner. They remain under the direct supervision of MR personnel at all times. Additionally, magnetic field warnings are in place in this zone, which must clearly indicate the presence of a strong magnet that is always on, as well as the potential for danger related to the magnetic field. The 5-G line must be clearly demarcated; it defines the perimeter within which the magnetic field exceeds 5 G and may interfere with electronic medical devices.

Zone IV represents the room in which the MR scanner is located and is the highest risk zone (Fig. 22.3). As in zone III, patients in zone IV remain under the direct

supervision of MR personnel at all times. Of note, zone IV is located within zone III by definition.

Magnetic Resonance Personnel

Appropriate training of MR personnel is critical in maintaining a safe MR environment. MR personnel serve as the most important means of avoiding MRI-related accidents and are divided into three distinct categories: level 1 MR personnel, level 2 MR personnel, and non-MR personnel.

Level 1 MR personnel must complete minimal MR safety educational requirements on an annual basis to ensure their own safety while working in zones III and IV. The training requirements ensure a basic level of understanding of safety issues such as projectile effects, common objects that should be restricted from the MR environment, and emergency protocols. Level 1 MR personnel may include transport staff, radiology nurses, physicians such as anesthesiologists and cardiologists, and other staff members who occasionally work in the MR environment.

Level 2 MR personnel must complete more extensive MR safety training on an annual basis to ensure their own safety as well as the safety of others while working in the MR environment. The training requirements ensure a deeper and broader understanding of MR safety issues, such as the risk of tissue heating and burns from the RF transmitters and peripheral nerve stimulation from rapidly changing gradients. Level 2 personnel may include MR technologists, medical physicists, and radiology residents, fellows, and attending physicians.

Individuals who have not completed the MR safety requirements on an annual basis, such as patients, accompanying family members, and staff who have not completed level 1 or 2 training, are considered non-MR personnel. Non-MR personnel must always be screened prior to entering zone III and must remain under the direct supervision of MR personnel at all times while in zones III and IV. Of note, level 1 MR personnel may accompany non-MR personnel into zone III, but only level 2 MR personnel may accompany non-MR personnel into zone IV.

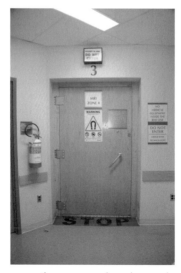

FIG. 22.3 The magnetic resonance imaging environment is divided into four distinct zones, with increasingly restricted access from zone I to zone IV. Zone IV represents the room in which the magnetic resonance scanner is located and is the highest-risk zone.

Screening

A comprehensive screening process for patients and devices is essential in maintaining a safe MR environment.

Effective patient screening consists of an MR safety screening form to be completed by the patient, a discussion between the patient and MR personnel in which the screening form is reviewed and any potential questions or concerns are addressed, and physical screening. A thorough screening form includes information pertaining to the presence of implanted medical devices, surgical history, prior metal work exposure, complications related to prior MR exams, allergies, claustrophobia, and pregnancy status. In addition, for patients in whom contrast will be or potentially will be administered, medical conditions that would preclude the administration of MR contrast agents should also be discussed. Depending on the information provided on the screening form, various measures may be required before a patient can safely enter zone III. For example, if the patient provides a history of prior metal work requiring medical attention, further investigation with radiographs and/or computed tomography (CT) scans may be necessary to exclude a foreign body. Additionally, if the patient provides a history of an implanted medical device, the device must be identified as MR safe, MR conditional safe, or MR unsafe. Some patient populations, such as those with intraocular metallic foreign bodies or certain models of cardiac pacemakers, may not be able to safety enter zone III under any circumstances.

After the patient and MR personnel have reviewed the screening form and all of the patient's questions and concerns have been addressed, the patient is physically screened for metallic objects such as keys, coins, jewelry, piercings, clothing with metallic zippers or fibers, tattoos, permanent makeup, and portable monitors or oxygen tanks. Patients must remove all removable metallic personal belongings and devices and change into a hospital-supplied dressing gown as deemed necessary. The use of ferromagnetic detection devices or strong handheld magnets (>1000 G) for the detection of metallic objects external to the patient is recommended by the ACR. In the future, the use of ferromagnetic detection devices may also be recommended for implanted medical devices. Of note, the use of conventional metal detectors is not recommended, as they vary in sensitivity and may not detect small ferromagnetic foreign bodies and do not differentiate between ferromagnetic and nonferromagnetic metallic objects, among other reasons.

When a metallic object is identified, it must be assessed for the potential for safety risks. In the case of implanted medical devices, such as cochlear implants, cardiac pacing devices, or neurostimulator devices, the potential for temporary interference with or permanent damage to the device must also be investigated. Additionally, in the case of implanted medical devices or metallic foreign bodies, the potential for image artifacts must be assessed. All metallic objects and devices must be classified as MR safe, MR conditionally safe, or MR unsafe and marked with FDA-specified labels prior to entering zone IV (Fig. 22.4). MR safety information can be determined from published written or electronic resources, product manufacturers, and/or peer-reviewed publications.

MR-safe objects pose no known safety risk in all MRI environments. They have no metallic components and are nonferromagnetic and nonconducting. Examples of MR-safe objects include devices composed of plastic or alloys such as Phynox (Elgiloy), titanium, titanium alloy, MP35N, and nitinol.

MR–conditionally safe objects pose no known safety risks in the MR imaging environment as long as appropriate safeguards are followed. MR–conditionally safe objects will be characterized by a maximum static magnetic field strength, spatial gradient, time-varying magnetic field (dB/dt), and SAR. Some MR–conditionally safe objects are only considered safe when scanning specific body parts and/or with specific MR coils (e.g., some vagal nerve stimulators or bladder stimulators are only MR conditionally safe when scanning the head using a send-receive coil and following additional safeguards). MR-unsafe objects pose known safety risks in all MRI environments. They have metallic components that are conducting and potentially ferromagnetic. MR-unsafe objects are generally contraindicated in zones III and IV, although as mentioned earlier, a handful of centers are beginning to image some of these devices in specific situations and with appropriate safeguards.

Of note, the term *MR compatible*, which was previously intended for objects that did not interfere with diagnostic quality, is no longer recommended by the FDA because the term was often confused with MR safe.

Occasionally, questions arise as to whether a patient who previously had an MRI can safely have an MRI again. However, caution needs to be taken in screening the patient, because differences in MRI scanners, the coils used, and the body part being scanned can all influence whether an MRI can safely be performed.

Determining whether an MRI can be performed safely in an individual with an implanted object is a complex process that requires a detailed understanding of MR physics

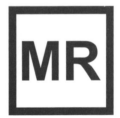
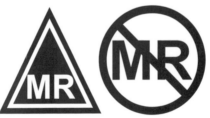

MR safe   MR conditionally safe   MR unsafe

FIG. 22.4 All objects and devices must be appropriately screened and labeled by magnetic resonance (MR) personnel as MR safe, MR conditionally safe, or MR unsafe prior to entering the MR imaging environment. Additionally, equipment used in the area should be labeled with one of these three labels.

and information about a specific device, in conjunction with an understanding of FDA and device recommendations and institution-specific MR safety protocols. It is best to think of this as a process whereby the risks and benefits are considered, rather than a simple yes or no question that needs to be answered. Sometimes the answer can change as we learn more about the nuances of MR safety; moreover, as the patient's clinical picture changes, the question as to why the MRI is being conducted can also change.

Pregnant Patients

MRI is able to provide important diagnostic information with regard to obstetric, placental, and fetal pathology that cannot be obtained with other imaging modalities. Fetal MRI has been performed for over 2 decades, and there remains no documented case of an adverse outcome for the fetus. Nevertheless, there are theoretical safety issues, and some animal studies have reported various adverse outcomes. Because of the lack of sufficient data to adequately characterize potential risks to the fetus, the ACR recommends avoiding MRI of pregnant patients if possible (e.g., a nonurgent MRI that could wait until after the delivery). But MRI has an important role in the evaluation of the fetus as well as the mother, especially in the hopes of avoiding CT and its associated ionizing radiation.

As with general safety issues related to MRI, safety considerations with respect to imaging pregnant patients can also be related to the three primary components of the MR scanner. For example, the RF system may result in tissue heating that could interfere with fetal stem cells and organogenesis. The gradient system has the potential to produce acoustic injury to the fetal ear. It has also been suggested that the static magnetic field may interfere with cell migration, proliferation, and differentiation. Despite these theoretical risks, there is no conclusive evidence to support these claims. Because of these theoretical concerns, the risks and benefits of MRI of pregnant patients must be considered by the radiologist and ordering physician. Multiple factors should be taken into consideration. For example, MRI of pregnant patients should be avoided if another imaging modality, such as ultrasound, is able to adequately address the clinical indication; it should be avoided if the examination can be safely postponed until after delivery; additionally, MR contrast agents should not be administered if they are not essential for the clinical indication. Finally, the gestational age of the fetus should be taken into account as well. If possible, MRI should be avoided during the first trimester, which is certainly possible if the evaluation is of the fetus itself, but may not be avoidable if there are clinical concerns in the mother.

Pediatric Patients

MRI is a particularly attractive option for pediatric patients given the lack of ionizing radiation. However, there are unique safety issues associated with MRI of pediatric patients, in addition to the previously discussed risks that apply to children and adults alike. These risks are due to the fact that pediatric patients are often unable to follow instructions and remain still in the bore. Under these circumstances, the patient may require sedation and/or an accompanying family member.

Recently, there has been increasing attention to the possibility that anesthetics may have consequences in terms of cognitive development in addition to the well-known risks of cardiac and respiratory drive suppression associated with anesthesia. For those patients who may be able to obtain a CT without sedation but for whom an MRI would require sedation, the risk of CT with ionizing radiation versus MRI with anesthesia must be considered; however, this calculus is not well understood and comparing risks and benefits in this situation is challenging. For those patients requiring anesthesia regardless, the consideration is then based on diagnostic accuracy of the two modalities for the specific clinical question and is a much easier, more understandable calculus for most radiologists.

With some pediatric patients, there is an additional alternative. Although many patients may not be able to tolerate a routine examination taking anywhere from 20 to 60 minutes or longer, even young children may be able to tolerate a short examination, for example, 5 minutes. Many strategies exist in this situation; deciding on a strategy requires taking into consideration the clinical question, having an understanding of the MR sequences needed to answer the clinical question, potentially modifying the imaging protocol, and developing strategies that might allow the patient to understand and cope with the MR environment. In pediatric hospitals, a child life specialist, someone who specializes in understanding child development and is trained to help children navigate the medical environment, can help prepare the child for the MRI scan. This involves making sure the child understands, at an age-appropriate level, what to anticipate when he or she enters the MRI. This can be facilitated with pictures and familiarizing the child with the noises of the MRI environment (with apps now available to help with this process). Even in hospitals without child life specialists, the technologists can work with children to show them the MRI scanner ahead of time and let the children see what the environment is like so it does not seem as frightening. For those institutions that have the ability, functional MRI equipment can be used to show a child a movie, which can help decrease patient movement. At the very least, most institutions are able to play music for children, which can also be calming.

Once the child is in the MR environment, obtaining the minimum number of sequences as fast as possible can also facilitate MR scan acquisition. For example, a number of articles have been published on the use of a single-shot T2 technique (a 30- to 45-second sequence) in the evaluation of patients with ventriculostomy catheters to assess the size of the extraaxial spaces. Most MRI scanner vendors have additional sequences that can be obtained rapidly (in 1 minute or less). Use of a PROPELLER (periodically rotated overlapping parallel lines with enhanced reconstruction) sequence (also known as a BLADE or MultiVane sequence) involves a radial sampling method that acquires images through k-space using rotary acquisition, thereby oversampling the center of k-space (signal amplitude and image contrast) and undersampling the periphery of k-space (high spatial frequency information). Although this method provides a way to compensate for patient motion, it usually takes 50% longer to acquire. Thus, although it helps with motion compensation, if the goal is to reduce scan length, this method is less useful.

Finally, although the diagnostic benefit of intravenous gadolinium contrast needs to be considered in each patient, in unsedated children, the difference between a high-quality acquisition and one with significant motion degradation can hinge on whether intravenous contrast is administered. Children can respond more adversely to needles and intravenous line placement than adults, and while a child may be able to tolerate a noncontrast MRI scan, there can be significant motion degradation if the child starts crying after intravenous contrast is administered.

Unconscious or Incapacitated Patients

MRI is an important diagnostic tool in the evaluation of patients, even those who are unconscious or unresponsive. However, this patient population creates new challenges in the screening, monitoring, and performance of an MRI examination.

If an MRI is deemed clinically necessary and cannot wait until a reliable screening history can be obtained, then an evaluation must be performed to determine if a foreign object exists that might preclude an MRI examination or at the very least may require further investigation. To this end, an institution may consider evaluating the patient with imaging and/or a clinical evaluation. The clinical evaluation consists of identifying any scars or deformities on a patient that might indicate an implant and would then require additional radiographs or CT images. At the very least, images (either radiographs or CT) through the orbits/head and chest should be obtained. Additional images through the neck and/or abdomen/pelvis should also be considered (some institutions require these additional films whereas others rely on a clinical evaluation of the patient). If this evaluation is negative, it is still recommended that the patient be imaged at 1.5 T or less. Some devices may not be identified on the clinical or imaging evaluation but could still be present in the patient. Devices that may go unrecognized are almost certainly MR safe or MR conditionally safe at 1.5 T but may not be MR conditionally safe at higher magnetic strengths.

Some objects that are infrequently related to burns (e.g., a tattoo or implanted foreign object) are easily monitored in the conscious patient who can communicate if he or she begins to experience any symptoms related to these objects and then be removed from the MRI environment. However, in an unconscious patient who is noncommunicative, this becomes more problematic. For objects that are recognized, such as a tattoo, a cold cloth can be placed on top prophylactically. Additionally, the patient's vitals can be monitored during the MRI scan to provide an additional safeguard. But despite these precautions, a small risk does remain, which is why the benefits/risks of the procedure must be assessed. Finally, during the MRI examination, monitoring equipment also becomes a concern, because the equipment must be MR safe or MR conditionally safe, with attention to minimizing complications by ensuring that no loops are created (with leads and by using appropriate cushions).

MAGNETIC RESONANCE QUALITY ASSURANCE

Although quality assurance (QA) is important in all aspects of radiology, it is especially important in performing a high-quality MRI examination. The nature of the equipment and physics of MRI result in innumerable variables that need to be evaluated and optimized. There are many levels where quality needs to be assessed, from the purchase and installation of MRI equipment, design and implementation of MRI protocols, training of MRI technologists, to continued maintenance of the equipment and execution of the imaging studies. Although general QA and quality control (QC) procedures in radiology can be applied to MRI, this section focuses on issues that are specific to MRI.

A number of people are involved in the QA and QC procedures needed to ensure adequate quality in MRI, including the radiologist, technologist, and medical physicist, as well as application specialists and engineers from the MRI scanner vendor. Each has an important role in maintaining the integrity of the MRI system and ensuring that appropriate image quality is obtained.

Quality Control in Magnetic Resonance Imaging

Both the radiologist and technologist must be ever vigilant in assessing the quality of each imaging sequence and study. But while some changes in quality may be abrupt and thus noticeable early, other issues may be subtle or gradual and may require QC testing to be detected. It is important for every interpreting radiologist to ensure that established imaging protocols are followed and to follow established procedures when images are of poor quality (to notify the supervising technologist or radiologist that a problem is detected and whether a patient may need to return for additional images).

QC testing begins with frequent (daily or weekly) testing of a number of parameters by a designated QC technologist(s) using an MRI phantom, including table position accuracy, center frequency, transmitter gain or attenuation, geometric accuracy, high-contrast spatial resolution, low-contrast detectability, and artifact evaluation, as well as QC of any film printer, if applicable.

Center frequency refers to the resonance frequency that corresponds to the magnetic strength of the MRI system, as given by the Larmor equation (63.87 for a 1.5-T MRI scanner; 127.74 for a 3-T MRI scanner); any drift may require the service engineer to evaluate the MRI system. Transmitter gain or attenuation is a measure of the power needed to nutate the bulk magnetization by 90 degrees, and issues detected raise concern for a problem in the RF transmitter and/or its associated coils, including problems in the RF transmission field, degradation of the B0 magnetic field homogeneity, and noise generated by the receiver chain electronics.

Geometric accuracy assesses any potential distortion that occurs as a result of displacement of a displayed point within an image or improper scaling of the distance between two points. Most modern-day scanners should achieve less than ±1% geometric distortion, which corresponds to a diameter measurement of ±2 mm and a length measurement of ±1.5 mm. Geometric distortions can result from gradient amplifiers that have been powered down and have not been adequately warmed up; sequences with low bandwidth, which accentuates B0 inhomogeneities; and a number of factors that lead to B0 field inhomogeneity: gradient offsets, passive and/or active magnet shims, and ferromagnetic objects in the magnetic bore.

High-contrast spatial resolution can be impaired by a number of factors including inappropriate filtering of the MRI signal, poor eddy current compensation (must be resolved by a service engineer), geometric errors (as described earlier), and gradient power supply instability. Low-contrast detectability depends on accurate positioning and adequate signal to noise. Finally, a number of common imaging artifacts can be evaluated on the phantom including gross geometric distortion, ghost images, receiver saturation errors, image blurring, truncation artifacts, as well as unusually high or low intensities of the lines or pixels that make up the phantom. These MRI artifacts are discussed in more detail in the next sections.

In addition to frequent QC performed by the technologist, a medical physicist or MR scientist should perform additional QC procedures annually, including assessment of magnetic field homogeneity, slice position accuracy, slice thickness accuracy, and RF coil checks (including evaluation of the signal-to-noise ratio [SNR], percent image uniformity, and percent signal ghosting). The magnetic field is prone to inhomogeneities, which result from a number of factors including imperfections in the magnet manufacturing, external ferromagnetic structures, and the presence of a patient in the field (which can be compensated for by shimming and/or gradient coils). These inhomogeneities can result in geometrical distortions, nonuniformity of signal, incomplete fat suppression, severity of wrap artifacts, and decreased SNR in some imaging sequences acquired rapidly. Slice position and thickness accuracy tests whether the acquired slices differ from the prescribed location and thickness, because this can result in failure to obtain the intended image and can affect image contrast and SNR. The RF coils used in MRI are designed to maximize image uniformity and enhance SNR but, given their constant movement and use, require periodic assessment to determine that they are functioning appropriately.

Quality Improvement in Magnetic Resonance Imaging

Although it is important to have a QC process in place to ensure that the MRI scanner and equipment are functioning properly, it is also important to both improve and monitor image quality. MRI scanners are constantly improving; new sequences are added each year and improvements are made to older sequences. These improvements can boost image quality (in terms of image contrast, SNR, resolution, decreased artifacts, etc.) as well as increase the efficiency of scan acquisition. Thus, it is important to work with the scanner vendor and their application specialists to implement new and improved sequences as they become available. This means that old protocols must be updated periodically and radiologists must learn how to interpret the new sequences as they are introduced.

In addition to implementing new and improved sequences as they become available, it is also important to monitor the quality of sequences that have already been implemented. Although it is important to understand MRI

artifacts (discussed in the next section), it is just as important to identify when a sequence does not appear as expected. Because there are numerous artifacts in MRI, some of which are not easily understood, identification becomes the starting point for troubleshooting. Although this starts in the radiology department with the radiologist, technologist, and/or medical physicist, it frequently requires involvement of the service engineer and application specialists but may need to be elevated to the MRI vendor.

Some artifacts only affect certain sequences (e.g., diffusion-weighted imaging), whereas others might affect all sequences. Some artifacts can be easy to troubleshoot and are frequently corrected at the scanner by the technologist. For example, the technologist may recognize that an error was made in truncating the nose resulting in a wrap artifact. If the sequence is repeated, the staff may not send the sequence with the artifact to the picture archiving and communication system, and the radiologist will not realize that there was a sequence with an artifact. Other artifacts may be identified, but despite numerous people being involved in troubleshooting, it can take a long time to identify the source of the problem. For example, at our institution, we identified a zipper artifact on images, but it was only after a long period of time that we recognized that the artifact was being produced by an incompatible battery in a cardiac pump in the MRI scan room. Thus, not only the MRI scanner itself but also any equipment in the room needs to be assessed for potential interference with the MR scan acquisition.

Finally, when interpreting images, it is important to be vigilant in scanning parameters and differences in scan acquisition. These are not strictly noninterpretive skills.

Errors can also occur if a sequence is not set up correctly. For example, it is common to allow the TR of a T1 sequence to vary. This is because as the TR increases, more slices can be acquired, which may allow better coverage. But as the TR increases, so does the imaging time. Therefore, to balance acquisition time versus maximizing coverage, one can allow the TR to vary. However, if the parameters are not set up correctly, the TR can vary too much. Fig. 22.5 demonstrates a T1 image where the TR crept up to 1500 ms, which is much higher than a typical T1 sequence (TR of 600 ms, although it can vary from 500 to 800 ms). Thus, this sequence has proton density weighting.

Fig. 22.6 shows images in a patient with neurofibromatosis type 2 (NF-2) who, in addition to having a resected medulloblastoma, had an enhancing mass related to the right sphenoid wing, which is believed to represent a schwannoma. Over 2 years, this lesion has been stable in size but has waxed and waned in terms of the avidity of contrast enhancement. However, this change in enhancement corresponds to the timing of the postcontrast sequences. Therefore, although one could interpret the increase in contrast avidity as concern for tumor progression, it in fact reflects a change in the imaging parameters and on subsequent images obtained with a similar contrast injection to imaging time frame, looks unchanged.

Magnetic Resonance Imaging Artifacts

As described earlier, an understanding of MRI artifacts is essential in troubleshooting image quality. The following section is not meant to be comprehensive but rather to familiarize the reader with some of the most common artifacts encountered and ways to minimize these artifacts.

Motion Artifact

A motion artifact occurs when a structure being imaged is at different locations across spatial localization steps. Common sources of motion artifacts include blood vessel

pulsation, respiratory motion, cardiac motion, bowel peristalsis, and conscious patient motion. Periodic motion, such as blood vessel pulsation, results in ghost artifacts of moving structures propagating along the phase-encoding dimension of the image, with the intensity of the artifact dependent on the amplitude of motion and signal intensity of the moving structure (Fig. 22.7). Nonperiodic motion, such as conscious patient motion, results in image blurring. Motion artifacts may occasionally mimic pathology, as in the case of ghosting of the abdominal aorta over the left hepatic lobe, which could be confused with a liver lesion (see Fig. 22.7A).

Motion artifacts most often occur along the phase-encoding dimension of an image, because the phase-encoding gradient is turned on during the whole TR interval, whereas the frequency-encode gradient occurs as the signal is being acquired. Additionally, spatial localization along the frequency-encoding dimension occurs in a much shorter time scale as compared to physiologic motion. Conversely, spatial localization along the phase-encoding dimension occurs on the order of seconds, which is generally a longer time scale than physiologic motion.

Various measures may be taken to minimize motion artifacts. For example, conscious patient motion can sometimes be reduced by instructing the patient to remain still throughout the exam, although methods such as sedation, anesthesia, or physical restraint may be necessary for uncooperative or anxious patients. Because motion artifacts are a result of insufficient imaging speed, imaging parameters can be adjusted to decrease image acquisition time, such as using a shorter TR or longer echo train. Faster imaging techniques can also be used such as single-shot sequences and parallel imaging. For thoracic or abdominal imaging, a respiratory motion artifact can be minimized with techniques such as breath hold imaging or respiratory gating. Similarly, gating techniques are used to eliminate motion artifacts in cardiac MRI. Finally, data acquisition techniques such as PROPELLER have also been shown to reduce motion artifacts, although this acquisition takes longer than traditional imaging sequences.

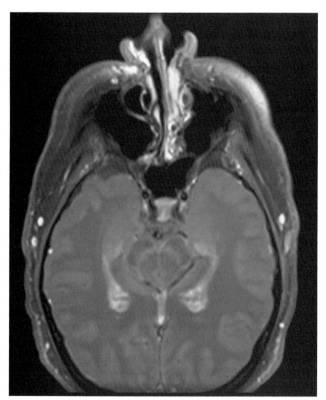

FIG. 22.5 INAPPROPRIATE IMAGING PARAMETERS. Axial image through the midbrain, which was intended to be T1-weighted, demonstrates proton density-weighted imaging features, such as hyperintense cerebrospinal signal. The time to repetition of this sequence was approximately 1500 ms.

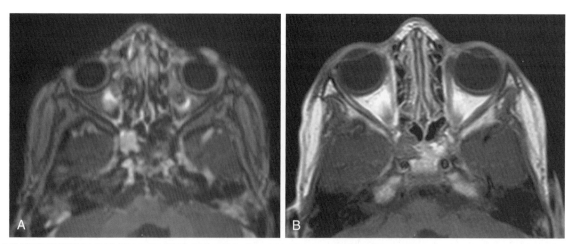

FIG. 22.6 INCONSISTENT IMAGING TIMING RELATIVE TO CONTRAST ADMINISTRATION. Axial postcontrast T1-weighted images demonstrate a variable pattern of contrast enhancement of a right sphenoid wing mass, with relatively homogeneous contrast enhancement on the (A) initial exam and a relative lack of contrast enhancement on the (B) follow-up exam, which was the result of differences in imaging timing relative to contrast administration. The differences in timing were a result of variability in whether a brain or spine magnetic resonance imaging scan was performed and whether the postcontrast spine imaging was performed before the brain magnetic resonance or afterward.

Finally, saturation bands can be placed over tissue outside the area of concern that might result in a motion artifact (e.g., a saturation band over the heart or bowel for a spine MRI). Because most of this motion artifact occurs in the phase-encoding direction, saturation bands should be placed so that they reduce motion along the phase-encoding direction; in some cases, it may be useful to place the saturation band outside the image to reduce motion artifacts that would wrap into the image (e.g., for a sagittal cervical spine MRI if the phase-encoding direction is superior-inferior, the saturation band should be placed over the esophagus, lungs, and/or heart; depending on the curvature of the spine, this might be angled along the inferior aspect of the image or be placed inferior to the field of view).

Aliasing

Aliasing (also known as the wraparound or fold-over artifact) refers to the misplacement of signal in an image due to undersampling, which occurs when the field of view is smaller than the excited slice (Fig. 22.8).

To briefly review, the field of view is determined by gradient magnetic field strength, which specifies a range of frequencies represented along a dimension of the image, and receiver bandwidth, which specifies a range of frequencies that are sampled during the application of the frequency-encode gradient. Additionally, the receiver bandwidth is inversely proportional to the sampling time. Regardless of the field of view, all protons within an excited slice generate signal that is detected by the receiver coil. If the receiver bandwidth is reduced and the field of view becomes smaller than the excited slice, there is an insufficient sampling rate to accurately represent precessional frequencies of protons peripheral to the field of view, which precess at higher frequencies because they experience a greater gradient magnetic field strength. Signal originating from outside of the field of view is undersampled, converted to a lower frequency in the Fourier transform, and misplaced in the image. Aliasing can occur in both phase and frequency directions.

Spatial locations in the frequency-encoding dimension of an image correspond to precessional frequencies along a gradient magnetic field. Accurate spatial localization requires a sufficient analog signal sampling rate to generate a representative digital signal. The Nyquist sampling theorem states that the sampling rate of an analog-to-digital converter must be at least twice the highest frequency contained in the signal to accurately reflect the native signal; a sampling rate less than the Nyquist rate will result in undersampling and cause aliasing.

Although increasing the field of view to include the entire excited slice would eliminate aliasing, it would also decrease spatial resolution, because voxel size would increase with a constant matrix size. To prevent aliasing in the frequency-encoding dimension while maintaining spatial resolution, the sampling rate can be increased, a technique known as oversampling. Because all of the samples

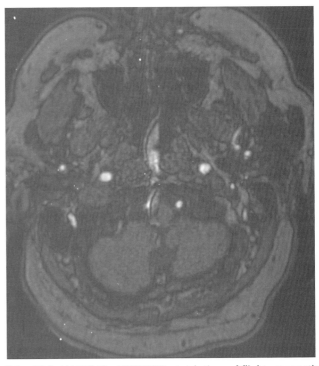

FIG. 22.8 **ALIASING ARTIFACT.** Axial time-of-flight magnetic resonance angiogram image demonstrates an aliasing artifact of the right earlobe, which was outside of the field of view. This could be misinterpreted as a vascular malformation if it is not understood as an artifact.

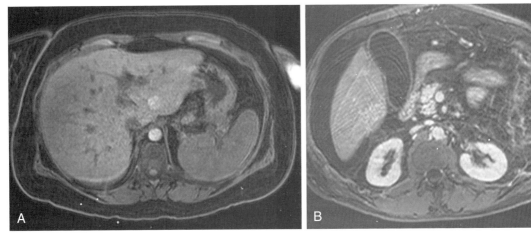

FIG. 22.7 **PERIODIC MOTION ARTIFACT.** Axial fat-saturation T1-weighted images demonstrate periodic motion artifacts along the phase-encoding dimension of the image related to (A) aortic pulsation and (B) respiratory motion.

in the frequency-encoding dimension are acquired during the sample time, oversampling in the frequency-encoding dimension does not increase imaging time (although it may decrease the SNR). Therefore, MR scanners perform oversampling by default, and aliasing is rarely problematic in the frequency-encoding dimension.

Spatial locations in the phase-encoding dimension of an image correspond to relative phase shifts ranging from −180 degrees to +180 degrees. Signal originating from outside the field of view, with a phase shift less than −180 degrees or greater than +180 degrees, is misplaced in the image by the Fourier transform. For example, signal originating from a location corresponding to a phase shift of +200 is assigned a phase shift of −160 and *wrapped around* to the opposite side of the image. As with the frequency-encoding dimension, oversampling can be performed to reduce aliasing in the phase-encoding dimension. However, because each phase-encoding step requires a new TR, oversampling in this dimension results in increased imaging time. For this reason, the phase-encoding dimension is typically selected as the shorter dimension of the image. To reduce aliasing in the phase-encoding dimension while maintaining a constant imaging time, oversampling can be performed while decreasing the number of signal averages, with only the central portion of the field of view being reconstructed. Although this technique eliminates aliasing while preserving spatial resolution, it leads to a reduction in the SNR. Finally, surface coils and presaturation bands may also be used to minimize signal detection from outside the field of view.

Chemical Shift Artifact

Chemical shift refers to the difference in precessional frequencies of protons in different tissues due to their unique molecular environment. Although the chemical shift between protons in most tissues is too small to affect an image, a significant chemical shift exists between protons in fat and other soft tissues, because fat protons have a relatively large electron cloud that shields them from the static magnetic field, causing them to precess at lower frequencies as compared to those in other soft tissue. The chemical shift between protons in fat versus other soft tissue varies with static magnetic field strength and is approximately 225 Hz at 1.5 T and 450 Hz at 3 T. The absolute chemical shift is 3.5 ppm. Because spatial location along the frequency-encoding dimension is determined by precessional frequency, signal originating from fat protons is misregistered along this dimension by a distance corresponding to the chemical shift and in a direction corresponding to the polarity of the frequency-encoding gradient magnetic field. Within large areas of uniform fatty tissue, the misregistered signal from fat is replaced with a signal from fat from the adjacent protons and therefore cannot be perceived. However, at interfaces between fat and other soft tissue, such as the kidneys and perinephric fat, the signal from fat is misregistered in relation to the soft tissue signal, which may result in a chemical shift artifact depending on the imaging parameters (Fig. 22.9). On the side of the interface with lower precessional frequencies, the signal from fat is misregistered in the direction of the soft tissue

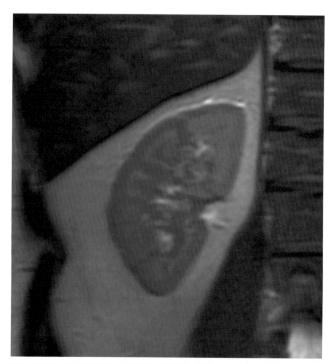

FIG. 22.9 **CHEMICAL SHIFT ARTIFACT.** Coronal T2-weighted turbo spin echo image demonstrates a chemical shift artifact propagating along the frequency-encoding dimension of the image at the kidney–perinephric fat interface.

signal, and a chemical shift artifact may appear as a thin hyperintense band along the interface. On the side of the interface with higher precessional frequencies, the signal from fat is misregistered away from the soft tissue signal, and a chemical shift artifact may appear as a thin hypointense band along the interface.

At a given static magnetic field strength, a chemical shift artifact is largely influenced by voxel size along the frequency-encoding dimension, which in turn is determined by receiver bandwidth and matrix size. If the range of frequencies represented in a single voxel is less than the chemical shift, the signal from fat is misregistered into the adjacent voxel, and a chemical shift artifact is accentuated. If the range of frequencies represented in a single voxel is greater than the chemical shift, some of the misregistered signal from fat remains in the same voxel, and the chemical shift artifact is diminished. Therefore, chemical shift artifacts can be reduced by increasing bandwidth and decreasing matrix size along the frequency-encoding dimension. Finally, chemical shift artifacts can also be reduced with fat suppression techniques or by imaging at lower static magnetic field strengths.

Susceptibility-Induced Signal Loss and Geometric Distortion

Magnetic susceptibility is introduced into the static magnetic field when a patient enters the MR scanner due to the varying magnetic properties of human tissues and any implanted device or foreign body. As discussed previously, diamagnetic substances such as calcium, cortical bone, and most other human tissues have a negative susceptibility in the presence of an external magnetic field, produce a relatively weak magnetic field in the opposite

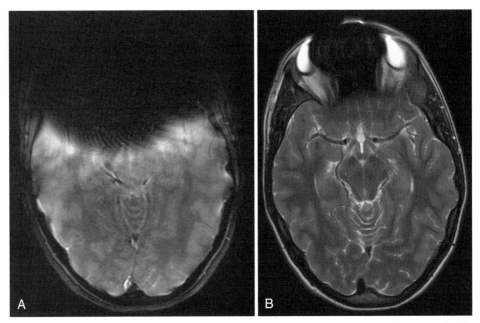

FIG. 22.10 **SUSCEPTIBILITY-INDUCED SIGNAL LOSS AND GEOMETRIC DISTORTION.** (A) Axial T2*-weighted image demonstrates a large area of susceptibility-induced signal loss related to dental hardware, which obscures the anterior portion of the head. (B) An axial T2-weighted image through the same level demonstrates a smaller area of susceptibility-induced signal loss with geometric distortion of the globes.

direction of an applied magnetic field, and slightly reduce the strength of the local magnetic field; paramagnetic substances such as air, some metallic ions, and some blood products have a relatively small positive susceptibility and produce a relatively weak magnetic field in the direction of an applied magnetic field, thereby slightly increasing the local magnetic field; and ferromagnetic substances containing iron, nickel, or cobalt, including implanted devices or foreign bodies, have a relatively large positive magnetic susceptibility and produce a relatively strong magnetic field in the direction of an applied magnetic field. Because of inhomogeneities in the static magnetic field, protons within a given volume can experience a range of static magnetic field strengths centered on B0 and therefore precess at a range of frequencies centered on the Larmor frequency. Field inhomogeneities cause protons to lose their phase coherence at a rate defined by T2*. This loss of coherence causes a loss in signal, because an echo is only formed when protons are spinning in phase. For example, hardware such as orthodontic braces may produce a large area of susceptibility-induced signal loss, with a less prominent susceptibility artifact occurring at tissue interfaces, for example, involving the skull base or paranasal sinuses (Fig. 22.10).

The severity of signal loss related to susceptibility artifacts increases with the magnitude of susceptibility, increasing static magnetic field strength and increasing echo time (TE), and decreases with receiver bandwidth. These parameters can be adjusted to increase or decrease susceptibility artifacts. For example, removing the paramagnetic object would be the easiest way to eliminate the artifact. However, if this is not possible, several techniques could be employed to decrease susceptibility, such as (1) using a spin echo sequence with a 180-degree refocusing pulse, which will rephase spins and help overcome susceptibility, (2) using a short TE, which allows less time for

dephasing to occur, and thus reduces signal loss, or (3) using a long echo train with multiple 180-degree refocusing pulses, which will also help overcome dephasing. Finally, imaging at a lower static magnetic field strength or using a broader bandwidth may be useful in minimizing susceptibility artifacts. Conversely, a gradient echo sequence can be used to accentuate dephasing and facilitate the detection of small amounts of blood products or calcification.

Gibbs Artifact

The Gibbs artifact (also known as the truncation or ring artifact) is a form of undersampling related to edge definition, which appears as multiple thin lines of alternating signal intensity parallel to a high-contrast interface. In contrast to periodic motion artifacts, the Gibbs artifact trails off over a short distance from an interface rather than propagating along the entire dimension of an image. The Gibbs artifact may also cause blurring, widening, and distortion of high-contrast interfaces, as well as distortion of the adjacent tissues. An edge in an MR image is characterized by an instantaneous change in signal intensity along one dimension at the interface between two tissues with different signal characteristics. Therefore, an infinite sampling rate would be necessary to accurately define an edge. Because the Fourier transform uses a finite number of spatial localization steps, the signal is truncated, or undersampled, and misplaced in the image. Gibbs artifacts are sometimes problematic in spinal imaging where there is a high-contrast boundary between the cerebrospinal fluid and the spinal cord, with an increased signal from the cerebrospinal fluid overlying the spinal cord, where it may mimic a syrinx (Fig. 22.11).

As with aliasing, Gibbs artifacts can be minimized by increasing the number of spatial localization steps, or oversampling, which results in improved edge

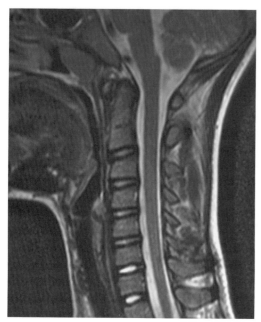

FIG. 22.11 **GIBBS ARTIFACT.** Sagittal T2-weighted image of the cervical spine demonstrates a linear hyperintense signal parallel to the cerebrospinal fluid–spinal cord interface, compatible with a Gibbs artifact.

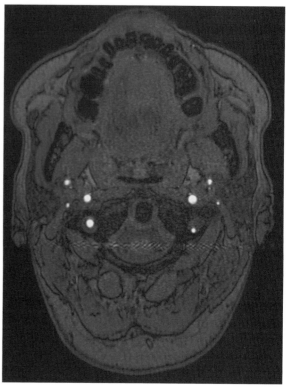

FIG. 22.12 **ZIPPER ARTIFACT.** Axial time-of-flight magnetic resonance angiogram image demonstrates a thin linear band of heterogeneous signal along the phase-encoding dimension of the image known as a zipper artifact.

definition. Additionally, because Gibbs artifacts are a result of undersampling and are more problematic in the phase-encoding dimension, because oversampling in this dimension is not routinely performed due to an increased imaging time. In addition to increasing spatial resolution, correction techniques such as Gegenbauer reconstruction or extrapolation methods may be used to recover data that have been truncated. Finally, fat-suppression techniques can effectively reduce Gibbs artifacts at interfaces involving fat.

Zipper Artifact

The zipper artifact (also known as the RF leak artifact) occurs when RF energy from sources extrinsic to the patient is detected by the receiver coil. Electronic equipment such as radios, computers, mobile devices, monitoring equipment, and faulty light bulbs may emit RF waves within the bandwidth of the receiver coil. MR scanner rooms are therefore shielded from outside RF energy by a Faraday cage, which consists of a wall of electrically continuous, grounded, conductive material surrounding the room. Additionally, cables, pipes, and other structures entering the room pass through penetration panels, which filter RF energy from their current. If the Faraday cage or penetration panels fail, or if the door is left open to the MR scanner room, RF noise may be detected by the receiver coil and incorporated into the image. Zipper artifacts may also be caused by electronic equipment inside the MR scanner room, such as pulse oximeters or faulty light bulbs. Narrowband RF energy appears as a linear band of alternating signal intensity in the phase-encoding dimension at a specific frequency corresponding the contaminating RF energy (Fig. 22.12). Conversely, broadband RF energy appears as a diffuse increase in image noise. Zipper artifacts may also occur in the frequency-encoding

dimension, typically as the result of computing issues and inadequate RF transmission. Eliminating zipper artifacts often requires servicing of the Faraday cage, MR scanner, and evaluating equipment in the MRI scanner room.

Corduroy Artifact

Corduroy artifacts (also known as herringbone or spike artifacts) occur when there is one or more aberrant data points in k-space. For example, a data point may have an abnormally high signal amplitude as a result of an electrical discharge during data acquisition. Because each point in k-space contains information related to all spatial locations in the image, the corduroy artifact is uniformly propagated throughout the image, typically as a series of obliquely oriented bands of alternating signal intensity. If the artifact compromises the diagnostic quality of the exam, the exam is usually repeated, because k-space corruption is the result of uncommon, randomly occurring events. However, special software can also be used to eliminate the aberrant k-space data points, and the image can then be reconstructed.

Cross-Talk and Cross-Excitation Artifact

The cross-excitation artifact occurs as a result of an imperfect frequency profile of RF pulses, which does not stimulate a single slice homogeneously and without affecting adjacent tissue but rather with potentially overlapping side lobes. If adjacent slices are sequentially excited during a single TR, protons in the overlapping tissue of the second slice are saturated at their

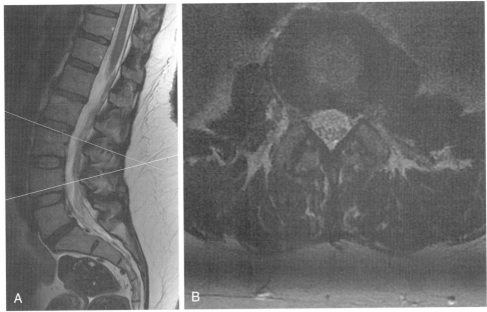

FIG. 22.13 **CROSS-TALK ARTIFACT.** (A) Sagittal T2-weighted image of the lumbar spine demonstrates intersecting slices resulting in a cross-talk artifact, which is seen in the axial plane as a horizontal band of hypointense signal in the paraspinal soft tissues at the level of slice intersection (B).

TE, which will manifest as an area of low signal on the image; this is known as cross excitation (Fig. 22.13). As excited nuclei start to relax back to equilibrium after the application of the RF pulse, their energy can dissipate to nuclei in the adjacent slice, thereby affecting the signal and contrast in that slice; this is known as cross excitation. In multiangle acquisitions, intersection of slices that are not parallel may also lead to saturation of protons in overlapping tissue, which manifests as a cross-talk artifact.

To prevent cross-excitation artifacts, interleaved image acquisition can be performed, in which odd-numbered slices are imaged, followed by even-numbered slices or vice versa, allowing protons in the overlapping tissue enough time to recover their longitudinal relaxation between acquisitions. Slices can also be spaced slightly apart such that their side lobes do not overlap (with modern-day scanners, 10% of the slice thickness is usually sufficient). Cross-talk artifacts frequently occur outside of the area of interest and thus may not be problematic for the diagnostic test. When necessary, to prevent cross-talk artifacts, angled stacks of images can be acquired separately or angulation can be removed.

CONCLUSION

Although MR safety and QA are noninterpretive skills vital to the proper performance of MRI, they also influence the interpretation of MRI, and the knowledge needed to perform each of these different pieces overlaps significantly. For example, a solid understanding of MRI artifacts influences both the interpretation of MRI as well as the QA processes that should be implemented. Thus, these noninterpretive skills are vital to the proper interpretation of MRI.

SUGGESTED READINGS

Ahmed S, Shellock FG. Magnetic resonance imaging safety: implications for cardiovascular patients. *J Cardiovasc Magn Reson*. 2001;3(3):171–182.

American College of Radiology. *Magnetic Resonance Imaging Quality Control Manual*. Reston, VA: American College of Radiology; 2015.

Bushberg JT, Seibert JA, Leidholdt EM, Boone JM. *The Essential Physics of Medical Imaging*. 3rd ed. Philadelphia, PA: Lippincott Williams & Wilkins; 2012.

Chaljub G, Kramer LA, Johnson RF, Johnson RF, Singh H, Crow WN. Projectile cylinder accidents resulting from the presence of ferromagnetic nitrous oxide or oxygen tanks in the MR suite. *AJR Am J Roetgenol*. 2001;177:27–30.

Coskun O. Magnetic resonance imaging and safety aspects. *Toxicol Ind Health*. 2011;27(4):307–313.

Dill T. Contraindications to magnetic resonance imaging. *Heart*. 2007;94:943–948.

Hardy PT, Weil KM. A review of thermal MR injuries. *Radiol Technol*. 2010;81:606–609.

Huang SY, Seethamraju RT, Patel P, et al. Body MR imaging: artifacts, k-space, and solutions. *Radiographics*. 2015;35:1439–1460.

Joint Commission on Accreditation of Healthcare Organizations. USA. Preventing accidents and injuries in the MRI suite. *Sentinel Event Alert*. 2008;14(38):1–3.

Kanal E, Barkovich AJ, Bell C, et al. ACR guidance document on MR safe practices. *J Magn Reson Imaging*. 2013;2013(37):501–530.

Lipton ML. *Totally Accessible MRI: A User's Guide to Principles, Technology, and Applications*. New York, NY: Springer Science & Business Media; 2008.

McJury M, Shellock FG. Auditory noise associated with MR procedures: a review. *J Magn Reson Imaging*. 2000;12(1):37–45.

Morelli JN, Runge VM, Ai F, et al. An image-based approach to understanding the physics of MR artifacts. *Radiographics*. 2011;31(3):849–866.

Schaefer DJ, Bourland JD, Nyenhuis JA. Review of patient safety in time-varying gradient fields. *J Magn Reson Imaging*. 2000;12(1):20–29.

Schenck JF. Safety of strong, static magnetic fields. *J Magn Reson Imaging*. 2000;12(1):2–19.

Shellock FG. Biomedical implants and devices: assessment of magnetic field interactions with a 3.0-tesla MR system. *J Magn Reson Imaging*. 2002;16:721–732.

Shellock FG, Crues JV. MR procedures: biologic effects, safety, and patient care. *Radiology*. 2004;232(3):635–652.

Shellock FJ. Radiofrequency energy-induced heating during MR procedures: a review. *J Magn Reson Imaging*. 2000;12(1):30–36.

Stecco A, Saponaro A, Carriero A. Patient safety issues in magnetic resonance imaging: state of the art. *Radiol Med*. 2007;112(4):491–508.

Tremblay E, Thérasse E, Thomassin-Naggara I, Trop I. Guidelines for use of medical imaging during pregnancy and lactation. *Radiographics*. 2012;32(3):897–911.

Tsai LL, Grant AK, Mortele KJ, Kung JW, Smith MP. A practical guide to MR imaging safety: what radiologists need to know. *Radiographics*. 2015;35:1722–1737.

Wang PI, Chong ST, Kielar AZ, et al. Imaging of pregnant and lactating patients: part 1, evidence-based review and recommendations. *AJR Am J Roentgenol*. 2012;198(4):778–784.

Zhuo J, Gullapalli RP. AAPM/RSNA physics tutorial for residents: MR artifacts, safety, and quality control. *Radiographics*. 2006;26:275–297.

Chapter 23

Optimizing Radiation Dose for Computed Tomography

Atul M. Padole and Mannudeep K. Kalra

EVOLUTION OF COMPUTED TOMOGRAPHY TECHNOLOGY

Computed tomography (CT) plays a major role in the practice of medicine. CT was invented by the British scientist Sir Godfrey Hounsfield in 1972 at Electric and Musical Industries research laboratories. Since its invention, CT has evolved rapidly and transformed the field of medicine. The first CT scanners were dedicated to acquiring head images. With development of subsequent scanners, it became possible to acquire images of other parts of the body. The first-generation scanners were *axial* (or step and shoot) CT scanners with a pencil x-ray beam (with a single or double row of detectors). These early axial CT scanners required around 5 minutes for acquisition of a single slice with reconstruction time of about 1.5 minutes per slice.

The second-generation axial CT, with a fan x-ray beam, took around 20 seconds for acquisition of a single slice. The first- and second-generation CT scanners used complex translation and rotation motion of the x-ray tube and detector elements for acquisition of images, which limited their scanning speed. Subsequent research in CT technology led to development of the fourth-generation axial CT (with a wider fan x-ray beam) in the early to mid-1970s. For axial scanning, the x-ray tube revolves 360 degrees around the patient in one direction to acquire a single slice, then the gantry table moves forward and the x-ray tube revolves 360 degrees around the patient in the opposite direction to acquire a second slice.

There were several limitations of the first- and second-generation axial CT scanners, including long scan times, inability to generate volumetric datasets, and inferior spatial and temporal resolution. In 1989, invention of slip-ring technology allowed continuous gantry (x-ray tube and detector array) rotation while the gantry table moved through the rotating gantry for acquisition of volumetric data. This slip-ring technology gave birth to continuous *spiral* or *helical* CT scanning, which helped overcome several limitations of axial CT. Helical CT scanning revolutionized the field of CT. With helical scanning, the entire chest or abdomen could be scanned within 20 to 30 seconds. Also, volumetric data acquisitions in helical scanning enabled generation of three-dimensional images for visualization of complex anatomic structures such as the heart, blood vessels, and fractures.

The first helical CT scanners were single-detector-row CT (SDCT) scanners in which a single detector row was placed along the patient's length or z-axis. Due to limitations of the single detector row along the z-axis, SDCT scanners were not able to efficiently use the entire fan x-ray beam. Spatial (slice thickness about 1 mm) and temporal (speed) resolution of SDCT were also limited. With the advancement of CT technology, multidetector row CT (MDCT) scanners were introduced to maximize the use of the fan x-ray beam. In 1992, the first MDCT scanners with dual-slice capabilities (with two detector rows) were introduced. Four-slice MDCT scanners were introduced in 1997, 64-slice scanners in 2004, and 320-slice scanners in 2007.

Due to an increase in the number of detector rows along the z-axis, a wider area (up to 16 cm) can be scanned in a single rotation within a fraction of a second. Modern MDCT scanners can complete a single x-ray tube revolution in as little as 0.25 seconds. Use of thinner detector elements led to improvement in the spatial resolution of MDCT, which can now generate a slice thickness of 0.5 mm through the entire volume of a scanned body region. The current MDCT scanners are also extremely dose efficient and capable of using up to 98% of the x-ray beam per rotation to generate CT images. The latter has enabled a substantial radiation dose reduction in recent years. Not unintentionally, advancements in MDCT capabilities have been associated with development of dose reduction technologies such as automatic exposure control (AEC), automatic kilovoltage selection, prepatient beam collimation, and iterative reconstruction techniques (IRTs).

With changes in CT technologies, substantial growth in the use of CT was reported. For each individual in the United States, the annual effective dose from medical imaging (mostly from CT) increased from 3.6 mSv in 1980 to 6.2 mSv in 2006. The increased radiation dose contribution from medical imaging was accompanied by evidence of large variations in scanning preferences and radiation doses for the same body regions in similarly sized patients across different hospitals in the United States. CT radiation dose optimization is vital to ensure that the radiation dose to each patient is as low as reasonably achievable (ALARA). This chapter discusses how various CT protocols can be tailored for radiation dose optimization based on the appropriateness or clinical indication for the exam and the patient's body region, age, and size.

APPROPRIATENESS OF COMPUTED TOMOGRAPHY

A major step in optimizing CT radiation dose is making sure that all CT exams are performed for appropriate clinical reasons. CT exams that are ordered based on clinical indication have a higher likelihood of providing information regarding a diagnosis (or disease process). However, if such information can be obtained from other low-radiation (plain radiograph) or nonradiation (ultrasound and magnetic resonance imaging [MRI]) imaging tests without compromising the clinical care of the patient, then CT should not be performed.

It is very important to avoid duplicate CT exams, which can substantially reduce radiation dose. The radiation dose information for all exams should be maintained and audited. There are various guideline resources and tools (websites, software) available for assessing the appropriateness of CT. Several clinical decision support (CDS) software systems are available to check the appropriateness of ordering CT. Overall, the appropriateness criteria for CT can avoid unnecessary CT exams and help reduce radiation dose imaging costs. Avoiding unnecessary exams can also reduce the anxiety among patients due to incidental findings of uncertain significance and avoid adverse effects due to contrast media.

Guidelines for use of CT scanning have been developed by several organizations including the American College of Radiology (ACR) Appropriateness Criteria, the European Commission Referral Guidelines for Imaging, the Royal College of Radiologists radiological investigation guidelines tool, and the Royal College of Radiologists of Australia, and New Zealand Diagnostic Imaging Pathways. Many other institutions and private organizations have also provided guidelines for appropriateness of CT and other imaging tests. The ACR Appropriateness Criteria help ordering physicians to choose the best imaging test for a given clinical indication. It provides a rating on a scale of 1 to 9 (where score 1 is the least useful imaging test and score 9 is most likely useful for a given clinical indication). It also provides the relative radiation level of an imaging test to help determine the benefit of the test (from the score) against its radiation level. The European Commission also provides comprehensive referral guidelines for physicians for imaging modalities. In the United Kingdom, the Royal College of Radiologists tool helps physicians determine the best available practices involving imaging tests for patient referral. In Australia, the Diagnostic Imaging Pathways tool provides guidelines for different organs or systems based on disorders and clinical features.

The various online software and CDS systems, such as radiology order entry, help physicians order imaging studies. Some decision support systems follow the ACR Appropriateness Criteria guidelines while others include input from the subspecialty physicians and radiologists. At Massachusetts General Hospital, the CDS system displays all available imaging studies (radiograph, ultrasound, CT, MRI, fluoroscopy, and nuclear medicine) to the ordering physician. In the system, the ordering physician logs in, enters the patient's medical record number, and selects the particular imaging test (such as CT head) based on the patient's clinical findings (such as headache, Fig. 23.1A). The system then requests more specific information regarding the imaging test and signs and symptoms (type of headache, such as cough headache, and sinusitis, see Fig. 23.1B and C). Based on the chosen imaging tests and clinical findings, the system provides scores from 1 to 3 (low utility), 4 to 6 (intermediate utility), and 7 to 9 (high utility) along with the expected usefulness in providing relevant information (see

Fig. 23.1D). The system provides alternate imaging studies with their utility scores so that if appropriate, the ordering physician can change and select an imaging test with a higher utility score (see Fig. 23.1D). If two imaging tests (such as chest radiograph and CT) receive similar scores, the ordering physician can consider ordering an inexpensive exam or an exam with a lower radiation dose, such as a chest radiograph instead of a chest CT first, unless that test has already failed to clarify the clinical picture.

The system also alerts physicians and radiologists to the patient's prior imaging studies to avoid ordering duplicate or redundant examinations. The systems also provide a radiation alert message if there are prior radiation-based tests for the patient. The radiation alert message informs the physician about the need to perform CT only when essential and limit the exposed area to the minimum required for diagnosis. When possible, outside imaging studies should be obtained if they can help avoid a new study.

Prior publications have reported the effect of implementation of appropriateness-based CDS systems. Sistrom et al. analyzed the effect of a CDS system (or radiology order entry) on the growth of outpatient imaging studies and reported a significant decrease in outpatient CT and ultrasound exams following implementation of the CDS. Raja et al. analyzed the effect of a CDS system on the use and yield of CT pulmonary angiography in the emergency department and reported a significant decrease in use and increase in yield of CT for assessment of acute pulmonary embolism. Dunne et al. reported similar findings in an inpatient population with use of a CDS system associated with decreased (12%) use of CT pulmonary angiography.

The Radiation Protection of Patients website of the International Atomic Energy Agency has outlined 10 guidelines related to appropriate referrals for CT:

1. Avoid unnecessary imaging examinations.
2. Discuss the choice of imaging test with radiologists to strengthen the justification process.
3. Discuss the benefits and risks of the examinations with patients.
4. Use appropriateness criteria and referral guidelines in daily practice.
5. Consult the radiologist or medical physicist and seek information about guidelines for referring medical practitioners.
6. Be careful to avoid inappropriate pediatric examinations because pediatric tissues are more sensitive to radiation, and they have a longer lifespan over which cancer effects may be expressed.
7. The number of CT scans, especially in children, must be decreased to make use of CT safer.
8. Before imaging tests, always ask if women of childbearing potential could be pregnant.
9. If CT is not indicated, then discuss the reasons for not performing the examination with the patient if the patient asks.
10. Always look for similar prior exams performed in patients to avoid needless repeat scanning.

STRATIFICATION OF COMPUTED TOMOGRAPHY PROTOCOLS

Body regions (head, chest, abdomen, etc.) are anatomically different, and therefore require different CT radiation

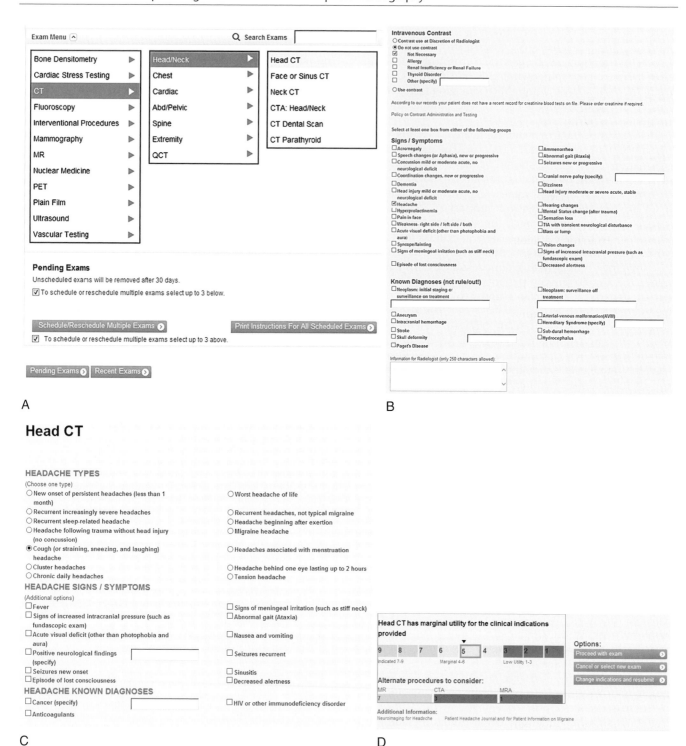

FIG. 23.1 Radiology order entry for ordering computed tomography (CT) scans at Massachusetts General Hospital. After logging in, the physician selects the desired imaging procedure for the patient and then selects the clinical reason. The decision support system provides feedback for the appropriateness of the requested examination for specified clinical indication on a 9-point scale.

doses. For all body regions, CT protocols should be named, dated, and archived on scanners. Modification or adjustment of protocols can be done at the time the CT exam is performed. However, spontaneous or *on the fly* creation of protocols is not optimal because valuable time can be wasted for urgent CT and not all operators have similar levels of training and understanding, which can result in errors. It is difficult to achieve consistency in protocols if they are created on the fly, which can make it harder to assess radiation doses for different clinical indications and patient sizes.

When creating scan protocols, one should make sure that all scan protocols have specific clinical indications for their use. First, body region–specific protocols should be created based on clinical indications. Each protocol (except for head CT) can be then subdivided based on patient size or weight, although with use of AEC techniques and automatic kilovoltage selection techniques, modern scanners can automatically optimize radiation dose and achieve a specified image quality according to body habitus determined from the planning radiographs.

These automatic techniques need modifications for very small or very large body habitus and for different clinical indications. Next, each scan protocol must have specific guidelines on the number of scan phases, scan range for each phase, and scan parameters for each phase, based on patient size or weight. The following sections present key scanning aspects of CT protocols based on body region.

HEAD COMPUTED TOMOGRAPHY

The head is one of the most frequently scanned body regions. Brain MRI has replaced head CT for several clinical indications, although the head CT is still used quite frequently for evaluation of trauma and stroke. When creating head CT protocols, users must take into account distinctive aspects of the head region. The skull base is the densest bone in the body and has a tendency to cause beam hardening artifacts on CT. Versus other body regions, the head anatomy changes rapidly from the skull base to the vault. Subtle differences between attenuation of gray and white matter in the brain lead to extremely low contrast in CT images, which may be adversely affected by the presence of high image noise on inadvertently low radiation dose images. Certain head CT exams for evaluation of paranasal sinuses, craniostenosis, and ventricular shunt patency can be performed at substantially reduced doses due to relatively high tissue contrast. Other head CT, such as for stroke and CT angiography of head and/or neck, require relatively higher doses. When appropriate and possible, brain MRI should be acquired.

Pediatric head CT should be acquired at a reduced radiation dose compared to adult head CT. When creating protocols, one should make sure that head CT doses are well under the recommended regional or national reference dose levels (RDLs). The ACR recommends an RDL of 75 mGy and an achievable dose level of 57 mGy for adult head CT (both values represent CT dose index volume [CTDIvol] using a 16-cm phantom size). The corresponding recommended levels for pediatric head CT examinations are 40 and 31 mGy, respectively. The RDL implies that 75% of the surveyed institutions use a radiation dose below the specified dose level, whereas achievable doses represent a dose limit for 50% of the surveyed institutions.

Routine Head Computed Tomography

Common indications for performing routine head CT include acute head trauma, suspected intracranial hemorrhage, and altered neurologic or mental status. Routine head CT can be performed with axial scanning mode (with gantry tilt) or helical scanning mode (without gantry tilt). Helical scanning is fast and can generate multiplanar images with diagnostic image quality at CTDIvol of 45 to 60 mGy. However, helical scanning can lead to higher eye dose. Some studies report that eye doses from helical CT are greater than tilted axial scanning of the head. A gantry tilt is also not possible with helical scanning. However, axial scanning is slow and has higher chances of motion artifacts. Many hospitals prefer axial scanning over helical CT, although at Massachusetts General Hospital, routine head CT is performed with the helical acquisition technique. Prior studies have suggested that image quality of narrow collimated helical CT is similar to that of wide collimated axial CT.

When using helical mode for head CT scanning, an overlapping pitch (~0.5:1) should be used to decrease artifacts from rapidly changing anatomy, particularly at the skull base. Also, narrow beam collimation should be used to decrease the radiation dose from overranging at the beginning and end of the helical mode. Motion artifacts can be minimized with faster gantry rotation speed. For uncooperative patients, faster scanning is preferred. It is important to ensure that the head is well positioned and isocentered. Scan length should be targeted on the region of interest.

As stated earlier, routine head CT can be performed with fixed milliamperage or AEC techniques. Because brain parenchyma has lower inherent tissue contrast, a comparatively higher tube current is often needed for scanning. Prior studies have reported the potential for substantial dose reduction for head CT with fixed milliamperage and with AEC techniques. Application of IRTs decrease image noise and artifacts and allow scanning at lower tube current compared to the conventional filtered backprojection (FBP) method of image reconstruction.

Typically, routine adult head CT is performed at 120 kV. Only essential or minimum scan series should be acquired. Lower doses should be used for acquisition of localizer radiographs. Scanning of the same regions (head and temporal bone, face and sinuses) should be avoided. Extraneous hardware must be removed before scanning to avoid artifacts and improve image quality. For head CT, shielding can be used to reduce the dose to the eyes, although it may cause artifacts over orbits. Scan parameters for adult and pediatric routine head CT are summarized in Table 23.1.

Head Computed Tomography Perfusion and Angiography

The head CT perfusion protocol is often performed for evaluation of acute ischemic stroke. As a rule of thumb, CT perfusion should only be performed at 80 kV. The lower kilovoltage maximizes sensitivity for detection of iodine-based contrast agent in the brain. Lower kilovoltage (80 kV) also helps reduce the radiation dose substantially compared to higher kilovoltage (120 kV).

TABLE 23.1 Scan Parameters for Adult and Pediatric Routine Head Computed Tomography

Scan Parameters	Adult	Pediatrics
Scan coverage	Base to vault	Base to vault
Mode	Helical or axial	Helical preferred
Rotation time	1 s	0.5 s
Pitch	Overlapping (~0.5:1)	0.5:1
Table speed	Faster is better	Faster is better
Reconstruction thickness	5 mm for viewing	5 mm for viewing
Detector collimation	Narrow is more efficient	Narrow is more efficient
Kilovolts	120 kV	80–120 kV
AEC or fixed milliamperage	Either	AEC

AEC, Automatic exposure control.

CT angiography for head and neck can also benefit from use of lower kilovoltage (80–100 kV). Smaller vessels are better seen at lower kilovoltage due to higher iodine contrast, which can enable use of less injected contrast volume. Lower kilovoltage also helps reduce the radiation dose in exams that frequently requires acquisition of multiple image series in precontrast, dynamic arterial, and delayed phases. A softer reconstruction kernel should be preferred for evaluation of CT angiography to reduce the extent of image noise in thin-section images. Contrary to the routine head CT, most CT angiography examinations are performed with helical scanning to avoid venous contamination.

Optimal scan triggering techniques should be employed for all CT angiography protocols using the automatic bolus tracking technique. Poor contrast injection can lead to nondiagnostic image quality and should be avoided. It is always important to ensure that there is good intravenous (IV) access for injecting contrast. Contrast injection volume and rate should be appropriate to create good contrast-enhanced studies.

PARANASAL SINUSES COMPUTED TOMOGRAPHY

Paranasal sinuses can be scanned at a very low radiation dose due to high tissue contrast between bones and air. Prior studies have shown the radiation dose reduction potential for paranasal sinuses CT. The sinuses can be sufficiently seen at 40 to 50 mAs and 100 to 120 kV. Paranasal sinus CT performed in helical mode allows isotropic image reconstruction without the need to acquire additional series in the coronal plane.

CHEST COMPUTED TOMOGRAPHY

The reason for creating indication-based clinical chest CT protocols is that certain structures can be assessed at a lower dose (such as lung nodules), but other structures (such as mediastinal lymph nodes) need higher doses. Prior studies have reported that lung structures and lesions can be assessed at extremely low radiation dose levels (1.5–2 mGy) without affecting diagnostic confidence. Radiation dose adjustment for chest CT protocols should be based on the clinical indication and patient size. Lung cancer screening and lung nodule follow-up protocols should be the lowest dose chest CT protocols followed by routine postcontrast chest CT, postcontrast pulmonary embolism CT, and routine noncontrast chest CT (when assessing extrapulmonary findings). Table 23.2 summarizes the stratification of chest CT protocols based on clinical indications with specific instructions on acquisition of additional images and scan lengths for each protocol.

AEC techniques should be preferred over fixed tube current for acquisition of chest CT. The arms should be raised above the shoulders for acquisition of planning radiographs and chest CT because AEC dose adjustment takes into account the arm position in the planning radiographs. If the patient is unable to raise the arms above the shoulders for any reason, AEC will increase the dose because the arms increase the regional attenuation and noise. Good patient centering is essential for optimal functioning of AEC. Like AEC, automatic kilovoltage selection

can enable dose reduction for chest CT. Automatic kilovoltage selection allows the scanner to automatically pick up the optimal kilovoltage based on body habitus (planning radiograph), exam type (noncontrast, bone, standard contrast, vascular), and tube current. The scanner automatically picks up kilovoltage values and corresponding milliamperage values.

Wider beam collimation should be preferred for chest CT, because it is more dose efficient for longer scan range. For variable detector array systems, the choice depends on the need for specific slice thickness. For example, when 1-mm or thinner slices are needed on a 16-channel MDCT scanner, detector configuration of 16 × 0.75 mm should be used, whereas if only 1.5-mm or thicker slices are acceptable, it is prudent to use the detector configuration of 16 × 1.5 mm. Gantry rotation speed should be fast for chest CT to minimize motion artifacts. A pitch equal to or greater than 1:1 is generally sufficient for chest CT. Lower pitch (<1:1) can be used in large patients. Higher pitch (>1:1) and faster scan times should be used in uncooperative patients and children. Reconstruction kernels do not directly affect dose, but it is important to note that softer kernels are better for a very low-dose CT or very thin images, unless the scan is looking for diffuse lung diseases where sharper kernels may be required.

Most chest CT must be performed with one scanning phase only. For routine chest CT, a single phase pre- or postcontrast CT is sufficient. Noncontrast CT should not be performed prior to contrast-enhanced CT. It is advisable to acquire chest CT with thin slices, which can then be

TABLE 23.2   Clinical Indications and Specific Instructions for Different Chest Protocols

Protocol	Clinical Reasons	Specific Instructions
Lung cancer screening CT	High-risk individuals for early detection of cancer	Noncontrast Lung apices to bases
Lung nodule follow-up CT	Follow-up nodule without known malignancy	Noncontrast Lung apices to bases
Routine chest CT with IV contrast	Masses, infections, trauma to lungs, mediastinum, pleural	Lung apices to adrenals
Routine chest CT without IV contrast	Elevated creatinine for above, follow-up nodule (cancer patient)	Lung apices to adrenals
Diffuse lung disease CT	Sarcoid, bronchiolitis obliterans, ILD, pulmonary fibrosis	Expiratory and prone images with reduced dose Lung apices to bases
Tracheal protocol CT	Tracheal stenosis and tracheobronchomalacia	Inspiration: helical skull base to lung bases Expiration: skull base to lung hila
CT pulmonary embolism	Suspected or known PE	Lung apices to bases

CT, Computed tomography; *ILD*, interstitial lung disease; *IV*, intravenous; *PE*, pulmonary embolism.

reconstructed at thicker sections, which have lower image noise. Various IRTs from different vendors can allow radiation dose reduction of up to 30% to 50% compared to FBP images. Decreased image noise can be seen with increased IRT strengths. Lower-strength IRTs should be used initially, and strength can be gradually increased with dose reduction. For evaluation of lungs and airways, lower image noise at higher radiation dose does not really translate into increased diagnostic performance.

Lung Cancer Screening Computed Tomography

Recent studies have reported a mortality benefit of low-dose chest CT (LDCT) for lung cancer screening in high-risk individuals. The study reported fewer (20%) deaths in patients who received LDCT compared to patients who did not receive LDCT. The US Preventive Services Task Force also recommends LDCT for lung cancer screening for individuals aged 55 to 80 years with a 30 pack-year smoking history (current smoker or quit within the past 15 years). Joint guidelines from the American College of Radiology and Society of Thoracic Radiology recommend LDCT at CTDIvol of up to 3 mGy for average-sized patients. Other studies have reported that LDCT for lung cancer screening can be performed at a fraction of this dose.

To achieve a low radiation dose for LDCT, the tube current (in milliamperes) should be adjusted. Although American College of Radiology and Society of Thoracic Radiology guidelines recommend use of AEC over fixed tube current, several studies have reported substantial dose reduction with the use of fixed milliamperage. Also, lower kilovoltage should be preferred (80–120 kV) based on the size of patients. The kilovoltage selection can be manual or automatic on scanners that have automatic kilovoltage selection. The scan coverage should be limited to the area from the lung apex to the lung bases for lung cancer screening (Fig. 23.2). Scan parameters for lung cancer screening CT are summarized in Table 23.3.

Lung Nodule Follow-up Computed Tomography

Demonstration of nodule stability or progression is a major reason for follow-up chest CT. The Fleischner society recommends follow-up chest CT for a lung nodule (based on size) detected incidentally on nonscreening CT. These recommendations for lung nodule follow-up are summarized in Table 23.4. Recent studies also show the benefit of lung nodule follow-up CT based on nodule size. The chest CT protocol for lung nodule follow-up should follow the principles of lung cancer screening CT (see Table 23.3). Multiple prior studies have shown that lung nodules can be seen adequately at low radiation doses. Similar to lung cancer screening CT, the dose for nodule follow-up can be achieved through low fixed milliamperage based on patient size; however, the AEC technique should be preferred.

Routine Chest Computed Tomography

Routine chest CT is the most commonly performed CT of the thorax. Clinical indications for performing routine chest CT are summarized in Table 23.2. Acquisition of both pre- and postcontrast images for routine chest CT protocols must be discouraged. Routine chest generally extends from the lung apex to the adrenal glands. Due to high inherent contrast, major lung findings can be evaluated at substantially low radiation doses. Relative to the lungs, mediastinal contrast on CT is lower, so higher radiation dose is often needed for mediastinal structures as compared to CT protocols for lung cancer screening and lung nodule follow-up. Routine chest CT doses should still be less than routine abdominal CT. It is also important to ensure that routine chest CT doses are well below the recommended RDLs and achievable doses. For an average-sized patient, the recommended RDL and achievable dose for chest CT are 21 and 14 mGy, respectively. Table 23.3 summarizes the scan parameters for the routine chest CT protocol.

For routine chest CT, AEC should be preferred over fixed milliamperage. In general, adult patients less than 80 kg can be scanned at lower kilovoltage (≤100 kV) for contrast-enhanced chest CT. Use of IRTs can allow lower kilovoltage in larger patients. Prior studies have reported that IRTs (such as Safire and Admire, Siemens; ASIR and MBIR, GE; iDose and IMR, Philips; and AIDR and AIDR three-dimensional, Toshiba) can allow substantial dose reduction for routine chest CT compared to FBP. The dose reduction with IRT stems from use of lower tube current and/or tube potential when using IRT-based image reconstruction methods.

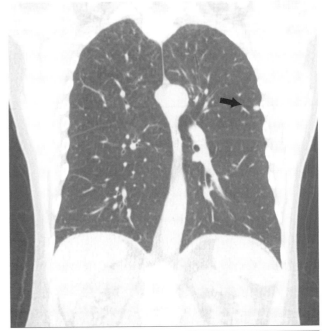

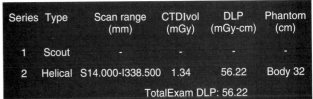

Series	Type	Scan range (mm)	CTDIvol (mGy)	DLP (mGy-cm)	Phantom (cm)
1	Scout	-	-	-	-
2	Helical	S14.000-I338.500	1.34	56.22	Body 32
				TotalExam DLP: 56.22	

FIG. 23.2 Lung cancer screening computed tomography (CT) exam of an elderly patient (70 kg, 120 kV, 48 mAs, CT dose index volume [CTDIvol] of 1.3 mGy, dose length product [DLP] of 56 mGy-cm) was performed on a 64-slice multidetector row CT scanner. Coronal CT images depict a solid pulmonary nodule in the left upper lobe (*black arrow*).

TABLE 23.3 **Scan Parameters for Different Chest Computed Tomgraphy (CT) Protocols**

Scan Parameters	Lung Cancer Screening and Nodule Follow-up CT	Routine Chest CT	CT Pulmonary Angiography
Scan coverage	Apex to base	Apex to adrenals	Apex to base
Mode	Helical	Helical	Helical
Time	≤0.5 s	≤0.5 s	≤0.5 s
Pitch	Pitch ≥1	Pitch ≥1	Pitch ≥1
Detector collimation	Wider is more dose efficient and quicker	Wider is more efficient	Wider is more efficient
Table speed	Faster is better	Faster is better	Faster is better
Reconstruction thickness	<1.5 mm	1.5–3 mm	<1.5 mm
Kilovolts	80–120 kV	80–120 kV	80–100 kV
AEC or fixed milliamperage	AEC preferred	AEC	AEC

AEC, Automatic exposure control.

TABLE 23.4 **Fleischner Society Recommendations for Follow-up of Solid Pulmonary Nodules Detected Incidentally on Chest Computed Tomography (CT) (Patients Age ≥35 y)**

Nodule Size	High-Risk Patients (History of Smoking, Other Risk Factors)	Other Patients Without High Risk Factors
≤4 mm	CT at 12 mo; if stable, no further follow-up	No follow-up is recommended
>4–6 mm	Initial CT at 6–12 mo; if stable, repeat CT at 18–24 mo	LDCT at 12 mo
>6–8 mm	Initial CT at 3–6 mo; if stable, repeat CT at 9–12 mo and 24 mo	LDCT at 6–12 mo then 18–24 mo if no change
>8 mm	CT at 3, 9, and 24 mo, consider PET or biopsy	If co-morbidities and negative PET, LDCT at 3, 9, and 24 months

LDCT, Low-dose chest CT; *PET,* positron emission tomography.

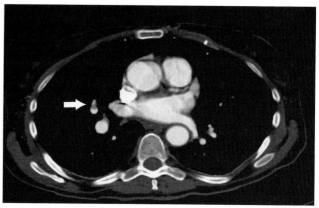

FIG. 23.3 Computed tomography (CT) pulmonary angiography in an elderly patient (50 kg) performed with a low radiation dose technique (80 kV, automatic exposure control, CT dose index volume of 3.2 mGy, dose length product of 106 mGy-cm) on a 128-row multidetector row CT scanner. Transverse CT image depicts a pulmonary embolus in the right middle lobe pulmonary artery *(white arrow).*

Computed Tomography Pulmonary Angiography

The scan range for computed tomography pulmonary angiography (CTPA) should extend from the lung bases to the apices. Some have argued that the dome of the diaphragm to the top of the aortic arch is sufficient for evaluation of pulmonary embolism up to the segmental pulmonary arteries. At Massachusetts General Hospital, CTPA for pulmonary embolism extends from the lung apices to the bases because some of these patients have other chest ailments that can be simultaneously detected while imaging for pulmonary embolism, such as consolidation, atelectasis, and pleural effusions.

When it comes to dose optimization for CTPA, the two most important aspects are construction and instruction. The former pertains to use of good IV access, a reasonable rate of contrast injection, and scan triggering, which are important for obtaining sufficient pulmonary arterial enhancement and avoiding repeat imaging. Bolus tracking or test bolus techniques should always be used over empirical scan delay. From an instructional point of view, users must ensure that proper breath hold instructions are provided and demonstrated. Motion artifacts are frequent in patients undergoing CTPA. If the patient cannot hold his or her breath as needed for scanning, asking him or her not to hold the breath may be the best option. The latter is now feasible on several wide-area detector CT and high-pitch scanners (dual-source CT), which can cover the entire scan range for CTPA in a second or less. Patients should be instructed not to perform the Valsalva maneuver as a lead up to their breath hold. To minimize motion artifacts regardless of breath-holding capabilities, the fastest scan time should be employed for CTPA protocols unless it is contraindicated by large patient size, which warrants slowing down to avoid excessive image noise and artifacts.

Scanning duration can be abbreviated with use of fast gantry rotation time, wider beam collimation, nonoverlapping pitch, and faster table movement.

CTPA is one protocol where dose reduction in at least the nonobese patients should primarily come from controlled scan range and use of lower kilovoltage (Fig. 23.3). The latter enables dose reduction while enhancing contrast conspicuity on CT images. Most patients undergoing CTPA should be scanned at 80 to 100 kV with the exception of patients over about 100 kg, which may require 120 kV. A notable exception to this could be scanners (such as Siemens Definition Force) that are capable of generating tube current as high as 1300 mAs, which can enable CTPA at lower kilovoltages (≤100 kV).

TABLE 23.5 Clinical Indications and Specific Instructions for Different Abdominal Protocols

Protocol	Clinical Indications	Specific Instructions
Routine abdomen CT	Masses, infections, pain, cancer staging (nonabdominal primary)	No noncontrast CT before contrast CT Dome of diaphragm to pubic symphysis
Kidney stone CT	Suspected or known renal colic	Scan from top of kidneys to pubic symphysis
CT urography	Hematuria	<40 7y: noncontrast CT only, if stone seen >40 y: noncontrast and postcontrast regardless of stone
CT adrenal protocol	Characterize adrenal nodule seen on chest or routine abdominal CT	All phases through adrenal region only
CT colonography	Screening exam, completion colonography	Lowest dose abdominal CT Scan range dome of diaphragm to symphysis
Multiphase liver CT	When MR cannot be performed in patients with suspected liver malignancies	No routine noncontrast images Arterial: liver only, lower kilovoltage Portal venous: entire abdomen Delays: through lesion only (not entire liver)
Appendix CT	Suspected appendicitis	Children: first ultrasound and/or MR. Suboptimal or doubtful: CT Adults: ultrasound or CT Limited scan coverage: L3 to symphysis

CT, Computed tomography; *MR,* magnetic resonance.

Due to better spectral separation capability, dual-energy CT (DECT)-based CTPA protocols are being increasingly used over single-energy CT. Prior studies have shown that some DECT-capable scanners can provide dose parity with single energy–based CTPA, although others may increase radiation dose compared to single-energy CT. Typically, the former group of scanners enables use of AEC with DECT, whereas the latter do not allow use of AEC with their DECT protocols. Radiation dose considerations should be taken into account, especially for young patients undergoing CTPA.

Diffuse Lung Disease Computed Tomography

For the diffuse lung disease protocol, scanning is often performed in both inspiratory and expiratory phases and at times in the prone position. Several scanning techniques have been described for assessing patients with suspected diffuse lung disease. Most often, helical scanning mode is used to acquire images in the inspiratory phase. For expiratory phase scanning, some prefer helical scanning at very low tube current, whereas others prefer axial scanning mode (1-mm slice at 10- to 20-mm intervals) to subsample the lungs in expiration for air trapping. Prone images must be acquired only when needed and with a dose reduction approach similar to expiratory phase imaging. At Massachusetts General Hospital, expiratory phase and prone images are acquired in axial scanning mode with acquisition of 1-mm sections at 20-mm section intervals through the entire chest for expiration and mid-chest to lung bases for prone images.

ABDOMEN COMPUTED TOMOGRAPHY

Currently in the United States, the predominant region imaged with CT is the abdomen for a large number of abnormalities such as cancer follow-up, kidney stone workup, appendicitis, abdominal pain, distention, and hematuria. Certain abdominal structures and abnormalities can be visualized at substantially lower radiation dose due to high inherent contrast such as kidney stones and CT colonography. Paradoxically, others (e.g., liver, renal parenchyma, and pancreas), with a propensity for subtle or low-contrast lesions, require lower-noise images, which requires a correspondingly higher radiation dose. These regions frequently need multiphase scanning through the same region. The abdominal CT protocols should meet the basic standard and ensure the reference dose levels.

On MDCT scanners, abdominal CT examinations are generally acquired in helical acquisition mode. AEC techniques should be used for performing abdominal CT and modified to adjust the milliamperage for different clinical indications. Prior studies have reported substantial dose reduction with IRTs for abdominal CT. The kilovoltage selection in abdomen CT can be manual, fixed, or automatic. In abdominal CT, lower kilovoltage (≤100) can be used in smaller patients and children. Scan length should be adjusted based on clinical indications. Most abdomen CT examinations should be performed with wider beam collimation and nonoverlapping pitch unless thin sections cannot be generated from legacy CT systems for specific CT protocols such as CT angiography. Table 23.5 summarizes stratification of abdominal CT protocols based on clinical indications with specific instructions.

Kidney Stone Computed Tomography

High-contrast lesions such as kidney stones can be seen on reduced-dose CT (Fig. 23.4). Several prior studies have reported that kidney stones can be assessed at substantially reduced radiation dose compared to routine abdominal CT. Thus, the routine abdominal CT protocol should not be used for evaluation of kidney stones. Table 23.6 summarizes the scan parameters for kidney stone CT protocol.

Although the kidney stone protocol is commonly performed at 120 kV, lower kilovoltage (100 kV) can be used in small to average-sized patients. Massachusetts General Hospital uses a single kilovoltage with a single helical run to scan the entire abdomen and pelvis for kidney stone CT protocol. Only a few institutions use different kilovoltages

(100 kV for abdomen and 120 kV for pelvis) for kidney stone protocol CT with two helical acquisitions. The tube current should be adjusted to make sure that lower milliamperage is used compared to routine abdomen CT for patients of similar size. AEC techniques should be used with the kidney stone protocol rather than to fixed milliamperage. Tube current can be further reduced when using the IRT to obtain additional dose reduction compared to conventional FBP-based image reconstruction methods. The scan range for kidney stone protocol CT extends from the top of the kidneys instead of the dome of the liver. Patients with urinary calculi often undergo follow-up CT, which should be performed at lower radiation dose.

Routine Abdomen Computed Tomography

Radiation doses for routine abdominal CT protocol should be well under the recommended RDL (25 mGy) and achievable doses (17 mGy) for an average-sized patient with a

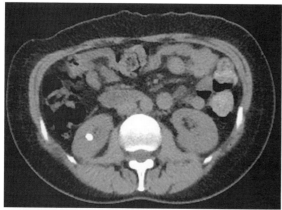

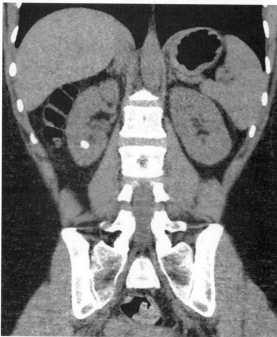

FIG. 23.4 Transverse and coronal low-dose computed tomography (CT) images (CT dose index volume of 2.8 mGy, dose length product of 147 mGy-cm) of an adult patient (58 kg) with suspected renal calculi demonstrate a right renal calculus without evidence of hydronephrosis.

lateral dimension of 38 cm. This implies that smaller patients should have even lower radiation dose and larger patients will require higher radiation doses. Table 23.6 summarizes the scan parameters for the routine abdomen CT protocol.

A routine noncontrast CT should not be performed prior to postcontrast routine abdominal CT. AEC techniques should be used for optimization of tube current relative to patient size. Although some AEC techniques need tweaking for patients at size extremes, others do not require such manipulations. For example, for the Auto mA technique (GE Healthcare), we prescribe different noise indices (image quality metric for this AEC) for different size patients and control the extent of tube current modulation with size-specific minimum and maximum tube current. For others, like Care Dose 4D (Siemens), for very large patients often a higher-quality reference milliampere-second value (image quality metric for this AEC) is used. This technique also allows users to separately control the extent of milliamperage decrease for smaller patients and the extent of increase in tube current for larger patients, which helps avoid aggressive changes in tube current for patients at size extremes. Traditionally, routine abdominal CT is performed at 120–140 kV. In general, unless the patient is morbidly obese, use of 140 kV should be avoided because it negatively affects the level of contrast enhancement. Lower kilovoltage with contrast-enhanced abdominal CT can be used in smaller patients, particularly when employing IRT for image reconstruction. Scan coverage for routine abdominal CT generally extends from the top of the dome of the liver to the pubic symphysis. When needed, delayed images should only be acquired in the region of abnormality rather than the entire abdomen or the organ of interest.

Multiphasic Liver Computed Tomography Protocol

Multiphasic scanning is more common in the abdomen, especially for evaluation of focal liver and renal lesions. Typically, scanning is performed in noncontrast, arterial,

TABLE 23.6   Scan Parameters for Kidney Stone and Routine Abdomen Computed Tomography (CT)

Scan Parameters	Kidney Stone CT	Routine Abdomen CT
Scan coverage	From top of kidneys to pubic symphysis	From top of liver dome to pubic symphysis
Mode	Helical	Helical
Gantry rotation time	Faster is better (0.4–0.5 s)	Faster is better (0.4–0.5 s) unless large patient body habitus
Pitch	Pitch ≥1	Pitch ≥1
Recon. thickness	5 mm for viewing	5 mm for viewing
Detector collimation	Wider is more efficient	Wider is more efficient
Kilovolts	100–120 kV	100–120 kV
AEC or fixed milliamperage	AEC (lower mAs compared to routine abdominal CT)	AEC

AEC, Automatic exposure control.

portal venous, and delayed phases of contrast enhancement for focal liver lesions. Increasingly, magnetic resonance (MR) is being used for such studies because it allows better lesion characterization and imaging at multiple additional time points without multiplying the associated radiation dose.

To reduce radiation dose, noncontrast CT images can be skipped before acquisition of postcontrast CT images without losing substantial information. Arterial phase CT should be limited to the liver only and can often be performed at lower radiation doses with use of lower kilovoltage (100 kV), which also helps increase the conspicuity of enhancing liver lesions. In the portal venous phase, low-attenuation liver lesions can be hard to visualize at lower radiation doses. Typically, the entire abdomen and/or pelvis are imaged in the portal venous phase. When performing multiphase CT exams, it is important to check the clinical reason for each scan phase. Without any apparent clinical indication or reason, unnecessary scan phases should be avoided. For the delayed phase, the scan length should be limited to the lesion only instead of the entire organ. Prior studies with IRTs have reported that lower kilovoltage can be used for arterial phase imaging because IRT can help reduce image noise.

Computed Tomography Urography

CT urography is performed for evaluation of hematuria. It is also a multiphase CT exam. Noncontrast and postcontrast (nephrographic and excretory) phases are often acquired. For this exam, the low-dose noncontrast phase (which can often be similar to the kidney stone protocol CT) should be acquired as the main goal to rule out urinary tract calculi or stone. There are considerable variations in CT urography protocols between different institutions. Some institutions acquire separate nephrographic and excretory phases, which makes the protocol a three-phase CT, whereas others, including Massachusetts General Hospital, combine the nephrographic and excretory phases into one phase with a split bolus contrast injection technique. The contrast injection bolus is split over 10 to 15 minutes beginning with a 50-mL IV contrast bolus, followed by 250 mL of saline drip infusion for about 15 minutes, followed by 80 to 100 mL of IV contrast at 3 mL/s. The patient is then scanned in a prone position at 100 s after injection of the second contrast bolus. The first contrast bolus provides excretory phase information, and the second contrast bolus allows nephrographic enhancement of the kidneys in a single CT acquisition.

Computed Tomography Colonography

The American Cancer Society suggests CT colonography (once in every 5 years) as an option for screening colon cancer or polyps. CT colonography can be performed at a significantly reduced dose due to high inherent contrast between air-filled colon, colonic wall, and lesions. CT colonography can be performed at a CTDIvol of 2 to 4 mGy in nonobese patients. With IRTs, these radiation doses can be reduced even further. Generally, low tube current (using AEC) and high nonoverlapping pitch are used to obtain CT colonography datasets.

PEDIATRIC COMPUTED TOMOGRAPHY

Children vary tremendously in size, from less than 1 kg to adult body habitus. Small children should be scanned at lower doses as compared to larger children and adults. Small children can also move during scanning and often need immobilization, sedation, and/or faster scanning to reduce motion artifacts. A radiologist or CT technologist should explain the scanning procedure to the patient and/or accompanying person to reduce the anxiety associated with the CT exam. Painful procedures such as IV access should be performed in advance of CT, outside the scanning room. For older children, breathing instruction should be demonstrated. Contrast-enhanced exams should be well planned. Contrast extravasation can lead to a repeat exam and can be prevented.

Several pediatric illnesses can be assessed with safer nonradiation (ultrasound, MRI) or low-radiation (plain radiographs) imaging tests. Compared to adults, children rarely need multiphase CT. Creation of on the fly protocols should be avoided in children. All pediatric protocols should be predefined and archived on CT. The best way to reduce the radiation dose in pediatric CT is to ensure that the clinical indications for the study are appropriate and alternative imaging tests cannot provide the required clinical information. Unnecessary repeat CT exams should also be avoided. The scanning should cover the required anatomic region of interest only. Scan parameters must be preset on the scanner based on patient size, body region, or indication. Certain clinical indications, such as craniosynostosis (Fig. 23.5), ventriculoperitoneal (VP) shunt patency (Fig. 23.6), scoliosis, and kidney stones, can be assessed at substantially reduced radiation dose levels. Table 23.7 summarizes some pediatric CT protocols that can be assessed with reduced radiation dose.

At our institution, use of pediatric head CT is limited to head injury, craniosynostosis, and VP patency. When indicated, head CT in children is performed at reduced radiation doses with use of AEC and low kilovoltage, particularly in little children. The intent of head CT in patients with suspected head injury is confined to assessing hemorrhage and bony fractures. Most other head conditions in the absence of known contraindications are assessed with MR.

For craniostenosis, CT is performed at 80 kV and low fixed milliamperage (50 mAs) (see Fig. 23.5). For the VP shunt patency protocol, a low-kilovoltage and fixed low-milliamperage protocol are sufficient for assessing ventricular size (see Fig. 23.6). Recent studies have shown that an extremely fast (in few minutes) MR protocol can be used for shunt patency evaluation in children.

Centering is very important in children. Off-centering can disturb the estimation of milliamperage with the AEC technique. It can also disturb the function of beam-shaping filters, which can lead to asymmetric distribution of noise and artifacts in the image. The surface doses to vital organs such as breasts and thyroid can be increased with off-centering.

Pediatric chest and abdomen CT can be performed with reduced doses (Fig. 23.7). As in adult patients, the AEC technique should be used instead of fixed milliamperage for scanning the chest and abdomen in children. Automatic kilovoltage selection should be used for pediatric CT when available. For manual kilovoltage selection, lower

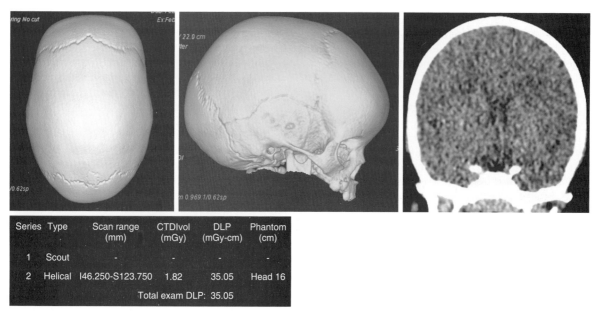

Series	Type	Scan range (mm)	CTDIvol (mGy)	DLP (mGy-cm)	Phantom (cm)
1	Scout	-	-	-	-
2	Helical	I46.250-S123.750	1.82	35.05	Head 16
				Total exam DLP: 35.05	

FIG. 23.5 Ultralow-radiation-dose computed tomography (CT) (80 kV, 25 mAs, CT dose index volume of 1.8 mGy with 16-cm phantom size) of the head for evaluation of an infant with suspected craniosynostosis. Images demonstrate premature fusion of the sagittal suture with scaphocephaly. The transverse image demonstrates high noise content but still allows exclusion of coexistent ventricular enlargement.

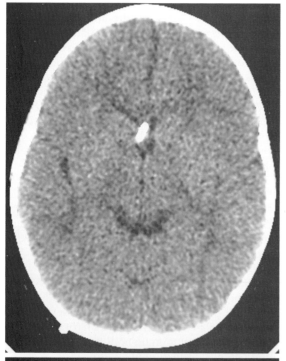

Series	Type	Scan range (mm)	CTDIvol (mGy)	DLP (mGy-cm)	Phantom (cm)
1	Scout	-	-	-	-
2	Helical	I4.500-S145.500	7.24	124.91	Head 16
				Total exam DLP: 124.91	

FIG. 23.6 Low-radiation-dose computed tomography (80 kV, 50 mAs, CT dose index volume [CTDIvol] of 7 mGy) of the head in a 7-year-old child demonstrates a ventricular shunt in place without evidence of hydrocephalus. Assessment of shunt patency can be established at extremely low-radiation-dose computed tomography or with a short magnetic resonance examination. *DLP*, Dose-length product.

TABLE 23.7 Clinical Indications for Reduced Dose Head, Chest, and Abdomen Computed Tomography (CT) in Children

Reduced-Dose Head CT	Reduced-Dose Chest CT	Reduced-Dose Abdomen CT
Ventriculoperitoneal shunt patency	Airway assessment	Kidney stones
Craniosynostosis	Lung abnormalities	CT enterography
Paranasal sinuses	Pleural effusion/ empyema	Follow-up abdominal CT
Facial trauma	Chest wall deformities	Bony abnormalities
Follow-up head CT	Scoliosis	
	Chest trauma	
	Follow-up chest CT	

kilovoltage should be used in small children. Infants can be scanned adequately at 70 to 80 kV. Lower kilovoltage should also be used for CT angiography in children. Most children up to 80 kg can be scanned at 80 kV, particularly for contrast-enhanced CT, whereas using IRTs to reduce image noise for heavier children, 100 to 120 kV may be needed. Most if not all chest and abdominal CT must be performed with a single-phase imaging protocol (with or without contrast, but not both). Prior studies reported substantial CT radiation dose reduction with IRTs in pediatric patients.

Prior studies have described use of the Broselow-Luten color-coded system for radiation dose optimization in pediatric chest and abdominal CT. This system uses the height and weight of children for optimization of radiation dose. Other studies have described use of a multifactorial color-coded system using information pertaining to patient weight, body region, clinical indication, number of prior exams, and AEC to adapt the radiation dose for chest and abdominal CT. In this color-coded system (Table 23.8), CT protocols are initially binned into a color zone (pink, green, red, and gray) based on clinical indications,

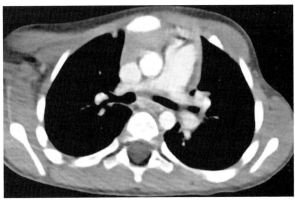 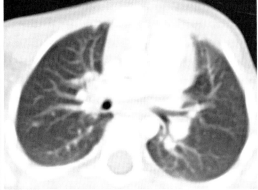

FIG. 23.7 Chest computed tomography (CT) (100 kV, 80 mAs, CT dose index volume of 2.6 mGy) in a 2-year-old child (16 kg) who underwent chest CT with contrast enhancement for assessment of vascular rings. CT images demonstrated no vascular anomalies.

TABLE 23.8 Color Coding Zones Based on Clinical Indications and Protocols (Decreasing Order of Radiation Dose)

Clinical Indications and Protocols	Color Zone	Radiation Dose
Routine abdomen CT	Pink	Standard ⇆
Follow-up abdomen CT, first chest CT	Green	↓
Multiple prior chest and abdomen CT, bone abnormalities	Red	↓↓
Kidney stone	Yellow	↓↓↓
CT angiography	Gray	↓↓↓↓

CT, Computed tomography.

body region, and availability of prior CT examination. Each color zone is then subdivided into subzones based on the weight of the child. Each weight subgroup has different settings for milliamperes, kilovolts, and AEC to optimize radiation dose. This color-coded system requires radiologists to review the indications for each pediatric CT and specify the appropriate color zone for CT technologists. This also gives radiologists an opportunity to assess the appropriateness of the clinical indications for CT and possible triage to other imaging studies.

When different CT scanners are available, a faster CT scanner and one with IRT should be chosen for pediatric CT. For example, dual-source CT scanners are faster than single-source CT, particularly when the latter has less than 128 detector rows. The faster gantry rotation speed should be used to reduce scan time and minimize motion artifacts in little children. Nonoverlapping pitch should be used for faster scanning (minimized scan duration and motion artifacts) in children. On certain scanners (such as some GE scanners), overlapping pitch (<1:1) can increase the associated radiation dose if all other scan parameters are held constant. On other scanners (e.g., Siemens scanners), pitch does not affect radiation dose because any change in pitch is offset by a concomitant change in tube current to keep a constant radiation dose. A wider beam collimation or detector configuration should be used for scanning longer regions such as the chest, abdomen, and spine. The width of detector configuration also depends on the need

for specific slice thickness, particularly for scanners with variable detector row thicknesses.

Scan length should be limited to the region of interest only. Pediatric chest CT should be limited to a scan range from the lung apices to the lung bases. When scanning two adjacent regions, such as the chest and abdomen, both regions should be scanned in a single run to avoid overlapping image acquisitions. Thick sections have lower image noise than thinner sections if all other acquisition and reconstruction parameters are kept constant. Low-contrast organs such as the liver can be assessed with thicker sections to lower image noise. High-contrast structures such as the chest and contrast-enhanced blood vessels can be assessed with thinner sections because these structures can tolerate higher image noise. Softer reconstruction kernels also have lower image noise and are particularly helpful for abdominal CT. Sharper or high spatial frequency reconstruction kernels increase image sharpness at the cost of increased image noise; their use should thus be limited to situations that are less affected by an increase in image noise.

As in adult patients, kidney stone protocol CT in children should be performed at a reduced radiation dose. For evaluation of appendicitis on CT, the scan range (from the top of the L3 vertebral body to the pubic symphysis) should be decreased to reduce radiation dose. Prior to resorting to CT, ultrasonography should be attempted. At Massachusetts General Hospital, an inclusive ultrasound is followed by MR to assess for appendicitis. CT is used as a modality of last resort when both ultrasound and MR are inclusive and/or unavailable. Prior simulation studies have reported that appendicitis can be assessed with low tube current to reduce radiation dose.

CONCLUSION

In summary, use of CT in appropriate clinical indications avoids misuse and overuse of CT and other imaging studies. Understanding CT image quality requirements for different clinical indications helps adapt radiation doses for CT protocols in the most appropriate manner. AEC and automatic kilovoltage selection techniques help adapt radiation dose for patients with different body sizes. IRTs allow users to reduce radiation dose while maintaining constant diagnostic quality.

SUGGESTED READINGS

Albert GW, Glasier CM. Strategies for computed tomography radiation dose reduction in pediatric neuroimaging. *Neurosurgery*. 2015;77:228–232.

American Association of Physicists in Medicine. Adult brain perfusion CT. <https://www.aapm.org/pubs/CTProtocols/documents/AdultBrainPerfusionCT.pdf>.

American Association of Physicists in Medicine. Lung cancer screening CT. <http://www.aapm.org/pubs/CTProtocols/documents/LungCancerScreeningCT.pdf>.

American Cancer Society. American Cancer Society recommendations for colorectal cancer early detection. <http://www.cancer.org/cancer/colonandrectumcancer/moreinformation/colonandrectumcancerearlydetection/colorectal-cancer-early-detection-acs-recommendations>.

American College of Radiology. practice parameters and technical standards. <http://www.acr.org/Quality-Safety/Standards-Guidelines> 2015.

American College of Radiology. ACR-AAPM practice guideline for diagnostic reference levels and achievable doses in medical x-ray imaging. <http://www.acr.org/~/media/0DAB1CD6FFC44F09A05E0BD0FCA175F8.pdf>.

American College of Radiology and Society of Thoracic Radiology. ACR-STR practice parameter for the performance and reporting of lung cancer screening thoracic computed tomography (CT). <http://www.acr.org/~/media/ACR/Documents/PGTS/guidelines/LungScreening.pdf>.

American College of Radiology. Computed tomography accreditation. <http://www.acr.org/Quality-Safety/Accreditation/CT>.

Andrabi Y, Pianykh O, Agrawal M, Kambadakone A, Blake MA, Sahani DV. Radiation dose consideration in kidney stone CT examinations: integration of iterative reconstruction algorithms with routine clinical practice. *AJR Am J Roentgenol*. 2015;204:1055–1063.

Andrabi Y, Saadeh TS, Uppot RN, Arellano RS, Sahani DV. Impact of dose-modified protocols on radiation doses in patients undergoing CT examinations following image-guided catheter placement. *J Vasc Interv Radiol*. 2015;26:1339–1346.

Baldwin DR, Duffy SW, Wald NJ, Page R, Hansell DM, Field JK. UK Lung Screen (UKLS) nodule management protocol: modelling of a single screen randomized controlled trial of low-dose CT screening for lung cancer. *Thorax*. 2011;66:308–313.

Barrett T, Bowden DJ, Shaida N, et al. Virtual unenhanced second generation dual-source CT of the liver: is it time to discard the conventional unenhanced phase? *Eur J Radiol*. 2012;81:1438–1445.

Bauer RW, Kramer S, Renker M, et al. Dose and image quality at CT pulmonary angiography-comparison of first and second generation dual-energy CT and 64-slice CT. *Eur J Radiol*. 2011;21(10):2139–2147.

Berlin SC, Weinert DM, Vasavada PS, et al. Successful dose reduction using reduced tube voltage with hybrid iterative reconstruction in pediatric abdominal CT. *AJR Am J Roentgenol*. 2015;205:392–399.

Brem MH, Zamani AA, Riva R, et al. Multidetector CT of the paranasal sinus: potential for radiation dose reduction. *Radiology*. 2007;243(3):847–852.

Brenner DJ, Hall EJ. Computed tomography—an increasing source of radiation exposure. *N Engl J Med*. 2007;357:2277–2284.

Brink JA. Radiation dose reduction in renal colic protocol CT: are we doing enough to ensure adoption of best practices? *Radiology*. 2014;271:323–325.

Brook OR, Gourtsoyianni S, Brook A, Siewert B, Kent T, Raptopoulos V. Split-bolus spectral multidetector CT of the pancreas: assessment of radiation dose and tumor conspicuity. *Radiology*. 2013;269:139–148.

Brown JH, Lustrin ES, Lev MH, Ogilvy CS, Taveras JM. Reduction of aneurysm clip artifacts on CT angiograms: a technical note. *AJNR Am J Neuroradiol*. 1999;20:694–696.

Bulla S, Blanke P, Hassepass F, et al. Reducing the radiation dose for low-dose CT of the paranasal sinuses using iterative reconstruction: feasibility and image quality. *Eur J Radiol*. 2012;81:2246–2250.

Buls N, Van Gompel G, Van Cauteren T, et al. Contrast agent and radiation dose reduction in abdominal CT by a combination of low tube voltage and advanced image reconstruction algorithms. *Eur Radiol*. 2015;25:1023–1031.

Caoili EM, Cohan RH. CT urography in evaluation of urothelial tumors of the kidney. *Abdom Radiol (NY)*. 2016;41:1100–1107.

Chen CY, Chen CH, Shen TC, et al. Lung cancer screening with low-dose computed tomography: experiences from a tertiary hospital in Taiwan. *J Formos Med Assoc*. 2016;115:163–170.

Chen CY, Hsu JS, Jaw TS, et al. Split-bolus portal venous phase dual-energy CT urography: protocol design, image quality, and dose reduction. *AJR Am J Roentgenol*. 2015;205:W492–W501.

Chen CY, Tsai TH, Jaw TS, et al. Diagnostic performance of split-bolus portal venous phase dual-energy CT urography in patients with hematuria. *AJR Am J Roentgenol*. 2016;2:1–10.

Corwin MT, Bekele W, Lamba R. Bony landmarks on computed tomographic localizer radiographs to prescribe a reduced scan range in patients undergoing multidetector computed tomography for suspected urolithiasis. *J Comput Assist Tomogr*. 2014;38:404–407.

de Leon AD, Xi Y, Champine J, Costa DN. Achieving ideal computed tomographic scan length in patient with suspected urolithiasis. *J Comput Assist Tomogr*. 2014;38:264–267.

Didier RA, Vajtai PL, Hopkins KL. Iterative reconstruction technique with reduced volume CT dose index: diagnostic accuracy in pediatric acute appendicitis. *Pediatr Radiol*. 2015;45:181–187.

Diederich S, Wormanns D, Semik M, et al. Screening for early lung cancer with low-dose spiral CT: prevalence in 817 asymptomatic smokers. *Radiology*. 2002;222:773–781.

Doğan H, de Roos A, Geleijns J, Huisman MV, Kroft LJ. The role of computed tomography in the diagnosis of acute and chronic pulmonary embolism. *Diagn Interv Radiol*. 2015;21:307–316.

Dunne RM, Ip IK, Abbett S, et al. Effect of evidence-based clinical decision support on the Use and yield of CT pulmonary angiographic imaging in hospitalized patients. *Radiology*. 2015;276(1):167–174.

Ellmann S, Kammerer F, Brand M, et al. A novel pairwise comparison-based method to determine radiation dose reduction potentials of iterative reconstruction algorithms, exemplified through circle of Willis computed tomography angiography. *Invest Radiol*. 2016;51:331–339.

Enchi Y, Imai K, Ikeda M, Takase I, Yamauchi-Kawaura C, Mori M. Arterial contour detectability in head CT angiography. *Int J Comput Assist Radiol Surg*. 2015;10:1–10.

Frush DP, Soden B, Frush KS, Lowry C. Improved pediatric multidetector body CT using a size-based color-coded format. *AJR Am J Roentgenol*. 2002;178:721–726.

Fuchs T, Kachelriess M, Kalender WA. Technical advances in multi-slice spiral CT. *Eur J Radiol*. 2000;36:69–73.

George KJ, Roy D. A low radiation computed tomography protocol for monitoring shunted hydrocephalus. *Surg Neurol Int*. 2012;3:103.

Georgiou A, Prgomet M, Markewycz A, Adams E, Westbrook JI. The impact of computerized provider order entry systems on medical-imaging services: a systematic review. *J Am Med Inform Assoc*. 2011;18:335–340.

Gervaise A, Gervaise-Henry C, Pernin M, Naulet P, Junca-Laplace C, Lapierre-Combes M. How to perform low-dose computed tomography for renal colic in clinical practice. *Diagn Interv Imaging*. 2015:S2211–S5684.

Goenka AH, Dong F, Wildman B, Hulme K, Johnson P, Herts BR. CT radiation dose optimization and tracking program at a large quaternary-care health care system. *J Am Coll Radiol*. 2015;12:703–710.

Goldman AR, Maldjian PD. Reducing radiation dose in body CT: a practical approach to optimizing CT protocols. *AJR Am J Roentgenol*. 2013;200(4):748–754.

Goldman LW. Principles of CT and CT technology. *J Nucl Med Technol*. 2007;35:115–128.

Goshima S, Kanematsu M, Noda Y, et al. Minimally required iodine dose for the detection of hypervascular hepatocellular carcinoma on 80-kVp CT. *AJR Am J Roentgenol*. 2016;206:518–525.

Greenwood TJ, Lopez-Costa RI, Rhoades PD, et al. CT dose optimization in pediatric radiology: a multiyear effort to preserve the benefits of imaging while reducing the risks. *Radiographics*. 2015;35:1539–1554.

Gulati S, Mulshine JL. Lung cancer screening guidelines: common ground and differences. *Transl Lung Cancer Res*. 2014;3:131–138.

Gupta A, Castellan M. Use of computed tomography (CT) for urolithiasis in pediatric patients. *Transl Pediatr*. 2015;4:33–35.

Hojreh A, Weber M, Homolka P. Effect of staff training on radiation dose in pediatric CT. *Eur J Radiol*. 2015;84:1574–1578.

Hopper KD, Neuman JD, King SH, Kunselman AR. Radioprotection to the eye during CT scanning. *AJNR Am J Neuroradiol*. 2001;22:1194–1198.

Hoxworth JM, Lal D, Fletcher GP, et al. Radiation dose reduction in paranasal sinus CT using model-based iterative reconstruction. *AJNR Am J Neuroradiol*. 2014;35:644–649.

Hwang I, Cho JY, Kim SY, et al. Low tube voltage computed tomography urography using low-concentration contrast media: comparison of image quality in conventional computed tomography urography. *Eur J Radiol*. 2015;84:2454–2463.

Iannaccone R, Laghi A, Catalano C, et al. Hepatocellular carcinoma: role of unenhanced and delayed phase multi-detector row helical CT in patients with cirrhosis. *Radiology*. 2005;234:460–467.

Ibrahim M, Parmar H, Christodoulou E, Mukherji S. Raise the bar and lower the dose: current and future strategies for radiation dose reduction in head and neck imaging. *AJNR Am J Neuroradiol*. 2014;35:619–624.

Imai K, Ikeda M, Kawaura C, et al. Dose reduction and image quality in CT angiography for cerebral aneurysm with various tube potentials and current settings. *Br J Radiol*. 2012;85:e673–e681.

International Atomic Energy Agency. 10 Pearls: appropriate referral for CT examinations. <https://rpop.iaea.org/RPOP/RPoP/Content/Documents/Whitepapers/poster-ct-appropriate-referrals.pdf>.

International Commission on Radiological Protection, Khong PL, Ringertz H, et al. ICRP publication 121: radiological protection in paediatric diagnostic and interventional radiology. *Ann ICRP*. 2013;42:1–63.

Ip IK, Schneider LI, Hanson R, et al. Adoption and meaningful use of computerized physician order entry with an integrated clinical decision support system for radiology: ten-year analysis in an urban teaching hospital. *J Am Coll Radiol*. 2012;9:29–136.

Iyama Y, Nakaura T, Yokoyama K, et al. Impact of knowledge-based iterative model reconstruction in abdominal dynamic CT with low tube voltage and low contrast dose. *AJR Am J Roentgenol*. 2016;206:687–693.

Jończyk-Potoczna K, Frankiewicz M, Warzywoda M, et al. Low-dose protocol for head CT in evaluation of hydrocephalus in children. *Pol J Radiol*. 2012;77:7–11.

Jones GS, Baldwin DR. Lung cancer screening and management. *Minerva Med*. 2015;106:339–354.

Juluru K, Shih JC, Raj A, et al. Effects of increased image noise on image quality and quantitative interpretation in brain CT perfusion. *AJNR Am J Neuroradiol*. 2013;34:1506–1512.

Juri H, Tsuboyama T, Kumano S, et al. Detection of bladder cancer: comparison of low-dose scans with AIDR 3D and routine-dose scans with FBP on the excretory phase in CT urography. *Br J Radiol*. 2016;89:20150495.

Kalender WA, Seissler W, Klotz E, Vock P. Spiral volumetric CT with single-breath-hold technique, continuous transport, and continuous scanner rotation. *Radiology*. 1990;176:181–183.

Kalender WA. X-ray computed tomography. *Phys Med Biol*. 2006;51:R29–R43.

Kalra MK, Maher MM, D'Souza R, Saini S. Multidetector computed tomography technology: current status and emerging developments. *J Comput Assist Tomogr*. 2004;28:S2–S6.

Kalra MK, Maher MM, Saini S. What is the optimum position of arms for acquiring scout images for whole-body CT with automatic tube current modulation?. *AJR Am J Roentgenol*. 2003;181. 596–567.

Kalra MK, Maher MM, Toth TL, et al. Strategies for CT radiation dose optimization. *Radiology*. 2004;230:619–628.

Kalra MK, Sodickson AD, Mayo-Smith WW. CT radiation: key concepts for gentle and wise use. *Radiographics*. 2015;35:1706–1721.

Kalra MK, Woisetschläger M, Dahlström N, et al. Radiation dose reduction with sinogram affirmed iterative reconstruction technique for abdominal computed tomography. *J Comput Assist Tomogr*. 2012;36:339–346.

Kalra MK, Woisetschläger M, Dahlström N, et al. Sinogram-affirmed iterative reconstruction of low-dose chest CT: effect on image quality and radiation dose. *AJR Am J Roentgenol*. 2013;201:W235–W244.

Karul M, Berliner C, Keller S, et al. Imaging of appendicitis in adults. *Rofo*. 2014;186:551–558.

Katsura M, Matsuda I, Akahane M, et al. Model-based iterative reconstruction technique for ultralow-dose chest CT: comparison of pulmonary nodule detectability with the adaptive statistical iterative reconstruction technique. *Invest Radiol*. 2013;48:206–212.

Kaul D, Grupp U, Kahn J, et al. Reducing radiation dose in the diagnosis of pulmonary embolism using adaptive statistical iterative reconstruction and lower tube potential in computed tomography. *Eur Radiol*. 2014;24:2685–2691.

Kaza RK, Platt JF, Goodsitt MM, et al. Emerging techniques for dose optimization in abdominal CT. *Radiographics*. 2014;34:4–17.

Kazerooni EA, Austin JH, Black WC, et al. ACR-STR practice parameter for the performance and reporting of lung cancer screening thoracic computed tomography (CT): 2014 (Resolution 4). *J Thorac Imaging*. 2014;29:310–316.

Kerl JM, Lehnert T, Schell B, et al. Intravenous contrast material administration at high-pitch dual-source CT pulmonary angiography: test bolus versus bolus-tracking technique. *Eur J Radiol*. 2012;81:2887–2891.

Khawaja RD, Singh S, Gilman M, et al. Computed tomography (CT) of the chest at less than 1 mSv: an ongoing prospective clinical trial of chest CT at submillisievert radiation doses with iterative model image reconstruction and iDose4 technique. *J Comput Assist Tomogr*. 2014;38:613–619.

Kim H, Park CM, Song YS, et al. Measurement variability of persistent pulmonary subsolid nodules on same-day repeat CT: what is the threshold to determine true nodule growth during follow-up? *PLoS One*. 2016;11(2):e0148853.

Kim SS, Hur J, Kim YJ, Lee HJ, Hong YJ, Choi BW. Dual-energy CT for differentiating acute and chronic pulmonary thromboembolism: an initial experience. *Int J Cardiovasc Imaging*. 2014;30:113–120.

Kim Y, Kim YK, Lee BE, et al. Ultra-low-dose CT of the thorax using iterative reconstruction: evaluation of image quality and radiation dose reduction. *AJR Am J Roentgenol*. 2014;204:1197–1202.

Kofler JM, Cody DD, Morin RL. CT protocol review and optimization. *J Am Coll Radiol*. 2014;11:267–270.

Kubo T, Lin PJ, Stiller W, et al. Radiation dose reduction in chest CT: a review. *AJR Am J Roentgenol*. 2008;190:335–343.

Kulkarni NM, Uppot RN, Eisner BH, Sahani DV. Radiation dose reduction at multidetector CT with adaptive statistical iterative reconstruction for evaluation of urolithiasis: how low can we go? *Radiology*. 2012;265:158–166.

Langner S. Optimized imaging of the midface and orbits. *GMS Curr Top Otorhinolaryngol Head Neck Surg*. 2015;14:Doc05.

Lehnert BE, Bree RL. Analysis of appropriateness of outpatient CT and MRI referred from primary care clinics at an academic medical center: how critical is the need for improved decision support? *J Am Coll Radiol*. 2010;7:192–197.

Lell MM, Wildberger JE, Alkadhi H, Damilakis J, Kachelriess M. Evolution in computed tomography: the battle for speed and dose. *Invest Radiol*. 2015;50:629–644.

Ley-Zaporozhan J, Ley S. [HRCT technique with low-dose protocols for interstitial lung diseases]. *Radiologe*. 2014;54:1153–1158.

Li ZL, Li H, Zhang K, et al. Improvement of image quality and radiation dose of CT perfusion of the brain by means of low-tube voltage (70 KV). *Eur Radiol*. 2014;24:1906–1913.

Lin CJ, Mok GS, Tsai MF, et al. National survey of radiation dose and image quality in adult CT head scans in Taiwan. *PLoS One*. 2015;10:e0131243.

Little BP, Duong PA, Knighton J, et al. A comprehensive CT dose reduction program using the ACR dose index registry. *J Am Coll Radiol*. 2015;12:1257–1265.

Little BP. Approach to chest computed tomography. *Clin Chest Med*. 2015;36:127–145.

Lubner MG, Pooler BD, Kitchin DR, et al. Sub-milliSievert (sub-mSv) CT colonography: a prospective comparison of image quality and polyp conspicuity at reduced-dose versus standard-dose imaging. *Eur Radiol*. 2015;25:2089–2102.

Luke FE, Allen BC, Moshiri ST, et al. Multiphase multi-detector row computed tomography in the setting of chronic liver disease and orthotopic liver transplantation: can a series be eliminated in order to reduce radiation dose? *J Comput Assist Tomogr*. 2013;37(3):408–414.

MacMahon H, Austin JH, Gamsu G, et al. Guidelines for management of small pulmonary nodules detected on CT scans: a statement from the Fleischner Society. *Radiology*. 2005;237:395–400.

MacMahon H, Bankier AA, Naidich DP. Lung cancer screening: what is the effect of using a larger nodule threshold size to determine who is assigned to short-term CT follow-up? *Radiology*. 2014;273:326–327.

MacRedmond R, Logan PM, Lee M, Kenny D, Foley C, Costello RW. Screening for lung cancer using low dose CT scanning. *Thorax*. 2004;59:237–241.

Maher MM, Kalra MK, Rizzo S, Mueller PR, Saini S. Multidetector CT urography in imaging of the urinary tract in patients with hematuria. *Korean J Radiol*. 2004;5:1–10.

Marin D, Nelson RC, Samei E, et al. Hypervascular liver tumors: low tube voltage, high tube current multidetector CT during late hepatic arterial phase for detection—initial clinical experience. *Radiology*. 2009;251:771–779.

Marin D, Nelson RC, Schindera ST, et al. Low-tube-voltage, high-tube-current multidetector abdominal CT: improved image quality and decreased radiation dose with adaptive statistical iterative reconstruction algorithm—initial clinical experience. *Radiology*. 2010;254:145–153.

Matsuki M, Murakami T, Juri H, Yoshikawa S, Narumi Y. Impact of adaptive iterative dose reduction (AIDR) 3D on low-dose abdominal CT: comparison with routine-dose CT using filtered back projection. *Acta Radiol*. 2013;54:869–875.

Mayo J, Thakur Y. Pulmonary CT angiography as first-line imaging for PE: image quality and radiation dose considerations. *AJR Am J Roentgenol*. 2013;200:522–528.

Mayo JR. CT evaluation of diffuse infiltrative lung disease: dose considerations and optimal technique. *J Thorac Imaging*. 2009;24:252–259.

McCollough C, Branham T, Herlihy V, et al. Diagnostic reference levels from the ACR CT Accreditation Program. *J Am Coll Radiol*. 2011;8:795–803.

McCollough CH, Chen GH, Kalender W, et al. Achieving routine submillisievert CT scanning: report from the summit on management of radiation dose in CT. *Radiology*. 2012;264:567–580.

McDermott A, White RA, Mc-Nitt-Gray M, Angel E, Cody D. Pediatric organ dose measurements in axial and helical multislice CT. *Med Phys*. 2009;36:1494–1499.

Mullins ME, Lev MH, Bove P, et al. Comparison of image quality between conventional and low-dose nonenhanced head CT. *AJNR Am J Neuroradiol*. 2004;25:533–538.

Murphy KP, Maher MM, O'Connor OJ. Imaging of cystic fibrosis and pediatric bronchiectasis. *AJR Am J Roentgenol*. 2016;206:448–454.

Murugan VA, Kalra MK, Rehani M, Digumarthy SR. Lung cancer screening: computed tomography radiation and protocols. *J Thorac Imaging*. 2015;30:283–289.

Nakaura T, Nakamura S, Maruyama N, et al. Low contrast agent and radiation dose protocol for hepatic dynamic CT of thin adults at 256-detector row CT: effect of low tube voltage and hybrid iterative reconstruction algorithm on image quality. *Radiology*. 2012;264:445–454.

National Lung Screening Trial Research Team. The National Lung Screening Trial: overview and study design. *Radiology*. 2011;258:243–253.

The National Lung Screening Trial Research Team. Reduced lung-cancer mortality with low-dose computed tomographic screening. *N Engl J Med*. 2011;365:395–409.

Nelson TR. Practical strategies to reduce pediatric CT radiation dose. *J Am Coll Radiol*. 2014;11:292–299.

New York Early Lung Cancer Action Project Investigators. CT screening for lung cancer: diagnoses resulting from the New York Early Lung Cancer Action Project. *Radiology*. 2007;243:239–249.

Ngaile JE, Uiso CB, Msaki P, et al. Use of lead shields for radiation protection of superficial organs in patients undergoing head CT examinations. *Radiat Prot Dosimetry*. 2008;130:490–498.

Nie P, Li H, Duan Y, et al. Impact of sinogram affirmed iterative reconstruction (SAFIRE) algorithm on image quality with 70 kVp-tube-voltage dual-source CT angiography in children with congenital heart disease. *PLoS One*. 2014;9:e91123.

Nievelstein RA, van Dam IM, van der Molen AJ. Multidetector CT in children: current concepts and dose reduction strategies. *Pediatr Radiol*. 2010;40:1324–1344.

Noël PB, Köhler T, Fingerle AA, et al. Evaluation of an iterative model-based reconstruction algorithm for low-tube-voltage (80 kVp) computed tomography angiography. *J Med Imaging (Bellingham)*. 2014;1:033501.

Ohana M, Labani A, Jeung MY, El Ghannudi S, Gaertner S, Roy C. Iterative reconstruction in single source dual-energy CT pulmonary angiography: is it sufficient to achieve a radiation dose as low as state-of-the-art single-energy CTPA? *Eur J Radiol*. 2015;84:2314–2320.

O'Neill BR, Pruthi S, Bains H, et al. Rapid sequence magnetic resonance imaging in the assessment of children with hydrocephalus. *World Neurosurg*. 2013;80:e307–e312.

Othman AE, Afat S, Brockmann MA, et al. Radiation dose reduction in perfusion CT imaging of the brain: a review of the literature. *J Neuroradiol*. 2016;43:1–5.

Pace I, Zarb F. A comparison of sequential and spiral scanning techniques in brain CT. *Radiol Technol*. 2015;86:373–378.

Padole A, Ali Khawaja RD, Kalra MK, et al. CT radiation dose and iterative reconstruction techniques. *AJR Am J Roentgenol*. 2015;204:384–392.

Padole A, Singh S, Ackman JB, et al. Submillisievert chest CT with filtered back projection and iterative reconstruction techniques. *AJR Am J Roentgenol*. 2014;203:772–781.

Patel DM, Tubbs RS, Pate G, Johnston Jr JM, Blount JP. Fast-sequence MRI studies for surveillance imaging in pediatric hydrocephalus. *J Neurosurg Pediatr*. 2014;13:440–447.

Patino M, Fuentes JM, Singh S, et al. Iterative reconstruction techniques in abdomino-pelvic CT: technical concepts and clinical implementation. *AJR Am J Roentgenol*. 2015;205:W19–W31.

Pedersen JH, Ashraf H, Dirksen A, et al. The Danish randomized lung cancer CT screening trial—overall design and results of the prevalence round. *J Thorac Oncol*. 2009;4:608–614.

Pegna AL, Picozzi G, Mascalchi M, et al. Design, recruitment and baseline results of the ITALUNG trial for lung cancer screening with low-dose CT. *Lung Cancer*. 2009;64:34–40.

Pontana F, Henry S, Duhamel A, et al. Impact of iterative reconstruction on the diagnosis of acute pulmonary embolism (PE) on reduced-dose chest CT angiograms. *Eur Radiol*. 2015;25:1182–1189.

Raja AS, Ip IK, Prevedello LM, et al. Effect of computerized clinical decision support on the use and yield of CT pulmonary angiography in the emergency department. *Radiology*. 2012;262:468–474.

Rapalino O, Kamalian S, Kamalian S, et al. Cranial CT with adaptive statistical iterative reconstruction: improved image quality with concomitant radiation dose reduction. *AJNR Am J Neuroradiol*. 2012;33:609–615.

Rivers-Bowerman MD, Shankar JJ. Iterative reconstruction for head CT: effects on radiation dose and image quality. *Can J Neurol Sci*. 2014;41:620–625.

Russell MT, Fink JR, Rebeles F, Kanal K, Ramos M, Anzai Y. Balancing radiation dose and image quality: clinical applications of neck volume CT. *AJNR Am J Neuroradiol*. 2008;29:727–731.

Ryu YJ, Choi YH, Cheon JE, Ha S, Kim WS, Kim IO. Knowledge-based iterative model reconstruction: comparative image quality and radiation dose with a pediatric computed tomography phantom. *Pediatr Radiol*. 2016;46(3):303–315.

Saul D, Mong A, Biko DM. Pediatric considerations in computed tomographic angiography. *Radiol Clin N Am*. 2016;54:163–176.

Schauer DA, Linton OW. NCRP Report No. 160, Ionizing radiation exposure of the population of the United States, medical exposure—are we doing less with more, and is there a role for health physicists? *Health Phys*. 2009;97:1–5.

Scott Kriegshauser J, Naidu SG, Paden RG, He M, Wu Q, Hara AK. Feasibility of ultra-low radiation dose reduction for renal stone CT using model-based iterative reconstruction: prospective pilot study. *Clin Imaging*. 2015;39:99–103.

Shin CI, Kim SH, Im JP, et al. One-mSv CT colonography: effect of different iterative reconstruction algorithms on radiologists' performance. *Eur J Radiol*. 2016;85:641–648.

Singh S, Kalra MK, Ali Khawaja RD, et al. Radiation dose optimization and thoracic computed tomography. *Radiol Clin N Am*. 2014;52:1–15.

Singh S, Kalra MK, Do S, et al. Comparison of hybrid and pure iterative reconstruction techniques with conventional filtered back projection: dose reduction potential in the abdomen. *J Comput Assist Tomogr*. 2012;36:347–353.

Singh S, Kalra MK, Gilman MD, et al. Adaptive statistical iterative reconstruction technique for radiation dose reduction in chest CT: a pilot study. *Radiology*. 2011;259:565–573.

Singh S, Kalra MK, Hsieh J, et al. Abdominal CT: comparison of adaptive statistical iterative and filtered back projection reconstruction techniques. *Radiology*. 2010;257:373–383.

Singh S, Kalra MK, Moore MA, et al. Dose reduction and compliance with pediatric CT protocols adapted to patient size, clinical indication, and number of prior studies. *Radiology*. 2009;252:200–208.

Singh S, Kalra MK, Shenoy-Bhangle AS, et al. Radiation dose reduction with hybrid iterative reconstruction for pediatric CT. *Radiology*. 2012;263:537–546.

Singh S, Khawaja RD, Pourjabbar S, Padole A, Lira D, Kalra MK. Iterative image reconstruction and its role in cardiothoracic computed tomography. *J Thorac Imaging*. 2013;28:355–367.

Sistrom CL, Dang PA, Weilburg JB, Dreyer KJ, Rosenthal DI, Thrall JH. Effect of computerized order entry with integrated decision support on the growth of outpatient procedure volumes: seven-year time series analysis. *Radiology*. 2009;251:147–155.

Sistrom CL. The ACR appropriateness criteria: translation to practice and research. *J Am Coll Radiol*. 2005;2:61–67.

Smith AB, Dillon WP, Gould R, Wintermark M. Radiation dose-reduction strategies for neuroradiology CT protocols. *AJNR Am J Neuroradiol*. 2007;28:1628–1632.

Smith EA, Dillman JR, Goodsitt MM, Christodoulou EG, Keshavarzi N, Strouse PJ. Model-based iterative reconstruction: effect on patient radiation dose and image quality in pediatric body CT. *Radiology*. 2014;270:526–534.

Sobue T, Moriyama N, Kaneko M, et al. Screening for lung cancer with low-dose helical computed tomography: anti-lung cancer association project. *J Clin Oncol*. 2002;20:911–920.

Song JS, Choi EJ, Kim EY, Kwak HS, Han YM. Attenuation-based automatic kilovoltage selection and sinogram-affirmed iterative reconstruction: effects on radiation exposure and image quality of portal-phase liver CT. *Korean J Radiol*. 2015;16:69–79.

Sui X, Meinel FG, Song W, et al. Detection and size measurements of pulmonary nodules in ultra-low-dose CT with iterative reconstruction compared to low dose CT. *Eur J Radiol*. 2016;85:564–570.

Sun Z, Al Ghamdi K, Baroum I. Multislice CT of the head and body routine scans: are scanning protocols adjusted for paediatric patients? *Biomed Imaging Interv J*. 2012;8:e3.

Tan JS, Tan KL, Lee JC, Wan CM, Leong JL, Chan LL. Comparison of eye lens dose on neuroimaging protocols between 16- and 64-section multidetector CT: achieving the lowest possible dose. *AJNR Am J Neuroradiol*. 2009;30:373–377.

Trattner S, Pearson GD, Chin C, et al. Standardization and optimization of CT protocols to achieve low dose. *J Am Coll Radiol*. 2014;11:271–278.

Udayasankar UK, Braithwaite K, Arvaniti M, et al. Low-dose nonenhanced head CT protocol for follow-up evaluation of children with ventriculoperitoneal shunt: reduction of radiation and effect on image quality. *AJNR Am J Neuroradiol*. 2008;29:802–806.

U.S. Preventive Services Task Force. Lung cancer: screening. <http://www.uspreventiveservicestaskforce.org/Page/Document/UpdateSummaryFinal/lung-cancer-screening>.

Vachha B, Brodoefel H, Wilcox C, Hackney DB, Moonis G. Radiation dose reduction in soft tissue neck CT using adaptive statistical iterative reconstruction (ASIR). *Eur J Radiol*. 2013;82:2222–2226.

van Straten M, Venema HW, Majoie CB, et al. Image quality of multisection CT of the brain: thickly collimated sequential scanning versus thinly collimated spiral scanning with image combining. *AJNR Am J Neuroradiol*. 2007;28:421–427.

Vardhanabhuti V, James J, Nensey R, Hyde C, Roobottom C. Model-based iterative reconstruction in low-dose CT colonography-feasibility study in 65 patients for symptomatic investigation. *Acad Radiol*. 2015;22:563–571.

Wiener RS, Gould MK, Arenberg DA, et al. An official American Thoracic Society/American College of chest physicians policy statement: implementation of low-dose computed tomography lung cancer screening programs in clinical practice. *Am J Respir Crit Care Med*. 2015;192:881–891.

Wille MM, Dirksen A, Ashraf H, et al. Results of the randomized danish lung cancer screening trial with focus on high-risk profiling. *Am J Respir Crit Care Med*. 2016;193:542–551.

Willemink MJ, Leiner T, de Jong PA, et al. Iterative reconstruction techniques for computed tomography part 2: initial results in dose reduction and image quality. *Eur Radiol*. 2013;23:1632–1642.

Yamada Y, Jinzaki M, Hosokawa T, et al. Dose reduction in chest CT: comparison of the adaptive iterative dose reduction 3D, adaptive iterative dose reduction, and filtered back projection reconstruction techniques. *Eur J Radiol*. 2012;81:4185–4195.

Yamada Y, Jinzaki M, Tanami Y, et al. Model-based iterative reconstruction technique for ultralow-dose computed tomography of the lung: a pilot study. *Invest Radiol*. 2012;47:482–489.

Yamamura S, Oda S, Imuta M, et al. Reducing the radiation dose for CT colonography: effect of low tube voltage and iterative reconstruction. *Acad Radiol*. 2016;23:155–162.

Yamashiro T, Miyara T, Honda O, et al. Adaptive iterative dose reduction using three dimensional processing (AIDR3D) improves chest CT image quality and reduces radiation exposure. *PLoS One*. 2014;9:e105735.

Yu L, Fletcher JG, Shiung M, et al. Radiation dose reduction in pediatric body CT using iterative reconstruction and a novel image-based denoising method. *AJR Am J Roentgenol*. 2015;205:1026–1037.

Yu MH, Lee JM, Yoon JH, et al. Low tube voltage intermediate tube current liver MDCT: sinogram-affirmed iterative reconstruction algorithm for detection of hypervascular hepatocellular carcinoma. *AJR Am J Roentgenol*. 2013;201:23–32.

Zarella C, Didier R, Bergquist C, Bardo DM, Selden NR, Kuang AA. A reduction in radiation exposure during pediatric craniofacial computed tomography. *J Craniofac Surg*. 2016;27:331–333.

Zhang WL, Li M, Zhang B, et al. CT angiography of the head-and-neck vessels acquired with low tube voltage, low iodine, and iterative image reconstruction: clinical evaluation of radiation dose and image quality. *PLoS One*. 2013;8:e81486.

Zhao YR, Xie X, de Koning HJ, Mali WP, Vliegenthart R, Oudkerk M. NELSON lung cancer screening study. *Cancer Imaging*. 2011;11:S79–S84.

Chapter 24

Interventional Radiology

Andrew J. Gunn and James R. Duncan

SAFETY CULTURE AND TEAMWORK IN INTERVENTIONAL RADIOLOGY

The practice of interventional radiology (IR) is distinct from that of diagnostic radiology (DR) in that IR is able to treat patients with a wide variety of vascular and nonvascular disorders. Inherent in these abilities is the responsibility to provide safe, evidence-based, and patient-centered care. One method of working toward this goal is creating a safety culture within the IR team. The safety culture requires a commitment at all levels of an organization, including hospital administration, physician leaders, physicians, managers, nursing, and technical staff. According to the American Board of Radiology, a safety culture encompasses these four features: (1) acknowledgement of the high-risk nature of an organization's activities and the determination to achieve consistently safe operations, (2) a blame-free environment, (3) encouragement of collaboration across ranks and disciplines to seek solutions to patient safety problems, and (4) organizational commitment of resources to address safety concerns. There are several validated resources available that aim to measure the safety culture within an institution or team, such as the Agency for Healthcare Research and Quality Patient Safety Culture Surveys and the Safety Attitudes Questionnaire.

Even though an improved safety culture can enhance patient care and reduce medical errors, there is still considerable work to be done in achieving sustainable increases in safety culture and addressing heterogeneity in perceived safety culture among team members. One potential reason for this heterogeneity may be due to steep *authority gradients*, in which team members who view themselves as lower in the hierarchy are hesitant to raise patient safety concerns. Overcoming such obstacles necessitates a team-oriented approach in which the contributions of all team members are acknowledged and valued. Teamwork is a critical component during preprocedure preparation, procedure performance, and postprocedure care. Teamwork relies on open, respectful communication. This is particularly evident during the preprocedure checklist or *time-out*. The time-out immediately precedes the procedure and serves as the last defense against wrong site, wrong patient, and wrong procedure events. To eliminate these *never events*, the time-out and other communications need to extend beyond simply broadcasting information. Rather, effective communication is defined by its ability to eliminate uncertainty in the message's recipients. All team members are encouraged to actively participate, raise concerns, and exchange information. When viewed from this perspective, communication depends on team members having shared mental models of not only the planned task but also its likely failure modes. High-performing teams will also share strategies for detecting and recovering from potential errors. As part of this preparation, the team anticipates communication errors and minimizes the impact of such errors through redundancy and closed feedback loops. For example, the use of multiple patient identifiers (name, date of birth, and/or medical record number) and reviewing the patient's allergies illustrate how redundancy can reduce communication breakdowns. Reconciling the consent form with the referring physician's order creates a feedback loop. Reviewing procedure-specific details such as plans for specimen handling, preprocedure antibiotics, and needs for special equipment and supplies serves to get the entire team on the same page.

A second barrier in achieving a safety culture is the tendency to blame individuals. In a culture of individual blame, excessive emphasis is placed upon the person who makes the error rather than focusing on the contributive systemic and environmental factors. This approach to patient safety often results in punitive or corrective actions toward the individual team member. Unfortunately, this has the untoward effect of making team members less likely to report mistakes and raise concerns. If errors are underreported, then the team misses an opportunity to address systemic patient safety issues, which increases the likelihood that the error will be repeated in the future. Therefore, when considering medical errors within a culture of safety, it becomes necessary to distinguish between *active errors* (mistakes that occur at the point of contact between a caregiver and patient, e.g., performing a percutaneous biopsy on the wrong kidney) and *latent errors* (systemic, design, or organizational failures that contribute to adverse events). However, it should be recognized that there are certain situations in which the specific actions of an individual team member need to be addressed. Therefore, the concept of a *just culture* has been introduced. A just culture does not punish team members when their actions are commensurate with their experience and training but does hold them accountable for negligent or reckless behavior. In a just culture, it is critical to distinguish *human errors* (also referred to as slips or mistakes) from *at-risk behavior* (e.g., not placing sharps within the appropriate container on the procedure table) from *reckless behavior* (e.g., proceeding with central line placement without performing the required time-out). In this model, any punitive measures to the individual would be based upon the type of behavior exhibited rather than the severity of the event or whether a patient was actually harmed by the incident.

PREPROCEDURAL CARE

Many of the noninterpretive skills necessary for IR occur before the patient ever enters the procedure suite. It is crucial that the interventionalist approaches each case with a thorough patient assessment including an evaluation of the patient's history, physical exam findings, imaging data, and review of pertinent laboratory values. The initial interaction between the IR service and the referring team should be viewed as a request for a consultation rather than an order for a procedure. As consultants, the IR team adds value to the patient's care. Such an approach will maximize the opportunities for success while minimizing the possibility of errors. Moreover, it allows the interventionalist a chance to determine the appropriateness of the requested procedure. In some instances, it may be necessary to offer an alternative treatment from that which was originally requested. The following section discusses several subsequent aspects of preprocedural care including determining the appropriateness of the procedure, establishing realistic patient expectations, planning for pain control and sedation, managing coagulation status, and obtaining informed consent.

Appropriateness

After gathering basic information about the patient's needs, the next question is whether the patient's condition might be best addressed by an image-guided procedure. This requires an understanding of the indications for the procedure as well as the identification of any potential contraindications. Certainly, it would be beyond the scope of the present chapter to adequately address all the indications and contraindications for the wide variety of procedures performed in IR. However, the American College of Radiology (ACR) has developed a set of guidelines, called the ACR Appropriateness Criteria, that can act as a valuable resource when trying to determine the correct course of action for a particular patient. These guidelines have been developed over the past 20 years by task forces consisting of recognized experts. The panels include radiologists and nonradiologists. The guidelines are meant to be seen as *living documents* that can change with new scientific discoveries. The Appropriateness Criteria are divided into 10 clinical imaging topics (breast, cardiac, gastrointestinal, musculoskeletal, neurologic, pediatric, thoracic, urologic, vascular, and women's), which are divided into clinical conditions, then further subdivided into variants of clinical conditions. The panel then uses the best scientific evidence available and, if lacking, expert opinion to determine the appropriateness of an intervention according to each clinical condition on a scale of 1 to 9. Ratings of 1 to 3 are defined as "usually not appropriate," 4 to 6 as "may be appropriate," and 7 to 9 as "usually appropriate." The panel may also opt to indicate that no consensus was reached. In a similar fashion to the Appropriateness Criteria, the ACR has also generated several Practice Parameters and Technical Standards documents that aim to give medical providers guidance toward best practices for their patients. Per the ACR, Practice Parameters describe recommended conduct in specific areas of clinical practice, whereas Technical Standards describe technical parameters that are quantitative or measureable. Importantly, when applying any guideline, one must remember that

each individual patient and situation is unique and a one size fits all approach may not be optimal for patient care. It is vital that differences in training and experience in addition to local practice patterns be taken into account when determining the appropriateness of any given treatment.

Establishing Reasonable Expectations

The interventionalist then needs to review the planned procedure with the patient. This conversation provides an opportunity to establish a rapport with the patient. Such discussions can have a marked impact on the perceived quality of care because patients tend to judge the quality of their healthcare experience by whether it met or exceeded expectations. Patient expectations vary widely, and time spent discussing reasonable predictions about when the procedure will occur, how long it might take, and its impact on the patient's condition is almost always time well spent. This conversation also touches on topics needed to complete the informed consent process, which are discussed later in this chapter.

Pain Control and Sedation

A chief concern for many patients is whether the procedure will be painful. The preprocedure discussion is an opportunity to gauge the patient's needs for analgesia and anxiolysis. This includes the patient's ability to tolerate proper positioning during the procedure. For example, a patient with compromised respiratory status may not be able to lie flat on the table for an extended period of time. Some situations may require the involvement of an anesthesiologist. This process is facilitated by familiarity with the American Society of Anesthesiologists (ASA) physical status classification score (Box 24.1). Patients who classify as ASA I or ASA II should qualify as candidates for sedation. Patients who are classified as ASA III or ASA IV may require further consideration before sedation, which could potentially include a formal consultation with an

---

BOX 24.1 American Society of Anesthesiologists Physical Classification Status

Class I: Normal healthy patient
- Example: Pheresis catheter placement in a healthy stem cell donor

Class II: Patient with mild systemic disease
- Example: Percutaneous abscess drain placement in a child for appendicitis

Class III: Patient with severe systemic disease
- Example: Chemoembolization of liver cancer in a cirrhotic patient

Class IV: Patient with severe systemic disease that is a constant threat to life
- Example: Thrombectomy and thrombolysis of a clotted dialysis graft in a patient with fluid overload, compromised respiratory status, and end-stage renal disease

Class V: Moribund patient that is not expected to live without the procedure
- Example: Splenic angiography and embolization in an unconscious, hypotensive patient with a grade IV splenic laceration after a motor vehicle collision

Class VI: Brain-dead patient being evaluated for organ transplant

anesthesiologist. Patients who are classified as ASA V or above should not be sedated without the assistance of an anesthesiologist. The Joint Commission (TJC) and ASA have described four levels of sedation, including minimal sedation, moderate sedation, deep sedation, and general anesthesia (Box 24.2). Most procedures in IR are performed with minimal or moderate sedation. Prior to administering sedation medications, one must inquire about the patient's NPO (nothing by mouth) status (most institutions require patients to be NPO for 6–8 hours to receive sedation), medication allergies, ability to protect his or her own airway (patients who are at significant risk for aspiration may require general anesthesia for airway protection during their procedure), and any history of obstructive sleep apnea (these patients may require continuous positive airway pressure during their procedure).

Coagulation Status and Hemostasis Risk

Coagulopathies and the use of anticoagulating medications represent one of the most commonly encountered contraindications to image-guided procedures in current practice. Thus, it is imperative that the interventionalist have a general idea about how to manage this complex issue, especially with the ever-increasing number of newer anticoagulants that are coming on the market. The Society of Interventional Radiology (SIR) has established practice guidelines for managing the coagulation status of patients undergoing image-guided interventions, which classifies procedures based on the anticipated bleeding risk (Table 24.1). The SIR has also issued guidelines regarding the use of anticoagulant and antiplatelet medications. The following are general guidelines:

1. A heparin infusion should be stopped or reversed when the activated partial thromboplastin time is 1.5 times normal.
2. One dose of low-molecular-weight heparin should be held for low- to moderate-risk bleeding procedures, and low-molecular-weight heparin should be held for 24 hours for high-risk procedures.
3. It is advisable that patients on warfarin have international normalized ratios within accepted limits (see Table 24.1) prior to the procedure.
4. Clopidogrel should be held for 5 days prior to elective procedures although a platelet transfusion may be appropriate in urgent or emergent circumstances.
5. Aspirin needs to be held for 5 days for high-risk procedures only.

BOX 24.2 Levels of Sedation According to The Joint Commission and American Society of Anesthesiologists

MINIMAL SEDATION
- Patient responds to verbal commands
- Cognitive function and coordination may be impaired
- Ventilatory and cardiovascular functions are intact
- Achieved with oral or intravenous medications

MODERATE SEDATION
- Minimal depression in the level of consciousness
- Patient retains protective reflexes, maintains a patent airway, and has the ability to be aroused by physical or verbal stimulation
- Achieved with intravenous medications

DEEP SEDATION
- Depression of consciousness
- Patients cannot be easily aroused but respond purposefully to repeated or painful stimuli
- Patient's ventilatory function and airway may be compromised but cardiovascular function is maintained
- Usually requires involvement of an anesthesiologist

GENERAL ANESTHESIA
- Controlled state of unconsciousness
- Complete loss of protective reflexes
- Do not respond appropriately to painful stimuli
- Requires involvement of an anesthesiologist

TABLE 24.1 Stratification of Image-Guided Procedures Based on Risk of Bleeding With Suggested Laboratory Cut-Off Values

	Low Risk	Moderate Risk	High Risk
TARGET LAB VALUES			
INR	≤2.0	≤1.5	≤1.5
Platelets (in K/mm³)	≥50	≥50	≥50
EXAMPLES			
Vascular	Dialysis access interventions, venography, central line removal, peripherally inserted venous catheter line placement, inferior vena cava filter placement	Angiography, venous interventions, chemoembolization, uterine fibroid embolization, transjugular liver biopsy, tunneled central venous catheter placement, port placement	Transjugular intrahepatic portosystemic shunt
Nonvascular	Catheter exchanges, thoracentesis, paracentesis, superficial aspirations and drainages, superficial biopsy	Intraabdominal or chest wall drainage or biopsy, lung biopsy, transabdominal liver biopsy, cholecystostomy tube, gastrostomy tube, radiofrequency ablation, spinal procedures	Renal biopsy, biliary interventions, nephrostomy tube placement, complex radiofrequency ablations

INR, International normalized ratio.
Modified from Malloy PC, Grassi CJ, Kundu S, et al. Consensus guidelines for periprocedural management of coagulation status and hemostasis risk in percutaneous image-guided interventions. *J Vasc Interv Radiol.* 2009;20:S240–S249.

6. Newer oral anticoagulants such as rivaroxaban should be stopped 1 to 2 days prior to the procedure.

Remember that these are only guidelines and that local practices may vary. Ultimately, it is best to discuss the withholding of anticoagulant or antiplatelet medications with the referring physician because it may not be possible to withhold such medication for some patients (e.g., recent cardiac stents) for any period of time. The consideration of patient-specific factors and overall care plan should be paramount in the decision-making process.

Informed Consent

The patient has a right to provide informed consent for any image-guided procedure and for the use of sedation. Because sedation has the ability to impair cognition, it is necessary to obtain informed consent prior to the administration of any sedation agents. The physician who is ultimately responsible for performing or supervising the procedure should be available to answer any questions or concerns that the patient may have, even though an appropriately trained midlevel provider or trainee with sufficient familiarity with the procedure may also obtain consent. The requirements for informed consent can vary from state to state, thus familiarity with local laws, regulations, and hospital policy is essential. At a minimum, informed consent should include a discussion with the patient regarding the purpose of the procedure, the method through which the procedure will be performed, its expected benefits, risks associated with the procedure (including the hazards of radiation exposure), any reasonable treatment alternatives, the risks of refusing treatment, and an acknowledgment of the patient's right to refuse treatment. The patient should demonstrate an understanding of the procedure and a willingness to proceed. This discussion should then be documented in the patient's medical record through a form signed by both the patient and the healthcare provider. Undoubtedly, there will be many instances in which patients may be temporarily or permanently incapable of making their own medical decisions. Under these circumstances, the medical team can obtain informed consent from the patient's authorized medical decision maker or appropriate family member. The scope of these conversations should be no less thorough than previously outlined. It is preferable to obtain informed consent from the patient's family or medical decision maker in person; however, it can also be obtained over the phone in certain situations. If telephone consent is obtained, the consent should be witnessed and attested to by a second healthcare provider on the consent form. For patients who have not yet reached the age of consent, informed consent can be obtained from their legal guardians in a similar fashion as detailed earlier. If the patient is incapable of making medical decisions in an emergent situation, the physician treating the patient can proceed with the procedure as long as it is medically necessary. The need for such emergent intervention and the inability to obtain informed consent in a timely manner should be well documented in the patient's chart.

INTRAPROCEDURAL CARE

After the patient has been deemed an appropriate candidate for the procedure, been fully evaluated, and provided informed consent, it is time to perform the procedure in a manner that maximizes the likelihood of success. One key to a successful procedure is the recognition by the interventionalist of the complexity of the patient and the myriad ways in which complications can arise while performing image-guided procedures. The following section introduces various noninterpretive skills necessary for IR during the actual performance of the procedure including the Universal Protocol for Preventing Wrong Site, Wrong Side, or Wrong Patient Surgery; infection prevention; radiation safety; executing a successful plan; and issues pertaining to the use of intraprocedural sedation.

Universal Protocol

Wrong-site/-side procedures and wrong implantable devices are considered *never events* by TJC. It is the responsibility of the performing physician to try to assure that these events do not take place despite the variety of causal factors likely at play. TJC's Universal Protocol for Preventing Wrong Site, Wrong Side, or Wrong Patient Surgery is a set of steps designed to help prevent these types of error throughout procedural areas in the hospital, including IR. According to the Universal Protocol, the healthcare team should perform a preprocedure verification process prior to entering the IR suite. This process should verify that the correct patient is about to enter the procedure suite using two patient identifiers. Furthermore, team members should ensure that everyone, including the patient, if possible, is clear about the procedure to be performed and the site of the procedure. Finally, team members should check that all necessary items to perform the procedure are readily available. The site of the procedure needs to be marked by the provider performing the procedure who, ideally, involves the patient in the site-marking process. Once in the procedural suite, a time-out involving all procedural personnel is performed prior to any invasive actions on the patient. The time-out process should be led by a designated member of the team, be standardized, and result in all team members agreeing on patient identity, procedure site, and the procedure to be performed. Using a checklist that is jointly developed by physicians, nursing, and technical staff can help with standardizing the time-out and making it a routine part of the everyday IR practice. Discrepancies discovered during the preprocedure verification process require resolution, and this may involve direct discussion with the referring physician to clarify details of the planned procedure.

Preventing Infection

The majority of procedures in IR entail some level of sterility. The first line of defense against procedure-related infection is the practice of good hand hygiene by all members of the team. It is well accepted that proper hand hygiene reduces nosocomial infections. Proper hand washing requires the use of an alcohol-based hand rub, antimicrobial soap and water, or plain soap and water. Alcohol-based hand rubs are preferred to soap and water given that they are more effective in reducing bacterial counts and provide a longer-lasting antimicrobial effect. However, one should remember that alcohol-based rubs are not recommended when hands are visibly soiled or after exposure to certain microorganisms. The use of aseptic technique for most procedures can also help reduce the risk of infection for the patient. This can be accomplished by cleaning the skin thoroughly with a 2% chlorhexidine-based agent, iodine, or a 70% alcohol-based solution. The skin should be allowed to completely dry, and a sterile drape should be placed over the patient. Certain procedures, such as central venous catheter placement, require the use of *maximum sterile barrier technique*, which is defined as the use of a cap, mask, sterile gown, sterile glove, a large sterile sheet, hand hygiene, and cutaneous antisepsis.

It is reasonable for the reader to become familiar with how the SIR has classified procedures with regard to their risk of infection, which follows the recommendations of the National Academy of Sciences/National Research Council. In this schema, a *clean procedure* does not pass through the gastrointestinal tract, genitourinary tract, respiratory tract, or an inflamed area. An example of this type of procedure in IR is the placement of a central venous catheter. A *clean-contaminated procedure* is where a noninfected/noninflamed gastrointestinal, biliary, or genitourinary tract is traversed. An example of this would be percutaneous gastrostomy tube placement. A *contaminated procedure* crosses through an inflamed or colonized gastrointestinal tract or genitourinary tract without evidence of frank pus. An example of this would be placement of a percutaneous nephrostomy tube in a patient with a urinary obstruction. Finally, a *dirty procedure* is one that involves entering a purulent site, such as with percutaneous abscess drainage. It is recommended that all clean and clean-contaminated procedures follow sterile technique as outlined earlier. With regard to periprocedural antibiotics, there is great variability in the IR community concerning their use for various procedures. For example, at some institutions, all patients receive a dose of prophylactic antibiotics prior to chest-wall port placement, whereas this is done more selectively at other institutions. An in-depth discussion of this topic is outside the scope of this chapter; however, the SIR has produced practice guidelines and recommendations for antibiotic prophylaxis for a number of commonly performed procedures. This document can be found in the Suggested Readings.

Radiation Safety

Imaging guidance is the cornerstone of IR. The majority of procedures involve exposing both patients and medical personnel to the ionizing radiation emitted from fluoroscopes or computed tomography (CT) scanners. The resulting images are used to plan the procedure as well as assess its progress. Although imaging provides clear and immediate benefits, the risks of skin injury and possible cancer induction necessitate a balanced approach. Physicians need to work with technologists and medical physicists to efficiently and effectively guide the procedure while minimizing the risks.

When considering radiation dose, there are two driving factors: the number of images necessary to complete the procedure and dose per image. As summarized in Table 24.2, dose per image can be further broken down into multiple components. Table 24.3 summarizes the factors that influence the number of images per procedure.

To a first approximation, the dose for medical personnel performing the procedure depends on the patient's dose. Reducing the patient's dose via the above factors will typically reduce the procedure team's dose. The procedure team can further reduce their doses via distance and shielding. The procedure team can also reduce their dose by understanding how their dose results from photons scattered within the patient. They should position themselves and any shielding material accordingly. The team can also employ additional dose optimization strategies. For example, operators should avoid acquiring high-dose images, such as spot images and digital subtraction angiography sequences, solely for the purpose of documentation when lower-dose alternatives, such as saving a single fluoroscopic image, would suffice. Interventionalists should also take an active role in reviewing and revising their current imaging protocols to find ways to minimize dose. The aim should be to create low-dose protocols with decreased frame rates and a diminished automatic exposure

TABLE 24.2 Factors Affecting Dose per Image

Factor	Control Point	Comment
Pixels/image	Image collimation	Collimation provides a reduced dose and improved images but at the cost of a diminished ability to monitor peripheral events.
Dose/pixel	Imaging protocol: setpoint for the automatic exposure control circuit	Automatic exposure control setpoint influences image quality through the number of photons available to populate each pixel in the image.
	Imaging protocol: beam intensity (peak kilovoltage) and energy profile (copper filtration)	Higher peak kilovoltage improves beam penetration but tends to reduce image contrast. Using copper filtration to preferentially attenuate lower-energy photons leads to lower skin dose but also leads to increased tube heating.
	Path length including the influence of angulation	Attenuation increases logarithmically with path length. Steep angulation typically increases path length.
	Material within the region of interest monitored by the automatic exposure control circuit	Attenuation also increases logarithmically with concentration of attenuating material (iodine, barium, metal, etc.)
	Magnification	As pixel size decreases, the intensity of the incident beam increases to maintain photons/pixels.
	Geometry: patient to detector distance	Reducing the distance between the patient and detector reduces the dose.
Skin dose/pixel	Geometry: x-ray source to patient distance	Increasing the air gap between the x-ray source and the patient reduces skin dose.

TABLE 24.3 Factors Affecting the Number of Images per Procedure

Factor	Control Point	Comment
Task difficulty	Planned procedure	All other factors being equal, simple procedures like central venous catheter placement have fewer decision points than complex procedures like biliary drainage or arterial embolization. As the number and complexity of intraprocedural decisions increase, more imaging data are needed. This typically leads to increases in images/procedure and pixels/image.
	Patient selection	Procedural complexity is also clearly influenced by patient factors. For example, central venous catheter placement becomes more difficult in patients with central venous stenoses or occlusions.
	Temporal resolution	High frame rates are needed to adequately assess rapidly changing situations (e.g., digital subtraction angiography at 6 fps in pulmonary angiography). On the other hand, a single image is sufficient for depicting static processes.
System capabilities	Team's skill in task planning and execution	Importance of prior experience with the same or similar tasks.
	Imaging tools	Last image hold, positioning tools, access to prior studies.
	Catheters, guidewires, devices and contrast agents	Differential attenuation of catheters, guidewires, devices, and contrast agents; operator familiarity with these tools.
Procedure documentation	Data capture tools	Ability to save individual fluoroscopy frames and fluoroscopy sequences.

control set point. Such low-dose protocols may be used as the starting point for the procedure with the ability to increase to higher-dose protocols if necessary.

Executing a Successful Procedure

Every voluntary action includes two phases: planning and execution. Planning is usually more than analyzing the problem at hand and selecting an appropriate action to achieve the desired goal. Planning often includes strategies for monitoring whether the planned action is proceeding toward the desired goal. Indeed, even simple actions such as advancing a needle toward a target include visual and/or tactile feedback loops that adjust arm and finger movements approximately 10 times per second. During image-guided procedures, the fluoroscopy, ultrasound, or CT images are analyzed to assess if the forces exerted on the external portion of a tool (needle or needle hub, guidewire, etc.) are having the desired effect on the other end of the tool. Each adjustment of the tool involves triggering the appropriate muscles and their motor units to accomplish the desired task.

Errors can occur during planning or execution. Execution errors cause one's hand to overshoot or undershoot the desired target. However, because task planning includes a monitoring strategy, such errors are readily identified and corrected. In contrast, planning errors are pernicious. They escape immediate detection and instead become apparent only after some delay. Planning errors are only apparent when successful completion of the desired set of actions does not yield the desired result. Errors in image interpretation are a type of planning error because reviewing a CT scan with a periappendiceal abscess and choosing a needle path that traverses the inferior epigastric artery will not yield the desired result. In this scheme, planning becomes more important than execution. Good plans anticipate problems with execution and include monitoring strategies that detect and act on execution errors before they cause irreparable harm.

Intraprocedural Sedation

A large majority of procedures in IR are performed with the patient receiving intravenous sedation. The interventionalist should have a sufficient background in the safe administration of sedation agents which, at many institutions, requires documented training in sedation, periodic evaluation of physician competency, and a current certification in both basic life support and advanced cardiac life support. Apart from the supervising physician, there must also be a nurse or otherwise qualified healthcare professional in the room at all times whose primary focus is that of monitoring the patient during the procedure. Continuous monitoring should include the level of consciousness, respiratory rate, pulse oximetry, blood pressure, heart rate, and cardiac rhythm. Similar monitoring is needed in the recovery period after sedation.

Most interventionalists use a combination of fentanyl (analgesic) and midazolam (anxiolytic) for sedation. A typical starting dose for midazolam and fentanyl would be 1 mg and 50 µg, respectively, which can be repeated approximately every 5 to 10 minutes until the desired level of sedation is achieved. If the patient's cardiorespiratory status becomes compromised from oversedation, then naloxone 0.4 mg IV every 2 to 3 minutes can be administered for the reversal of fentanyl while flumazenil 0.2 mg IV every 1 minute can be given to reverse the effects of midazolam. Many institutions require some sort of safety report if reversal agents are used during a procedure.

POSTPROCEDURAL CARE

One of the most important changes in the field of IR has been the development of the role of IR as a clinical specialty that can provide continuity of care to its patients. Providing responsible postprocedural care is another unique aspect of IR when compared with DR that requires the interventionalist to establish a treatment relationship with the patient and a clinical rapport with referring services. The following section focuses on critical postprocedural issues in IR including postprocedural monitoring, communication, specimen handling, and safety monitoring with regard to radiation doses and procedure-related complications.

Postprocedure Monitoring

There is variability among IR practices concerning the amount and timing of postprocedural monitoring that is required for a host of procedures. For example, some practices would admit all patients for a percutaneous gastrostomy tube or percutaneous abscess drain, whereas other practices may perform these procedures on an outpatient basis in certain circumstances. Additionally, various protocols exist for patient monitoring after percutaneous renal biopsies that range from overnight admission to a simple 2-hour postprocedure monitoring period. Certainly, many of these decisions must be tailored to local practice patterns and physician experience. Nevertheless, there are certain things that should be kept in mind when considering these issues such as the nature/invasiveness of the procedure, patient status, and the type of sedation used during the procedure. Clearly, invasive procedures that carry a high risk of bleeding or other complication (e.g., liver biopsy, renal biopsy, transjugular intrahepatic portosystemic shunt) require more monitoring than a routine exchange of a long-standing nephrostomy tube. Outpatients may require longer monitoring than inpatients for the same procedure, given that they will be discharged to home. Patients from intensive care units are typically best served by an immediate return to their inpatient bed after an IR procedure where they can benefit from a high level of care. Finally, patients who receive only local anesthesia may be discharged from IR almost immediately after their procedure, whereas patients who receive general anesthesia typically require an admission to the postanesthesia care unit for recovery. For outpatients who receive sedation, several conditions must be met prior to their discharge. First, they must have returned to a baseline level of consciousness. Second, they should have stable vital signs. Third, a responsible party should be with the patient to accompany him or her home because patients are unable to drive or make decisions after receiving sedation. Fourth, in accordance with recommendations from TJC, patients and their caregivers should be provided with written instructions regarding medications, activity, diet, follow-up (if necessary), and a phone number to call in case of questions or an emergency.

Communication

The traditional written radiology report is the most common form of communication between radiologists and the remainder of the healthcare team. It serves as both medical and legal documentation of care provided for practitioners in both DR and IR. Yet referring physicians do not generally read IR procedure reports on a routine basis given that the focus of IR is primarily providing treatment to patients rather than diagnostic information to referring physicians. Therefore, it is requisite for the IR team to ensure that treatment findings and future recommendations are communicated to the other medical teams involved in the patient's care. Problems with postprocedural communication and hand-offs are not unique to IR. According to TJC, poor communication during care transitions can result in treatment delay, increased cost, medical errors, and inefficiency from redundant activities. The Agency for Healthcare Research and Quality emphasizes the use of the acronym ANTICipate for effective patient sign-out, which signifies *a*dministrative data (e.g., name, date of birth), *n*ew clinical information, *t*asks that need to be performed by the receiving provider, *i*llness severity, and *c*ontingency plans for changes in the patient's clinical status. This communication can occur in person, over the phone, or even over email in some situations. However, even though direct communication with the other medical teams is vital for patient care, these conversations do not supplant the necessity of documenting findings and recommendations in the procedure report and in the patient's chart. Strong, consistent, and effective communication from the IR team will help foster camaraderie with other clinical services.

Specimen Handling

The large number of medical personnel from various departments who are involved in specimen acquisition, labeling, transport, and evaluation means that errors in processing and handling can occur at many points in the chain. These types of errors are not uncommon, and exact causes of any specific problem with specimens are difficult to pinpoint. Although intuitive, the best mechanism to deal with lost or mishandled specimens is to avoid the problem in the first place. This requires the IR team to have a clear discussion with the referring service prior to the procedure to determine what clinical information is desired and with the pathology department to ensure that the samples are prepared properly. For example, tissue samples for flow cytometry may need to be placed in normal saline rather than formalin. If there is any confusion about sample preparation or storage, the interventionalist should speak directly with the pathology department and document that conversation in the procedure report. Specimens should be placed in the appropriate solution or container and clearly marked with the following information: two patient identifiers, site of collection, date of collection, and time of collection. The accompanying pathology requisition form should be filled out with matching information in addition to any relevant clinical history that may guide the pathologist toward the correct diagnosis. Once labeled, the specimen needs to be delivered in a timely fashion to the laboratory. Many interventionalists choose to hand-deliver their specimens to increase the speed and reliability of delivery. Most pathology departments have a sign-in sheet to document when specimens were received. If such a log is not available, the interventionalist can document, in the patient's medical record, the time of specimen delivery and the name of the individual who received the specimen.

Monitoring Radiation Dose

Data-driven improvements in radiation safety require collecting data and analyzing them. Modern fluoroscopy units provide multiple measures of radiation use (Table 24.4).

TABLE 24.4 **Measures of Radiation Use During Procedures**

Metric	Units	Utility
Peak skin dose ($D_{skin,max}$)	mGy	Best predictor of possible skin injury
Reference point air kerma ($K_{a,r}$)	mGy	Surrogate for total skin dose
Kerma area product (P_{KA})	Gy cm^2	X-ray energy deposited in field of view and potential for future neoplastic transformation
Fluoroscopy time	Seconds or minutes	Procedure difficulty

TABLE 24.5 **Key Dose Metric Thresholds for Fluoroscopically Guided Procedures**

Dose Metric	Initial Alert	Substantial Radiation Dose Level[a]
Peak skin dose	2 Gy	3 Gy
Reference point air kerma	3 Gy	5 Gy
Kerma area product	300 Gy cm^2	500 Gy cm^2
Fluoroscopy time	30 min	60 min

[a]Procedures where the dose metric exceeds these Substantial Radiation Dose Levels warrant notification of the referring physician, patient, and follow-up per recommendations from the National Council on Radiation Protection and Measurements (NCRP).

The usefulness of these measures varies. Although older units might only provide fluoroscopy time, fluoroscopy time is not a useful measure of radiation exposure because it does not take into account dose per image or images per second.

One of the chief aims of monitoring radiation exposure is to avoid radiation-induced skin injuries. These are most common following complex procedures where an intense x-ray beam repeatedly passed through the same skin entry point. Tracking peak skin dose during a procedure requires not only assessing the intensity of the beam but also mapping the skin entry point. Reference point air kerma ($K_{a,r}$) serves as a surrogate measure of beam intensity at the skin entry point, but it must be combined with patient position, table position, beam angles, and field of view during each exposure to create skin dose maps. Newer systems are capable of aggregating this information and calculating maps of estimated skin doses. A second goal of monitoring radiation exposure is monitoring overall exposure. Kerma area product (P_{KA}) estimates the total x-ray energy deposited in the field of view. When P_{KA} is combined with information on which organs were within the field of view and the imaging angles, it can be used to begin estimating organ doses. Although such calculations are not yet routinely available, they provide the best insight into the possibility of future carcinogenesis.

Recording these dose metrics provides two benefits. First, it allows predictions at the level of individual patients, such as the probability of skin injury from the current procedure and how that risk might be compounded by subsequent procedures in the coming months. Indeed, the procedure team might use skin dose maps to plan beam position and orientation to avoid skin sites that received the highest dose in the prior procedure. The team might also use those skin dose maps to counsel patients about the delayed but observable consequences of the recent procedure on the patient's skin. Second, capturing dose metrics provides the data needed to drive improvement efforts. In the same way that image-guided procedures have an expected duration (e.g., 5 minutes for a central venous catheter or 60 minutes for a hepatic chemoembolization), fluoroscopic procedures should have expected values for the different radiation metrics. Quality improvement projects use deviations from expectation as signals of potential failures in efficient/effective use of radiation or the predictive model. A single large deviation (30 minutes for a central venous catheter where the $K_{a,r}$ was 200 mGy) is usually readily apparent. Smaller, but systematic deviations (routinely requiring 10 minutes for a central venous catheter with $K_{a,r}$ of 75 mGy) are best detected using control charts and other tools from statistical process control. Effective monitoring also requires flexibility as to who is monitoring. During procedures, the performing physician's attention is usually focused on catheters, needles, guidewires, and other devices, not the portion of the fluoroscopy screen where radiation metrics are displayed. As a result, the other team members, especially technologists, are usually better able to monitor radiation metrics. This includes acknowledging alarms that occur at preset thresholds and alerting the physician when key thresholds are crossed (Table 24.5).

After the procedure, radiation metrics should be recorded. The need to monitor dose metrics in CT has led many hospitals to invest in dose monitoring systems. These systems can also be used to capture, store, and help analyze dose metrics from fluoroscopic procedures. Patients whose procedure exceeds the substantial radiation dose level may have skin changes such as erythema in the coming days and weeks. More severe skin changes occur with higher doses, and patients and their referring physicians should be informed of the expected skin changes and need to avoid additional high-dose exposures that could cause further skin damage.

Monitoring Key Performance Indicators and Complications

Key performance indicators (KPIs) are measures that are selected to evaluate organizational and individual success. These measures could be related to patient safety, quality, and/or financial measures; however, an ideal KPI should reflect the ideals of the institution in addition to being well defined, measurable, and reproducible. In radiology, one of the most common KPIs employed is report turnaround time. In IR, KPIs could include relative value unit generation, patient satisfaction scores, central line infection rates, hospital readmission rates, number of sedation reversals, compliance with a preprocedural time-out, and/or complications. In academic centers, KPIs could also be related to educational and research activities. There are many mechanisms available for the monitoring of KPIs including *dashboards* (graphical visual representations of each relevant measure typically made available electronically on a single screen for easy viewing), *run charts* (graphical display

TABLE 24.6   Possible Trigger Events in Interventional Radiology

Event Category	Event Description	Trigger Tool
Oversedation	Sedation reversal	Pharmacy records of reversal agents
Procedural complication	Unplanned need for increased monitoring	Transfer to higher level of care
Procedural complication	Rescue	Calling rapid response or code team
Nondurable result	Earlier than expected return for additional procedure	Unplanned additional procedure
Radiation exposure	Potential skin injury	Dose reporting system identifies cases that exceed Substantial Radiation Dose Levels (see Table 24.5)

used in process variation analyses where data points are plotted to show the trend over time rather than focusing on any single data point), and *control charts* (graphical display used in process variation analyses, where data points are plotted to show trends over time but to also display the mean or median in addition to upper and lower limits for normal process variation). Apart from KPIs, other specialties have developed trigger tools to help monitor the current system's performance and estimate event frequency. These trigger tools are used to analyze objective data acquired during the course of normal operations. In many practices, a positive trigger tool prompts the need for further investigation as well as entering the investigation's results into an event reporting system. These trigger tools provide an additional layer of system surveillance. Several trigger tools for image-guided procedures are summarized in Table 24.6.

Although careful planning and skillful execution during each of a procedure's steps offer the highest probability of achieving the desired outcome, untoward outcomes will occur. It is important for interventionalists to track their complications and participate in regular morbidity and mortality conferences. The SIR has provided definitions of both major and minor complications by outcome to the patient to facilitate this tracking. In this classification scheme, minor complications result in no additional therapy/consequence or only nominal therapy or consequences. Extending the postprocedure observation period falls under this category as well. Major complications are then defined as resulting in death, permanent adverse sequelae, an unplanned increase in the patient's level of care, additional major therapy, prolonged hospitalizations (>48 hours), or additional therapy necessitating a minor hospitalization (<48 hours). Complications should also be tracked so that they can be compared against national benchmarks provided and used as a means to identify practice areas in need of improvement. Although the number and diversity of procedures performed by IR preclude an exhaustive discussion of every benchmark,

the ACR and SIR worked together to produce a set of practice parameters and technical standards for many procedures which, in most cases, includes the accepted rate of complications for the procedure and an additional complication rate that should trigger a review within the institution. Hopefully, these unpredicted events are infrequent, but when they do occur, they provide a learning opportunity. Only by recording such events and better understanding what factors caused these deviations from expectation can we hope to better understand the underlying system and improve its future performance. Event reporting systems are now commonly used to capture such occurrences, but unfortunately, they tend to underestimate event frequency.

SUGGESTED READINGS

American Board of Radiology. Noninterpretive Skills Resource Guide. <http://www.theabr.org/sites/all/themes/abr-media/pdf/Noninterpretive_Skills_Domain_Specification_and_Resource_Guide.pdf>.

American College of Radiology. ACR Practice Parameters and Technical Standards. <http://www.acr.org/~/media/ACR/Documents/PGTS/toc.pdf>.

Chan D, Downing D, Keough CE, et al. Joint practice guideline for sterile technique during vascular and interventional radiology procedures. *J Vasc Interven Radiol.* 2012;23:1603–1612.

Kandarpa K, Machan L, eds. *Handbook of Interventional Radiologic Procedures.* 4th ed. Philadelphia, PA: Lippincott Williams & Wilkins; 2011.

Kohi MP, Fidelman N, Behr S, et al. Periprocedural patient care. *Radiographics.* 2015;35:1766–1768.

Malloy PC, Grassi CJ, Kundu S, et al. Consensus guidelines for periprocedural management of coagulation status and hemostasis risk in percutaneous image-guided interventions. *J Vasc Interv Radiol.* 2009;20:S240–S249.

National Council on Radiation Protection and Measurements. *Radiation Dose Management for Fluoroscopically Guided Interventional Medical Procedures.* Bethesda, MD: National Council on Radiation Protection and Measurements; 2011.

Omary RA, Bettmann MA, Cardella JF, et al. Quality improvement guidelines for the reporting and archiving of interventional radiology procedures. *J Vasc Interven Radiol.* 2003;14:S293–S295.

Patel IJ, Davidson JC, Nikolic B, et al. Consensus guidelines for periprocedural management of coagulation status and hemostasis risk in percutaneous image-guided interventions. *J Vasc Interven Radiol.* 2012;23:727–736.

Patel IJ, Davidson JC, Nikolic B, et al. Addendum of newer anticoagulants to the SIR consensus guideline. *J Vasc Interven Radiol.* 2013;24:641–645.

Venkatesan AM, Kundu S, Sacks D, et al. Practice guideline for adult antibiotic prophylaxis during vascular and interventional radiology procedures. *J Vasc Interven Radiol.* 2010;21:1611–1630.

Chapter 25
Quality Considerations in Children

Michael M. Moore, Einat Blumfield, and Ramesh S. Iyer

Although many of the quality and safety discussions throughout this volume are applicable to all aspects of radiology including the imaging of children, there are several topics that are especially critical or unique to pediatric patients including radiation reduction, sedation, and selection of the optimal study.

RADIATION REDUCTION

In recent years, medical imaging has become a major source of ionizing radiation exposure, with the most significant contributor being computed tomography (CT) scans. In the United States, the annual number of CT scans has steadily increased from 3 million in 1980, to 26 million in 1998, to more than 70 million in 2008. Ionizing radiation in doses administered by CT scans may cause damage to DNA and increase the lifetime risk of cancer. The lifetime risk of developing cancer is cumulative and increases with repeated exposures. It is well accepted by the medical community that children are more sensitive to ionizing radiation than adults because their organs and tissues are still developing. Furthermore, because children have a longer life expectancy from the time of exposure, their lifetime cancer risk is higher.

It is therefore critical for every medical professional who orders or performs imaging studies to decrease the radiation exposure to the minimum required for the diagnosis and management of children. This is the central principle of the *as low as reasonably achievable* (ALARA) concept and is reflected in the guidelines of the Image Gently campaign that was launched in 2008 by the Alliance for Radiation Safety in Pediatric imaging.

Following a review of several basic measures of radiation, the emphasis of the discussion in this section will be the reduction of radiation exposure from CT, which is the major contributor of ionizing radiation. Additional modalities such as fluoroscopy are also discussed.

Basic Measures of Radiation

Absorbed dose: This term refers to the radiation dose concentration applied to a given unit or volume and is measured in grays (Gy).

Dose equivalent: This term, expressed in sieverts (Sv), refers to the biological effect of a given type of radiation in relation to the gamma or x-ray.

Effective dose: This term is a method of converting dose to specific organs to an equivalent risk to the whole body (measured in millisieverts [mSv]).

CT dose index (CTDI): This is a measurement of radiation dose based on a phantom (32 or 16 cm). This measurement takes into account the absorbed dose within a slice.

The measure of CTDI volume (CTDIvol) is more standard and takes into account the contribution of pitch: CTDIvol = CTDI/pitch. Pitch is defined as the distance of table translation in the *z*-axis per rotation of the scanner gantry.

Dose length product (DLP): This is the product of CTDIvol and the scan length in centimeters. DLP is the radiation dose of the entire scan, expressed in mGy•cm.

It is important to understand that CTDIvol and DLP are measures of radiation output and not of patient dose. The size-specific dose estimate is an estimate of the patient dose taking into consideration the thickness of the torso. This applies only to CT examinations of the torso.

Efforts to Reduce Radiation Exposure From Computed Tomography Scans

The Image Gently campaign recommends that radiologists take the lead and be committed to increase awareness and to work in collaboration with clinicians, technologists, and physicists to reduce radiation doses. In addition, it recommends revising CT protocols by eliminating multiphase scanning (because additional phases rarely add useful information in children), adjusting the doses administered in each scan, and limiting the scans to the area of interest.

Studies demonstrated that such interventions led to significant reductions in the number of CT scans and in the administered radiation doses. This was achieved by increasing the awareness of clinicians, radiology residents, and CT technologists through education and training. Introduction of alternative methods of imaging (e.g., ultrasound for acute appendicitis, magnetic resonance imaging [MRI] for headache) and daily interactions with the ordering clinicians, particularly in pediatric emergency departments where the majority of CT scans are ordered, played a significant role as well.

Revision of scanning protocols to reduce the administered dose of each scan may involve automatic tube current modulation, adjustment of the tube potential (peak kilovoltage), and use of modern algorithms that enable significant dose reduction while maintaining diagnostic image quality (e.g., Adaptive Statistical Iterative Reconstruction). This should be done in collaboration with medical physicists.

Efforts to Reduce Radiation Exposure From Digital Radiography

Digital radiography has largely replaced traditional film radiography and has become the standard in the United States. Although it has many advantages, there is a risk of exposure to higher radiation doses. It is therefore important to educate radiologists and radiographers to prevent unnecessary radiation exposure to children. As always, the ALARA principle should be applied, and only the clinically indicated region should be exposed. Grids should only be used when the body part thickness dictates their need. Technologists must properly collimate before the exposure rather than using electronic cropping of the image after the exposure. Automatic exposure control has many advantages, but it should be used cautiously because it may not work well for children.

Efforts to Reduce Radiation Exposure From Fluoroscopy

The Pause and Pulse campaign by Image Gently addresses the need to protect children from radiation exposure during fluoroscopy. It emphasizes the need to *child-size* the radiation exposure and use pulsed fluoroscopy at the lowest rate required for diagnostic imaging. Prior to the examination, the technologist should select the appropriate setting of the machine for the size of the child and for the examination.

During the examination it is recommended to use breast and gonadal shielding when possible. To decrease scatter and patient doses, it is important to lower the image intensifier, to use appropriate collimation, and to avoid magnification when not necessary. Furthermore, a last image hold can be used instead of a radiographic spot image, which administers a radiation dose about 10 times higher. The radiologist needs to pay attention to the duration of fluoroscopy and to reduce it to the minimum required.

Efforts to Reduce Radiation Exposure From Interventional Radiology

The Step Lightly campaign by Image Gently addresses radiation protection of children who undergo interventional procedures. Interventional procedures can be performed under CT or fluoroscopic guidance. The principles are similar to the other, previously discussed, modalities and apply the same steps that were discussed in the CT and fluoroscopy sections. These steps involve shielding, collimation, child-sizing the exposure, and using the lowest doses that are required for diagnosis and management.

Efforts to Reduce Radiation From Nuclear Medicine

Nuclear medicine tests may be essential for diagnosing illnesses in children. As in every other modality in which ionizing radiation is administered, it is important to follow the ALARA principle, to perform tests only when justified, and to consider alternative imaging modalities. When performing the tests it is important to child-size the doses of the administered radiopharmaceuticals. For specific doses, Image Gently provides the *2014 Update of the North American Consensus Guidelines for Pediatric Administered Radiopharmaceutical Activities*.

SEDATION

Sedation is a vital component for many diagnostic imaging studies and image-guided procedures in children. Its use has grown in recent years due to a variety of factors. There are newer, more effective agents with improved adverse effect profiles. As pediatric exam volumes increase, there is a premium placed on minimizing patient motion safely and efficiently. Keeping children comfortable and managing pain during examinations are also of utmost importance, particularly during interventional procedures.

The goals of sedation in the pediatric patient include (1) keeping the patient safe, (2) minimizing any pain or discomfort, (3) minimizing any anxiety or potential psychological trauma, (4) controlling behavior and motion to ensure a successful examination, and (5) returning the patient to a state in which he or she may be safely discharged from the department.

Managing sedation in radiology departments is a multidisciplinary task. This team of providers may consist of one or more radiologists, anesthesiologists, critical care physicians, nurse anesthetists, registered nurses, child life specialists, technologists, and other medical personnel. The area in which sedation is administered should be fully equipped to manage emergencies and/or resuscitation. Most major complications from sedation are adverse respiratory events, including airway compromise, hypoventilation, hypoxemia, and apnea. Cardiovascular complications such as hypotension or arrest may also occur. Rare complications from sedation include allergic reactions and seizures. To guard against these potential life-threatening events, sedation facilities should have emergency kits (crash carts) on hand and a protocol in place to recruit backup emergency services.

Sedation in a radiology department presents some unique challenges. It requires the coordination of multiple providers, services, and devices to be brought together simultaneously to administer sedation. These difficulties are often compounded by the need to allay fears of children and their families and by the nature of a busy schedule that prioritizes throughput. Radiology suites usually have bulky equipment that the sedation team must maneuver around to access the patient. Providers also must remain mindful of MRI safety when selecting their equipment. This can be particularly challenging if a severe adverse event occurs with a patient in the magnet. Finally, sedation for imaging often requires the child to be transported to and from a nonradiology location, such as a procedure room or postanesthesia care unit. This distance may be substantial depending on the department layout and the location of these resources. These considerations often impact where sedation can be initiated and when the patient is transported, which are the two periods associated with the greatest adverse event risk.

In general, healthy children 6 to 7 years and older can tolerate most diagnostic imaging examinations without sedation, including MRI. Most infants younger than 3 to 4 months can avoid sedation for MRI by feeding and then letting them fall asleep just prior to the examination. Young children between these age groups most often require sedation for diagnostic imaging. Older children who are developmentally delayed or who have physical impairments also may need sedation to minimize motion or reduce anxiety. The inherent risks and costs of sedation may be avoided through several alternative techniques. MRI-compatible video goggles, digital video disk players, wall-mounted television screens, and headphones playing patient-selected music may all be employed. Oral sucrose solution (e.g., Sweet-Ease), pacifiers, and swaddling are used to calm newborns. Child life or play specialists are often invaluable in distracting patients during imaging studies and may introduce anxious children to their upcoming exam through videos or toys (e.g., miniature plastic CT gantry).

Definitions

- *Minimal sedation (anxiolysis):* The patient is awake but calm and responds normally to verbal stimuli. Respiratory and cardiovascular functions remain normal.
- *Moderate sedation ("conscious sedation"):* The patient is drowsy but responds purposefully to verbal or light tactile stimulation. Respiratory and cardiovascular functions remain normal.
- *Deep sedation:* There is depressed consciousness, and the patient cannot be easily aroused; he or she may respond purposefully after repeated verbal or tactile stimulation. Respiratory and cardiovascular function may be impaired, and an artificial airway may be required. This state may be indistinguishable from general anesthesia.
- *General anesthesia:* There is complete loss of purposeful response to verbal and tactile stimuli. The patient's ability to maintain the airway is typically lost, and cardiovascular function may be impaired.

Despite these definitions, from a practical standpoint, sedation should be viewed as a continuum. It is frequently difficult to distinguish deeper levels of sedation clinically, and the patient may move between levels of sedation during an exam. At some institutions, the only levels of sedation generally used are mild sedation and general anesthesia.

Practitioners administering sedation should be appropriately licensed and credentialed to do so. They must be skilled in identifying the varying levels of sedation and be prepared to recover the patient from at least one level deeper than intended. Providers should be able to recognize loss of or impending airway compromise and be prepared to deliver respiratory support as warranted. They must be intimately familiar with the pharmacology of the administered sedative(s), its antagonist(s), and any rescue medications in the emergency kit.

Screening Assessment

The screening evaluation prior to sedating pediatric patients is of critical importance. Key components are a focused review of the child's current health, any chronic illnesses or underlying disorders, and a review of systems. The physical examination includes a complete upper airway assessment to identify possible intubation difficulties. The team will also elicit a complete medication history and note any allergies. Informed consent for sedation must be obtained and documented according to institutional policy.

TABLE 25.1 **American Society of Anesthesiologists Physical Status Classification System**

Class I	A normal healthy patient
Class II	A patient with mild systemic disease
Class III	A patient with severe systemic disease
Class IV	A patient with severe systemic disease that is a constant threat to life
Class V	A moribund patient who is not expected to survive without the operation
Class VI	A declared brain-dead patient whose organs are being removed for donor purposes

From American Society of Anesthesiologists (ASA) Physical Status Classification System (last approved 10/15/2014). http://www.asahq.org/resources/clinical-information/asa-physical-status-classification-system.

TABLE 25.2 **Fasting Requirements for Pediatric Patients Receiving Sedation**

Most Recent Intake	Fasting Time
Clear liquids	2 h
Breast milk	4 h
Infant formula	6 h
Nonhuman milk	6 h
Light meal	6 h

From Practice guidelines for preoperative fasting and the use of pharmacologic agents to reduce the risk of pulmonary aspiration: application to healthy patients undergoing elective procedures: an updated report by the American Society of Anesthesiologists Committee on Standards and Practice Parameters. *Anesthesiology.* 2011;114(3):495-511.

One common method to assign overall patient risk from sedation is the American Society of Anesthesiology classification (Table 25.1). Children who are American Society of Anesthesiology class I or II are considered appropriate to receive sedation. Patients in higher classes are at greater risk and should receive additional consideration on a case-by-case basis.

Children and their families should also be informed of fasting requirements at least the day prior to the examination (Table 25.2). The primary complication avoided by adequate fasting is pulmonary aspiration; prolonged fasting may lead to dehydration or hypoglycemia. Adherence to a fasting schedule will minimize these risks while keeping the patient as comfortable as possible. However, in the emergent setting, the risk of aspiration must be weighed against the benefits of rapid imaging and providing timely care.

Common Agents

A detailed review of the various pharmacologic agents available for pediatric sedation is beyond the scope of this textbook, but some of the more common medications will be reviewed. There is no single agent or combination regimen that is perfect. Published success rates for sedation are generally above 95%. Increasing the number of sedation agents may increase the probability of drug reactions and other adverse events. The ideal regimen would have rapid onset of action and cessation, a predictable duration, be easily titratable, feature multiple routes of administration, possess a wide therapeutic window, and have minimal interactions with other drugs.

Propofol is an intravenous (IV) anesthetic used primarily for general anesthesia. It is a highly potent sedative without providing analgesia. Because of its rapid onset of action, short recovery time, and high success rate, propofol has become the most popular choice for sedating children for imaging examinations, especially MRI. Like most other sedatives, the action of propofol involves positive modulation of the inhibitory neurotransmitter γ-aminobutyric acid (GABA). For shorter procedures (<15 minutes), intermittent boluses may be administered; for longer examinations, a maintenance infusion is recommended. Potential adverse effects include respiratory depression, apnea, and hypotension.

Pentobarbital is a short-acting barbiturate that has a long history of successful sedation in pediatric patients. It functions as a potent sedative-hypnotic without analgesia. As a single agent it has reported sedation success rates exceeding 95%. One attractive feature of pentobarbital is that it may be administered through oral, IV, or intramuscular routes. Given that sedation times may be 45 to 60 minutes or longer, pentobarbital is better suited as a sedative for MRI than CT. Adverse effects of pentobarbital include respiratory depression and paradoxical agitation.

Midazolam is a short-acting benzodiazepine that produces sedation, amnesia, and anxiolysis. It acts through GABA-mediated central nervous system inhibition, like other sedatives. Although IV administration is preferred, midazolam may be given via oral and intranasal routes as well. The main side effect of midazolam to be cautious of is respiratory depression. When administering midazolam and opioids in combination, the risks of hypoxia and apnea are greater due to synergistic effects than when either agent is given alone. Flumazenil is a benzodiazepine receptor antagonist that can successfully reverse the effects of midazolam.

Chloral hydrate is an alcohol-based sedative-hypnotic and one of the oldest medications used for sedating children for imaging studies. Historically it has been most successful in sedating young children younger than 3 years. However, it has largely fallen out of favor due to increased rates of adverse events and failed sedation compared to newer agents. Chloral hydrate suspension is no longer commercially manufactured in the United States.

Dexmedetomidine is a newer agent available to sedation practitioners. It is a highly selective α$_2$-adrenergic receptor agonist, similar in action to clonidine but with eightfold greater specificity. It stimulates α$_2$-adrenergic receptors in the locus ceruleus to provide sedation and in the spinal cord to augment analgesia. IV is the preferred route, although buccal, intramuscular, and intranasal administrations are all possible. The major adverse effects of dexmedetomidine are bradycardia and hypotension.

Opioids are the mainstay for analgesia during pediatric radiologic examinations. Fentanyl is the most common agent used and is approximately 100 times more potent than morphine. It is highly lipid soluble, which allows for rapid blood-brain barrier penetration. Fentanyl is a potent analgesic but also has mild sedative properties. Its duration of action for analgesia is 20 to 30 minutes, making it an ideal medication for shorter examinations. It is frequently used in combination with a sedative such as midazolam. Severe adverse events from opioid administration include respiratory depression and chest wall rigidity. Naloxone is a narcotic antagonist that effectively reverses analgesia, sedation, and ventilation depression.

Future Implications

In the last decade, a growing body of evidence suggests that many common sedatives that increase GABA receptor activity or block excitatory glutamate receptors (e.g., ketamine) produce profound neurotoxic effects in laboratory animals. For example, propofol has been shown to cause apoptosis of neurons and oligodendrocytes in the brains of fetal and neonatal macaque monkeys. These animal studies have been complemented by a smaller number of observational studies in children who received anesthesia early in life. Although there are several confounding factors, studies suggest that early anesthetic exposure may impact cognitive function and school performance. Since 2012, consensus statements from the Food and Drug Administration and the American Academy of Pediatrics have recommended avoiding elective surgeries requiring anesthesia in children younger than 3 years, calling for further research to better define the risks. Although much of the focus has been on surgical procedures requiring anesthesia, imaging sedation is a logical extension with similar risks. Well-designed clinical trials investigating anesthetic-induced neurotoxic effects will be vital in the coming years.

SELECTION OF THE OPTIMAL STUDY

One critical aspect of providing high-quality and safe imaging to children is performing the optimal study. Ideally, following careful acquisition of history and physical examination, if a persistent diagnostic question remains, appropriate imaging should be requested. Although in certain cases the best imaging choice may be straightforward, the decision to perform imaging and which type are often more difficult. This struggle in decision making may arise from several conflicting objectives including the desire to obtain the best diagnostic performance, reduce ionizing radiation exposure, reduce sedation, reduce exposure to contrast media, and depends upon institutional modality availability, technologist skill, and radiologist expertise. There are two main strategies for determining the *best test*, which are often complementary: the use of the pediatric radiologist as a consultative physician and the use of decision-support tools.

Pediatric Radiologist As Consultative Colleague

The radiologist as a consultant is not a new concept. In fact, it represents one of the cornerstones of our profession. Prior to the advent of picture archiving and communication systems, in-person consultation was a common component of radiology practice. Although the benefits of the widespread implementation of picture archiving and communication systems are numerous, one disadvantage is that direct communication is now a less common occurrence. Without direct interaction with referring physicians, the radiologist not only risks losing value as a member of the patient's care team, but decreased communication may, even more importantly, risk adverse effects in the patient's care. This is why American College of Radiology Imaging 3.0 includes physician consultation as a key feature. Within pediatric radiology, a prime example includes pediatric radiology-neonatology rounds. The radiographs of patients in the neonatal intensive care unit are one of the most challenging areas in radiology. Although the vast majority of neonatal patients have respiratory distress syndrome, detailed discussion will help decipher more subtle changes in chest radiographs and affect the daily management of ventilation strategies or fluid balances. In-person discussion also facilitates planning of fluoroscopic studies, particularly when necessary in newborn infants. Another of the closest collaborative relationships is often with pediatric surgical colleagues. Maintaining optimal communication is critical for patient care, not only in clear areas of collaboration such as intussusception management but also in selecting optimal imaging for myriad clinical situations and questions that will never occur with sufficient frequency to result in clinical practice guidelines. Other potential opportunities for pediatric radiologists to provide input include a tumor board with pediatric oncology, radiology–pediatric intensive care unit rounds, and clinical conferences with various referring services (e.g., gastroenterology, cardiology, pediatric emergency medicine). Not only do these settings facilitate patient care by providing an opportunity to recommend optimal imaging but they also provide information to facilitate imaging planning and interpretation and educational opportunities for colleagues and trainees. Although many of the strategies mentioned facilitate excellent patient care, certainly more can be done in terms of comprehensive evidence-based practice guidelines.

Utilization of American College of Radiology Appropriateness Criteria In Children

The most comprehensive clinical practice guidelines with the strongest underlying methodology to determine the appropriateness of imaging are the American College of Radiology Appropriateness Criteria, which are readily available at http://acr.org/ac. The Appropriateness Criteria cover many aspects of diagnostic radiology, interventional radiology, radiation oncology, and current pediatric radiology–specific appropriateness criteria, including development dysplasia of the hip, fever without a source, head trauma, headache, hematuria, limping child younger than 5 years, seizures, sinusitis, suspected physical abuse, urinary tract infection (UTI), and vomiting in infants up to 3 months of age (Box 25.1). Additional pediatric-specific appropriateness criteria are also expected in the future. Additionally, pediatric patients are covered in variant tables in topics that cover both adult and pediatric patients. Three examples are neck mass/adenopathy variants 6 and 7; right lower quadrant pain, suspected appendicitis variant 4; and Crohn disease variants 3, 5, and 7. Based on the best available evidence, the applicable radiology procedures and tests are categorized as "usually appropriate" (7-9), "may be appropriate" (4-6), and "usually not appropriate" (1-3). An additional feature of the variant tables that is particularly helpful when imaging children is the relative radiation level designation in the right column. Relative radiation level designations are based on the pediatric effective dose estimate range

---

> **BOX 25.1 Key Points From American College of Radiology Appropriateness Criteria in Children**
>
> - In pediatric patients, a head CT is usually not appropriate for minor head injury without neurologic signs or high-risk factors.
> - In a primary headache without permanent neurologic exam findings or signs of increased intracranial pressure, imaging is usually not appropriate.
> - Imaging is usually not appropriate in simple febrile seizures.
> - In the clinical setting of acute sinusitis without complications, imaging is generally not indicated.
> - With bilious vomiting in an infant, an upper gastrointestinal series is indicated to evaluate for intestinal malrotation.
> - In atypical UTI or recurrent UTI, VCUG is usually appropriate in addition to ultrasound.
> - In a child <5 years with a limp, in the absence of localization and without concern for infection, tibia/fibula radiographs are usually appropriate prior to additional radiographs.
> - In patients <4–6 months, hip ultrasound is usually appropriate in the scenarios of positive or equivocal physical exam findings, female infant with breech presentation, or positive family history without physical findings.
>
> *CT*, Computed tomography; *UTI*, urinary tract infection; *VCUG*, voiding cystourethrogram.

(categorized as 0 mSv, <0.03 mSv, 0.03-0.3 mSv, 0.3-3 mSv, 3-10 mSv, and 10-30 mSv). A comprehensive discussion of all recommendations is beyond the scope of this chapter and readily available from the American College of Radiology, but discussion of several key points within each is illustrative.

Development Dysplasia of the Hip

In patients younger than 4 to 6 months (prior to femoral head ossification), hip ultrasound is usually appropriate (rating 8) in the scenarios of positive or equivocal physical exam findings, female infant with breech presentation, or positive family history without physical findings. In patients younger than 4 to 6 months, pelvis radiographs are usually not appropriate (rating 2); however, in older patients with clinical suspicion for dysplasia of the hip, a pelvis radiograph is indicated (rating 8).

Fever Without a Source

In children with a fever of unknown origin, imaging studies are often of low yield; however, several scenarios warrant special attention. Infants younger than 1 month are at high risk for serious bacterial infection. In this age group, a chest radiograph is appropriate in the presence of respiratory symptoms (rating 8) and may be appropriate even in the absence of respiratory symptoms (rating 5). In a child with fever of unknown origin and neutropenia, particularly in the setting of bone marrow transplant, a chest CT may be appropriate (rating 6) even in the setting of normal chest radiographs.

Head Trauma

In pediatric head trauma, minor head injury (defined as Glasgow Coma Scale score >13) without neurologic signs or high risk factors (such as altered mental status or clinical evidence of basilar skull fracture), a head CT is usually not appropriate (rating 3). In the setting of moderate to severe head trauma (Glasgow Comma Scale score ≤13) or with high-risk factors, head CT receives the highest appropriateness rating level of 9. In the setting of suspected nonaccidental trauma, both head CT and head MRI receive a rating of usually appropriate at 9 and 8, respectively.

Headache

In the presence of headache in a child with positive neurologic exam findings or signs of increased intracranial pressure, MRI of the head is most appropriate (rating 8). Although quite rare in the pediatric setting, high-intensity headaches of sudden onset suggesting vascular rupture do occur, and head CT and CT angiography are usually appropriate. In the remaining settings of primary headache without permanent neurologic exam findings or signs of increased intracranial pressure, imaging is usually not appropriate (head MRI receives a rating of only 3).

Hematuria

In a child with hematuria, imaging is usually appropriate. The choice between ultrasound and CT, however, often depends of the clinical scenario. In the presence of isolated (not painful or traumatic) hematuria, ultrasound of the kidneys and bladder is the most appropriate imaging modality (rating 7). In the presence of nontraumatic painful hematuria (with concern for renal calculus), both CT and ultrasound are usually appropriate (ratings of 8 for both). In the presence of traumatic macroscopic hematuria, contrast-enhanced CT receives the highest rating of 9. Ultrasound is usually not appropriate except in the setting of follow-up (rating 3).

Limping Child

In the setting of a child younger than 5 years of age with a limp, a detailed clinical evaluation is critical to help determine the most appropriate imaging. If the clinician is able to determine the location of pathology, the presence or absence of trauma, and ascertain if there is concern for an infectious etiology, then the most effective imaging may be requested. In the absence of localization and without concern for infection, tibia/fibula radiographs are usually appropriate (rating 8) prior to additional radiographs of the pelvis, leg, or foot, which may be appropriate (rating 5), or MRI (rating 5). If localization is possible and there is a concern for infection, then focused radiographs are clearly warranted (rating 9). In the setting of concern for infection including septic arthritis, then hip ultrasound is most appropriate (rating 9), although pelvis radiographs and pelvis MRI are also deemed usually appropriate. Sedation risks should also be considered with MRI.

Seizures

Within the American College of Radiology Appropriateness Criteria for seizures in children, eight different variant scenarios are presented. Cranial ultrasound should be the first imaging in the setting of neonatal seizures (rating of 9). In neonatal seizures, MRI may also be appropriate (rating 5), particularly if congenital malformations or hypoxic ischemic encephalopathy are suspected. In the setting of posttraumatic seizures, head CT is the most appropriate modality (rating 9); otherwise, MRI is often the most appropriate modality. MRI is usually appropriate in partial seizures or generalized seizures with abnormal neurologic findings (rating 9). Imaging is usually not appropriate in simple febrile seizures.

Sinusitis

In the clinical setting of acute sinusitis without complications, imaging is generally not indicated. In children with persistent, recurrent, or chronic sinusitis, CT of the paranasal sinuses is usually appropriate (rating 9). If there is concern for orbital or intracranial complications, CT of the paranasal sinuses with contrast is the most appropriate imaging modality (rating 9). MRI of the paranasal sinuses and head is also usually appropriate (rating 7), particularly when evaluation for intracranial complications is warranted. Radiographs of the paranasal sinuses are typically not indicated in any of the above scenarios (rating 1).

Suspected Physical Abuse

Given the medical and legal importance of evaluation for suspected physical abuse, direct review of the American College of Radiology Appropriateness Criteria is encouraged. An important point provided within the summary is that a radiographic skeletal survey is always indicated in children younger than 24 months in the evaluation for suspected physical abuse; in older children, radiographs may be tailored to the area of injury. A head CT is always indicated (rating 9) in the setting of head trauma, neurologic signs, seizures, and should be strongly considered when other high-risk injuries are present. Additional discussion is beyond the scope of this chapter.

Urinary Tract Infection

In children younger than 3 years with a febrile UTI, ultrasound of the kidney and bladder is usually appropriate (rating 9). In children older than 3 years with febrile UTI and good response to treatment, renal ultrasound may be appropriate (rating 6), although yield decreases with age. In atypical UTIs (e.g., poor response to antibiotics, sepsis, elevated creatinine) or recurrent UTI, a voiding cystourethrogram is usually appropriate (rating 7) in addition to ultrasound.

Vomiting Infant

In an infant younger than 3 months, the American College of Radiology Appropriateness Criteria primarily depend on whether the vomiting is bilious or nonbilious. With *bilious* vomiting in an infant, an upper gastrointestinal series is indicated to evaluate for intestinal malrotation. In the newborn, a contrast enema is also usually appropriate if an abdominal radiograph suggests distal bowel obstruction. With new onset *nonbilious* vomiting, ultrasound of the pylorus is most appropriate (rating 9) to assess for hypertrophic pyloric stenosis. With intermittent *nonbilious* vomiting, imaging with an upper gastrointestinal series may be appropriate when anatomic evaluation is requested (rating 6).

In summary, close communication with clinical colleagues and use of clinical practice guidelines such as the American College of Radiology Appropriateness Criteria help facilitate the highest quality imaging of our pediatric patients.

SUGGESTED READINGS

Radiation Reduction

American Association of Physicists in Medicine. Report of AAPM Task Group 204. Size-Specific Dose Estimates (SSDE) in Pediatric and Adult Body CT Examinations. http://www.aapm.org/pubs/reports/detail.asp?docid=143; 2011.

Blumfield E, Zember J, Guelfguat M, Blumfield A, Goldman H. Evaluation of an initiative to reduce radiation exposure from CT to children in a non-pediatric-focused facility. *Emerg Radiol.* 2015;22(6):631-641.

Brenner DJ, Hall EJ. Computed tomography—an increasing source of radiation exposure. *N Engl J Med.* 2007;357:2277-2284.

Image Gently Alliance. <http://www.imagegently.org/>.

Image Gently Alliance. Update of the North American Consensus Guidelines for Pediatric Administered Radiopharmaceutical Activities. <www.imagegently.org/Portals/6/Nuclear%20Medicine/NA%20Guidelines%202014%20Update%20-%20Poster.pdf>; 2014.

Pearce MS, Salotti JA, Little MP, et al. Radiation exposure from CT scans in childhood and subsequent risk of leukaemia and brain tumours: a retrospective cohort study. *Lancet.* 2012;380:499-505.

Thaker A, Navadeh S, Gonzales H, Malekinejad M. Effectiveness of policies on reducing exposure to ionizing radiation from medical imaging: a systematic review. *J Am Coll Radiol.* 2015;12(12 Pt B):1434-1445.

Sedation

American Academy of Pediatrics. American Academy of Pediatric Dentistry, Coté CJ, Wilson S. Guidelines for monitoring and management of pediatric patients during and after sedation for diagnostic and therapeutic procedures: an update. *Pediatrics.* 2006;118:2587-2602.

Berkenbosch JW. Options and considerations for procedural sedation in pediatric imaging. *Paediatr Drugs.* 2015;17(5):385-399.

Edwards AD, Arthurs OJ. Paediatric MRI under sedation: is it necessary? What is the evidence for the alternatives? *Pediatr Radiol.* 2011;41(11):1353-1364.

Frush DP, Bisset III GS, Hall SC. Pediatric sedation in radiology: the practice of safe sleep. *AJR Am J Roentgenol.* 1996;167(6):1381-1387.

Macias CG, Chumpitazi CE. Sedation and anesthesia for CT: emerging issues for providing high-quality care. *Pediatr Radiol.* 2011;41(suppl 2):517-522.

Rappaport BA, Suresh S, Hertz S, Evers AS, Orser BA. Anesthetic neurotoxicity—clinical implications of animal models. *N Engl J Med.* 2015;372(9):796-797.

Selection of Studies

American College of Radiology. ACR Appropriateness Criteria. <www.acr.org/Quality-Safety/Appropriateness-Criteria>.

American College of Radiology. Imaging 3.0™. <www.acr.org/Advocacy/Economics-Health-Policy/Imaging-3>.

Chapter 26
Emergency Radiology

Ryan B. O'Malley, Tarun Pandey, Matthew T. Heller, Linda E. Chen, Anika L. McGrath, Prabhakar Rajiah, and Puneet Bhargava

COMMUNICATION IN EMERGENCY RADIOLOGY

Physician-to-Patient Communication

Physician-to-patient communication is a unique challenge for radiologists. Radiologists and patients often have isolated encounters, without any prior patient-physician relationship established. Most radiology services, including an emergency radiology service, do not schedule dedicated clinic time, and therefore meeting with patients may not be a set priority in the daily workflow. Additionally, radiologists often do not have enough information from the emergency medicine team to discuss detailed management plans with patients.

For radiologists in the emergency department (ED), the physician-to-patient communication can come with a different level of challenges. Being physically in the ED and having regular shift work, emergency medicine providers are usually easier to reach for communication of study results, and they are responsible for conveying study results and diagnosis to patients with their management plans. In this setting, radiologists do not commonly encounter opportunities to discuss difficult and stressful imaging results with patients. However, situations requiring radiologist-to-patient communication may still occur. For example, it may be important for a radiologist to communicate with a patient and family when performing a focused assessment with a sonography in trauma (FAST) scan at the bedside.

In emergency radiology, physician-to-patient communication may be useful for obtaining additional clinical information not provided in the imaging requisition. At Harborview Medical Center in Seattle, Washington, emergency radiologists are embedded in the trauma section of the ED and frequently speak with patients for additional clinical history or may even perform a focused physical exam to correlate with imaging findings. In some situations, a radiologist is best suited for directly correlating imaging findings with symptoms or physical examination findings. However, such interactions may be challenging, and specific guidelines are useful to consider.

Five Tips to Begin a Successful Radiologist-to-Patient Communication in the Emergency Department

To begin, it is important to be aware of the time constraint, especially in the busy setting in the ED. It can be useful to initiate communication by explaining the special role that radiologists play in patient care, which is significantly different from the roles of other clinicians that patients usually encounter. Following this introduction, discussion should center around the actual imaging results, without commenting too extensively on the treatment options. The following list of strategies will help radiologists improve communication skills with patients and family members in the ED.

1. Use AIDET (Acknowledge, Introduce, Duration, Explanation, and Thank You) for Patient and Family

In most interactions, including those between radiologists and patients, the first impression can set the tone for the entire conversation. AIDET, which stands for acknowledge, introduce, duration, explanation, and thank you, serves as a useful guideline in promoting effective communication with patients. The role of the radiologist in patient care is not well understood beyond the medical profession, so it is important to provide context to the patient at the start of the conversation. Having a standard scripted introduction can help radiologists begin the interaction smoothly and focus on the specific medical condition of each patient.

An equally important aspect in the first impression is to acknowledge the patient's family members, friends, or caregivers at the bedside. Many patients present to the ED accompanied by key caregivers who may have just as much clinical information or be directly responsible for decision making. Radiologists should also be mindful of the patient's privacy and always confirm whether the conversation should be conducted alone or in the presence of the other visitors.

Example for gathering additional clinical information: "Hi, I am Dr. Smith. I'm a radiologist here in the emergency department. Patients usually don't meet with me directly, but I work behind the scenes with your emergency medicine team to review your x-ray studies and help them make decisions based on the imaging findings. I am in the process of reviewing your foot x-rays and would like to perform a focused physical exam to help me better understand what these images mean."

Example for performing a FAST scan or other ultrasound study and addressing the patient's family members: "Hi, my name is Dr. Smith. I am a radiologist here in the emergency department. I understand that you are the sister. I usually work behind the scenes with your emergency medicine team to review imaging studies so that the team can use the results to decide on an appropriate treatment. Today, I'd like to perform a quick ultrasound study. After I complete the exam, I'd also like to share with you what I see."

2. Give Concise Information, Using Terminology the Patient Can Understand

Radiologists may need to explain medical terminology in simple phrases that are easier for the general public to understand. This can be substantially different from using standard medical jargon when talking to other colleagues in the medical field. In addition, it can be helpful to have images ready or to use hand gestures to provide visual context for the verbal explanation.

Example for gathering additional clinical information: "On your foot x-ray, there is a tiny crack in your bone at the same spot where I just pressed. It seemed like that is where you are having pain as well. From what you told me, this may be a stress fracture from increased running with the new marathon training program you recently started."

3. Provide a Radiology Plan

Describing a concrete plan can help reduce uncertainty for the patient and increase the level of trust between patients and physicians. However, this is particularly challenging in the ED because treatment plans are often in flux during emergent situations, and there are multiple teams involved in caring for any single patient. In this complex environment, radiologists can help reduce patient anxiety by outlining the process as clearly as possible. For example, if the radiologist is asked to perform a FAST exam at bedside, it is helpful to specify how the result will be communicated to the ED provider, whether via phone or in person. The radiologist can also inform the patient that ED providers and the patient's primary care providers will be able to access the images and the radiologist's interpretations.

Example for performing a FAST scan: "The study is normal. I am going to return to my work station and review it again carefully with my colleagues to confirm. Immediately afterward, I will speak to your emergency medicine team to tell them the final results so that they can discuss with you further regarding a treatment plan or other test options. I will also submit a report of the study results into your medical record, so your doctors will be able to access my impression along with the images we took."

4. Use Nonverbal Cues to Show Empathy

A major aspect of effective communication is making the patient feel comfortable through nonverbal cues. For example, physicians can show empathy for the patient by simply sitting down during their conversations together. This alone can convey that the physician has dedicated time to the patient and can foster an environment conducive to establishing trust.

It is equally important to perceive and respond to nonverbal cues from patients. Patients might indicate, through their body language, emotions that they do not feel comfortable expressing out loud. Being aware of these emotions and validating them verbally can be particularly useful in stressful environments like the ED.

5. Answer All Questions With Patience

Even with the limited time available, it is crucial to give patients a chance to ask questions. The radiologist should directly answer any questions pertaining to the imaging results but defer to the ED providers regarding management plans. In addition to answering questions patiently, the radiologist should reassure the patient that there will be future opportunities to ask questions.

Be Present and Add Value as a Radiologist in the Emergency Department

With recent healthcare reform, reimbursement will soon be tied to patient satisfaction. As such, effective radiologist-patient communications are critical for patient-centered value-based care. In one study, Kuhlman et al. showed that 64% of patients want to meet the radiologists who interpret their exams. Cabarrus et al. found that 85% of patients want to see images as part of the conversation when they receive results. Such data suggest tremendous opportunities for radiologists and emphasizes the increasing importance of effective conversation skills when delivering study results to patients. Radiologists must be cognizant and take advantage of such opportunities when they arise. Radiologists often overestimate the time needed to review images with a patient. In many instances, reviewing images can save time, because a visual explanation of the disease process or abnormality may convey more than even a lengthy verbal discussion. Increasing patient awareness of the radiologist's role in their care is a valuable way to incorporate radiology in patient-centered care.

The American College of Radiology (ACR) Imaging 3.0 initiative emphasizes radiologists' visibility and leadership. Providing optimal patient-centered care requires that radiologists employ effective communication skills with fellow physicians and providers and with patients. Using the five tips outlined earlier, radiologists can achieve brief but impactful conversations in the ED.

Physician-to-Physician Communication

Radiologists frequently find themselves professionally compelled to propose alternative imaging plans in discussions with physician colleagues in the ED. Unfortunately, the sensitive dynamics of these conversations all too often produce the conditions necessary for a hostile exchange, especially when the proposed alternative is to forgo imaging altogether. The source of this tension is rooted in some of the most common themes underlying medical staff conflict, namely, deficiency in communication, a lack of trust, and incorrect assumptions.

Despite the potential for conflict, up to 40% of referring providers note that they would like to discuss imaging protocols in advance, and up to 50% are interested in feedback regarding protocol selection. Working in a collaborative fashion can seem time-consuming in the midst of a busy shift; however, investing a small amount of effort initially will save time in the end. Communication skills, negotiation strategies, and a touch of charisma are essential. Radiologists must also be attuned to the needs and priorities of their ED colleagues, namely, assistance in rapidly triaging severity of pathology and provision of timely and accurate diagnoses. The following section lists several strategies that will help the radiologist mitigate conflict and deescalate confrontational interactions as they arise.

Four Key Steps in Mitigating Conflict

1. Ask for More Information

When an inappropriate imaging request is ordered, the first step is to call the provider and ask for more information. This is the most critical step in conflict mitigation and will break down barriers of incorrect assumptions and lack of trust. In most instances, acquiring additional information will prove that the study is indicated or aid in choosing a more appropriate study. In conversation, use the keywords "brief" and "quick" to demonstrate respect for their time and the frenetic nature of their specialty. For example, "Can you briefly describe what you're looking for?"

Case scenario: A noncontrast head computed tomography (CT) is ordered for the indication chronic headache. The radiologist asks for more information, and the ED provider replies, "Yes, the headache is chronic but has acutely worsened in the last couple of hours." This indication is now appropriate, and the radiologist prevented conflict by asking for more information and avoiding an incorrect set of assumptions.

2. Provide the Best Alternative

Assisting the ED provider in choosing the most appropriate study can be difficult at times, particularly if the alternative causes perceived delays in patient care. However, the radiologist has the responsibility of caring for the patient beyond the ED visit, often on an inpatient or outpatient basis as the patient's care evolves. The radiologist can leverage this knowledge to assist the ED provider in confidently selecting the best study in the larger context of a patient's care. In conversation, use the keywords, "Have you considered?" or "Have you thought about?" to demonstrate regard for their clinical judgment and expertise. Other key phrases such as "saves time in the end" or "best answers your question" connect with their fundamental need for rapid and accurate diagnoses.

Case scenario: A noncontrast head CT is ordered for the indication of chronic headache. The radiologist then proposes the best alternative: "Have you considered a brain magnetic resonance (MR) instead, possibly on an outpatient basis if the patient can be safely discharged tonight? This would ultimately yield the most information and is the best diagnostic test for chronic headache. Overall, this would save time in the end and best answer your question, as the head CT will add time and is unlikely to provide diagnostic value."

3. Provide Coaching

Myriad factors drive ED physicians in their request for inappropriate or suboptimal imaging studies. However, every instance in which a better alternative is available represents an opportunity for shared learning. Navigating these conversations begins with a thorough understanding of the American College of Emergency Physicians (ACEP) clinical practice guidelines. The ability to confidently reference these guidelines enables us to effectively educate our colleagues regarding these nationally developed standards

for clinical management of ED patients. One must initiate these opportunities deftly to avoid the air of condescension. Using the keywords "You're right, however ..." in conversation overall signifies agreement but allows for a small educational opportunity.

Case scenario: A noncontrast head CT is ordered with the indication syncope. The radiologist provides coaching: "You're right, it is important to rule out acute pathologies in the emergency setting. However, the ACEP guidelines actually state that head CT is not indicated in syncope unless there is focal neurologic deficit, significant head trauma, or some other factor guided by history or physical exam."

4. Arrive at a Resolution Together

Allow for the possibility that your clinical acumen and even widely accepted practice guidelines may not lead to the best solution for every patient. There are circumstances in which the best course may be to trust the ED physician to exercise clinical judgment and learn to trust his or her intentions. Practice guidelines are recommendations and not absolutes. However, the radiology department should track potentially nonindicated studies with quality improvement/quality assurance databases to link outcomes to provider feedback. Low overutilization rates will continue to be essential in keeping the cost of practicing radiology at reasonable levels, particularly in the transition to new payment models, such as value-based care.

How to Deescalate a Confrontational Situation

Confrontations will inevitably arise, and when they do, it is critical to artfully defuse the situation. One effective method is to redirect attention to the needs of the colleague so he or she feels accepted and understood. Take a moment, refocus one's perspective, and view the interaction for what it is fundamentally: an ED provider who is worried about a patient. Understanding their basic intent encourages warm and genuine responses, which are two of the key tenants in effective and charismatic communication. Maintaining a friendly temperament despite the conflict helps radiologists foster reputations as valued and accessible colleagues.

During disagreements, tone is everything—in voice and language. Tone is directly related to one's facial expressions, body language, and hand gestures, which unfortunately are absent in most provider conversations. Over the phone, words and intonation are increasingly important, because they are the radiologist's only form of communication. It is also important not to let emotions control the conversation. Learn to anticipate conflict, which allows one to *respond* positively, rather than *react* negatively.

Communication experts recommend having verbal *aikidos* that we should all feel comfortable using when necessary. The term is a reference to the martial arts technique of redirecting one's attacker and describes phrases we can use to defuse escalating tension. For example, phrases such as "you're right" or "I understand" are generic enough to be used abundantly and provide time to generate thoughtful responses. These phrases also represent a small form of flattery and can validate self-esteem, which may be important as hostile conversation often develops as a result of our colleagues feeling that their professional competence and reputation are under attack.

If the conversation becomes frankly confrontational, redirect attention back onto our shared common goal: the patient. The keywords "Let's take a step back…" allow for a swift, neutral change in the direction of a conversation and represent the subtle offering of an olive branch. Remind the provider of physician-patient shared decision making, in which informing patients of options, and explaining the risks and benefits, is the cornerstone of patient autonomy and respect. For example, "What do you think the patient would want, if we asked? Would he or she want a head CT now, knowing that it will not be helpful and expose the patient to radiation? Or would he or she be willing to wait for a brain MR sometime this week?"

Finally, if all else fails, reiterate one's commitment to partnership with the ED provider and formulate a resolution, even if it may occasionally represent a suboptimal solution. Emphasize your commitment to the relationship by stating, "I am happy to do what you feel is best, and from my point of view, this has been an educational and productive conversation." Medicine can be a contentious profession, and it is difficult not to take altercations personally. Long work hours and conflicting demands can lead to disrespectful behavior between medical professionals, and workplace depression causes inward self-focus, lack of empathy, and unwillingness to cooperate. Hopefully, by employing some of these tactics, such situations become the rare exception to what are largely cordial workplace relationships with ED providers.

Communication to Minimize Litigation

Inappropriate interpretation, transcription mistakes, or deficient documentation of communication and recommendation can lead to errors in radiology reports, which in turn may result in legal action against radiologists. A study of the Physicians Insurers Association of America from 1985 to 2000 demonstrates that radiology ranks sixth among all specialties in the number of lawsuits filed and closed. Medical specialties with higher numbers of malpractice suits compared to radiology include obstetrics and gynecology, internal medicine, family practice, general surgery, and orthopedics. However, this data represented the total number of legal cases, suggesting that radiologists actually encounter much higher litigation rates because they represent less than 4% of doctors in the United States. To minimize litigation risk and avoid anxiety related to malpractice suits, it is paramount that radiologists learn the legal ramifications of radiology reports.

Typical legal implications in radiology are related to a variety of deficiencies in interpretation and reporting. Observation errors and errors in interpretation include scanning errors (failure to focus on the area of lesion), recognition errors (focusing on the territory of the lesion but not detecting the lesion), and errors in decision making. Of the above, decision-related errors are the most common, accounting for approximately 45% of observation errors. Finally, satisfaction of search is an error that can occur after detection of an initial lesion, when radiologists can experience reduced perception of other abnormalities, resulting in false-negative interpretations of secondary lesions.

Communicating results and recommendations have also become an essential part of the daily workflow of radiologists. Four out of five malpractice lawsuits in radiology involve complications in communication. Radiologists can minimize the risk of lawsuits by clearly documenting when and how results are communicated to other providers and to patients. Documentation should include the date and time of communication, the name of the person spoken to, and the context in which the results were discussed. A common scenario in a teaching institution would be when an attending's final report contains a discrepancy with the overnight resident's preliminary impression. In some lawsuits, courts have ruled that the final report must be conveyed to the ordering providers and the patient, regardless of urgency.

ACR's Practice Guideline for Communication of Diagnostic Imaging Findings, published in 2010, states that follow-up studies to clarify or confirm initial findings should be suggested and documented in reports. In lawsuits, an ordering physician can claim ignorance of the proper actions following a radiology diagnosis, because the radiologist did not provide recommendations. Therefore, it is important for radiologists to include concrete follow-up instructions to clarify, confirm, or exclude the initial impression.

Four Must-Do's in Communicating Imaging Results

This section discusses the four key components of communicating imaging results (in the ED or elsewhere). This is an opportunity for radiologists to directly make a difference by ensuring quality patient care while minimizing litigation risk.

1. Physician-to-Physician Communication

For any critical result or incidental findings warranting further workup or change in management, the radiologist commonly makes a phone call to the ordering provider. When conveying the diagnosis, the conversation should be simple and to the point but ensure that pertinent information is understood. It is important to be very clear, especially when offering two or more diagnoses, and explain to the ordering provider why certain differential diagnoses are more or less likely. As discussed in the previous section on physician-to-physician communication, radiologists should remain professional but firm, even if the ordering providers disagree with the imaging diagnoses.

2. Physician-to-Patient Communication

Compared to the outpatient setting, needing to communicate an urgent finding directly to a patient when the ordering providers cannot be reached is less common in the ED because of the ready availability of dedicated ED providers and staff. However, direct radiologist-to-patient communication of imaging findings can occur in the ED when the radiologist is present for the examination (e.g., ultrasound) or is performing a procedure (e.g., esophagram for leak). Radiologists may also need to contact a patient directly when there is a discrepancy with a preliminary report, and the patient has already been discharged from the ED.

3. Documentation

Documenting communication accurately is a crucial component of the patient's medical record and for minimizing radiologists' litigation risk. Essential components include date, time, name of the person spoken to, and the information discussed. If any recommendation was conveyed verbally, it is helpful to include it in the communication section as well. Additionally, it is good practice to document multiple communications when multiple attempts were made or if a radiologist conveyed findings to multiple services on the same study. For example, "The above critical result of a large right-sided pneumothorax was communicated to Dr. Smith (ED resident) and Dr. Jones (surgery chief resident) by Dr. Lee at 1000 hours on 1/24/2017."

4. Further Recommendations

Recommendations, such as follow-up imaging or interventions, should be made and documented when appropriate. In the ED, this may include recommendations to consult other specialties, such as general surgery or interventional radiology, although radiologists should be careful that such subspecialty consultations are truly warranted. For example, "Recommend follow-up head CT in 6 hours and neurosurgery consult."

Communication Challenges in the Emergency Department

1. To Whom Should Results Be Communicated in a Busy ED Setting?

At a teaching institution, radiologists may need to decide between conveying results to the attending emergency medicine physicians or the residents. In these situations, one should consult the standard protocol in his or her institution's ED. Regardless, it is important to always document if a radiologist is unable to reach the ordering provider and the subsequent action taken if any. For example, "Unable to convey results to attending physician (Dr. Smith); the above critical finding was conveyed to the senior resident (Dr. Jones) in the ED."

2. How Should Nonurgent Incidental Findings Be Managed?

An incidental finding may not seem like a priority in the busy ED setting, but communication and documentation are still necessary to ensure needed outpatient workup. For example, "This is not an emergent finding, but further outpatient workup is recommended."

3. What Should Be Done During a Trauma Code?

During a trauma code, the emergency room is loud and frenetic with ongoing resuscitation and a large trauma team. At certain institutions, such as Harborview Medical Center, the emergency radiology reading room is embedded in the center of the trauma ED. This allows emergency radiologists to convey the trauma series results directly to the trauma team. In this chaotic environment, it is particularly important to make eye contact to ensure the person in charge of the trauma team receives and acknowledges the critical imaging results. Although difficult, interrupting

resuscitation is acceptable when the findings are emergent and will change management, but information conveyed should be concise and clear. Communicating nonurgent incidental findings should take place after the resuscitation is completed.

Awareness of key medicolegal concepts can help radiologists reduce the risk of errors and malpractice lawsuits and ensure optimal patient care. Improving communication skills and consistently documenting conversations are ways that radiologists can take direct action to minimize litigation risk.

PATIENT SAFETY IN EMERGENCY RADIOLOGY

Emergency radiology is a high-stakes environment with rapidly evolving situations and frequent complex decision making. Functioning in this type of high-risk environment creates continual threats to patient safety, and therefore ensuring safety must be a component of the system itself. Safety is a direct result of how an organization is designed, led, and managed. At its most effective, emergency radiology provides frictionless tools and support to allow emergency healthcare personnel to provide safe, effective, patient-centered care.

Most emergency radiology departments have adopted a systematic approach to patient safety such that the entire organization is constantly engaged in efforts to prevent and identify errors before they cause harm. Rather than focusing on individual errors, modern safety practices emphasize organizational elements that promote safety and use error to identify and analyze weaknesses in the system. It is crucial that there is buy-in from all team members to ensure that errors are reported without fear of repercussion and to encourage solutions to problems that arise. Individuals in this environment must be taught situational awareness and encouraged to detect potential adverse events before harm is caused. Standardization can help individuals detect variance and potential deviations. Having a systematic method for capturing safety events should encourage ongoing analysis, timely response, and data gathering for systematic review. Some examples of specific threats against patient safety in emergency radiology include scanning the wrong patient, imaging the wrong side or body part, order entry errors, discrepancies with preliminary interpretations, interruptions and distractions, faulty communication, ineffective handoffs, and fatigue.

To ensure the correct patient and correct body part are imaged, two patient identifiers are used prior to an examination as per Joint Commission requirements. Identifiers include name, date of birth, hospital identification number, or other person-specific identifier and can be verified directly with the patient or a family member, spouse, partner, or healthcare provider who has previously identified the patient. This may seem obvious and straightforward in an outpatient setting but can be quite challenging in a chaotic emergency or trauma setting with an unresponsive patient being actively resuscitated. Patient identifiers must also be cross-referenced with the examination order to ensure the correct examination type and site are performed. After the examination is performed, the technologist must verify that the scanned patient's images are imported into the matching patient's folder in the picture archiving and communication system (PACS). Finally, the radiologist must be vigilant and verify that the patient information in the dictated report matches the images reviewed. Each step in this process offers the potential for errors to occur.

Correct patient identification is particularly critical in emergency radiology where images are frequently viewed (by a radiologist or other provider) immediately after they are acquired. Portable radiographs are very common in emergency radiology and particularly prone to error. In a large retrospective review of near-miss wrong-patient events, Sadigh et al. found that portable chest radiography accounted for most mislabeling-misidentification events (69%) and wrong dictation events (44%). Mislabeled or misidentified images in PACS can quickly lead to incorrect decisions and inappropriate or delayed management. Most importantly, they are often difficult to recognize after the error has occurred. In one series, the mean time between when a mislabeling-misidentification event occurred and when it was detected was 100 hours, which could result in severely compromised patient care. Standard procedures are required to minimize such occurrences. For example, the radiology information system (RIS) may link the dictation software and images in PACS. Acquiring facial photographs simultaneously with radiographs has also been reported to increase detection of mislabeled examinations without sacrificing interpretation time.

Effective communication is critical for patient safety in emergency radiology, and specific strategies have already been discussed. Failure to communicate results of radiologic examinations is reportedly the second most common cause of malpractice litigation with communication problems a causative factor in up to 80% of cases. It is insufficient to simply communicate findings and results. Radiologists must communicate results in a comprehensive and timely fashion to the appropriate person with acknowledgment of receipt and understanding of the information. In emergency radiology, it is helpful to have access to an ED whiteboard that is updated in real time to minimize time wasted contacting the incorrect provider. Ensuring that the patient's care team and contact information are readily available helps to ensure that critical results can be communicated quickly to the appropriate provider.

Handoffs are ubiquitous in emergency radiology, occurring whenever patient information and responsibility are transferred between healthcare providers, and are among the greatest threats to patient safety. For example, a radiologist shift change may include information regarding examinations in progress, patients receiving premedication or intravenous (IV) hydration, protocols on hold, or pages awaiting a return call. In a root cause analysis (RCA), handoffs and resultant patient safety events have been shown to be particularly prone to error when information is exchanged via the telephone, which is especially applicable to emergency radiologists. Ineffective handoff events result in uncertainty regarding the care plan, near misses, or failure to effectively communicate the most important piece of information about a patient, even when the parties involved believe the handoff was effective. Because the resultant errors can have major implications for care, high-quality handoffs must be addressed on an organizational level with directed strategies for providers to ensure effective transfer of critical information. It is critical that participants understand that many handoff errors occur even when both parties believe the handoff is effective; thus specific skills must be taught and acquired.

In general, major discrepancies between resident preliminary and final faculty interpretation are infrequent, with published rates ranging from 0.8% to 2.6% in many large series. Nonetheless, standard practices must be implemented to ensure that discrepancies that do occur are managed in a timely and routine fashion to minimize any adverse effects on patient care. The first step is to ensure consistent reporting of discrepancies, among resident preliminary reports and also discrepancies among other faculty. Participants in a peer-review process must understand and accept that the purpose of the process is to improve safety and is not punitive, to encourage uniform participation and meaningful intervention. Second, emergency radiologists and emergency care providers need a consistent closed-loop process for reporting and tracking discrepancies. This process must include a follow-up mechanism to ensure that discrepancies requiring additional workup or management are tracked until the loop is closed and do not "fall through the cracks." Periodic review of discrepancy data is also mandatory to identify trends and intervene early before safety is compromised on a larger scale.

In a busy emergency radiology practice, interruptions and distractions are frequent and can increase the possibility of errors. In this setting, radiologists (including trainees, faculty, and practicing radiologists) are constantly shifting attention between medical (e.g., image interpretation, communicating with emergency providers) and nonmedical tasks (e.g., answering phone calls or pages), particularly during off hours when nonphysician support personnel may be less available. Telephone calls are one of the most frequent workflow interrupters and were shown in one series by Balint et al. to raise the probability of a significant error by a radiology resident by 12%. Although telephone calls are a common distraction, they are by no means the only type of interruption that can increase errors and detrimentally affect safety. Any unscheduled workflow disruption can force the radiologist to disengage from his or her interpretive tasks and, in the process, forget the context and mindset that existed prior to the disruption. Returning to the prior mindset is costly, requires added time and effort, and introduces the potential for serious error. Nonetheless, distractions in an emergency radiology reading room are the norm and may be mitigated but not eliminated entirely. For example, nonradiologists can support the radiologist by managing nonmedical tasks and ensuring that interruptions, when they occur, are warranted and time sensitive. As such, efforts to optimize patient safety must balance minimizing interruptions and distractions with maintaining radiologist availability for emergency practitioners. Providing optimal patient care in the ED often relies on time-sensitive consultations, and in this setting, interrupting the radiologist may be appropriate and outweigh the risk of error.

RISK MANAGEMENT FOR ERRORS IN EMERGENCY RADIOLOGY

Risk, Medical Error, and Risk Management

At its core, medical care is a balance of risk and benefit. Risk is defined as a chance or possibility of danger or incurring

TABLE 26.1 Risk Management Scenarios With Possible Solutions and Recommendations

Type of Error	Error/Scenario	Comments/Recommendation
Mistake, false-positive error	1. Radiologist reads a normal variant as a fracture. 2. Radiologist recommends computed tomography instead of magnetic resonance imaging to rule out foot osteomyelitis. 3. A noncontrast computed tomography is ordered to rule out pulmonary embolism. 4. Consistent poor-quality magnetic resonance imaging exam on weekends.	These indicate lack of radiologic/technical skills, experience, knowledge, or insufficient training. Reducing the likelihood of mistakes typically requires more training, supervision, or occasionally disciplinary action (in case of negligence).
Slip, false-negative error	1. Radiologic finding missed on chest x-ray on a busy call day. 2. Emergency department technician incorrectly labeled the wrong side on a busy day. 3. Resident forgot to document critical results on a case due to constant phone calls from the emergency department on a busy night shift.	Slips are lapses in concentration and failure of schematic behavior due to fatigue, stress, or emotional distractions, unlike mistakes that represent failure during attentional behavior.
Latent error	1. Incorrect diagnosis was made because old films were not available to review at the time of reading. 2. Cardiac magnetic resonance imaging on a patient with constrictive pericarditis was prelimed as normal by the on-call resident. 3. Patient sued clinic for missed Lisfranc fracture on a digitized radiograph. 4. Incorrect contrast dose was administered because the tech who programmed the injector confused it with a different model used in the department.	Latent error refers to less apparent failures of organization or design that contribute to errors. They are typically related to a faulty institutional policy, equipment failure, organizational/management flaws, work and team environment, lack of proper staffing, and other reasons. This is also called a blunt-end error, as opposed to an active or sharp-end error, where the source of error lies with the personnel or parts of the healthcare system in direct contact with patient.
Close call (near-miss incidents)	1. Patient with a contrast allergy gets a contrast computed tomography but has no reaction. 2. The radiologist recognizes a wrong side marker based on a review of old studies.	No injury happened as a result of this event, due to the robustness of the patient or a fortuitous and timely intervention from a member of the healthcare team.
Adverse event	1. Patient with no prior risk factor develops reaction to intravenous iodinated contrast. 2. Pneumothorax from central venous line placement	These are undesirable clinical outcomes resulting from some aspect of diagnosis or therapy, not from the underlying disease process. An adverse event does not imply *error* or poor quality of care.

loss or injury. Medical error is the failure of a planned action to be completed as intended or the use of a wrong plan to achieve an aim. In the United States, an estimated 44,000 to 98,000 deaths per year may be attributable to medical errors and cost $17 to $29 billion.

It is important to understand that risk is not limited to the patient and also affects the medical practitioner and the healthcare system as a whole. The highest risk for errors exists in high-acuity settings, such as the intensive care unit (ICU), operating room (OR), and ED, and emergency radiology departments interface with all of these departments. Therefore, it is important that emergency radiology departments adopt forward-thinking risk management strategies to identify areas of weakness and reduce the sources of error.

In the simplest terms, radiology risk management includes systems and processes that ensure that medical images are acquired and reported in accordance with agreed protocols, by competent staff working within a defined scope of practice, and with advance identification and addressing of potential problems. This process involves all those who are responsible for the delivery of healthcare, not just the clinician who is directly caring for the patient.

The key to risk management is to acknowledge that mistakes happen and even the best processes and procedures will fail. All participants must be willing to evaluate all actions with transparency and openness, including appropriate efforts to remedy failures and alter practices

where needed. A summary of possible errors, scenarios, and recommendations are summarized in Table 26.1.

Lapses in the standards of care in emergency radiology may present in several ways:

1. A completely unexpected *error* in radiologic reporting that results in harm to the patient.
2. A *service* performing suboptimally over a period of time producing unsatisfactory outcomes.
3. An individual *practitioner* whose performance is impaired due to inadequate knowledge or skills or dysfunction related to health and behavioral problems.

Risk Management in Emergency Radiology: Considerations and Challenges

Errors in Reporting

This is one of the key components of the patient's overall care in the department. However, for risk management, it must be noted that the radiologist is ultimately responsible for the final report, but reporting is highly dependent on other quality measures in the department and cannot be viewed in isolation. Also, in spite of best efforts and standard reporting practices, variation will exist among radiologist reporting and interpretations. A study of ED plain radiograph reporting showed that disagreement can range from 5% to 9%.

False-positive errors. This error occurs when an abnormality is incorrectly described but is normal or a normal variant. It can also occur when a finding is attributed to the wrong cause. False-positive or cognitive errors are more likely to be related to a lack of experience or knowledge, rather than external factors. However, incomplete clinical data and unavailability of old examinations may also contribute. Risk management issues may involve repeated examinations to assess for change, seeking outside comparison examinations, and comparison with the opposite side, especially in cases of pediatric trauma. False-positive errors in emergency radiology can result in inappropriate treatment initiated for an abnormality that does not exist and treatment complications that may ensue. False-positive errors can also delay the correct diagnosis, because the patient's symptoms are incorrectly attributed to an alternate diagnosis.

False-negative errors. False-negative errors result from underreporting, where a finding is missed or incorrectly dismissed, and are five times more common than false-positive errors. This includes findings that were not present on the original image due to an inadequate exam. False-negative errors in emergency radiology can have the drastic negative effect of delaying diagnosis and management.

Intrinsic and Extrinsic Factors

Several intrinsic (related to radiologist) and extrinsic factors (not directly related to radiologist) may be responsible for producing errors:

Poor-quality examinations. This can be due to inadequately trained staff, poor equipment, or suboptimal working conditions, such as when a technologist is overwhelmed and unsupported. Poor-quality examinations may result from failure to use correct imaging parameters (radiographic technique, sequence parameters, sonographic gain/frequency, etc.), performing inappropriate views, improper centering of anatomy, failure to mark the region of interest, and so on. It is also important to consider patient factors, such as size, body habitus, inability to stay still, and inability to reposition, which can all be responsible for poor exam quality. This requires staff to be educated about how to identify barriers with directed strategies for how to overcome limitations. Regardless of the source of error, if a radiologist identifies a poor-quality or nondiagnostic exam, he or she should clearly state the technical limitation and request a repeat or alternate procedure and, in most cases, defer interpretation until exam quality is sufficient. The exam should also be flagged for internal review so that a proper risk assessment can be undertaken, and the source of the poor quality can be addressed.

Failure to consult previous studies or reports. The importance of reviewing old studies cannot be understated. Using a comparison examination to establish temporal stability can help make an indeterminate finding more likely benign, which can help prevent unnecessary workup. Similarly, establishing a timeline during which findings developed can help narrow the differential diagnosis or gauge whether findings are getting better or worse. For radiologists, this is analogous to *history taking* and should be standard practice for all radiologic reporting. To support the radiologist in this effort, hospitals and radiology departments must ensure that there is a robust system for archiving and storage of old studies, such that pertinent comparison exams are readily available when needed. This includes hiring adequate clerical and information technology staff, software support to upload outside studies, and investing in short-term and long-term storage. Achieving such a system requires balancing costs and practicality of storage and retrieval of old images with the risk of a lesion being missed or misinterpreted when old films are not available.

Clinical information. Accurate clinical information is a vital component of an imaging request or requisition. Lack of clinical information or inadequate/inaccurate clinical information has been shown to be a common source of reporting error. Ideally, the requisition will include pertinent clinical information that helps the radiologist focus on the area of concern and answer specific questions. However, it would be naïve to assume that all requisitions will include comprehensive accurate clinical information. In an ED setting, radiologists frequently receive incomplete or irrelevant clinical history, which can be a major source of error and inefficiency. In many cases, at the time the examination is ordered, data gathering is ongoing, so the emergency provider does not yet have all relevant information. Consequently, emergency radiologists should be prepared to search for relevant clinical information when necessary. To support the radiologists, emergency radiology departments should be proactive and establish frictionless mechanisms for accessing the medical record during the course of image interpretation. This can be achieved in a variety of ways, including direct integration of the electronic medical record (EMR) into the PACS, using support personnel to gather additional data, or launching an always-open EMR window on a separate computer or accessory monitor.

Multiple lesions. Failure to report multiple lesions has been previously described as a source of reporting error, commonly due to satisfaction of search. The missed lesions can be related or unrelated to the primary finding. Failure to diagnose an additional neoplastic lesion can change management (e.g., medical vs. surgical) or delay diagnostic workup.

Poor viewing conditions. Standard viewing conditions must be established for image interpretations to minimize error that can result from poor viewing conditions. Interpreting radiographs can be particularly sensitive to viewing conditions, especially for subtle findings. Emergency radiology departments should have standard practices with periodic review of workstations and viewing conditions. Radiologists should also be taught how to establish optimal viewing conditions so that they can report suboptimal conditions if they arise.

Fatigue. Resident and/or staff fatigue is another cause of errors, and several studies have demonstrated how overwork affects accuracy and its medical-legal implications. Strategies for minimizing fatigue can include limiting workload to only truly emergent cases while on call, having overlapping or short call shifts, and providing more coverage to high-volume areas like ED CT.

Service Failure

Some errors are due to failure of the systems or the service line in a hospital or radiology department. Potential areas of service failure include the following:

Inadequate staffing. Hospitals may be inadequately staffed to provide quality emergency radiology services on a 24-hour basis. If 24-hour in-house radiologists are not feasible, then it is imperative to define what services are provided during the daytime and on a 24-hour basis. During holidays and weekends, some specialized services may need to be temporarily withdrawn or arrangements may need to be made with other healthcare providers. In areas where an in-house radiologist is not available, a robust remote access network can be used to allow radiologists elsewhere to remotely view and report studies. Remote interpretations can be provided by radiologists within the department or outsourced to other groups (e.g., teleradiology). Some departments require periodic night shifts for staff and/or residents for ED calls.

Miscommunication. If not addressed on a system level, miscommunication can result in an inappropriate investigation being performed, incorrect treatment initiated, or the wrong patient or wrong side being imaged. Emergency radiology departments need standard practices for communication of urgent results or unsuspected findings to minimize deviation and errors. Many departments use internal codes that flag the study, in addition to documenting verbal communication. All such verbal communication should be followed with documentation in the patient chart or radiology report, indicating the time and the person with whom the information was shared.

Preliminary interpretations. Use of electronic or verbal preliminary reports is a common strategy for providing 24-hour emergency radiology but should be acknowledged as a potential source of system failure, especially if radiologists use them inconsistently or have different expectations for what constitutes a preliminary report. Although it facilitates prompt communication between a busy emergency radiology department and the ED, a hasty verbal impression or incorrect preliminary report can result in serious error, especially when the case was not reviewed comprehensively. Emergency radiology departments must have standard policies regarding what is expected and appropriate for preliminary interpretations so that radiologists and emergency providers have consistent expectations. Reading of preliminary reports by attending and/or subspecialty radiologists should be performed in a timely fashion, with consistent expectations regarding the time from preliminary to final interpretation.

Excess workload/inadequate workflow. Overworked radiology departments with suboptimal workflow will tax all components of the system and are a setup for system-related errors. The department should have mechanisms for dynamically responding to increased workload (e.g., major disaster or trauma), including how to appropriately allocate and assign resources and personnel where needed. Examination volumes should also be periodically evaluated so that longitudinal trends can be identified and increasing workload can be anticipated.

Machine and equipment error. Paperless and filmless departments have been revolutionary but have contributed to another category of errors. Examples include incorrect patient identifiers in the PACS, assigning images to the wrong patient in a RIS-PACS system, dictated reports that are not pushed to PACS and/or the EMR, incorrect examination timestamps that do not match the report, incorrect accession numbers resulting in reports with the wrong header or assigned to the wrong patient, and examinations not completed by technologists that never populate the radiology worklists. The role of the RIS-PACS administrator is critical in anticipating and identifying such errors before they affect patient care.

Practitioner Performance

Lack of subspecialty training. The ever-increasing complexity of radiology coupled with the massive scope of the specialty means that diagnostic imaging is used for a myriad of conditions from head to toe. This presents significant challenges for radiologists and technologists alike. As part of their practice, emergency radiologists often become proficient in the most common examinations performed in the ED, regardless of whether they have received subspecialty training. However, emergency radiologists may encounter examinations for which they do not feel properly trained or have not maintained their expertise, which can lead to errors and suboptimal care. Subspecialty training may be beneficial or required in certain areas, and it is important that radiologists acquire such subspecialty training when it is needed. It is also important that radiologists recognize their limitations and consider subspecialty backup, if available. In large departments, having many radiologists with a variety of subspecialty interests may be feasible, but this may not be possible in small departments.

Lack of continuing medical education. It is imperative that physicians keep abreast of changes in their specialty and within their scope of practice. This is required to provide good patient care and for maintaining hospital credentials, board certification, and licensing. Medical knowledge evolves quickly, and radiologists must include continuing education as a necessary component of their practice.

Inappropriate conduct and psychological or medical problems. Physical and mental health are a critical component of practitioner performance and, when impaired, can result in serious errors and dangerous situations. An impaired physician or staff member poses a risk to him or herself, his or her coworkers, and his or her patients. Continuously assessing practitioner wellness is crucial for maintaining a functional department and should be a priority. Resources must be available so that practitioners know how to recognize impairment, in themselves and others, and how to seek help.

Risk Management Paradigm

The risk management paradigm involves several components, all sharing the common goal of providing safeguards for the patient, personnel, and the organization (Fig. 26.1).

Prevention and Foresight

There is no better place to implement the "prevention is better than cure" philosophy than risk management. Defining potential problems in advance and implementing appropriate protocols and procedures goes a long way toward successful risk management. It helps all members of the team determine how to operationalize goals

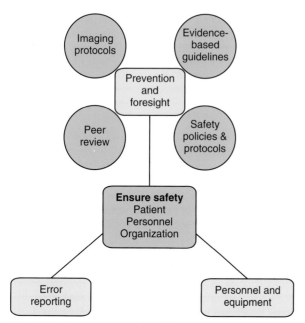

FIG. 26.1 Components of the risk management paradigm.

and intentions. Strategies can include appropriate imaging protocols, use of evidence-based guidelines for imaging algorithms, and peer-review activities. It also includes designing safety systems that will identify, eliminate, or reduce complications from radiologic examinations. This component relies on performance indicators, quality metrics, audits, and quality maps to function effectively. An accreditation program can also be used to ensure safety and quality.

Good policies are the product of research, collaboration with important stakeholders, and ongoing dynamic reviews. A good policy or procedure is useless if not understood or effectively implemented, so policies should be made user-friendly and widely available. Effective implementation generally requires interactive staff training when a new policy is rolled out so that participants understand the rationale and can ask questions. Displaying some policies in a visual format in the department or patient care areas may also be useful to encourage compliance and diminish barriers to use.

Error Reporting

In spite of the best efforts, risk in healthcare cannot be completely eliminated. Hence, prompt acknowledgment of risk and maintaining transparency are key elements of risk management. This includes recognizing the limits of the radiologic diagnosis and establishing systems that ensure proper timely disclosure of errors, documentation of actions taken, and participation in discrepancy review meetings. It is critical that the explicit objective of error reporting is to share knowledge and learn from mistakes or near misses to prevent future incidents. An effective error reporting process requires that participants understand and accept that it is conducted in an anonymous nonpunitive fashion without fear of retribution. A 2012 Agency for Healthcare Research and Quality (AHRQ) hospital survey showed that most respondents, including physicians, felt that

their mistakes were held against them. An environment that is punitive or does not allay such fears will lead to higher overall risk.

Personnel and Equipment

The radiologist and the radiologic equipment form another critical component of risk management. To ensure the highest quality and radiologic accuracy, radiologists must maintain professional competence, and the department/hospital should invest in high-quality equipment and properly trained staff. This also includes maintaining appropriate workload, funding, and recruitment.

Addressing Errors in Emergency Radiology

First, it is important to understand how to correctly label an error, which implies that a mistake was made, such as a missed finding or incorrect diagnosis. This also implies that a correct diagnosis or interpretation was possible and could have been achieved. Previous studies have shown that many factors can cause interobserver variation in reporting or differences in opinion, especially in subtle cases, which should not be labeled as an error. Similarly, all discrepancies between retrospective review of images and the original report should not automatically be viewed as an error. Reviewing images in hindsight offers perspective and information that was not available during the initial review. Imaging is only part of the patient's diagnostic information and may be undertaken early in the course of an illness when findings are subtle. Radiology is not histology, and the process of risk management recognizes that there will be cases where accurate radiologic diagnosis is not possible. Once error occurs and is correctly identified, there must be standard practices for documentation, education, and follow-up. The three essential steps include the following:

Informing the Patient and Provider

Patient safety comes first, and it is necessary that the essential details of a significant error be explained to the patient and provider so that appropriate treatment or workup can be initiated, if applicable. This communication must be undertaken in a sensitive manner after discussion between the radiologist and the clinical team. In emergency radiology, errors may only be discovered in retrospect, long after the patient has been discharged from the ED, so such communication is generally more appropriate for a primary provider than an emergency medicine provider. Patients have a right to know about errors that have adversely affected their management. However, if the error is not an immediate threat to the patient, then communication can be deferred until the root cause investigation has been completed. This may allow a more informative discussion with the patient in which the entire process can be described, including how the error was discovered, how it was evaluated, and what steps will be taken to prevent similar errors. In some cases, this discussion should take place in conjunction with hospital or department risk management personnel.

Notifying the Hospital of Critical Incidents

What constitutes a radiologic critical incident needs to be clearly defined in advance and not on a case-by-case basis. Typically, errors that lead to mismanagement and/or cause significant morbidity or mortality should be recorded as critical incidents. Hospital risk management personnel should be informed of such errors so that they can initiate further analysis and have advance knowledge of potential claims against them.

Root Cause Investigation and Error Reporting

RCA is a structured method used to analyze serious adverse events. A central tenet of RCA is identifying underlying problems that increase the likelihood of errors while avoiding the trap of focusing on mistakes by individuals. The goal of RCA is thus to identify both active errors (errors occurring at the point of interface between humans and a complex system) and latent errors (the hidden problems within healthcare systems that contribute to adverse events). RCA can be performed by assigned personnel or by a peer-review committee per the department policy. RCAs should generally follow a specified protocol that begins with data collection and reconstruction of the event in question through record review and participant interviews.

For adequate risk management, it is necessary to have a forum to report and discuss discrepancies, errors, near misses, and so on. Many departments conduct mortality and morbidity (M&M) or difficult diagnosis conferences. Emergency radiology departments may struggle with the logistics of such conferences because radiologists work variable shifts with minimal or no overlap. To encourage error reporting, the department should create an atmosphere of trust in which staff are encouraged to report problems but are still held accountable. When possible, anonymity should be maintained with images and reports anonymized. To reduce bias, individuals conducting consensus peer review should be given the same information as the original reporting radiologist. The process should be educational, nonpunitive, and involve a clear no-blame culture. A confidential record of the cases discussed should be made identifying the perceived reporting discrepancy. The original reporting radiologist should be informed of the case in a confidential fashion, and the clinical team should be informed of the discrepancy, if they are not already aware, to ensure that harm to the patient is avoided or appropriate workup can be pursued. If process or system factors contributed to or caused the discrepancy, they should be recorded along with the steps taken to rectify them. Any general lessons learned should be promulgated throughout the department.

INFORMED CONSENT IN EMERGENCY RADIOLOGY

Informed Consent Defined

Although a signed consent form is commonly used to document the physician's discussion with the patient, informed consent is a shared discussion regarding the risks, benefits, and alternatives for an imaging examination or procedure. The ACR-SIR (Society of Interventional Radiology) Practice

Parameter on Informed Consent for Image-Guided Procedures states that "informed consent is a process and not the simple act of signing a formal document." Informed consent can also be documented with a note in the patient's medical record or recorded on videotape or another similar permanent modality.

Need for Informed Consent

Informed consent is required for invasive image-guided procedures and may be required (or at least advisable) for some diagnostic imaging procedures. Specific procedures for which informed consent is required may be determined at a national level such as by The Joint Commission or locally by state law or local institution policy. Furthermore, patients have the right to be informed about the procedures they undergo, even if they are noninvasive or do not expose them to ionizing radiation, and may request to speak with a radiologist even when local policy does not require an informed consent process.

Elements of Informed Consent

Elements of informed consent include a detailed discussion of the proposed procedure, including its benefits, potential risks, and reasonable alternatives to the procedure. The information provided must be timely, accurate, and understood by the patient. It is not necessary to relay every conceivable risk to the patient, but radiologists should be prepared to describe likely and unlikely complications. It is also important that patients understand that they have a right to refuse the procedure or examination and should be informed about alternatives and the risks of not performing the procedure or examination. It should be ensured that the consent is given without duress and obtained in a noncoercive manner. To this end, some radiologists prefer that informed consent take place in a neutral setting, such as a consultation room, rather than the procedure suite or nursing holding area. In obtaining consent, radiologists must also ascertain whether the patient is competent to give consent. As a corollary, consent must be obtained before procedure-related sedation is administered.

Informed Consent in Special Situations

Pregnant Patients

In the ED, situations will arise where pregnant patients may require imaging that could expose the fetus to ionizing radiation. This includes fluoroscopic procedures, radiographs of the abdomen and pelvis, CT of the abdomen or pelvis, and CT-guided interventional procedures. In such situations, the first step is to confirm that the examination is medically necessary and that there are no suitable alternatives, which generally requires a discussion with the ordering provider. Once confirmed, informed consent should include a discussion regarding the risks to the fetus weighed against the risk of not performing the examination, including misdiagnosis or delayed diagnosis. For detailed guidance and risk assessment, radiologists and departments should consult the ACR-SPR Practice Parameter for Imaging Pregnant or Potentially Pregnant Adolescents and Women With Ionizing Radiation.

Other situations that warrant informed consent may include a pregnant patient who needs contrast-enhanced magnetic resonance imaging (MRI). Because it is unclear how gadolinium-based contrast media (GBCM) affect the fetus, they are relatively contraindicated in pregnant patients. GBCM are known to pass through the blood-placental barrier into the fetal bloodstream, then be excreted via the fetal kidneys into the amniotic fluid. Prolonged stay in the amniotic fluid has a potential for the GBCM to dissociate into the free gadolinium ion. Therefore, GBCM should only be used in pregnant patients if the contrast-enhanced MRI may provide critical results and the potential benefits outweigh the unknown risk to the fetus. Similar to ionizing radiation in a pregnant patient, a risk-benefit discussion should take place between the radiologist and ED personnel prior to proceeding with the examination. The ACR recommends that this discussion be documented in the patient's medical record or radiology report, including specific language that the diagnostic information cannot be obtained without GBCM, that the information needed affects the patient and/or fetus during the pregnancy, and that the referring physician believes it is not prudent to wait until after the patient is no longer pregnant. Informed consent with the patient should include a similar discussion regarding the unknown risks to the fetus weighed against the risk of not performing the examination, including misdiagnosis or delayed diagnosis.

Language Barriers

Language barriers may present unique challenges for performing informed consent. Specifically, informed consent and the ED setting have been identified as two of the five high-risk clinical areas where immediate attention is needed to prevent adverse events among limited-English-proficient patients. Nearly 9% of the US population is at risk for an adverse event because of language barriers, according to the AHRQ. Recent research suggests that adverse events that affect limited-English-proficient patients are more frequently caused by communication problems and more likely to result in serious harm compared to English-speaking patients. Three recommendations address these high-risk scenarios and are necessary for informed consent: requiring the presence of qualified interpreters, providing translated material in plain language, and using "teach-back" to confirm patients' understanding of care processes. Radiologists should avoid using family members/friends or nonqualified staff as interpreters. Radiologists with basic or intermediate foreign language skills may attempt to get by without the use of a competent interpreter, but this can increase patient risk by introducing uncertainty and misunderstanding.

A few hospitals have used translation apps, such as Canopy, and web-based services such as Google Translate in such situations. Although these technologies are promising and effective in casual use, they have not been validated in healthcare environments and are not advised for informed consent. A study testing Google Translate in various European languages found only a 57.7% accuracy rate on a number of medical phrases.

Fortunately, The Joint Commission has developed a new set of standards on patient-centered communication that emphasizes the importance of language, cultural competence, and patient-centered care. Hospitals seeking accreditation will be expected to comply with these recommendations, which were adopted in 2012.

CLINICAL DECISION SUPPORT

Clinical decision support tools have their origins in the 1950s and serve the important function of addressing both over- and underutilization. Clinical decision support can enable the integration of established guidelines in patient care and can act as a mechanism to curtail and standardize the use, cost, and radiation dose of emergent imaging examinations. Clinical decision support tools offer a favorable alternative to radiology business managers, which have been associated with inefficiencies and lack of transparency that have burdened the national healthcare system. As the Centers for Medicare and Medicaid Services seek incentives to reduce inappropriate imaging, clinical decision support will play an ever-increasing role in the delivery of healthcare. Since 2003, the US federal government began requiring quality reporting programs for healthcare. By 2006, the Physician Quality Reporting Initiative was introduced and focused on quality metrics of physician reporting. For radiology, reporting entities such as comparison examinations, radiation exposure, and pertinent positive and negative imaging findings were tied to financial incentives. In 2008, the Medicare Improvements for Patients and Providers Act included the Medicare Imaging Demonstration project to develop support tools to assist ordering of the 12 costliest imaging examinations. By 2009, the American Recovery and Reinvestment Act was created and included financial incentives for adoption of EMRs that were paid for meaningful use based on quality measures. Moving forward, decision support mechanisms will be required for any advanced imaging examination ordered for Medicare patients beginning in 2017 to reach the goal of tying 90% of Medicare fee-for-service payments to quality metrics by 2018. Throughout the evolution of clinical decision support, the ACR has lobbied for inclusion of clinical decision support in the hopes of increasing the value of radiology in medicine.

The process of integrating clinical decision support into daily ED patient care will require acceptance and buy-in by the emergency medicine physicians who most utilize imaging. Despite the establishment of the ACR Appropriateness Criteria in 1993, a survey of physicians from various specialties indicated that only a minority of referring physicians seek out and refer to these criteria when choosing an imaging technique. However, several clinical decision support options with commercially available software that use the ACR Appropriateness Criteria have been developed in the past several years, because it has been argued that appropriate use criteria can be most effective when they are embedded into electronic order entry clinical decision support tools. The ACR Appropriateness Criteria were created to address the relative appropriateness of imaging in various clinical situations. The usefulness of the ACR Appropriateness Criteria is that they are based on clinical scenarios for which literature evidence and expert consensus opinion are applied to determine the likelihood that an imaging examination would result in meaningful information for a given indication. The ACR Appropriateness Criteria provide a score of 1 through 9, corresponding to the likelihood that an imaging examination will provide useful information. The ACR Appropriateness Criteria provide evidence-based guidelines for 211 topics with more than 1050 variants to assist referring physicians. The Appropriateness Criteria address topics in diagnostic and interventional radiology and radiation oncology. In addition to the appropriateness score and its justification, the Appropriateness Criteria provide information on the relative amount of radiation.

Several studies have shown that incorporating clinical decision support for imaging into the electronic physician order entry system leads to decreased inappropriate imaging. For clinical decision support to be successful in the ED, it must be comprehensive and seamlessly integrated into the EMR or web-based portals. Clinical decision support can act as a stand-alone reference or be integrated with the computerized physician order entry system. The advantage of integrating clinical decision support with computerized physician order entry is that it promotes use at the point of care, which is crucial in the ED. In this scenario, the referring physician has decided that an imaging examination is needed and is in the process of selecting and ordering an examination from a list based on the body part and indication for imaging. The clinical decision support software uses an algorithm to match the combination of imaging examination choice and indication with all possible combinations of examinations and indications and computes an appropriateness score. Imaging examinations that are given higher scores are more likely to result in clinically useful information. Although the system allows for clinical judgment and exceptional circumstances, the ordering physician is typically prompted for more information or to reconsider ordering imaging examinations that are assigned low appropriateness scores. Although clinical decision support software does not typically provide a hard stop or prevent a referring physician from ordering a particular imaging examination in an individual case, the referring physician's utilization performance can be tracked over time. This data can then be used to identify physicians who routinely deviate from accepted imaging utilization standards and allow directed feedback and education. Additionally, the collection of national data can be used for creation of transparent comparative statistics for utilization and cost, health system and individual performance reports, and clinical decision support benchmarking nationwide. In addition to providing an appropriateness score for an imaging examination for a particular clinical indication, some clinical decision support tools can suggest appropriateness scores for alternative examinations aimed at the same clinical problem.

Another benefit of clinical decision support is the scaffold it provides for ongoing learning and improved patient care. Emergency medicine providers can rely on clinical decision support to manage demanding patients who desire unnecessary imaging examinations. Such decision support may also help increase ED throughput by offering better alternatives that can be performed on an outpatient basis. These physicians can find reassurance that their recommendations are in compliance with national consensus guidelines. Mechanisms can also be built into clinical decision support to alert the referring physician to allergies, renal function prior to contrast media administration, and evaluation of implanted devices prior to MRI.

> **BOX 26.1 Important Factors for Successful Integration of Clinical Decision Support**
>
> - Allows seamless integration into the electronic medical record at the site of physician order entry
> - Provides real-time, evidence-based/consensus recommendations for imaging utilization
> - Provides a mechanism for feedback from referring physicians
> - Helps eliminate the need for preauthorization
> - Generates quality data that can be longitudinally tracked against national benchmarks
> - Leads to consistency in imaging utilization and payments

In summary, appropriate use of imaging should be a goal for all physicians. Box 26.1 provides a summary of the important factors needed for a successful clinical decision support system. One way to achieve this is through use of clinical imaging support that is grounded in evidence-based appropriateness for common diagnoses that is integrated into the EMR at the site of physician order entry. Clinical decision support mechanisms will continue to gain acceptance if radiologists increase collaboration with emergency physicians and prevent such support tools from being viewed as obstructionist. As physician leaders, radiologists can use their administrative roles to develop and incorporate guidelines and clinical decision support tools. There is much opportunity to be had through harnessing technology to increase meaningful interactions with referring physicians.

TRANSFER OF OUTSIDE IMAGING

Cross-sectional imaging examinations, such as CT, MR, and ultrasound, have become essential to an ED patient's diagnosis and workup. Due to the sometimes limited specialization and resources of the hospital to which the patient initially presents, many patients require transfer to another ED for further evaluation and definitive care, particularly in the trauma setting. Focusing only on patients being evaluated in EDs, it is estimated that there are more than 2 million patient transfers annually. A critical component of this process is the transfer of outside imaging. An outside imaging examination is defined as one that was performed at a hospital or imaging center other than the hospital to which the patient has been transferred for definitive care. If the process of transfer of outside imaging is neglected or inefficient, the imaging examinations may need to be repeated and can lead to delays in care, increased cost, and higher radiation dose.

Although many institutions, especially tertiary care and academic medical centers, receive and use outside imaging examinations, there is a general lack of consensus regarding the process of integrating outside imaging into the radiology department and the patient's care. For example, a patient may arrive with an outside imaging examination copied to a compact disc (CD) in one of several formats. The recipient institution can use one of several software packages to open and view the contents of the disc. In some instances, the examinations must be reviewed by using the included image viewer applications. Because the outside examination is on a disc and not integrated into the recipient institution's PACS, the outside images are often initially viewed on lower-resolution, nondiagnostic monitors. These factors may partly contribute to the significant percentage of patients who undergo repeat imaging despite having been transferred with their outside imaging examinations. In a previous study, it was estimated that most of the transferred ED patients (36% of total ED patients) were rescanned because of inefficiencies and technical difficulties associated with the process of handling outside imaging examinations.

The inconsistencies associated with the transfer of outside imaging can lead to miscommunication due to the lack of consensus regarding the reporting process. A final report typically does not accompany the previously performed outside imaging examination despite the practice parameter recommendations made by the ACR that state, "When feasible, a copy of the final report should accompany the transmittal of relevant images to other health care professionals, when such images are requested." Additionally, the Emergency Medical Treatment and Active Labor Act states that the referring hospital must provide the receiving institution with the portion of the patient's medical record that is pertinent to the reason for transfer, including the radiologist's report for an imaging study. However, Sung et al. found that verbal or written reports for outside imaging examinations were available for only 16% of transferred ED patients; of the available reports, they noted a 12% discrepancy rate when the examinations were reinterpreted at the recipient institution. In numerous medical centers that have a radiology residency program, interpretation of imaging examinations for trauma patients who were transferred after hours was reviewed only by a radiology resident; there was a variable degree of written documentation and eventual attending radiologist overread for these outside examinations. Even in centers where an attending radiologist initially reviews the outside imaging, he or she may provide only a verbal consult, whereas others may be required to generate a written report for inclusion in the medical record. Because verbal reports are subject to hearsay and recall error, an erroneous report may be recorded in the patient's EMR and propagated to other clinical services that are consulted. For these reasons, a written report is the preferred method of communicating a formal interpretation of outside imaging examination. However, the generation of formal, written reports can lead to liability concerns because the outside imaging examinations may be of lower quality or performed according to a protocol that is unfamiliar to the radiologist at the recipient institution. Additionally, the requirement for a formal dictation on every outside examination can lead to a significantly increased workload for some institutions. The increased workload may be a point of contention if the recipient radiologist's state or practice does not permit reimbursement for reviewing the outside examinations and time spent consulting with the referring clinical service.

The inconsistencies and inefficiencies associated with the process of transferring outside imaging may also lead to delay in patient triage and treatment. The two main bottlenecks include the copying of patient imaging data into a suitable medium, such as a CD or DVD, and the uploading of the images at the recipient institution. As suggested by Sung et al., radiology departments may consider several avenues to standardize and expedite the outside imaging

---

BOX 26.2 Suggested Methods to Transfer Outside Imaging

- Develop a remote imaging network of hospitals in a geographic region
- Import outside imaging into the receiving institution's picture archiving and communication system
- Standardize compact disc viewing software
- Create central image repositories
- Standardize format (digital imaging and communications in medicine)
- Standardize reporting with generation of a written report

---

transfer process (Box 26.2). One example is the development of remote access capabilities for hospitals within a defined geographic region. Development of a hospital network can facilitate earlier consultation, more efficient patient triage, and initiation of treatment; if initiated early enough, the remote consult can even lead to a decrease in unnecessary patient transfers. Additionally, hospital networks with integrated radiologic computer networks have been shown to decrease the number of repeat imaging examinations and CT use rates for transferred patients. If such a network does not exist, the uploading of outside imaging examinations into the recipient institution's PACS serves to preserve the images and permit universal viewing by multiple specialists throughout the institution. Uploading the outside examination into the PACS eliminates the risk of potential misplacement or damage of the disc but requires that the technologist or file room clerk manually reconcile differences in the image headers and data in the RISs of both institutions. Another advantage of this is that the uploaded study can be viewed using familiar PACS hardware and navigation tools; in the setting of a web-based PACS, multiple subspecialty radiologists and surgeons can view the images simultaneously from the radiology department, remote locations, or the operating room. It is also possible for the recipient institution to create reformatted images from the uploaded outside examination.

There are several additional means to facilitate and improve the transfer of outside imaging. From a technical standpoint, transfer of imaging between institutions could be more efficient if there was increased uniformity of the format used for recording imaging examinations. For example, the Integrating the Healthcare Enterprise initiative endorses a set of technical specifications referred to as the Portable Data for Imaging profile; this is meant to standardize the archiving and expression of digital imaging and communications in medicine format (DICOM) on physical media so that diagnostic imaging studies are interchangeable across PACS vendors. Universal acceptance of this standardization could make transfer of outside imaging more seamless across institutions. In addition to the format, standardization of the embedded viewing software would also enable the process of image sharing. Creation of large image repositories and universal patient identifiers could permit numerous facilities to access patient imaging data simultaneously. Assuming that these technical logistics of image transfer are successfully implemented, creation of an outside imaging examination service can allow referring physicians to have their imaging studies sent to the referral center for uploading into the PACS prior to the patient's arrival in the ED. In this model, a written report can be generated and made available even before the patient's arrival, which can allow for more efficient management in the ED. In some instances, the professional fee for reinterpreted examinations can be reimbursed by insurers.

Referral centers that deal with transfer of outside images should be familiar with the regulations stated in the Health Information Technology for Economic and Clinical Health Act, which is a component of the American Recovery and Reinvestment Act of 2009. Although this act endorses electronic transmission and sharing of images, it also describes security regulations for the storage of images on CD-ROMs and during Internet transfer that align with the regulations issued under the Health Insurance Portability and Accountability Act (HIPAA).

In summary, efficient transfer of outside imaging has become a critical process for patient care and an important component of emergency radiology departments associated with referral centers. If a standard process has not been established, the associated workload and medicolegal ramifications can become a significant burden for radiology departments. Because technical issues are commonly barriers to successful transfer of outside imaging, it behooves radiology departments to invest in information technologies and personnel who are adept in integrating outside imaging examinations into the department's existing PACS. Issues with reporting and miscommunication should be addressed by creating a standard set of expectations used by all emergency radiologists who evaluate outside imaging examinations.

INFORMAL/CURBSIDE CONSULTS ON OUTSIDE READS: LEGAL RAMIFICATIONS

Imaging examinations performed at another institution prior to the patient's transfer to another ED are generally referred to as "outside imaging." There are many reasons for an emergency radiologist to provide a second opinion on an outside imaging examination. For one, reinterpretation at academic centers is an avenue for dedicated emergency or subspecialty radiologists to provide added value in patient care. Next, subspecialty interpretations have been shown to alter clinical management in a significant percentage of patients. Third, imaging utilization has been shown to be significantly lower for patients whose outside imaging was successfully imported to the receiving medical center compared to those whose transfer of imaging failed.

However, a consult for outside imaging poses an interesting dilemma for radiologists: the radiologist is asked to balance the need to be a collegial and responsive consultant against the medicolegal responsibilities of interpreting an examination that may be of suboptimal quality or performed according to an unfamiliar protocol. There are many reasons why it is often undesirable to repeat an imaging examination for a transferred patient: repeat examinations are associated with increased cost, increased radiation dose, increased exposure to contrast agents, delayed initiation of treatment, increased length of stay, and increased morbidity and mortality. Indeed, although the consulted radiologist wants to facilitate patient care, he or she must navigate through an imaging study without

having control over the scan parameters, appropriateness, protocol selection, or image quality.

In an urgent setting, the secondary interpretation of outside imaging may be done in a casual, informal manner in which the full patient history and prior imaging examinations are not disclosed. Such interactions between the consultant radiologist and the referring physician are often colloquially referred to as "wet reads" or "curbside" consults. These interactions are typically verbal exchanges that lack documentation except for an occasional cursory chart note written by the referring clinician. Unfortunately, despite the informal and courteous exchange between physicians, providing an opinion for the outside imaging examination is enough to establish a "doctor-patient relationship" and to potentially hold the consulted radiologist legally responsible for a proper interpretation. These ramifications hold true despite the perceived level of informality and lack of written documentation.

Another nebulous and potentially costly entity is the note regarding the outside imaging interpretation that is placed into the patient's chart or EMR by the referring clinician. In many cases, the notes of some referring clinicians act to substantiate the informal consultation that occurred with the radiologist and can be beneficial to the radiologist in the medicolegal arena. However, the referring clinician's note of a radiologist's second opinion regarding an imaging study can also be subject to recall bias, incompleteness, and misunderstanding. Therefore, it behooves the radiologist to place his or her own documentation in the patient's medical record or to avoid casual, curbside consultations altogether.

Several institutions rely on radiology residents to manage the emergency radiology department after hours. Residents may be the only radiology personnel available for consultation on outside imaging examinations. Due to the complexity of some transferred patients and the need to make medical decisions within a short time frame, radiology residents may find themselves in the awkward position of reinterpreting an imaging examination that has been already read by a more experienced board-certified radiologist at another institution. However, this may be the only second opinion that is rendered on an outside imaging examination; a survey of residency program directors revealed that in 45% of responding institutions, residents review outside trauma examinations without final review by an attending radiologist. Despite the relatively high accuracy of resident interpretations while on call, allowing residents to provide the only reinterpretation may expose them to unnecessary medicolegal issues because this practice has raised concerns over proper supervision and credentials. However, some departments have successfully developed processes to include attending oversight over outside imaging examinations that were initially reviewed by residents.

In an effort to standardize the process of integrating outside imaging into the transferred patient's care plan, some referral centers have developed guidelines and resources within their radiology departments. One example is the development of an algorithm designed to provide subspecialty-level interpretations of outside imaging examinations when requested; the algorithm includes assessment of technical adequacy, consideration for reinterpretation, and creation of a plan for completion of

BOX 26.3   Suggestions to Avoid Medicolegal Ramifications of Curbside Consults for Outside Imaging Examinations

- Avoid informal, undocumented verbal consultations regarding outside imaging examinations; offer to provide a written report instead.
- If a second opinion is required for an outside examination, the radiologist places a note in the medical record to document the interpretation.
- Develop an algorithm that requires a referring clinician's order to be placed prior to interpretation of any outside imaging examination.
- Develop an algorithm that mandates that a formal, written report is generated for the interpretation of any outside imaging examination.
- Mandate that all resident interpretations of outside imaging examinations be approved and signed by an attending radiologist within a defined time period.
- If an outside examination is technically suboptimal, this should be emphasized in the second opinion report with a statement that the report can be modified if repeat imaging is sought.

imaging. If reinterpretation of an outside imaging examination is requested, a dictated, formal report is issued. If imaging examinations need to be repeated at the receiving institution, then the reinterpretation of outside imaging of the same body part is deferred. By following such an algorithm, the need for informal, curbside consults is obviated.

In summary, there are several strategies that emergency radiologists and their departments can undertake to mitigate potential medicolegal issues that could arise from informal, curbside consultations in the ED (Box 26.3). These strategies may become more important in the future as healthcare payment structures continue to evolve; it is conceivable that interpretation of outside imaging may be relied upon more if repeat imaging becomes more restricted. Although requests for curbside consultations will never completely go away, the manner in which they are handled can be crafted to benefit the radiologist instead of creating exposure to medicolegal risk.

CHAPERONES

Imaging examinations of sensitive areas, such as pelvic ultrasound, scrotal ultrasound, contrast enema, and urethrography, may warrant the presence of an appropriate chaperone. However, practice patterns in the United States are often inconsistent with no standard guidelines from major societies. As such, most institutions develop local policies that may or may not be consistently applied. This is in stark contrast to the United Kingdom where chaperones are standard practice, with the General Medical Council, the Royal College of Physicians, the Royal College of Obstetricians and Gynaecologists, and the Royal College of Radiologists specifying that a chaperone must be offered to all patients who undergo an "intimate exam."

Although patient preferences regarding chaperones during intimate physical examinations in the ED and outpatient setting have been examined, very little data exist regarding patient preferences for the presence of chaperones during sensitive imaging examinations. A recent survey of patients undergoing pelvic ultrasound found that 46% of women preferred a chaperone if their sonographer was male compared to only 12% if their sonographer was female. Notably, the subset of patients (10%) who felt that a chaperone would be embarrassing was comparable to those who desired one with a female sonographer (12%). These findings are similar to other specialties where female patients generally prefer a chaperone when being examined by a male practitioner, but a minority of male and female patients desire a chaperone when being examined by a practitioner of the same gender. Importantly, most patients feel that it is important that they are offered a chaperone and are able participate in the decision making.

Chaperones serve as impartial observers to protect both the operator and patient by ensuring that inappropriate action does not occur. In some cases, chaperones may also provide reassurance for anxious patients. In addition to standard procedures to ensure patient comfort and privacy, patients should be offered a chaperone of the same gender, regardless of whether the operator is of the same gender. Ideally, the chaperone should be a fellow healthcare provider who is familiar with the procedure performed and, therefore, can recognize appropriate and inappropriate behavior. Potential chaperones include technologists, sonographers, medical students, radiologists, nurses, and other members of the care team. The chaperone should be comfortable observing the procedure and staying for its entirety. For medicolegal purposes, the identity and presence of the chaperone should also be clearly documented. Although it may also be helpful to have a patient's family member or friend present, they should not be considered a chaperone because they are not an impartial observer and may lack technical familiarity with the procedure. Care should also be taken to identify and respect religious or cultural preferences when appropriate.

In a busy emergency radiology department, many barriers exist that may make routine use of chaperones difficult. However, the presence of a chaperone is a critical component of patient and employee safety and, as such, standard department policies are encouraged for certain procedures. Based on existing preference data, patients should always be offered a chaperone. Every effort should be made to ensure the presence of a chaperone when requested, including delaying an examination, as long as it does not compromise patient care. For departments with male sonographers and technologists performing sensitive examinations, having a chaperone available should be anticipated for female patients.

CONTRAST EXTRAVASATION IN THE EMERGENCY DEPARTMENT

Extravasation of iodinated contrast media is uncommon, with a reported incidence of 0.1% to 0.9%. However, certain patients in an emergency setting are at higher risk for extravasation, including patients with altered consciousness, severe debilitation, and abnormal circulation in the limb injected. For these patients, technologists must

Contrast Extravasation QA Form

Tech Names: _____ Date: _____

Patient Name: _____ Hospital number: _____ Accession# _____

Patient Phone Contact - ***REQUIRED:*** _____ Inpatient or Outpatient - *Circle One*

CT Study: _____ Amount of Extravasation: _____

IV Gauge: _____ IV Site: _____ Injection Rate: _____

Who placed IV? *Circle One* **Nurse** *Pick One*   **Tech**   **ICU**   **ED Physician**   **Other** Explain_____

Floor

Radiology

ED

ICU

Please Note Patient's Symptoms; Check All that Apply:

☐ Swelling   ☐ Blistering
☐ Redness   ☐ Skin Color Changes Other than Redness
☐ Tendemess   ☐ Patient Unable to Communicate
☐ Burning/Stinging   ☐ No Symptoms
☐ Other_____

Check the Following when Completed:

     On-line Incident Report   ☐
     Post Extravasation Instructions Given to Patient (Pink Card) or
     Nurse (White Sticker Placed on Front of Chart).   ☐

If the Contrast Extravasation is 75ml's or Greater, the Patient Must Remain in Radiology for 2 to 4 Hours for Re-Evaluation by Radiologist. Contact Radiology Nursing Care Coordinator @ 2512 or Radiology Nurse if NCC is not Available. After Hours Techs Must Notify the Day Shift Lead at Shift Change for Follow-Up.

Plastic Surgery Must Evalute the Patient if the Following Conditions Exist:
     a. Skin Blistering
     b. Evidence of Altered Perfusion - Decreased Capillary Refill
     c. Increasing Pain
     d. Change in Sensation at or Distal to the Extravasation Site

FIG. 26.2 Sample contrast extravasation quality assurance form.

carefully assess the injection site for edema, erythema, and tenderness because the patient may be unable to report the symptoms of extravasation. Extravasations can occur following hand or power injection and are independent of the injection flow rate. The antecubital fossa is preferred for most contrast injections. Distal sites, such as the hand, foot, ankle, or wrist, have a higher risk of extravasation and should be avoided.

Once recognized, a radiologist should be notified to examine the patient. The initial focused evaluation should assess for swelling, erythema, tenderness, burning/tingling, blistering, capillary refill, and weakness. To facilitate follow-up and for internal quality assurance, a standard form should be completed for every extravasation, which includes the radiologist's evaluation and details regarding the IV gauge, injection site, and the amount of extravasation (Fig. 26.2). In the absence of signs of severe injury, management of an extravasation is usually conservative. Such measures attempt to promote resorption of the extravasated fluid and may include elevation and warm or cold compresses, noting that there is no consensus regarding the most effective treatment. Some advocate aspirating the fluid via an inserted needle or injecting local agents, such as hyaluronidase or corticosteroids, but evidence demonstrating clear efficacy is lacking.

Most symptoms are mild and resolve spontaneously, but radiologists must be able to recognize a rare severe injury, such as compartment syndrome or tissue necrosis. If there are signs of altered perfusion (e.g., decreased capillary refill), neurologic compromise (e.g., tingling, altered sensation), blistering, or ulceration, the patient should be evaluated by a surgeon. Even when there are no signs of severe injury on initial evaluation, patients should be observed for several hours to identify delayed worsening. For patients being evaluated in the ED, continued observation usually occurs in the ED or an inpatient unit if they are being admitted. For patients who are ultimately discharged from the ED, patients and caregivers should be given written instructions and contact information about how to seek additional care if their symptoms worsen following discharge. A follow-up phone call from a radiology nurse or radiologist within 24 hours may also be warranted for large-volume extravasations or patients who are still symptomatic at the time of discharge. The patient's final disposition and the care provider notified should also be documented in the standard extravasation evaluation form.

IMAGING THE OBESE PATIENT

Imaging the obese patient is a challenge that is encountered by emergency physicians and radiologists. Obesity is defined as a body mass index (BMI) greater than 30; morbid obesity carries a BMI greater than 40 and super obesity, a BMI greater than 50. There has been an epidemic of obesity in several countries, especially in the United States. Thirty-five percent of adults (78.6 million people) and 17% of youth in the United States are obese. Approximately two-thirds (69%) of US adults are either overweight or obese. The annual medical cost of this obesity in the United States was $147 billion in 2008, with the obese patients generally costing $1428 more than those with normal weight. There has been a significant increase in the imaging of these obese patients, due to the overall general increased utilization of imaging procedures and the need to image the diseases that are caused by obesity, such as cardiovascular disease, stroke, diabetes mellitus, and cancer.

An emergency radiology department should be well prepared to handle the challenging task of imaging the obese patient, which is important to obtain a prompt diagnosis and initiate appropriate treatment. The ED should be equipped for safe transport and imaging of obese patients, and the staff should be well trained in the logistics and operations. One major challenge is how to fit these patients inside the scanners. A study showed that 25% of US EDs were unable to perform CT, two-thirds were unable to perform MRI in patients weighing more than 350 pounds, and 90% were unable to perform CT or MRI in patients weighing more than 450 pounds. Scanning patients who do not fit in the scanner or are too heavy may result in device malfunction, damage to the equipment, and injury to patients. Radiation doses are also typically higher in these patients due to changes in scanning parameters. Even if the patient can be scanned, many studies are suboptimal and provide limited information. There are image quality issues and artifacts that are specific to each imaging modality, which will be discussed in detail in subsequent sections (Table 26.2). Studies that are difficult to interpret have doubled over the last 15 years. All of these challenges, including additional time taken for transporting and moving the patient to and from the scanner and for optimizing imaging parameters, result in lower throughput and higher health costs. In addition, suboptimal imaging can result in inadequate diagnosis, longer hospital stay, multiple procedures, higher cost, dissatisfaction, anxiety, and complications. An emergency radiology department must be aware of these challenges and adopt specific strategies for managing them.

General Strategies

A comprehensive program should be in place in the ED to address the challenge of imaging obese patients. Equipment to image the obese patient, such as scanners with larger bores, higher weight limits, and bariatric tables, should be purchased. The personnel involved in scanning and the referring physicians should be aware of the weight and gantry limitations so that patients who will not fit in the scanner are not unnecessarily sent to the scanner, resulting in delays and anxiety. The staff should be trained in transporting and moving these patients safely in and out of the scanner, to protect themselves and the patient. The ED and radiology department should be equipped with adequate manpower and devices for transportation and handling of these patients, such as stretchers, wheelchairs, beds, scales, lifts, safety straps, and hover mats. Appropriately sized waiting and dressing rooms should be available. There should be nurses who are adequately trained in obtaining IV access in these patients and handling extravasation issues. Radiologists and technologists should be trained in optimizing the image parameters to obtain diagnostic-quality images, while limiting radiation dose. Having a comprehensive protocol in place for imaging obese patients will also improve the throughput in the scanner and avoiding extra costs.

Radiographs

Challenges of radiographs in obese patient include difficulty in positioning, x-ray attenuation, scatter, low image contrast, long exposure time, motion artifact, poor anatomic landmarks, and higher radiation dose.

Due to the increased patient thickness, there is *increased x-ray attenuation and poor image quality*. This may be solved by using appropriate higher kVp and mAs to penetrate the tissues. However, these higher exposure factors also increase the radiation dose. Automatic exposure control can be used to select optimal exposure factors without undue increase in radiation dose.

Scatter radiation is generated in obese patients due to the increased body thickness. Other factors that affect scatter radiation include field of view (FOV) and kVp, both of which are high in obese patients and hence worsen the scatter. The scatter radiation reaches the image receptor and reduces tissue contrast. Scatter can be reduced by using a tight collimation and reducing the FOV. Use of an antiscatter grid with a high grid ratio between the body and image receptor can also improve image quality. The use of a grid increases radiation dose and also causes motion artifact due to longer exposure time. A stationary system with a mobile grid is more effective than a portable system in reducing scatter. For portable films, the cassette can be lined with lead, with a grid placed between the patient and cassette.

Image contrast is low in an obese patient due to generation of scatter radiation and the use of high kVp for penetration. *Motion artifacts* are seen due to longer exposure times. *Positioning* is another challenge because the maximum cassette size is 14 × 17 inches, and it is often not possible to get the images in a single film. Hence multiple films may be used and then fused together digitally. With cassette mapping, the number of cassettes and their orientation can be planned ahead of time. In addition,

TABLE 26.2 **Strategies for Imaging an Obese Patient**

Modality	Challenge	Solution
Radiograph	Increased x-ray attenuation	High kVp, high mAs
	Scatter	Tight collimation to reduce FOV, antiscatter grid
	Motion artifact from long exposure time	Minimize exposure time; use higher kilovoltage and milliamperage
	Low image contrast	Antiscatter measures
	Poor coverage	Use multiple films to cover area of interest
	Poor anatomic landmarks	Use indirect landmarks
Fluoroscopy	Table weight limit	Newer systems, upright positioning, overhead films, CT
	Table to image intensifier distance	Newer systems, supine positioning
	Table width	Newer systems
	Poor penetration	Proper positioning, higher x-ray tube capacity
	Inadequate coverage	Largest FOV, tight collimation, no magnification, overhead films
CT	Table weight limit	New scanner with higher limit
	Gantry diameter limit	New scanner with bigger bore
	Smaller scanning FOV	Proper positioning in FOV, extrapolation algorithm
	Smaller reconstruction FOV	Extrapolation algorithm
	Truncation artifact	Extrapolation algorithm, truncation artifact correction algorithm, bundling
	Photon starvation	Higher tube power, dual source, higher mAs, higher kVp, tube current modulation, lower pitch, increased gantry rotation time, iterative reconstruction algorithm, thicker slices, adaptive filters
	Poor contrast	Higher dose, rate of contrast
	Radiation dose	Optimal dose, automatic tube current modulation, iterative reconstruction algorithms
Ultrasound	Increased attenuation	Different position (lateral decubitus, prone, coronal oblique), lower-frequency transducer, tissue harmonic imaging, compound imaging, speckle-reduction filters, processing filters, penetrate mode
MRI	Scanner limitation, table weight limitations	New scanners have higher limits
	Small bore	Open MRI, open bore
	Patient discomfort	Open MRI, open bore
	FOV limitations	Use smallest possible FOV, phase oversampling to reduce artifact, large coils
	Low signal-to-noise ratio	High magnetic field strength, high strength gradients
	Radiofrequency deposition burns	Padding between skin and gantry

CT, Computed tomography; *FOV,* field of view; *MRI,* magnetic resonance imaging.

anatomical localization is a challenge because the conventional landmarks may be difficult to identify. Other landmarks can be used, such as elbow or iliac crest.

High radiation dose is seen due to increased use of higher exposure factors. Automatic exposure control can be used to limit radiation dose for appropriate image quality. Radiation dose can be reduced by placing the side of the patient with the thinnest fat layer close to the receptor.

Fluoroscopy

The challenges specific to fluoroscopy in an obese patient are table weight limitations, distance between the table and image tower, table width, x-ray capacity, and patient positioning.

The *table weight limit* for most fluoroscopy units is 350 pounds. Placing patients above this weight will damage the system and may harm the patient. Newer systems can take weight limits up to 500 pounds with tilt and 600 pounds without tilt. Another option is to perform the study in an erect position, although this may not be ideal in all situations because the patient may not be able to

stand. In addition, the girth increases in the upright position compared to the supine position, so the patient may no longer fit in the space. If he or she does fit, there is also higher radiation due to the use of higher exposure factors to penetrate the increased tissues. If it is not possible to fit the patient in the fluoroscopy table, overhead radiographs or CT can be performed.

The *distance between the table and the image intensifier* is also a limitation, usually 45 to 49 cm, although newer systems can have up to 60 cm distance. If the patient cannot fit in this distance, fluoroscopy cannot be performed. Due to tissue dispersion, it is easier to acquire an image in the supine rather than the upright position in obese patients. *The width of a fluoroscopic table* is small, usually 45 cm, and is also a consideration. Patients who are borderline or cannot fit will be uncomfortable, scared, and reluctant to move, thus limiting the study. Newer systems may be to 69–80 cm wide.

Poor penetration of tissues is a challenge due to increased soft tissue, which can be worsened by poor positioning, suboptimal exposure, and long exposure, all of which may result in blurry images. Higher x-ray tube capacity helps improve penetration in deeper tissues of obese patients. Exposures should be collimated adequately. Exposure factors are optimized to penetrate the tissues, either automatically or manually.

The largest possible FOV should be used, with no magnification. In patients with poor coverage with only a limited area seen, an alternative is to use overhead films instead of fluoroscopy. This is not ideal because the exact anatomy is not evaluated and multiple overhead films may be needed. Interpretation of the films is challenging, and it may miss critical information, without the dynamic information offered by fluoroscopy.

Computed Tomography

CT challenges include scanner size limitation (table weight, gantry width), FOV limitation (scanning and reconstruction), tube capacity, contrast modification, artifacts (truncation artifact and photon starvation), and radiation dose. Because CT may be the only feasible imaging option available in many of these patients, it is crucial that steps are taken to ensure that images can be adequately acquired.

There is an upper limit of table weight that each CT scanner can withstand. This limit should be followed; otherwise the table may not move at the appropriate speed, resulting in artifacts, damage to the table, and compromised patient safety. The technologist should be aware of this weight limit, and patients who are in excess of the prescribed weight limit should not be brought to the scanner. Most scanners have an upper limit of 450 pounds, but a few scanners are now available with weight limits up to 680 pounds, which should be considered in hospitals that have a high number of obese patients. Bariatric table tops are also available, and these should be changed for the patient, although this may slow the throughput.

Gantry width is another parameter that limits imaging of obese patients, even in patients who are within the weight limits. Typically, CT has a gantry diameter of 70 cm. However, the effective diameter of the scanner may actually be much smaller than this, due to the presence of the table, which may take up to 19 cm. Hence, these patients should be placed in the scanner to see if they can fit in the scanner. In such patients, if a larger gantry diameter is available, it should be preferentially used, because new scanners have diameters up to 90 cm.

Scanning FOV is usually smaller than the gantry aperture due to the presence of the table. Hence, the periphery of the patient, that is, the area between the gantry and the scanned FOV, is not included in the image. Because of this, critical findings may be missed on the periphery of the image (e.g., perforation or hernia of bowel loops). To minimize this, the patient is positioned so that the area of interest is directly in the scanned FOV on the table. In patients with a large chest, the feet-first position may be used to scan the abdomen. In some cases, extrapolation algorithms must be used to reconstruct with a wider FOV, although the image quality is compromised. Extrapolation algorithms can allow up to a 650-mm FOV compared to a scanning FOV of 500 mm.

Reconstruction FOV (the area of the reconstructed image) also has an upper limit to balance spatial resolution and coverage. This can vary from 50 to 82 cm. In patients larger than this, the projection data from beyond this are not included. Extrapolation techniques may be used to reconstruct these projections.

Truncation artifact is seen as a bright signal in the edge of the image. This is caused by the peripheral portion of the obese patient located between the scanning FOV and the gantry. Although this portion is outside the scanning FOV, the x-ray beam is attenuated by this tissue as well, but the scanner erroneously assumes that these data are coming from within the scanning FOV and hence, in the reconstruction, this appears as attenuation from within the scanning FOV, giving an artifactual bright appearance. Algorithms can be used to extrapolate the data outside the FOV, although this will have lower image quality. Truncation artifact correction is another solution.

Photon starvation is caused by higher photon attenuation through the thicker tissues of the obese patient, as a result of which, inadequate photons reach the detectors, producing quantum mottle, and thus low contrast-to-noise ratio (CNR) and poor low-contrast detectability. This is more often seen in the transverse dimension in the abdomen due to the larger diameter of this portion. This is also amplified in some reconstruction algorithms. To resolve photon starvation, the number of photons should be increased. This can be done by using higher power (60–100 kW), higher tube current, higher kVp (up to 140 kVp), lower pitch, increased rotation time, iterative reconstruction algorithms, adaptive filtration, thicker collimation, and thicker slices. Higher tube power may be used to increase the number of photons. With dual-source scanners, the two tubes can be operated simultaneously at high power and high kVp to improve penetration and reduce noise. However, the scanning FOV is small in one of the tubes. Tube current and kVp can be automatically modulated using automatic scanner software. Automatic tube modulation algorithms are based on the diameter and attenuation of the scout or by preset values based on BMI. However, this may increase the radiation dose. Increased reconstruction slice thickness reduces noise but lowers spatial resolution and increases partial volume averaging. Partial volume averaging can be reduced by reconstruction of overlapping sections and using coronal and sagittal reconstructions. Use of iterative reconstruction algorithms instead of filtered back projection helps lower noise and maintain spatial resolution. However, advanced iterative reconstruction algorithms require additional time for postprocessing.

The contrast in obese patients in vascular structures is often *suboptimal* due to increased body size and the use of higher kVp. This can be resolved by using a higher concentration, volume, and rate of contrast injection. The contrast dose can be calculated based on weight, but this is not accurate because fat does not disperse or dilute contrast. In addition, placing an IV cannula may be challenging in obese patients and may require placement of a peripherally inserted central catheter (PICC) and ultrasound guidance. Contrast extravasation is also a risk in these patients.

An *asymmetric profile* may be caused by asymmetric thickness of soft tissues. For example, in a female patient without a bra, the subcutaneous tissues and breasts are prominent on the side; this results in increased girth in the lateral dimensions, as a result of which, truncation and photon starvation are seen in the lateral CT. By bundling the tissues, that is, placing the patient in sheets, a bra, or commercial devices, a symmetrical profile is created, which reduces artifacts.

Obese patients receive a *higher radiation dose in* CT scans due to thicker soft tissues that must be penetrated and also require many of the parameter modifications described earlier. AEC causes a higher tube current rotation time product in larger patients and an upper limit of radiation dose may be set. Although the skin dose is higher, there is not a significantly higher radiation of internal organs because most of the radiation is absorbed by subcutaneous tissue and only a small amount reaches the internal organs. Iterative reconstruction algorithms can be used to minimize noise at acceptable radiation dose limits.

Ultrasound

The specific problems encountered in ultrasound of the obese patient are difficulty in positioning, beam attenuation, and an inability to reach deeper tissues.

The *ultrasound beam is attenuated* as the distance from the transducer increases; hence, in an obese patient, most of the beam is attenuated in the subcutaneous soft tissues before reaching the deeper organs of interest in the abdomen. The ultrasound beam attenuation also increases with the frequency of the ultrasound transducer. Therefore, in an obese patient, a lower-frequency transducer should be used to reach the deeper tissues.

Appropriate positioning of the patient can also help in reaching the tissues of interest. A modified lateral decubitus position can be used to displace the fatty pannus. The kidneys and the aorta can be scanned in the posterior oblique or coronal view.

Harmonic imaging, compound imaging, speckle-reduction imaging, and pre- and postprocessing filters can be used to improve the signal-to-noise ratio (SNR). *Tissue harmonic imaging* (THI) involves the generation of harmonic frequencies that are not present in the original wave; these frequencies are created by wave distortion, which is caused by nonlinear sound propagation. These harmonics increase with depth, unlike the fundamental frequency, which decreases with depth. It helps that fat has the highest nonlinearity coefficient, because the maximal intensity of harmonic waves is directly proportional to the nonlinearity coefficient. The generation of high-intensity harmonic waves in fat improves image quality compared to a conventional ultrasound beam. Using THI, images with increased penetration, improved resolution, and fewer artifacts such as reverberation and side lobe are obtained.

Compound imaging is a broad-bandwidth technology that combines multiple coplanar images obtained from different steering angles into a single real-time image. This improves image contrast resolution and edge detail and reduces speckle artifacts. *Speckle-reduction imaging* using filters is a postprocessing tool, where an algorithm is used to identify strong and weak signals, following which the weak signals (speckle) are eliminated and the strong signals are enhanced. The resolution is also improved. Other *processing filters* can also be used to improve the image quality. *Penetrate* mode should be used with any frequency to reach deeper tissues.

Magnetic Resonance Imaging

The specific challenges of MRI in an obese patient are scanner limitations, patient positioning, patient comfort, radiofrequency (RF) penetration, gradient strength, maximal FOV, and noise.

Scanner limitations include the table weight limit, bore diameter, bore length, coil, field strength, and gradients. The table weight limit for most scanners is 350 pounds, which is lower than that for CT. The bore diameter of a standard scanner is approximately 60 cm, but the effective diameter is smaller because of the space taken up by the table and coils. Hence, patients with large girth often cannot get into the scanners. It is less common to see patients with suboptimal images in MRI compared to CT, because many patients end up not having an MRI due to these limitations. Open scanners can take patients up to 500 pounds, but these scanners are typically of low field strengths and gradients, resulting in poor SNR and image quality. The latest open-bore scanners have larger bore diameters up to 70 cm. These scanners have shorter bore lengths (125 cm vs. 170 cm), as a result of which, the head is located outside the scanner, improving comfort and reducing claustrophobia. However, coronal FOV is reduced. Newer scanners can tolerate weights up to 550 pounds with availability of high field applications.

Optimal patient positioning in the center of the magnet and using an optimal coil are also a challenge. Body coils occupy more space and might reduce the space already available, while a surface coil may be too small for these patients. Due to tight fit in the scanner, *patient discomfort* is more of a challenge than in CT due to long scan times, and claustrophobia is aggravated. *Longer scan times* result from suboptimal positioning and the additional time required to optimize the image, both of which increase patient discomfort and motion artifacts. RF penetration and gradient strengths are technical factors.

The *maximal FOV* is limited to 40 to 50 cm. In obese patients, increasing the FOV beyond this range will result in lower spatial resolution. Hence, the FOV should be limited to the area of interest. However, the presence of tissues outside the FOV will result in wraparound artifacts. To avoid wraparound, phase oversampling can be used. Large coils are necessary to image the obese patient, but this will result in lower SNR and suboptimal images. Saturation bands can decrease noise from subcutaneous fat. There is a lower SNR in obese patients, because the tissues of interest are located farther from the coil. Use of surface coils is not possible due to the tissue size. The use of body coils lowers the SNR and CNR. High magnetic field strengths and gradients are required to increase SNR and CNR. RF deposition on the skin abutting the gantry will result in burns. To avoid this, the patient should be padded at areas of contact with the gantry.

DOSE REDUCTION IN THE EMERGENCY SETTING

In the ED, imaging has become an integral part of the increased use of modalities that involve ionizing radiation, including radiographs and CT scans. Particularly,

TABLE 26.3 **Radiation Dose Reduction Strategies**

Modality	Dose Reduction Strategies
Radiograph	Appropriate indication
	Reduce number of views
	Appropriate mAs
	Appropriate kVp
	Automatic exposure control
Computed tomography	Appropriate indication
	Appropriate protocol
	Virtual noncontrast in dual-energy scanner
	Higher noise images
	Optimizing scan
	Optimal scan length
	Overlap
	Adaptive z collimation
	Prepatient filtration and collimation
	Bismuth shielding
	Partial scanning
	Lower tube current
	Low mAs in some phases
	Anatomy-based tube current modulation:
	• Longitudinal tube current modulation
	• Angular tube current modulation
	• Combined tube current modulation
	ECG-based tube current modulation
	Prospective ECG triggering
	Prospective high pitch helical imaging
	Non-ECG gated
	Low kVp
	Pitch
	Reconstruction slice thickness
	Reconstruction FOV
	Postprocessing filters
	Iterative reconstruction algorithms

ECG, Electrocardiogram; *FOV,* field of view.

there has been an exponential increase in the use of CT scans due to their high diagnostic capabilities, rapid turnaround time, wide availability, and the need to make a diagnosis and avoid medicolegal issues. In 1990, the total number of CT scans performed in the United States was 13 million, which tripled by 2000 to 46 million and quadrupled by 2006 to 62 million. Although it has revolutionized medicine, this increasing use of CT has also brought concerns regarding the risks of ionizing radiation, particularly the development of radiation-induced cancer. Articles have been written in the lay and scientific press about the carcinogenic effects of low-dose radiation, largely based on data from atomic bomb survivors who faced a much higher dose of radiation. A linear no-threshold model has been proposed, which indicates that there is no threshold for developing cancer, and the risk increases with increasing radiation dose. Although there have been no solid data to prove this, the radiology community has risen to the challenge of alleviating these fears by actively proposing and developing many radiation dose reduction strategies. The commonly used radiation reduction strategies in the ED are discussed here and summarized in Table 26.3.

Appropriate Indication

One of the most important steps in reducing unnecessary radiation exposure is to scan only patients with appropriate indications for the CT scan. The CT scan should be performed only if the scan is justified and if the scan will provide information that will contribute to the management of the patient. This involves education of the referring physicians and good communication and discussion between the radiologist and the referring physician. National and locally established guidelines can be used, for example, the ACR appropriateness criteria. If there is an alternative test that provides similar information without the use of ionizing radiation, it should be preferred, especially in younger patients.

Appropriate Protocol

All patients who are getting a CT scan should be scanned with an optimized appropriate protocol. Dedicated protocols should be established for specific indications, with specific parameters based on patient size. The aim should be to obtain a diagnostic-quality scan with the least possible radiation dose, and the ALARA (as low as reasonably achievable) principle should be followed. Although there are no established upper limits of radiation dose, the least possible radiation dose should be used.

Virtual Noncontrast Images From a Dual-Energy Scanner

Virtual noncontrast (VNC) images are material composition images that are obtained from dual-energy scanners and have comparable appearance and attenuation numbers compared to a true noncontrast scan. VNC can be used to replace the true noncontrast phase in multiphasic studies and thus reduces the radiation dose associated with it. For example, VNC images are thought to be equivalent to conventional true noncontrast images in the evaluation of renal masses, endovascular aortic repair, and solitary pulmonary nodules.

Higher Noise Images

Although it is essential to obtain high-quality images with minimal radiation dose, occasionally it may be acceptable to obtain images that have some or a moderate amount of noise without losing diagnostic capability. This allows the use of low tube current, which reduces radiation dose. This has been validated for several clinical indications such as renal colic and acute appendicitis. Alternatively, low tube current and hence images with more noise can be used in some phases of multiphasic studies. For example, in a trauma protocol, it may be acceptable to have some noise in the delayed phase. Similarly, noise may be acceptable in the delayed phase of studies for follow-up of endovascular repair or in the noncontrast phase of renal and hepatic mass evaluation.

Scan Length

The scan length should be limited to only the required portion. Unnecessary exposure of regions outside the area of interest should be avoided. In some studies, especially in younger patients, the scan range can be restricted. For example, in pulmonary embolism, the lung bases and apical regions could be excluded. Limited abdominal CT can be performed in acute appendicitis. Although the topogram is used to determine the scan length, the scanning can be stopped if the required area has been scanned.

Overlap

When scanning different portions of the body, it is preferable to do continuous helical scanning instead of separate scanning of the different parts of the body in a segmental approach because the radiation dose is lower with the former approach than the latter, where some parts of the body may be scanned twice due to longitudinal axis overlap. A 17% dose saving can be obtained using a single helical acquisition compared to a segmented approach, especially in trauma protocols.

Dynamic Adaptive Section Collimation in the z-Direction

In helical scanning, it is not uncommon to scan the areas above and below the area of interest to obtain helical reconstruction, a phenomenon called z-scan overranging. The amount of extra tissue scanned depends on the pitch, collimation, and section width. The radiation dose of this excess scanning can be reduced up to 38% by using prepatient adaptive section collimators.

X-Ray Filters and Prepatient Collimators

Filters can be placed beneath the x-ray tube to attenuate low-energy photons that do not contribute to image formation but add to radiation dose. There are various filter sizes and the choice of filter affects the FOV and radiation dose. The smallest filter that allows the entire region of interest (ROI) to be imaged within the FOV should be used. Prepatient collimators are placed close to the x-ray tube, allowing the width of the beam to be altered. This limits radiation to the area to be scanned and avoids unnecessary radiation.

Bismuth Shielding

Bismuth shielding consists of placing a bismuth-impregnated latex over radiosensitive organs, which attenuates the photons before reaching organs such as the breast and thyroid. When placed over the breast, this shielding reduces the dose reaching the breast from the anterior direction. There will still be radiation that reaches the breast from the posterior aspect, but the intensity of this radiation is less because it is attenuated by the table and patient. Using bismuth shielding, radiation savings of up to 57% have been reported. If automatic tube current modulation (ATCM) is used, the bismuth shield must be placed after acquisition of the topogram so that the ATCM can use the topogram to calculate the dose settings. It has been shown that bismuth shielding can increase the noise and pixel values in the thorax due to beam hardening, thus diminishing image quality. Hence, it is generally not recommended for cardiovascular imaging. A spacer placed between the bismuth shield and the skin may reduce artifacts.

Partial Scanning

Radiation dose can be minimized by using a partial scanning technique, in which 180 degrees of projection plus

the fan angle are used to reconstruct the images, rather than the entire 360 degrees of projection. The tube current is on only for this duration and off for the remaining time, thus saving radiation dose. When exposing the breasts, the radiation can be turned off when the tube is in the anterior projection and the breasts exposed only when in the posterior aspect, because the x-ray beam is attenuated before it reaches the breasts.

Optimization of Exposure Parameters: Tube Current

The tube parameters (i.e., mAs [tube current-time product] and kVp) should be optimized to provide the best diagnostic image quality at the lowest possible radiation dose. The tube current is the number of electrons accelerated across the x-ray tube per unit of time, and the tube current-time product is the product of the tube current and time. Radiation dose is directly proportional to the tube current, and noise is inversely proportional to the square root of the tube current. Hence, lowering the tube current decreases the radiation dose proportionally but increases the image noise. Preset mAs values can be used for each protocol and also based on the BMI, with lower values for a lower mass index.

Anatomy-Based Tube Current Modulation

With tube current modulation, also called ATCM or automatic exposure control, the tube current can be modulated based on patient size and anatomic shape, with higher radiation used for larger patients and thicker body parts. The patient size can be determined based on visual inspection, BMI, width of the topogram, or noise measurement from a cross-sectional prescan. Online tube current modulation during the scan is performed based on the thickness of the body part along the path of the x-ray as measured by the tomogram. The tube current is reduced for body projections where the body part is thin and increased where the body part is thick. This technique can reduce radiation dose by 20% without increasing noise in thoracic CT.

Longitudinal Tube Current Modulation

In this technique, the tube current is automatically modulated along the z-axis, depending on the body part. For example, the chest contains air, which has poor attenuation, whereas the pelvis has bone and soft tissue, which has strong attenuation. Several scanners have automatic algorithms that depend on attenuation values obtained from the topogram to vary the tube current to achieve uniform noise throughout the body.

Angular Tube Current Modulation

The tube current is modulated during the rotation of the tube around the body to achieve uniform image quality. For example, the shoulder attenuates more photons in the lateral direction than in the anteroposterior direction. Hence, less tube current can be applied in the anteroposterior direction than in the lateral direction to achieve uniform image noise in all directions. This is achieved by using real-time online projection data lagging 180 degrees from the x-ray generation angle (Siemens); or based on the last topographic image (GE) and modulating the tube current in each of the four projection ranges; or selecting a noise index level to approximate the noise, which is equal to the standard deviation in the central region of the image when a uniform phantom is scanned and reconstructed using a standard reconstruction algorithm (GE).

Combined Tube Current Modulation

This is a combination of longitudinal and angular techniques. Using these various tube modulation techniques, doses can be reduced, especially to organs like the breasts. The noise level can also be controlled depending on the comfort level of the radiologists. For example, for an abdominal scan in an obese patient, a higher noise level may be acceptable. For children and small patients, a lower noise level (i.e., higher mAs) is preferred. The dose reduction is higher in small patients, and this technique may result in higher radiation exposure for larger patients.

Electrocardiogram-Based Tube Current Modulation in a Retrospective Gated Scan

This technique is used in cardiovascular acquisitions to reduce radiation dose. Retrospective electrocardiogram (ECG) gated helical acquisitions are associated with high radiation dose because the scanner is on for the entire cardiac cycle and generally not preferred. However, they are used if the heart rate is high and irregular or if functional information is required. In such circumstances, the radiation dose can be minimized by modulating the tube current along the R-R interval so that the maximum tube current is delivered in only one or two phases of the cardiac cycle, and for the rest of the time, the tube current is ramped down to 20% to 25% of the peak tube current. This technique can reduce radiation dose up to 50%. Images with lower radiation have higher noise levels but are still diagnostic. This technique also requires a regular and low heart rate, because the tube current modulation may not work at irregular heart rates.

Prospective Gated Electrocardiogram Triggering

Prospective ECG-triggered axial acquisition reduces radiation dose by as much as 68%. In this technique, data acquisition is triggered based on the R-wave and is acquired only in one phase of the cardiac cycle R-R interval. This should be the default mode of acquisition of cardiovascular CT due to the low radiation dose. However, this requires a steady and slow heart rate, and hence beta blockers are necessary to decrease the heart rate. Another disadvantage of this technique is that if there is an ectopic beat or if the heart rate goes up during the scan and an artifact appears in the image, the scan has to be repeated because data from other cardiac phases are not available. Functional information cannot be obtained.

Prospective High-Pitch Helical Mode

Prospective high-pitch helical mode is available in select scanners, especially the latest generation of dual-source scanners. A pitch of 3.4 can be used, and the gaps in image

data that are expected with a high-pitch scan can be filled by data from the second tube. This reduces the radiation dose and allows acquisition of images with prospective triggering in shorter acquisition time.

Non-Electrocardiogram Gated Acquisitions

Although most of the cardiac scans are performed using ECG gating, occasionally the scans can be performed without ECG gating to minimize radiation dose. A few such examples include CT for evaluation of pulmonary veins and evaluation of thoracic endovascular stent graft repair. Motion artifacts are rare in these parts of the anatomy.

Reducing Tube Voltage

Tube potential is the voltage across the x-ray tube, which determines both the energy and intensity of the x-ray beam. The number of photons is proportional to the square of the kVp, and hence reducing the kVp has a significant effect on radiation dose reduction. The lowest possible kVp should be used to minimize radiation dose. Reducing the kVp from 140 to 120, 100, and 80 kVp reduces the dose by a factor of 2.1, 3.3, and 5.1 times, respectively, because lower energy means there is lower penetration. The kVp can be preset based on BMI values, with 100 kVp used for a BMI less than 30, and 120 kVp for a BMI greater than 30 for most applications. A setting of 80 kVp can be used in children and small patients and 140 kVp reserved only for obese patients or in the presence of metal such as a stent or extensive calcium. In addition, at low kVp, there is higher attenuation of the x-ray beam and hence improved image contrast, particularly from within the vasculature. Hence for vascular studies, it is advantageous to use a low kVp. In addition, low doses of contrast can be used. Although with low kVp the mAs automatically increases if ATCM is used, the overall dose is still decreased. The noise increases by up to 26% with the use of the low kVp technique.

Pitch

Pitch is the ratio of the table movement to the detector width per gantry rotation of helical acquisition. Pitch values of less than 1 indicate overlapping acquisitions that are typically used in cardiovascular studies, whereas pitch values greater than 1 are associated with gaps between acquisitions. There is an inverse relationship between pitch and radiation dose. The highest possible pitch for obtaining the image should be used. As mentioned earlier, using the latest dual source scanner in high-pitch helical mode, a lower radiation dose can be achieved. Pitch does not affect the noise, but affects the z-axis spatial resolution depending on the type of reconstruction algorithm.

Reconstructed Slice Thickness

Reconstructed slice thickness does not directly affect radiation dose, but it does indirectly. This determines how many photons contribute to the final image. If thicker slices are used, the noise is lower, which means that lower tube potential or tube current can be used, although this comes at the expense of spatial resolution. If thinner slices are used, the noise is higher, which requires higher tube potential and tube current although the spatial resolution is higher with thinner slices. Hence, protocols should have the maximum reconstructed slice thickness that will provide clinical information.

Reconstruction Field of View

The reconstruction FOV is the area that is used to reconstruct the image. This typically does not affect the radiation dose. As mentioned earlier, the acquisition FOV is generally smaller than the gantry size. The area to be scanned should be located within this area to obtain good images.

Postprocessing Filters

After the scan is acquired, several postprocessing filters can be used to reduce radiation dose. Most of these filters reduce the noise in the image, which means that low-dose protocols can be used. Adaptive nonlinear filters reduce noise by analyzing the entire image and removing random noise but preserving edge sharpness based on the local pixel orientation. This allows the radiation dose to be lowered by up to 80% (De Geer). For evaluation of liver lesions, these filters have shown 30% radiation dose reduction without affecting image quality.

Iterative Reconstruction Algorithms

Filtered back projection (FBP) used to be the most commonly used type of image reconstruction algorithm. Currently, there are several different iterative reconstruction algorithms available; these are statistical methods that predict the projection data based on an assumption about the initial attenuation coefficients of all the voxels. The measured data are then compared to the projected data, and the attenuation values are modified until an acceptable level of error is achieved between the predicted and measured data. These methods can be image or projection based and have different names based on the vendor. The iterative techniques are useful in reducing the noise in the image. This can be used to adapt low-dose techniques (low mAs, low kVp) because iterative reconstruction can remove noise or use the same radiation dose but obtain improved image quality and spatial resolution.

Establishing a Radiation Dose Program

A robust program to optimize radiation dose should be established in every hospital, with involvement of all the parties, particularly the physicians, surgeons, radiologists, physicists, and technologists. The clinical indications and appropriateness should be clearly established. The imaging protocols should be optimized and updated every year. There should be continuous monitoring of radiation doses and comparison with established acceptable radiation dose, for example the ACR Registry. Any scans with abnormal radiation doses should be reviewed and corrective actions taken.

Reducing Radiation Dose From Radiographs

Radiographs are often used in emergency rooms. The ALARA principle should be used for radiographs as well.

Radiographs should be ordered only when it is clinically appropriate and the use of radiographs is justified. The minimal views required for making a diagnosis and the optimal tube current and tube voltage required for the study should be used. Automatic exposure control is used to set the optimal exposure factors to obtain good quality images.

SUGGESTED READINGS

Agency for Healthcare Research and Quality. *Hospital Survey on Patient Safety Culture.* Available at <http://www.ahrq.gov/professionals/quality-patient-safety/patientsafetyculture/hospital/index.html>.
Agency for Healthcare Research and Quality. *Improving Patient Safety Systems for Patients With Limited English Proficiency: Executive Summary.* Available at <http://www.ahrq.gov/professionals/systems/hospital/lepguide/lepguide-summ.html>.
American Board of Radiology. *Non-Interpretive Skills Resource Guide.* <http://www.theabr.org/sites/all/themes/abr-media/pdf/Noninterpretive_Skills_Domain_Specification_and_Resource_Guide.pdf>.
American College of Radiology. *Best Practice Guidelines on Imaging Clinical Decision Support Systems.* Available at <http://www.acr.org/~/media/ACR/Documents/PDF/Economics/Managed%20Care/Best%20Practices%20Guidelines%20for%20Imaging%20Clinical%20Decision%20Support%20Systems1.pdf>.
American College of Radiology. *ACR Practice Parameter for Communication of Diagnostic Imaging Findings.* Available at <http://www.acr.org/%7E/media/C5D1443C9EA4424AA12477D1AD1D927D.pdf>.
American College of Radiology. *ACR-SIR-SPR Practice Parameter on Informed Consent for Image-Guided Procedures.* <http://www.acr.org/~/media/ACR/Documents/PGTS/guidelines/Informed_Consent_Image_Guide.pdf>.
American Institute of Ultrasound in Medicine (AIUM). American College of Radiology (ACR), American College of Obstetricians and Gynecologists (ACOG), Society for Pediatric Radiology (SPR), Society of Radiologists in Ultrasound (SRU). AIUM practice guideline for the performance of ultrasound of the female pelvis. *J Ultrasound Med.* 2014;33(6):1122–1130.
Ashman CJ, Yu JS, Wolfman D. Satisfaction of search in osteo-radiology. *Am J Roentgenol.* 2000;175:541–544.
Baber JA, Davies SC, Dayan LS. An extra pair of eyes: do patients want a chaperone when having an anogenital examination? *Sex Health.* 2007;4(2):89–93.
Bagg SA, Steenburg SD, Ravenel JG. Handling of outside trauma studies: a survey of program directors. *J Am Coll Radiol.* 2008;5:657–663.
Balint BJ, Steenburg SD, Lin H, et al. Do telephone call interruptinos have an impact on radiology resident diagnostic accuracy? *Acad Radiol.* 2014;21(12):1623–1628.
Bautista AB, Burgos A, Nickel BJ, et al. Do clinicians use the American College of Radiology Appropriateness Criteria in the management of their patients? *Am J Roentgenol.* 2009;192:1581–1585.
Bechtold RE, Chen MYM, Ott DJ, et al. Interpretation of abdominal CT: analysis of errors and their causes. *J Comput Assist Tomogr.* 1997;21:681–685.
Beinfeld MT, Gazelle GS. Diagnostic imaging costs: are they driving up the costs of hospital care? *Radiology.* 2005;235:934–939.
Berbaum KS, Franken Jr EA, Dorfman DD, et al. Satisfaction of search in diagnostic radiology. *Invest Radiol.* 1990 Feb;25(2):133–140.
Berbaum KS, Franken Jr EA, Dorfman DD, et al. Time course of satisfaction of search. *Invest Radiol.* 1991;26:640–648.
Berlin L. Curbstone consultations. *Am J Roentgenol.* 2011;197.W191.
Berlin L. Liability of interpreting too many radiographs. *Am J Roentgenol.* 2000;175:17–22.
Berlin LM. Failure of radiologic communication: an increasing cause of malpractice litigation and harm to patients. *Appl Radiol.* 2010;39(1–2):17–23.
Bischoff B, Hein F, Meyer T, et al. Impact of a reduced tube voltage on CT angiography and radiation dose. Results of the PROTECTION I study. *JACC Cardiovasc Imaging.* 2009;2:940–946.
Blackmore CC, Mecklenburg RS, Kaplan GS. Effectiveness of clinical decision support in controlling inappropriate imaging. *J Am Coll Radiol.* 2011;8(1):19–25.
Boland GW, Duszak R. Imaging appropriateness and implementation of clinical decision support. *J Am Coll Radiol.* 2015;12(6):601–603.
Boland GWL, Duszak R, Dreyer K. Appropriateness and patient preparation. *J Am Coll Radiol.* 2014;11:225–226.
Brenner DJ, Hall EJ. Computed tomography: an increasing source of radiation exposure. *N Engl J Med.* 2007;357(22):2277–2284.
Burwell SM. Setting value-based payment goals—HHS efforts to improve U.S. health care. *N Engl J Med.* 2015;372(10):897–899.
Cabarrus M, Naeger DM, Rybkin A, Qayyum A. Patients prefer results from the ordering provider and access to their radiology reports. *J Am Coll Radiol.* 2015;12:556–562.
Cannavale A, Santoni M, Mancarella P, Passariello R, Arbarello P. Malpractice in radiology: what should you worry about? *Radiol Res Pract.* 2013;2013:219–259.
Carucci LR. Imaging obese patients: problems and solutions. *Abdom Imaging.* 2013;38(4):630–646.
Centers for Disease Control and Prevention. *Adult Obesity Facts.* <www.cdc.gov/obesity/data/adult.html>.

Chae EJ, Song JW, Seo JB, Krauss B, Jang YM, Song KS. Clinical utility of dual-energy CT in the evaluation of solitary pulmonary nodules. Initial experience. *Radiology.* 249;671-681.

Chandarana H, Godoy MC, Vlahos I, et al. Abdominal aorta: evaluation with dual-source dual-energy multidetector CT after endovascular repair of aneurysms: initial observations. *Radiology.* 249;692-700.

Chandy J, Goodfellow T, Vohrah A. Clinical governance in action: radiology. *Hosp Med.* 2000;61:326-329.

Chen LE, Bhargava P. The two-minute radiologist. *Curr Probl Diagn Radiol.* 2016;45(2):149-150.

Cooper VF, Goodhartz LA, Nemcek AA, Ryu RK. Radiology resident interpretations of on-call imaging studies: the incidence of major discrepancies. *Acad Radiol.* 2008;15:1198-1204.

Cotton VR. Legal risks of "curbside" consults. *Am J Cardiol.* 2010;106:135-138.

Davenport MS, Brimm D, Rubin JM, Kazerooni EA. Patient preferences for chaperone use during transvaginal sonography. *Abdom Radiol (NY).* 2016;41(2):324-333.

De Geer J, Sandborg M, Smedby O, Persson A. The efficacy of 2D, nonlinear noise reduction filter in cardiac imaging: a pilot study. *Acta Radiol.* 2011;52:716-722.

Deak PD, Langner O, Lell M, Kalender WA. Effects of adaptive section collimation on patient radiation dose in multisection spiral CT. *Radiology.* 2009;252:140-147.

Diamond LC, Schenker Y, Curry L, Bradley EH, Fernandez A. Getting by: underuse of interpreters by resident physicians. *J Gen Intern Med.* 2009;24(2):256-262.

Divi C, Koss RG, Schmaltz SP, Loeb JM. Language proficiency and adverse events in U.S. hospitals: a pilot study. *Int J Qual Health Care.* 2007;19(2):60-67.

Duong PA, Pastel DA, Sadigh G, et al. The value of imaging part II: value beyond image interpretation. *Acad Radiol.* 2016;23:23-29.

Eakins C, Ellis WD, Pruthi S, et al. Second opinion interpretations by specialty radiologists at a pediatric hospital: rate of disagreement and clinical implications. *Am J Roentgenol.* 2012;199:916-920.

Ellenbogen PH. Imaging 3.0: what is it? *J Am Coll Radiol.* 2013;10:229.

European Society of Radiology. *Risk Management in Radiology in Europe.* Available at <http://www.myesr.org/sites/default/files/ESR_brochure_04_2.pdf>.

Fitzgerald R. Error in radiology. *Clin Radiol.* 2001;56:938-946.

Flores G, Rabke-Verani J, Pine W, Sabharwal A. The importance of cultural and linguistic issues in the emergency care of children. *Pediatr Emerg Care.* 2002;18(4):271-284.

Fricke BL, Donnelly LF, Frush DP, et al. In-plane bismuth breast shields for pediatric CT: effects on radiation dose and image quality using experimental and clinical data. *Am J Roentgenol.* 2003;180:407-411.

Ginde AA, Foianini A, Renner DM, Valley M, Camargo Jr CA. The challenge of CT and MRI imaging of obese individuals who present to the emergency department: a national survey. *Obesity (Silver Spring).* 2008;16(11):2549-2551.

Goh KY, Tsang KY, Poon WS. Does teleradiology improve inter-hospital management of head-injury? *Can J Neurol Sci.* 1997;24:235-239.

Golub RM. Curbside consultations and the viaduct effect. *JAMA.* 1998;280:929-930.

Gore RM, Miller FH, Pereles FS, Yagmai V, Berlin JW. Helical CT in the evaluation of the acute abdomen. *Am J Roentgenol.* 2000;174:901-913.

Graser A, Johnson TR, Hecht EM, et al. Dual-energy CT in patients suspected of having renal masses: can virtual non enhanced images replace the non-enhanced images? *Radiology.* 2009;252(2):433-440.

Grogan MJ, Marn C. My PQI project—medical legal issues with outside trauma studies: are you opening yourself up to liability? *J Am Coll Radiol.* 2011;8:528-529.

Gunn MLD, Kohr JR. State of the art: technologies for computed tomography dose reduction. *Emerg Radiol.* 2010;17:209-218.

Gupta A, Ip IK, Raja AS, et al. Effect of clinical decision support on documented guideline adherence for head CT in emergency department patients with mild traumatic brain injury. *J Am Med Inform Assoc.* 2014;21:e347-e351.

Hall J, Roter DL, Rand CS. Communication of affect between patient and physician. *J Health Soc Behav.* 1981;22:18-30.

Hopper KD, King SH, Lobell ME, TenHave TR, Weaver JS. The breast: in plane x-ray protection during diagnostic thoracic CT: shielding with bismuth radioprotective garments. *Radiology.* 1997;205:853-858.

Huber T, Gaskin C, Krishnaraj A. Early experience with implementation of a commercial decision support product for imaging order entry. *Curr Probl Diagn Radiol.* 2016;45(2):133-136.

Ip IK, Gershanik EF, Schneider LI, et al. Impact of IT-enabled intervention on MRI use for back pain. *Am J Med.* 2014;127:512-518. e1.

Jakobs TF, Becker CR, Ohnesorge B, et al. Multislice helical CT of the heart with retrospective ECG gating. Reduction of radiation exposure by ECG-controlled tube current modulation. *Eur Radiol.* 2002;12:1081-1086.

Jena AB, Seabury S, Lakdawalla D, Chandra A. Malpractice risk according to physician specialty. *N Engl J Med.* 2011;365(7):629-636.

Kallen JA, Coughlin BF, O'Loughlin MT, Stein B. Reduced z-axis coverage multidetector CT angiography for suspected pulmonary embolism could decrease dose and maintain diagnostic accuracy. *Emerg Radiol.* 2009;17:31-35.

Katz DS, Jorgensen MJ, Rubin GD. Detection and follow up of important extra-arterial lesions with helical CT angiography. *Clin Radiol.* 1999;54:294-300.

Keen CE. The clinical decision-support mandate: now what? *Radiol Bus J.* Available at <http://www.radiologybusiness.com/topics/policy/clinical-decision-support-mandate-now-what?nopaging=1>.

Khorasani R. What you should know about handling digital studies generated outside your practice. *J Am Coll Radiol.* 2006;3:954-955.

Kirkpatrick AW, Brenneman FD, McCallum A, Breeck K, Boulanger BR. Prospective evaluation of the potential role of teleradiology in acute interhospital trauma referrals. *J Trauma.* 1999;46:1017-1023.

Kreichelt R, Hilbert ML, Shinn D. Minimizing the legal risk with "curbside" consultation. *J Healthc Risk Manag.* 2008;28:27-29.

Kuhlman M, Meyer M, Krunpinski EA. Direct reporting of results to patients: the future of radiology? *Acad Radiol.* 2012;19(6):646-650.

Leape LL, Shore MF, Dienstag JL, et al. Perspective: a culture of respect, part 1: the nature and causes of disrespectful behavior by physicians. *Acad Med.* 2012;87(7):845-852.

Linda K, Janet C, Molla D, eds. *To Err Is Human: Building a Safer Health System.* Washington, DC: Committee on Quality of Health Care in America, Institute of Medicine, National Academy Press; 2000.

Mahoney E, Agarwal S, Li B, et al. Evidence-based guidelines are equivalent to a liberal computed tomography scan protocol for initial patient evaluation but are associated with decreased computed tomography scan use, cost, and radiation exposure. *J Trauma Acute Care Surg.* 2012;73(3):573-578.

Martinsen AC, Saether HK, Olsen DR, Skaane P, Olerud HM. Reduction in dose from CT examinations of liver lesions with new post processing filter: a ROC phantom study. *Acta Radiol.* 2008;49:303-309.

McCollough CH, Primak AN, Braun N, et al. Strategies for reducing radiation dose in CT. *Radiol Clin North Am.* 2009;47(1):27-40.

McGrath AL, Bhargava P. The charismatic radiologist. *J Am Coll Radiol.* 2015;12(11):1234-1236.

McNeeley MF, Martin ML, Robinson JD. Transfer patient imaging: current status, review of the literature, and the Harborview experience. *J Am Coll Radiol.* 2013;10:361-367.

Miller RA. Medical diagnostic decisions support systems—past, present, and future: a threaded bibliography and brief commentary. *J Med Inform Assoc.* 1994;1(1):8-27.

Modica MJ, Kanal KM, Gunn ML. The obese emergency patient: imaging challenges and solutions. *Radiographics.* 2011;31:811-823.

Mossanen M, Johnson SS, Green J, Joyner BD. A practical approach to conflict management for program directors. *J Grad Med Educ.* 2014;6(2):345-346.

Mulkens TH, Bellinck P, Baeyeart M, et al. Use of an automatic exposure control mechanism for dose optimization in multi-detector row CT examinations: clinical evaluation. *Radiology.* 2005;237:213-223.

Niemann T, Kollmann T, Bngartz G. Diagnostic performance of low-dose CT for the detection of urolithiasis: a metanalysis. *Am J Roentgenol.* 2008;191:396-401.

Oestmann JW, Green R, Kushner DC, Bourgouin PM, Linetsky L, Llewellyn HJ. Lung lesions: correlation between viewing time and detection. *Radiology.* 1988;166:451-453.

Ogden CL, Carroll MD, Kit BK, Flegal KM. Prevalence of childhood and adult obesity in the United States, 2011-2012. *JAMA.* 2014;311(8):806-814.

Paladini D. Sonography in obese and overweight pregnant women: clinical, medico-legal and technical issues. *Ultrasound Obstet Gynecol.* 2009;33:720-729.

Patil S, Davies P. Use of Google Translate in medical communication: evaluation of accuracy. *BMJ.* 2014;349:g7392.

Perry DJ, Kwan SW, Bhargava P. Patient-centered clinical training in radiology. *J Am Coll Radiol.* 2015;12:724-727.

Physician Insurers Association of America. *Claim Trend Analysis Study.* Rockville, MD: Physician Insurers Association of America; 2004.

Pinto A, Brunese L. Spectrum of diagnostic errors in radiology. *World J Radiol.* 2010;2(10):377-383.

Pitts SR, Niska RW, Xu J, Burt CW. National Hospital Ambulatory Medical Care Survey: 2006 emergency department summary. *Natl Health Stat Rep.* 2006;7:1-38.

Platon A, Jlassi H, Rutschmann OT, et al. Evaluation of low-dose CT protocol with oral contrast for assessment of acute appendicitis. *Eur Radiol.* 2009;19:446-454.

Psoter KJ, Roudsari BS, Vaughn M, Fine GC, Jarvik JG, Gunn ML. Effect of an image-sharing network on CT utilization for transferred trauma patients: a 5-year experience at a level I trauma center. *J Am Coll Radiol.* 2014;11(6):616-622.

Ptak K, Rhea JT, Novelline RA. Radiation dose is reduced with a single-pass whole-body multi-detector row CT trauma protocol compared with conventional segmented method: initial experience. *Radiology.* 229:902-905.

Rajiah P, Halliburton SS, Flamm SD. Strategies for dose reduction in cardiovascular computed tomography. *Appl Radiol.* 2012:10-15.

Reis SP, Lefkovitz Z, Kaur S, Seiler M. Interpretation of outside imaging studies: solutions from a tertiary care trauma center. *J Am Coll Radiol.* 2012;9:591-594.

Renfrew DL, Franken EA, Berbaum KS, Weigelt FH, Abu-Yousef MM. Error in radiology: classification and lessons in 182 cases presented at a problem case conference. *Radiology.* 1992;183:145-150.

Robinson PJA, Wilson D, Coral A, Murphy A, Verow P. Variation between experienced observers in the interpretation of accident and emergency radiographs. *Br J Radiol.* 1999;72:323-330.

Royal College of Radiologists. *Intimate Examinations and the Use of Chaperones.* Available at <https://www.rcr.ac.uk/sites/default/files/bfcr154_intimateexams.pdf>.

Royal College of Radiologists. *Workload and Manpower in Clinical Radiology.* London: The Royal College of Radiologists; 1999.

Sadigh G, Loehfelm T, Applegate KE, et al. Journal Club: Evaluation of near-miss wrong-patient events in radiology reports. *AJR Am J Roentgenol.* 2015;205(2):337-343.

Schindera ST, Nelson RC, Yoshizumi T, et al. Effect of automatic tube current modulation on radiation dose and image quality for low tube voltage multidetector row CT angiography: phantom study. *Acad Radiol.* 2009;16:997-1002.

Scott J. Utilizing AIDET and other tools to increase patient satisfaction scores. *Radiol Manage.* 2012;34:29-33.

Sectra. *How Radiology Can Improve Communication With Referring Physicians.* Available at <https://sectra.com/medical/press/pdf/Report%202013%20How%20radiology%20can%20improve%20communication%20with%20referring%20physicians_%20.pdf>.

Sipe CY, West RW. Risks associated with outside radiographs. *J Am Coll Radiol.* 2005;2:859-861.

Sistrom CL, Dang PA, Weilburg JB, Dreyer KJ, Rosenthal DI, Thrall JH. Effect of computerized order entry with integrated decision support on the growth of outpatient procedure volumes: seven-year time series analysis. *Radiology.* 2009;251:147-155.

Smart DR. *Physician Characteristics and Distribution in the US.* Chicago, IL:American Medical Association; 2010;30-31, 97-149.

Sodickson A, Baeyens PF, Andriole KP, et al. Recurrent CT, cumulative radiation exposure, and associated radiation-induced cancer risks from CT of adults. *Radiology.* 2009;251:175-184.

Sodickson A, Opraseuth J, Ledbetter S. Outside imaging in emergency department transfer patients: CD import reduces rates of subsequent imaging utilization. *Radiology.* 2011;260:408-413.

Srinivasa BA, Brooks ML. The malpractice liability of radiology reports: minimizing the risk. *Radiographics.* 2015;35(2):547-554.

Stevens KJ, Griffiths KL, Rosenberg J, Mahadevan S, Zatz LM, Leung AN. Discordance rates between preliminary and final radiology reports on cross-sectional imaging studies at a level 1 trauma center. *Acad Radiol.* 2008;15:1217-1226.

Sung JC, Sodickson A, Ledbetter S. Outside CT imaging among emergency department transfer patients. *J Am Coll Radiol.* 2009;6:626-632.

Teague R, Newton D, Fairley CK, et al. The differing views of male and female patients toward chaperones for genital examinations in a sexual health setting. *Sex Transm Dis.* 2007;34(12):1004.

Thrall JC. Appropriateness and imaging utilization: computerized provider order entry and decision support. *Acad Radiol.* 2014;21:1083-1087.

Uppot RN. Impact of obesity on radiology. *Radiol Clin North Am.* 2007;45(2):231-246.

van Hecke O, Jones KM. The attitudes and practices of general practitioners about the use of chaperones in Melbourne, Australia. *Int J Family Med.* 2012;2012(466):1-6.

van Ooijen PM, Guignot J, Mevel G, Oudkerk M. Incorporating outpatient data from CD-R into the local PACS using DICOM worklist features. *J Digit Imaging.* 2005;18:196-202.

Vollmar SV, Kalendar WA. Reduction of dose to the female breast in thoracic CT: a comparison of standard-protocol, bismuth-shielded, partial and tube-current modulated CT examinations. *Eur Radiol.* 2008;18:1674-1682.

Wakeley CJ, Jones AM, Kabala JE, Prince D, Goddard PR. Audit of the value of double reading magnetic resonance imaging films. *Br J Radiol.* 1995;68:353-360.

Walker ST, Goodenberger MH, Devries MJ. On-call resident outside study overreads: our department's experience streamlining workflow and improving resident supervision while providing a new source of revenue. *Curr Probl Diagn Radiol.* 2015;44:118-121.

Whang JS, Baker SR, Patel R, Luk L, Castro 3rd A. The causes of medical malpractice suits against radiologists in the United States. *Radiology.* 2013;266(2):548-554.

Wijetunga R, Tan BS, Rouse JC, et al. Diagnostic accuracy of focused appendiceal CT in clinically equivocal cases of acute appendicitis. *Radiology.* 2001;221:747-753.

Yousem DM. Establishing an outside film reading service/dealing with turf issues: unintended consequences. *J Am Coll Radiol.* 2010;7:480-481.

Zafar HM, Mills AM, Khorasani R, Langlotz CP. Clinical decision support for imaging in the era of the Patient Protection and Affordable Care Act. *J Am Coll Radiol.* 2012;9(12):907-918.

SECTION IV
Special Topics

Chapter 27
Malpractice and Radiology: A Hapless Relationship

Leonard Berlin

PROLOGUE

To gain a more meaningful understanding of the current state of affairs with regard to medical malpractice litigation in the United States, we begin by looking back at certain events that have brought us to the present.

England, 1765

British legal scholar Sir William Blackstone published *Commentaries on the Laws of England*, in which "neglect or unskillful management of a physician or surgeon" was referred to as "mala praxis." It is from this term that the modern word "malpractice" is derived.

Connecticut, 1832

A state supreme court establishes the Standard of Care (SOC) for a physician: "A physician and surgeon is liable for injuries resulting from the want of ordinary diligence, care, and skill.… Ordinary means usual, common. If you were to draw a line of distinction just halfway between the eminently learned physicians and those grossly ignorant, you would hit exactly on those who are ordinary."

Pennsylvania, 1853

A state supreme court added the following: "The law requires physicians to possess reasonable skill and diligence… not extraordinary skill such as belongs only to few men of rare genius and endowments."

Colorado, 1896

One year after Roentgen's discovery of the x-ray, an x-ray image showing a bone fracture was offered as legal evidence for the first time in an American court. Disagreeing with a lawyer's arguing against admitting the x-ray, the judge stated: "We have been presented with a photograph showing a femur bone which is surrounded with tissues and therefore is hidden…. Modern science has made it possible to look beneath the tissues of the human body and has aided in telling hidden mysteries. The photograph will be admitted in evidence."

United States: First Half of the 20th Century

In the decades prior to the end of World War I, most malpractice cases focusing on radiology involved alleged x-ray and radium burns. For the entire first half of the 20th century, most malpractice lawsuits filed against all physicians focused on errors of *commission*: that is, the doctor did something wrong.

United States: Second Half of the 20th Century

Beginning in the early 1950s, allegations of malpractice evolved from errors of *commission* to errors of *omission;* that is, the doctor failed to do something right: they failed to make a timely diagnosis. In the last 3 decades of the 20th century, allegations of malpractice against radiologists focused mainly on failure to diagnose; that is, the radiologist missed an abnormality on the radiographic images. By the mid-1980s, missed lung and breast cancers became the most frequent reason radiologists were sued for malpractice.

United States: The Present

Of all radiology medical malpractice lawsuits, 57% to 67% are diagnosis related. Failure to diagnose accounts for most of these. Only 2% of all patients sustaining adverse events file malpractice lawsuits.

HOW OFTEN ARE RADIOLOGISTS SUED FOR MALPRACTICE?

A recent review of malpractice records of more than 8400 radiologists found that 50% of radiologists would be sued by age 60. A later survey disclosed that 75% of radiologists were sued for malpractice at least once in their lifetime. A recent report focusing on all medical malpractice cases reported to the National Practitioner Data Bank between 2005 and 2014 revealed that internists accounted for 15% of all cases; obstetrician-gynecologists, 13%; general surgeons, 12%; orthopedic surgeons, 7%; and radiologists, 6%. Other studies have disclosed that the number of malpractice lawsuits filed in the United States has decreased 10% to 15% over the past several years, but payment per case has increased (Medical Protective Insurance Company unpublished report).

Radiologic Errors

Causes of error in radiology are multifactorial: poor technique, failure of perception, lack of knowledge, poor judgment. Numerous research studies reported over the past 60 years have disclosed an average 30% "miss rate" in the retrospective evaluation of general radiographic, computed tomography (CT), magnetic resonance, and ultrasound examinations. This means that if 100 radiologic examinations containing abnormal findings are given blindly to radiologists, an average of 30% of the abnormalities will be missed. Such studies, however, do not reflect the everyday practice of radiology, where the number of normal examinations far exceeds those that are abnormal. Various studies and performance improvement data derived from radiologists' interpretations under ordinary working conditions of both normal and abnormal radiologic studies disclose an average error rate of 3% to 4%. Fortunately, most of these errors are not injurious to the patient or are corrected by review of radiologic studies before they become injurious.

Seventy percent of missed radiologic diagnoses are perceptual in nature; that is, the radiologist fails to "see" the abnormality. The remaining 30% are cognitive errors; that is, the radiologist "sees" an abnormality but attaches the wrong significance to what is seen, either through lack of knowledge or lack of judgment. Diagnostic errors are also caused by the phenomenon known as "satisfaction of search"; that is, an imaging study may contain several abnormalities. The radiologist notes one or perhaps two abnormalities but then tends to "stop looking" for additional abnormalities; his or her "search" has been "satisfied" prematurely. Another cause of errors is the "alliterative" error, also termed "diagnosis momentum." Here, the radiologist looks at a previous study and previous report rendered by the same or another radiologist before interpreting the new follow-up study, and if the previous diagnosis was erroneous, the radiologist interpreting the new study has a tendency to repeat the same error.

Errors Versus Differences of Opinion

Variations in diagnosis are thought to imply the presence of error, but this is not always the case. Variation may reflect error but can be a genuine difference of opinion. Variability can occur as inconsistencies in practice by the same radiologist on different occasions or discrepancy between radiologists. Radiology researchers have found that experienced radiologists miss 30% of radiographs positive for evidence of disease and, furthermore, will disagree with themselves 20% of the time. A study by Harvard University radiologists disclosed that radiologists disagree on interpretation of chest radiographs as much as 56% of the time. Another academic study disclosed that up to 90% of all lung carcinomas were missed by radiologists when interpreting radiographs. A University of Arizona study found that in 75% of mammograms initially interpreted as normal, breast carcinomas were seen on retrospective evaluation.

The main reason for studying medical errors is to try to prevent many, if not most, of them. Physicians feel a sense of guilt as a result of making an error and may fear suffering professional and economic consequences and being isolated by their colleagues. Unfortunately, a friendly and confidential reporting culture does not exist in medicine. The current "blame culture" in healthcare inhibits error reporting. To lower the miss rate, we need to develop a safety culture so that we can bring errors to our colleagues' attention in a sensitive and constructive fashion. Such a culture will exist only when radiologists who make errors use such feedback positively as a learning experience and know that punitive action will not be taken against them.

Unfortunately, errors of perception are an unavoidable hazard of the human condition. Although technology has made enormous progress in the last century, there is no evidence of similar improvement in the performance of the human eye and brain.

Radiology diverges from the normal path of most other medical specialties in that it depends entirely on visual perception. However, lest nonradiologic physicians believe that radiologists' error rates are considerably higher than their own; in fact, studies that date back as far as the 1950s reveal a 20% to 30% error rate in clinical medicine. For example, medical researchers have found clinicians to be unreliable in their assessment in 32% of physician examination skills. Accuracy in the physical diagnosis of abdominal ascites was as low as 56% among good clinicians. Pediatricians were 50% accurate in clinical diagnosis of acute otitis media; otolaryngologists were 73% accurate.

Autopsies revealed a major missed diagnosis 25% of the time; despite more modern diagnostic techniques, the number of missed major diagnoses has not changed over 30 years. A meta-analysis of 53 autopsy articles published over a 40-year period disclosed a major finding median error of 23.5%, with a range of 4% to 50%. "The error rate has been strikingly unchanged," emphasized the authors.

False-Positive Radiologic Findings

Although almost all radiologic diagnostic errors are false-negative errors, occasionally there are false-positive errors. A review of claims occurring in the United Kingdom between 1995 and 2006 disclosed that 7% were due to false-positive radiologic findings.

A very sad medical malpractice lawsuit from Massachusetts is an unfortunate illustration of a false-positive rather than a false-negative radiologic error. A 4-month-old infant was admitted to the hospital with symptoms of urinary tract infection and started on intravenous (IV) antibiotics. Although improving, a precautionary sonogram was done and showed a "lesion" in the upper pole of the right kidney, suspicious for Wilms tumor. A CT scan confirmed a positive right renal Wilms tumor. The patient was taken to surgery, during which the surgeon felt a subtle enlargement of the kidney and proceeded to perform a nephrectomy. Postsurgical study of the kidney revealed chronic pyelonephritis but no evidence of tumor. A malpractice lawsuit was filed and eventually settled for $500,000.

In the 70 years since radiologic errors were first acknowledged, the error rates have not decreased appreciably. This must not dissuade us from making every effort to reduce them, however. Yes, to do so is a daunting challenge, but radiologists cannot simply shrug their shoulders and walk away. Will computers help us decrease errors? A recently published study suggests that the answer is likely no. In a study comparing the results of 496,000 women whose screening mammograms were interpreted with the aid of computer-assisted detection (CAD) with 130,000 women whose mammograms were interpreted without CAD over a period from 2003 to 2009, no statistical difference in sensitivity and specificity was found. The researchers' conclusion was that CAD does not improve diagnostic accuracy in mammography interpretations.

It is highly unlikely that radiologists will ever be able to eliminate radiologic interpretive errors, but we can reduce them by adhering to the following suggestions:

- Possess sufficient knowledge of the modality by which the image being interpreted was obtained.
- Ensure prompt transmission of imaging reports to the ordering physician and possibly to the patients themselves.
- Expend sufficient time interpreting and reporting.
- Be cautious about voice recognition and templates.
- Proofread dictated reports.
- Because poor image quality increases the likelihood of missing an abnormality, insist that patient positioning and radiographic exposure be adequate before interpretation.
- Have available as much patient information as possible, along with previous radiologic examinations and reports for comparison, but take care not to be overinfluenced by this information.
- Considering all possible diagnostic possibilities is far preferable to making hasty conclusions.
- When interpreting studies that are follow-ups from previous studies, ask the following: "Could the findings represent anything different from the previously suggested diagnosis?"
- When asked by a referring physician, "What did you find on the radiologic examination of my patient?" instead of recalling what was diagnosed, if time permits a much better answer would be, "I interpreted the study as normal (or as showing specific pathology), but let's look at it again together" (if physician is present) or "let me look at it again" (if physician is not present). A second look by the radiologist with or without a referring physician or colleague can reveal a radiographic finding that was initially overlooked or misinterpreted.
- Occasionally the patient's physical condition or other circumstances may prevent technologists from obtaining all required views or using optimal exposure techniques. In such circumstances, state in the report that the examination was incomplete because of the patient's condition and that additional or follow-up views need to be obtained when the patient's condition permits.
- Consultation with radiology colleagues and referring physicians before rendering final reports is encouraged.
- Make recommendations for additional or follow-up studies when indicated.
- Making instant or rapid diagnoses may be acceptable goals in film-interpreting conferences at medical meetings, but doing so in everyday practice may cause radiologists to limit diagnostic possibilities and may increase the likelihood of error. Taking sufficient time during radiologic interpretation for deliberation and reflection is essential for good judgment.

- "If you don't think of it, you won't diagnose it" is a basic axiom in diagnostic radiology. Radiologists must constantly reinforce and expand their reservoir of radiology knowledge by reading current scientific publications and attending continuing medical education programs.

As we look toward the future, the major issue about which we should be concerned is electronic medical records (EMRs). Mistyped words, reversed numbers, inaccurate information, or other data entry mistakes are often "cut and pasted" repeatedly in the patient record; templates are often repeated even though minor imaging changes may occur. Every time an exam or image is reviewed on a monitor, it is accurately timed and permanently recorded; EMRs are anticipated to cause an increase in the number of medical malpractice lawsuits, although data are not yet available.

Proving Malpractice

To prevail in a medical malpractice lawsuit involving a defendant-radiologist, the plaintiff must prove that (1) the radiologist had a physician-patient relationship with the patient, (2) the radiologist committed a negligent act, (3) the negligent act caused an injury to the patient (proximate cause), and (4) the patient sustained injury directly from the defendant's alleged negligent conduct. In almost all cases, items 1, 3, and 4 are obvious and therefore rarely challenged. As for the physician-patient relationship, anytime the radiologist interprets a radiologic study on a patient, whether that interpretation is written and included in a formal medical record or was given by conversing with a referring physician who later, in his own chart, writes a notation of his conversation with the radiologist, a physician-patient relationship has been legally established. Thus, in almost all medical malpractice lawsuits, the single point to be debated and argued is whether the defendant acted in a negligent manner. How is the word *negligence* defined? What constitutes physician negligence? Let us go back to an 1860 medical malpractice lawsuit when physician negligence was argued for the first time before the Illinois State Supreme Court. In that case, a farmer named Richie sustained a fracture of the wrist and was treated by Dr. West, a general practitioner. Dr. West applied a plaster cast to the wrist, but for some inexplicable reason, Mr. Richie's wrist became permanently deformed. He sued Dr. West, alleging malpractice. Dr. West retained a Springfield, Illinois, attorney by the name of Abraham Lincoln. A trial was held, and a jury rendered a verdict in favor of Mr. Richie; Dr. West appealed the matter to the Illinois Supreme Court, which issued a decision affirming the jury verdict:

> *When a person assumes the profession of physician and surgeon, he must be held to employ a reasonable amount of skill and care. For anything short of that degree of skill, the law will hold him responsible for any injury which may result. While he is not required to possess the highest order of qualification, to which some men attain, still he must possess and exercise that degree of skill which is ordinarily possessed of the profession, and whether the injury results from a want of skill, or the want of its application, he will, in either case, be equally liable.*

At about the same time, the Georgia Supreme Court issued a similar opinion:

> *The physician must exercise a reasonable degree of care and skill. He does not undertake to use the highest possible degree of skill, for there may be persons who, for having enjoyed a better education and greater advantage, are possessed of greater skill in our profession; but he undertakes that he will bring a fair, reasonable and competent degree of skill.*

Over the next several decades, appellate or supreme court decisions in all American states rendered opinions using similar wording. In other words, the courts have stated that an accused physician's performance must be compared to a "standard" performance that does not need to be ideal, perfect, extraordinary, excellent, or match that of an expert witness. Rather, it is compared to a standard of performance that is *ordinary* and/or *reasonable*. Herein lies one of the basic problems that has always existed in medical malpractice litigation, namely, how the words *reasonable* and *ordinary* are defined. Defining the exact meaning of these two words might seem simple, but it is not. Webster's dictionary defines *reasonable* as "not extreme, not excessive, moderate, not demanding too much, possessing good sound judgment, well-balanced, sensible." The word *ordinary* is defined as "common, lacking in excellence, not distinguished in any way from others, not above but rather below average, somewhat inferior level of quality." Thus, clear-cut definitions of these two words unfortunately have never been spelled out by the courts. If radiologists, who are trained to precisely pinpoint radiologic abnormalities and render interpretations in specific terms, feel perplexed at the vagueness of the words *reasonable* and *ordinary*, they are not alone. More concrete definition of these words remains elusive. Some light was shed on the term *reasonable person* in a decision of a Canadian malpractice case:

> *The reasonable person is not an extraordinary or unusual creature; he is not superhuman; he is not required to display the highest skill of which anyone is capable; he is not a genius who can perform uncommon feats, nor is he possessed of unusual powers of foresight. He is a person of normal intelligence who makes prudence a guide for his conduct. He acts in accord with general and approved practice.*

Notwithstanding the words of the court, every juror and every jury in every medical malpractice lawsuit will have their own opinion regarding whether a defendant-radiologist acted reasonably under the circumstances described during a malpractice trial.

Defending the Missed Diagnosis

The question to be answered by a jury in a medical malpractice lawsuit involving a missed radiologic diagnosis is theoretically not "Has the radiologist missed an x-ray finding, or made an erroneous interpretation?" Rather, it should be "Has the radiologist missed an x-ray finding, or made an erroneous interpretation, which could have been missed, or made by an ordinary radiologist, practicing in a reasonable (average) manner?" There are several major issues that exacerbate a jury's difficulty in determining whether

a radiologist's conduct was negligent or not. One is *hindsight bias*, defined as "the tendency for people with knowledge of the actual outcome of any event, to believe falsely that they would have predicted the outcome." Researchers have repeatedly pointed out that the retrospective reader has new information regarding the clinical course and later x-ray findings showing advanced disease that were not available at the time of the original interpretation. This improves the ability to perceive subtle abnormalities that were not seen on the previous study. Perception is better if you know where to look. The courts do attempt to minimize the effect of hindsight bias. One typical instruction to a jury states:

> *I charge you that in a medical malpractice action, physicians cannot be found negligent for assessing a patient's condition which only later or in hindsight proved to be incorrect, as long as the initial assessment was made in accordance with the then-reasonable standards of medical care. The concept of negligence does not encompass hindsight.*

An Illinois Appellate Court decision included the words, "In hindsight, almost everything is foreseeable, but that is not the test we should employ."

One other inherent problem in medical malpractice litigation that especially involves radiology is *outcome bias,* which is defined as "[t]he tendency for people to attribute blame more readily when the outcome of an event is serious than when the outcome is comparatively minor." In other words, hypothetically, if a radiologist is accused of negligence for missing a rib fracture that can be plainly seen in retrospect, most jurors and others would conclude that there was no negligence, because the injury was so minimal. On the other hand, if a radiologist is accused of negligence for missing an extremely subtle fracture of the cervical spine that probably would be missed by well over 95% of radiologists, but the patient is now quadriplegic, most jurors and physicians would agree that the radiologist was negligent, because the injury, that is, the outcome, was so serious and debilitating.

It is very difficult, but certainly not impossible, to convince a jury that a radiologist who is well paid and is supposed to be well trained to find all abnormalities on a radiologic study should be excused for failing to perceive a radiologic abnormality that in retrospect can be readily perceived by medical and nonmedical observers alike. However, solid defense-supporting data are available that may at times be presented to a jury that can assist in achieving vindication for the defendant-radiologist. These data include statistics regarding the frequency of errors committed by radiologists and other physicians during the course of an ordinary everyday practice, the factors that limit conspicuity of radiographic densities, limitations of normal human visual perception, and evidence that the process by which the radiologist originally rendered the interpretation was free of deficiency.

Occasionally juries can be successfully educated by defense attorneys and expert witnesses as to psychovisual phenomena and other human limitations affecting the visual process, and radiologists are exonerated for failing to observe and report radiologic abnormalities. A good working relationship between the defendant-radiologist and the defense attorney increases the chances of achieving a satisfactory jury verdict.

also how many radiologic studies he read per hour and the amount of his income per hour of work paid to him by the company. In short, the plaintiff's argument was that reading too fast was the cause of the radiologist's error.

The defense experts countered that many radiologists would have missed the CT finding under myriad different conditions and that the speed of reading had nothing to do with the failed interpretation. The jury returned a defense verdict, but another jury hearing the same testimony could well have returned a plaintiff's verdict.

Although it is intuitive to believe that the faster radiologists read the more mistakes they will make, there are no hard data in the literature to substantiate this. There is no SOC that specifies how much time a radiologist should spend interpreting a radiologic study. There are fast readers, and there are slow readers. All radiologists must depend on their conscience to tell them how much time they should take to render an accurate radiologic interpretation. And they should not forget that picture archiving and communication systems do record the exact length of time radiologists have the images displayed on the computer screen and the exact length of time taken for their dictation.

MAMMOGRAPHY

As already mentioned, the leading cause of medical malpractice litigation involving radiologists is the allegation of missed or delayed diagnosis of breast cancer. A recently published survey of radiologists interpreting mammography showed that radiologists believe that the likelihood of getting sued for malpractice for misinterpretation of mammograms is 4 times the actual incidence of litigation. Nevertheless, radiologists must be especially vigilant in this area. Women's expectation of near perfection in the interpretation of mammography is high. Unfortunately, a delay in diagnosis of breast cancer as short as a period of 3 months, although perhaps not being clinically significant, can well result in substantial indemnification to the patient from a legal point of view.

Screening Versus Diagnostic Mammography: A Potential Pitfall

The distinction between screening mammography and diagnostic mammography is important. Performing a screening mammogram and interpreting it as normal, when instead a diagnostic mammogram was indicated because of the patient's history or physical findings, can lead to a malpractice lawsuit. A plaintiff's argument that had a diagnostic mammogram been done it would have shown evidence of a malignancy that was not apparent on a screening mammogram is likely to result in a verdict against the defendant-radiologist and/or radiology facility.

Notwithstanding various obligations imposed on the patient, referring physician, and the technologist to supply and authenticate clinical information, radiologists must keep in mind that it is ultimately their legal duty to apprise themselves of all pertinent clinical data relevant to the patient before rendering an interpretation of a screening mammogram. Thus, radiologists should review the patient intake form before interpretation, and if the form is missing, the radiologist should request that the patient complete another one.

Several Other Risk Management Issues Regarding Mammography

Reasonable efforts should be made to recover prior mammograms, especially when a potentially significant mammographic abnormality is detected. If such radiographs are not immediately available, radiologists should note in their reports their inability to compare current findings with previous studies. If the previous mammograms become available, an addendum report may be issued. Attempts made to retrieve previous studies should be documented.

Although supplementary imaging of the breast by magnetic resonance imaging (MRI), ultrasound, and scintimammography is not yet generally acceptable for screening purposes, these modalities are useful as an adjunct to diagnostic mammography. Radiologists should keep abreast of indications and standards regarding the use of these ancillary modalities, because they are evolving quickly.

Will Breast Density Laws Result in More Malpractice Lawsuits?

The MQSA that became effective in 2001 required that density information be included in screening mammography reports, but it did not define how density should be quantified. The 5th edition of the ACR's Breast Imaging Reporting and Data System (BI-RADS) lexicon lists four categories of breast density: (1) breasts are almost entirely fatty; (2) scattered areas of fibroglandular density; (3) breasts are heterogeneously dense, which could obscure small masses; and (4) breasts are extremely dense, lowering the sensitivity of mammography. There is no evidence that breast density actually causes cancer, but its presence may obscure a small cancer on a screening mammogram.

In October 2009, Connecticut became the first state to adopt a law requiring radiologists to report the presence and extent of breast density directly to patients. At present, 22 states have passed breast density notification laws, and 13 states, as well as the US Congress, are considering doing so.

As of the writing of this chapter, there is no record of any malpractice lawsuit having been filed alleging a radiologist's negligence related to the reporting of breast density. However, it is of course possible that malpractice lawsuits could appear that allege that the radiologist (1) miscategorized the degree of density, (2) failed to communicate the degree of density to the referring physician or the patient, or (3) failed to suggest follow-up ultrasound, radionuclide, or MRI for patients with category c breasts.

AMERICAN COLLEGE OF RADIOLOGY PRACTICE PARAMETERS AND TECHNICAL STANDARDS

Because the ACR is clearly recognized as the preeminent professional society of radiologists, its Practice Parameters and Technical Standards unquestionably exert more influence than those of any similar organization on what the medical and legal communities may perceive to be the radiology SOC. Notwithstanding the fact that the ACR precedes each written practice guideline with a disclaimer that states that the guidelines are neither "rules" nor "legal standards of care or conduct" but rather are intended to set a "minimum level of acceptable technical parameters and equipment performance," they have been used as evidence in the courtroom more often against a defendant-radiologist (inculpatory) rather than in support of the defendant-radiologist (exculpatory). In recent years, the ACR Guidelines seem to be playing an increasingly important role in influencing jurors and appeals court justices in their determination of whether a defendant-radiologist in a given situation has or has not met the SOC. The trend toward more widespread use of the ACR Guidelines by the courts is likely to continue.

Some judges permit published parameters to be introduced as evidence, and some even allow jurors to take copies of the printed parameters into the deliberation room at the end of the trial. Jurors know that expert witnesses lie and may not believe much of what a specific expert witness may testify. However, jurors are not likely to question the accuracy or reliability of a written parameter published by the ACR or other respectable medical specialty college.

All US hospitals accredited by The Joint Commission are required to have policies regarding the operations of its radiology department. Among the first documents requested by a plaintiff's attorney after initiation of a medical malpractice lawsuit involving a hospital-based radiologist are the radiology department policies. Hospital-based radiologists should be familiar with their local department's policies and assure themselves that they are adhering to all such policies. If a radiologist is not able to adhere to every facet of the policy, the radiologist should attempt to change the policy so that it can be followed completely.

RISK MANAGEMENT SUGGESTIONS REGARDING AMERICAN COLLEGE OF RADIOLOGY PARAMETERS AND GUIDELINES

- All radiologists should be familiar with the ACR Practice Parameters and Technical Standards and have them available for easy reference.
- When reading national or local radiology guidelines or policies, radiologists should pay strict attention to verbs such as "may," "recommend," "should," and "must." The two former words are more advisory and allow flexibility in implementation. The two latter words tend to preclude flexibility.
- Radiologists should be cautious about deviating from the written practice parameters. Radiologists who find they must depart from such guidelines in a specific case should document contemporaneously their reasons for so doing in the radiology report, the patient's chart, or a log kept in the radiology department.
- Radiologists can adopt policies that differ from those of other radiology facilities in their local community or from practice parameters issued by professional societies. Any such minority position, however, should comply with the "two schools of thought doctrine," which holds that a minority view must be recognized by not just one or several but rather by a respectable number of similarly trained and practicing physicians.

DISCLOSING MISTAKES AND SAYING "I'M SORRY"

Patients who are injured by medical errors do not look kindly on physicians who commit them. Surveys indicate that a substantial percentage of such patients believe medical malpractice litigation is warranted and that disciplinary action should be imposed on the errant physician. Nevertheless, medical errors must be disclosed. However, although many published surveys of physicians find that most physicians agree that all errors should be disclosed, in reality the number who do disclose is quite low. A study of house staff physicians disclosed that 90% admitted making serious clinical errors, but only 25% made disclosures to their patients. Reports reveal that the percentage of physicians who respond in surveys that they actually do disclose errors to patients lies in the low 30% range.

A research study involving radiologist-mammographers who hypothetically failed to report breast cancer on a screening mammogram because the films were labeled incorrectly were asked whether they would disclose their error to patients in whom the cancer diagnosis was delayed. The radiologists specifically were asked to indicate whether (1) they would definitely disclose the error and reasons why it occurred to the patient; (2) probably disclose it; (3) disclose it only if asked by the patient; (4) disclose part but not explain the reasons for the error; or (5) not disclose the error at all. Only 15% answered that they would have told the truth, the whole truth, and nothing but the truth. The remaining 85% would have remained silent or would not have told the whole truth or would have simply lied to the patient.

State Apology Laws

Ethical standards, moral value, and mandates of The Joint Commission and virtually all professional societies call for full disclosure of medical errors to patients who have been subject to them. Many states have passed legislation that grants immunity to physicians' apologies or expressions of regret; however, a radiologist's admission of wrongdoing or fault can be considered as an *extrajudicial admission* that can be used against the radiologist in a court of law. Whether disclosure and/or apologies and expressions of regret will increase or decrease the likelihood of a medical malpractice lawsuit is uncertain. In a recent survey of radiologists who had been sued for malpractice, when asked whether saying "I'm sorry" to a patient who had sustained an injury due to the radiologist's error would have helped avoid or mitigate a malpractice claim, 87% answered "no." Baker has pointed out that in most instances where there is conversation between the hospital's staff and the patient regarding an error that occurred, the radiologist is not involved. The stage is set for the referring physician to apologize, but the radiologist has little opportunity to do so unless he has performed an interventional procedure. It is more likely that the radiologist becomes the odd man/woman out in any prospective apology-colloquy. Having little occasion to confess to the patient either that "I am sorry you were harmed" or "I am sorry I harmed you," the radiologist is more apt not to be forgiven but rather to be made a scapegoat. Thus, apology laws may be a trap for radiologists. Referring physicians, while they are our colleagues, are also not necessarily our allies when an effective apology can reduce their liability, contends Baker. He concludes that as our practices are currently constituted, radiologists cannot really enjoy a close relationship with their patients.

In any event, if a radiologist is advised to speak directly and apologize to a patient who has been subjected to the radiologist's error, it would be prudent for the radiologist to consult with his or her hospital risk manager or professional liability insurance claims representative beforehand for guidance regarding the manner in which such disclosure and expression of sorrow and apology should be made.

Reporting an Abnormal Radiologic Finding Missed on a Previous Exam

One of the most frequently asked questions by radiologists at continuing medical education (CME) meetings is: "What should a radiologist do when, while interpreting a current radiologic study, he or she sees an abnormal finding that is visible in retrospect on the patient's previous study but was not reported?" There is no single *correct* answer to this question, but a brief discussion is in order.

A direct statement in a radiology report that a carcinoma was overlooked on a previous study can be a *red flag* or *smoking gun* to an attorney who may find no other medical grounds in a patient's chart on which to file a malpractice lawsuit. Furthermore, on occasion, various hospital personnel (nurses, secretaries, clerks, medical records librarians) may be informants or finders who pass on information about potentially adverse events.

When radiologists interpret a radiologic exam and they know there was a previous similar exam, then some mention of the comparison between the two studies should be made. The ACR Communication Parameter states that comparisons with previous exams and reports should be made when possible. If the radiologist chooses not to document a comparison and thus ignores a missed diagnosis, it could appear to be a breach of the standard of the care. The Code of Medical Ethics of the American Medical Association (AMA) calls for physicians to deal honestly with patients. Clearly, the preponderance of legal opinion and, from an ethical point of view, almost every commentary on the subject agree that failure to disclose errors and mistakes constitutes unethical, if not illegal, conduct. To deliberately ignore radiologic misdiagnoses could give the appearance of a lack of integrity at the very least. The report of a misdiagnosis should be succinct, matter-of-fact, and nonjudgmental. One possible example is a single statement such as "In retrospect, the abnormality was present on the previous radiograph" may be sufficient.

If an abnormal finding is now seen but was not reported previously, some radiologists state, "In retrospect, a lesion is seen on the previous study." Others may say, "The current study is compared with the previous study … study now shows a lesion …," without mentioning whether the finding was present on the previous study. If, for example, a radiologist finds a 10-mm lung lesion that was present on a prior study where it measured 5 mm, a "preferred statement" might be, "a 10-mm nodule has grown from 5 mm on the prior study." This statement

avoids drawing too much attention to the missed finding but without being evasive. Such words as "missed," "error," or "mistake" or such phrases as "should have been diagnosed" or "was obviously present but not seen" should be avoided.

Academic Centers Disclose Adopt/Apologize/ Compensate Policies

In an effort to be more patient sensitive and transparent with regard to iatrogenic errors, many academic medical facilities have instituted "admit-apologize-indemnify" policies. Medical centers' medical and nursing staffs are asked to report all major or minor errors to a designated department. Each error is immediately investigated, patients are then apprised of the error, explanations are given, apologies are made, and compensation is offered. Virtually all centers that have implemented such disclosure policies have found them very successful. California's Stanford University reported that its admit-apologize-indemnify program has resulted in 50% reduction in the frequency of malpractice lawsuits and 40% reduction in indemnification payouts.

There is considerable speculation and debate about the impact of disclosure on litigation. The actual effect may never be known. By apprising a patient of the details of a mistake that has been made on his or her radiologic test, the radiologist might increase the likelihood of precipitating a malpractice lawsuit. On the other hand, patients may be more likely to institute litigation if they believe that the radiologist has not been honest and forthcoming in admitting mistakes. When discussing a complication or error with a patient's family, radiologists should be honest and truthful. They should not speculate about the cause of the complication or error. They should be cautious about casting blame on others or on themselves. Nevertheless, if the radiologist believes he or she has definitely made a mistake that has resulted in a patient injury, he or she is ethically and professionally bound to divulge this fact to the patient.

Occasionally a radiologist may consult with a colleague for a second opinion regarding a questionable finding. Some researchers believe that naming colleagues who are consultants, and books and articles that were used, as references in the report strengthens the radiologist's defense against a malpractice claim. I strongly disagree with this; names of colleagues and books consulted should not be included in radiology reports.

COMPLICATIONS OF RADIATION EXPOSURE

Exposure to imaging involving ionizing radiation and the hazards related to such exposure have myriad medicolegal ramifications. Americans were exposed to more than 7 times as much ionizing radiation from diagnostic medical procedures in 2006 than they were in the early 1980s. Whereas in 1980 medical imaging was responsible for only 15% of the total radiation exposure to the US population, now the proportion has risen to 50%. This is alarming to much of the public at large, because there has been considerable publicity given to reports linking the development of cancer to exposure to radiation. It has been proven that *overexposure* to ionizing radiation utilized in radiologic diagnostic procedures can lead to soft tissue injury. However, there are insufficient data available from the scientific community to justify an unequivocal determination that cancer can develop from diagnostic-level radiation used in radiologic imaging. Thus far there has never been a successful medical malpractice lawsuit alleging development of cancer or genetic defects resulting from diagnostic x-ray examinations. Nevertheless, it is quite possible that lawsuits alleging such adverse effects arising from diagnostic imaging using today's ionizing radiation levels may be forthcoming.

Radiologists should make every effort to ensure that diagnostic and therapeutic radiologic equipment are calibrated and operating correctly. Radiologists should also attempt to minimize radiation exposure from diagnostic radiologic procedures and examinations by adhering to the ACR's "as low as reasonably achievable" (ALARA) policy of radiation control when performing or supervising such procedures.

EPILOGUE: MALPRACTICE LAWSUITS, TORT REFORM, AND DEFENSIVE MEDICINE

How long will the medical malpractice problem continue in the United States? The only reliable answer is "indefinitely." Tort reform legislation, that is, placing caps on malpractice indemnification, has been passed and has been successful in decreasing the frequency of malpractice lawsuits in some states but has been ruled unconstitutional in many other states. It has never even come close to being adopted by the US Congress. Malpractice litigation will continue. Although the number of suits has decreased somewhat in the past several years, many professional liability insurance companies predict that the Accountable Care Act and the increased use of electronic health record (EHRs) will result in a rise in such litigation.

There is little doubt that the most noteworthy offshoot of malpractice litigation has been defensive medicine: physicians ordering too many (or not enough) imaging and laboratory studies, or performing too many (or not enough) procedures, for the purpose of protecting themselves from malpractice litigation rather than for the benefit of their patients. Clearly, malpractice litigation gave birth to defensive medicine, but defensive medicine is now an independent entity and has a life of its own. Several generations of physicians have grown up, been trained, and have practiced defensive medicine, and they know no other way to practice. Even if tort reform were to occur, and even if malpractice lawsuits were eliminated, physicians' manner of practicing would not change. Lawsuits would be replaced by numerous local medical facility and state medical board review bodies that would investigate most if not all adverse events to determine whether the physician involved met the SOC in the matter. Remedial and/or punitive action would be taken if a physician was found to have acted in a subpar manner. Defensive medicine will remain for the foreseeable future.

Radiologists and all other physicians will continue to be sued for malpractice, sometimes without a valid reason, sometimes for a valid reason. In either event, the now-defendant-radiologist or nonradiologist should heed, and perhaps be somewhat consoled by, the following words of a state appeals court decision:

> We can sympathize with a physician or any other person who, confronted with an unwarranted and unfounded lawsuit, must still expend time, money, and suffer anxiety. … This unfortunately is a price that must necessarily be paid to keep the courts open to the people. It remains a valid truism that such ordinary trouble and expense that arrive from the legal controversy should be endured by the law-abiding citizen as one of the inevitable burdens which men must sustain under civil government…. The importance of free access to the courts demands that this access be maintained even though occasionally some innocent person must suffer.

SUGGESTED READINGS

Abujudeh HH, Boland GW, Kaewlai R, et al. Abdominal and pelvic computed tomography (CT) interpretation: discrepancy rates among experienced radiologists. *Eur Radiol.* 2010;20:1952.

ACR. *Practice Parameter for Communication of Diagnostic Imaging Findings. Revised (Resolution 11).* Reston, VA: American College of Radiology; 2014.

Arland v. Taylor, OR 131, Canada (1955).

Ashman CJ, Yuj S, Wolfman D. Satisfaction of search in osteoradiology. *AJR Am J Roentgenol.* 2000;175:541.

Babu AS, Brooks ML. The malpractice liability of radiology reports: minimizing the risk. *Radiographics.* 2015;35:547-554.

Baker SR, Whang JS, Luk L, Clarkin KS, Castro 3rd A, Patel R. The demography of medical malpractice suits against radiologists. *Radiology.* 2013;266:539-547.

Baker SR. The role of apology in radiology. In: Abujudeh HH, Bruno MA, eds. *Quality and Safety in Radiology.* New York, NY: Oxford University Press; 2012:104-110.

Barnes v. Wall, 411 SE 2d 270 (Ga App 1991).

Berbaum KS, Franken EA, Dorfman DD, et al. Tentative diagnoses facilitate the detection of diverse lesions in chest radiographs. *Invest Radiol.* 1986;21:532-539.

Berbaum KS. Difficulty of judging retrospectively whether a diagnosis has been "missed." *Radiology.* 1995;194:482-483.

Berlin L, Berlin J. Malpractice and radiologists in Cook County, IL: trends in 20 years of litigation. *AJR Am J Roentgenol.* 1995;165:781-788.

Berlin L. Accuracy of diagnostic procedures. Has it improved over the past 5 decades? *AJR Am J Roentgenol.* 2007;188:1172-1178.

Berlin L. Alliterative errors. *AJR Am J Roentgenol.* 2000;175:925.

Berlin L. Hindsight bias. *AJR Am J Roentgenol.* 2000;175:597-601.

Berlin L. Outcome bias. *AJR Am J Roentgenol.* 2004;183:557-560.

Berlin L. Perceptual errors. *AJR Am J Roentgenol.* 1996;167:301.

Berlin L. Proximate cause. *AJR Am J Roentgenol.* 2002;179:569-573.

Berlin L. Reporting the missed radiologic diagnosis: medicolegal and ethical considerations. *Radiology.* 1994;192:183-187.

Berlin L. The mea culpa conundrum. *Radiology.* 2009;253:284-287.

Berlin v. Nathan, 381 NE2d 1367 (Ill App 1978).

Berquist TH. From the editor's notebook: communication: the needs of the patient come first. *AJR Am J Roentgenol.* 2009;192:557-559.

Blendon RJ, DesRoches CM, Brodie M, et al. Views of practicing physicians and the public on medical errors. *N Engl J Med.* 2002;357:1933-1940.

Borgstede JP, Lewis RS, Sunshine JH. RADPEER quality assurance program: a multifacility study of interpretive disagreement rates. *J Am Coll Radiol.* 2004;1:59-65.

Borngesser v. Jersey Shore Medical Center, 774 A2d 615 (NJ 2001).

Brennan TA, Sox CM, Burstin HR. Relation between negligent adverse events and the outcomes of medical malpractice litigation. *N Engl J Med.* 1996;335:1963-1967.

Brenner DJ. Medical imaging in the 21st century: getting the best bang for the rad. *NEJM.* 2010;362:943-945.

Code of Medical Ethics of the American Medical Association Council on Ethical and Judicial Affairs, 2014-2015 Edition. Chicago, IL: American Medical Association; 2015: xv.

Corteau v. Dodd, 773 SW 2d 436 (Ark 1989).

D'Orsi CJ, Mendelson EB, Ikeda DM, et al. *Breast Imaging and Reporting System: ACR BI-RADS.* 5th ed. Reston, VA: American College of Radiology; 2013.

Dick 3rd JF, Gallagher TH, Brenner RJ, et al. Predictors of radiologists' perceived risk of malpractice lawsuits in breast imaging. *AJR Am J Roentgenol.* 2009;192:327-333.

Eliot DL, Hickam DH. Evaluation of physical examination skills: reliability of faculty observers and patient instructors. *J Am Med Assoc.* 1987;258:3405-3408.

Fitzgerald R. Radiological error: analysis, standard setting, targeted instruction and team working. *Eur Radiol.* 2005;15:1760-1767.

Gallagher TH, Cook AJ, Brenner RJ, et al. Disclosing harmful mammography errors to patients. *Radiology.* 2009;253:443-452.

Garland LH. On the scientific evaluation of diagnostic procedures. *Radiology.* 1949; 52:309-328.

Garland LH. Study on the accuracy of diagnostic procedures. *AJR Am J Roentgenol.* 1959;82:25-38.

Haas JS, Kaplan CP. The divide between breast density notification laws and evidence-based guidelines for breast cancer screening-legislating practice. *J Am Med Assoc Int Med.* 2015;175:1439-1430.

Halpin SFS. Medico-legal claims against English radiologists: 1995-2006. *Brit J Radiol.* 2009;82:982-988.

Harvey HB, Tomov E, Babayan A, et al. Radiology malpractice claims in the United States from 2008 to 2012: characteristics and implications. *J Am Coll Radiol.* 2016;13:124-130.

Harvey JA, Fajardo LL, Innis CA. Previous mammograms in patients with impalpable breast carcinoma; retrospective versus blinded interpretation. *AJR Am J Roentgenol.* 1993;161:1167-1172.

Herman PG, Gerson DE, Hessel SJ, et al. Disagreement in chest roentgen interpretation. *Chest.* 1975;68:278-282.

Hyams AL, Brandenburg JA, Lipsitz Shapiro DW, Brennan TA. Practice guidelines and malpractice litigation: a two-way street. *Ann Int Med.* 1995;122:450-455.

Kushner DC, Lucey LL. Diagnostic radiology reporting and communication: the ACR Guideline. *J Am Coll Radiol.* 2005;2:15-21.

Landon v. Humphrey, 9 Conn 209, 1832.

Landro L. Hospitals learn to say "I'm sorry" to patients. *Wall Street J.* 2016:D1-D3.

Lehman CD, Wellman RD, Buist DS, et al. Diagnostic accuracy of digital screening mammography with and without computer-aided detection. *J Am Med Assoc Int Med.* 2015;175:1828-1837.

Levine v. Rosen, 616 A2d 623 (Pa 1992).

Levinson W. Physician-patient communication: a key to malpractice prevention. *J Am Med Assoc.* 1994;272:1619-1620.

Localio AR, Lawthers AG, Brennan TA, et al. Relation between malpractice claims and adverse events due to negligence: results of the Harvard Medical Practice Study III. *N Engl J Med.* 1991;325:245-251.

Lowrey JJ. Vicarious liability. In: Zaremski MJ, Goldstein LS, eds. *Medical and Hospital Negligence.* Deerfield, IL: Callaghan; 1988:1-20 (13).

Loy CT, Irwig L. Accuracy of diagnostic tests read with and without clinical information. *J Am Med Assoc.* 2004;292:1602-1609.

Malpractice Verdicts, Settlements, and Experts, April 2010. Published by Triple L Publications, Selma, AL.

Mazor KM, Simon SR, Yood RA, et al. Health plan members' views about disclosure of medical errors. *Ann Intern Med.* 2004;140:409-418.

McCandless v. McWha, 22 Pa 261, 1853.

Mohr JC. American medical malpractice litigation in historical perspective. *J Am Med Assoc.* 2000;283:1731-1737.

Muhm JR, Miller WE, Fontana RS. Lung cancer detected during a screening program using four-month chest radiographs. *Radiology.* 1983;148:609-615.

Newman B, Callahan MJ. ALARA (as low as reasonably achievable) CT 2011—executive summary. *Pediatr Radiol.* 2011;41(suppl 2):S453-S455.

Peckham C. Malpractice and medicine: who gets sued and why? Medscape Malpractice Report 2015. <http//www.medscape.com/viewarticle/855229_print>.

Physician Insurers Association of America and American College of Radiology. *Practice Standards Claims Survey.* Rockville, MD: Physician Insurers Association of America; 1997.

Pichichero ME, Poole MD. Assessing diagnostic accuracy and tympanocentesis skills in the management of otitis media. *Arch Pediatr Adolesc Med.* 2001;144:1137-1142.

Pinto A, Brunese L. Spectrum of diagnostic error in radiology. *World J. Radiol.* 2010;2:377.

Richie v. West, 23 Ill 329 (1860).

Roosen J, Frans E, Wilmer A, Knockaert DC, Bobbaers H. Comparison of premortem clinical diagnosis in critically ill patients and subsequent autopsy findings. *Mayo Clin Proc.* 2000;75:562-567.

Sandor AA. The history of professional liability suits in the United States. *J Am Med Assoc.* 1957;163:459-466.

Schauer DA, Linton OW. National Council on radiation protection and measurement report shows substantial medical exposure increase. *Radiology.* 2009;252:293-296.

Shojania KG, Burton EC, McDonald KM, Goldman L. Changes in rates of autopsy-detected diagnostic errors over time: a systematic review. *J Am Med Assoc.* 2003;289:2849-2856.

Smith v. Overby, 30 Ga 241 (1860).

Studdert DM, Bismark MM, Mello MM, Singh H, Spittal MJ. Prevalence and characteristics of physicians prone to malpractice claims. *N Engl J Med.* 2016;374:354-362.

Studdert DM, Thomas EJ, Burstin HR, Zbar BI, Orav EJ, Brennan TA. Negligent care and malpractice claiming behavior in Utah and Colorado. *Med Care.* 2000;38:250-260.

Vaughan v. Oliver, 822 So2d 1163 (Ala 2001).

Warren v. Burris, 758 NE 2d 889 (Ill App 2001).

Webster's Third New International Dictionary of the English Language Unabridged. Springfield, MA: Merriam-Webster; 1993:1592.

Williams JW, Simel DL. Does this patient have ascites? *J Am Med Assoc.* 1992;267:2645-2648.

Withers S. The story of the first roentgen evidence. *Radiology.* 1931;17:99-103.

Wu AW, Folkman S, McPhee SJ, Lo B. Do house officers learn from their mistakes? *J Am Med Assoc.* 1991;265:2089-2094.

Chapter 28

Leadership: A Manifesto for the Nonclinical Education of Radiologists Looking to Succeed in Difficult Times

Frank J. Lexa

INTRODUCTION

Historically, to be successful in their professional careers, radiologists must train intensively for years. They must master a daunting amount of clinical material, pass comprehensive tests, and meet a wide array of challenges in their training. That has not changed during my own career (now around a quarter-century in length) and, if anything, the amount of material that radiologists are expected to master keeps increasing as we develop new technologies and new clinical discoveries are made. In this book, you have read about the other critical nonclinical topics that you need to master in addition to all that you have already done on the clinical side. When we consider the list of things that radiologists and other physicians need to know to be successful that are *not* taught in a traditional medical school curriculum or during postgraduate training, it is unfortunately a daunting list of important topics. It is always surprising to some, particularly those who are outside the medical field, that these subjects are often absent in any serious form in internship, residency, or even in a fellowship curriculum. You should not need to wait until you are in your first or second real job to begin leadership training. These topics are so numerous and so important that a book like this is indispensable for all of us who are hoping to have a successful career in diagnostic radiology in the 21st century.

This chapter focuses on leadership and the role that it should play in the careers of radiologists and why and how you should pursue it. What radiologists need to know to lead is discussed, as well as the ways they can obtain this information. The ability to lead is one of the core nonclinical skills that usually distinguishes highly successful physicians from the rest of us. However, leadership skills are not and should not be limited to those in positions of alpha leadership. On the other hand, do not assume (because it is manifestly not the case) that all *leaders* in radiology have these capabilities and skills today. Unfortunately, not everyone who carries the title of leader in medicine is effective or even competent in that role. This chapter focuses on the essential skill sets that most of us, perhaps all of us, should have. Being able to lead will allow you to accomplish more in your career, regardless of whether you ever take on a significant leadership role.

LEADERSHIP: MYTH AND REALITY IN THE NATURE-VERSUS-NURTURE DEBATE

One of the obstacles to effective nonclinical education in radiology, and in medicine more broadly, is the misguided notion that skills like leadership cannot be taught. If you take the nihilistic view that leadership is not something that you can learn, then the idea follows that there is no point in teaching it or any point in expecting people to get leadership training. Instead of teaching physicians the leadership skills they need to excel in institutions, they are instead not taught anything or are merely taught how to function in an institution where others are the leaders and the physicians are the followers. The latter approach often devolves into a reductionist set of nonclinical things that someone thinks physicians should know but that do not help that radiologist understand how they might lead a group themselves. These nonleadership courses do not even give a physician the skills to lead at the level of a small group, let alone at the level of a department or hospital. That is not leadership training nor does it provide the building blocks to take even baby steps toward becoming proficient at leadership.

This misguided notion usually springs from the idea that leaders are made (or not made) long before their professional career begins and that leadership training during your career is therefore a waste of time. This is a deterministic view; apparently, your genes or your family interactions and/or upbringing determine your ability to be a leader. Furthermore, it falsely assumes that there are good tests of leadership potential. Much of the genuine value of a leader is proven by him or her in the moment, and although some people can be weeded out of leadership tracks, it is much harder to predict decades in advance who will be a great leader when the big challenges come. I strongly disagree with the myth of being born to leadership, and in my own work at Wharton and elsewhere I have, in fact, seen many examples of midcareer nonleaders turning (with the right training and mentorship and opportunities) into great leaders. In this chapter, I discuss what you can do to acquire these important nonclinical skills. However, I would like to provide a bit more information before closing this argument so that you have a clearer perspective on this debate. Although that could be

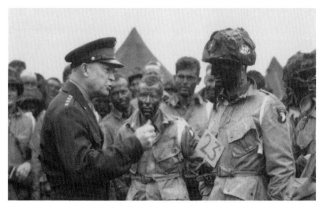

FIG. 28.1 General Dwight D. "Ike" Eisenhower, speaking to the troops who would soon storm the beaches at Normandy, France, on D-day in World War II. The invasion assured an allied victory but claimed 209,000 lives. Few people are ever thrust into a leadership role such as this. (From US National Archives and Records Administration.)

a chapter unto itself, there are two important caveats that I provide that can help answer the naysayers, perhaps give you a broader perspective on how to think about leaders and leadership, and help you get over your own doubts and concerns about seeking leadership training. The first caveat is that acquiring basic or even core leadership skills does not mean that you will then be ready to be an alpha leader on the scale of a chief executive officer of a Fortune 500 company, the US president, or perhaps the Pope or a powerful admiral in the navy (Fig. 28.1). Those rarefied positions require abilities that are much more advanced and far more specialized than what is available in general leadership training. Moreover, they require both highly specialized and often lengthy life experiences in addition to any other formal training and requirements for someone to be successful. So in that case, the people who are skeptical about the effectiveness of leadership education are technically correct when it comes to certain positions like those just noted. Leadership courses cannot prepare you for every type of leadership position.

The second caveat I would like to leave you with is that although leadership skills may help anyone who seeks them to become better leaders, this training cannot help people who really do not want to be leaders. You would not force someone to learn to ride a motorcycle against his will anymore than you would push someone out the door of an airplane for her first parachute jump if she does not want to learn to skydive. In both of those cases, success (and not getting seriously hurt or dead) depends on active learning. In the same way, forcing someone to be a leader is not a good idea, particularly if you push him or her too hard and too fast. If the person is so fearful or resistant to taking on a leadership role that he or she cannot learn it and/or could not do it, then he or she may well fail and provide yet another case study for those who denigrate leadership education. At a more practical level, you should not force this on would-be leaders, and if you insist, you (and they) probably will not be successful. I have met some very unhappy former leaders who feel that they failed in a leadership position because someone pushed them to do it when they were not ready or willing. Although wanting to be a good leader is not a sufficient factor—you need to do a lot more to succeed, as is discussed later in this chapter—it is a necessary factor to successfully lead. Like many of life's journeys, it begins with the desire and the will to take that first step.

LEADERSHIP: A CORE CURRICULUM OF NONCLINICAL SKILL SETS

What does a leadership curriculum look like? If you ask people in different fields, you will get different answers—being the head of an information technology start-up company is a bit different from being the head of a religious organization or being a US Senator—but there is a convergence that leads to a core set of skills that most leaders do need to master in their day-to-day work. When I was asked to be the chief medical officer for the Radiology Leadership Institute of the ACR, one of the things we did was to review the intellectual framework that we use to guide the nonclinical education of radiologists. The final product reflects the core skills that cut across leadership settings, the overlay of issues that are specific to medicine, and there is even more focus on the current and future practice of diagnostic radiology. Although leadership itself is an important topic, there is a manageable list of topics that are germane to leadership development. Some of these overlap topics that are listed elsewhere in this book. That is a good thing; it shows the convergence of how leading thinkers consider the central issues in leadership education. Following is a core curriculum that I proposed in an article on leadership in the *Journal of the American College of Radiology (JACR)* in 2011.

Core Curriculum for 21st Century Medical Leaders in the United States

1. Strategic challenges to the future of US medicine
2. Introduction to financial principles for healthcare professionals
3. Healthcare systems: how they operate in the United States [or other country], including how they get paid in the public and private sectors
4. Centers for Medicare and Medicaid Services (CMS), Relative Value Update Committee (RUC), work relative value units (wRUVs), Current Procedural Terminology (CPT), and other acronyms that you need to know so you can understand how we get paid and how to do coding, billing, and other bureaucratic work in healthcare
5. Negotiations 1: internal issues to your department or group
6. Negotiations 2: advanced issues for negotiations external to your group, including institutions, systems, and where appropriate, political work
7. Marketing, branding, and promoting health services to the many stakeholders we serve
8. Your first job after training: getting it, getting it right, making it work, and keeping it
9. Healthcare reform and change and its impact on US [or your nation's] medicine
10. Personal career management from hiring to retirement: how to manage your career, insights from successful leaders, service and quality issues in healthcare including putting patients at the center of high-quality healthcare while meeting mandates from institutions and organizations

11. Service and quality issues in healthcare: other medical professionals, administration, and other stakeholder groups
12. Professionalism in healthcare: staying true to your values and the oath you took when you decided to become a healthcare professional
13. Leadership: personal and local issues
14. Leadership: interacting with larger organizations and building influence outside your organization(s)
15. Accounting practices for medical professionals: what you need to know
16. Macroeconomics 101: why the dismal science matters to healthcare leaders and (at a minimum) what they need to know
17. What makes a medical group great and how to foster superior group dynamics and success in your group or department
18. Strategic planning for medical leaders: why this alien-sounding topic has become so important for us
19. Envisioning the future of healthcare: learning to anticipate change in the public and private sectors

OBTAINING THE SKILLS YOU NEED TO SUCCEED

If the list in the prior section represents the "what" of the nonclinical education of a radiologist leader should look like, we next need to discuss the "how." This is an important question. Although we have been trained in how to learn clinical issues, how to review for examinations like the maintenance of certification tests, and how to read the scientific literature to keep up with medical advances, most of us do not know where to start when it comes to obtaining nonclinical skills. What are the most effective ways to learn this material? Is a reading list of business books adequate for most people, or should some of this be done in an interactive fashion? Is a classroom or online course interaction going to be enough, or should you seek out a practicum type of experience where you can learn to lead groups and do projects in a practical setting with lots of opportunities to get guidance and feedback? Do you want to do topics à la carte or in a structured program or degree program?

Here are some of the advantages and disadvantages of each option. Books and passive webinars are easy-to-use tools and are also relatively cheap. You can do them at your own speed and pick and choose the topics that matter most to you. The bad news is that approach to the material may not provide the depth and level of complexity that you need as a leader. Much of leadership, at least the good kind, requires both depth and practicality, and that often requires practice and hands-on work. That depth may not be conveyed well in a single lecture, particularly if it is done in a passive fashion. That is one of the reasons that traditional business school education was and often still is done in an interactive, classroom setting that requires active preparation and participation in each session. Often this revolves around preassigned readings, projects, or preparing a case study. The point is it requires active learning. You cannot just memorize a set of bullet points; you have to work the material and make it your own. The leadership challenges that you face will not be exactly the same as the ones in the case

studies that you cover in a class, but those cases and how you work with them will help you get started in your own leadership journey. A higher level of intensity comes with doing adventure-based leadership training. These experiences are set up with facilitators who help with role playing and creating challenges within a learning team. The value and impact of the learning are often enhanced by doing it in a fun, challenging setting, like a strenuous hike or a survival trip. Participants learn to rely on each other, take turns leading, develop strategies, delegate tasks, and evaluate each other's responses to stressful situations. That type of situational learning can be very helpful in creating perspective on what is important and how to perform well despite a challenging environment.

Often a less expensive but high-impact learning setting is to do project-based learning with a team or a cohort of fellow students. These experiences are often facilitated by teachers and coaches who structure the coursework and help students learn leadership skills in controlled surroundings. The project approach more closely approximates the types of leadership projects that radiologists would have in their home institutions. The challenge can be modulated based on how well the team performs. The projects can be simulations or they can be real projects done with a high degree of supervision for corporate, government, or nonprofit clients. Again, the learners can take turns leading, can face stressful situations, and be evaluated by peers and professionals in a relatively safe setting before having to do leadership on their own in the real world.

For most of us the choice will probably be a blend of the above. Organizations such as the Radiology Leadership Institute (http://www.radiologyleaders.org/) are good places to look for opportunities to meet your needs and get started on serious leadership training.

LEAD OR BE LED: YOUR CHOICE

Talking about leadership may feel like one more challenge or burden that is being imposed on you during an already intense career. Like many of the other nonclinical topics in this volume, you may be feeling your "fight or flight" mechanism activating and have a desire to run from this. You may feel that it was enough to take call, master magnetic resonance physics, and pass your board exams. Why do you need to master leadership at this point in your career? I wish that I could tell you that there is an easy answer and that you can have a great career in the next decades without doing this, but I am afraid that I would be sending you down the wrong path. The starkest answer to that question is the header for this section: your choice is to lead or be led. Do you really want to be led by people who do not understand radiology, who are not professionals, and who are not dedicated to working for the best possible future for our profession? If so, then by all means hide in the dark and hope for the best. I hope that it works out for you, but if you want to have a career on *your* terms, to be part of a great profession, and to feel fulfilled and happy on the day you decide to retire, I predict that successful leadership will play a profound role in your accomplishments. I hope that this chapter helps you in taking the first steps in that direction.

SUGGESTED READINGS

Fisher R, Sharp A. *Getting It Done: How to Lead When You Are Not in Charge*. New York: HarperBusiness; 1998.

Lexa FJ. Deciding to lead. *J Am Coll Radiol*. 2008;5(1):60-62.

Lexa FJ. Qualities of great leadership. *J Am Coll Radiol*. 2008;5(4):598-599.

Lexa FJ. Educating leaders: a foundation curriculum for radiologists. *J Am Coll Radiol*. 2011;8(7):517.

Lexa FJ. Leading from below. *J Am Coll Radiol*. 2011;8(1):65-66.

Lexa FJ. Strive and…not to yield: a radiologist's response to hard times. *J Am Coll Radiol*. 2013;10(9):643-644.

Chapter 29

Imaging Appropriateness Guidelines and Clinical Decision Support

John P. Nazarian, Jeffrey J. Farrell, Franz J. Wippold II, and Christos Kosmas

Over the past few decades, diagnostic imaging has become a vital part of healthcare delivery in the United States and other developed nations. In many cases, medical imaging adds demonstrable value to patient care by improving diagnostic accuracy, providing prognostic information, guiding management decisions, and reducing the need for more invasive procedures. The rapid expansion of medical imaging has, however, been accompanied by heightened concerns about increasing healthcare costs and risks from radiation exposure. These concerns have led to various efforts by medical specialty organizations, government entities, and private insurers to slow the growth of medical imaging. Particular scrutiny has been drawn to the phenomenon of *overutilization*, which has been defined by Hendee and colleagues as "applications of imaging procedures where circumstances indicate that they are unlikely to improve patient outcome."

Familiarity with initiatives and tools developed to address overutilization of medical imaging is critically important for radiologists as our healthcare system transitions to value-based payment models. In this chapter, we specifically address the development and use of appropriate use criteria (AUC) for medical imaging applications, as well as the current and future role of the information technology tools known as clinical decision support (CDS).

AMERICAN COLLEGE OF RADIOLOGY APPROPRIATENESS CRITERIA

By the early 1990s, the growth of healthcare costs had begun to draw serious attention from policymakers. Spending on physician services was a significant driver of this growth, and it was evident that expenditures for radiology services were increasing at a faster rate than expenditures for most other physician specialties.

In April 1993, then-chairman of the American College of Radiology (ACR) Board of Chancellors K.K. Wallace Jr, MD, testified before the House of Representatives Ways and Means Health Subcommittee regarding the Clinton administration's proposed 1994 Medicare budget. Dr. Wallace stated that the ACR was prepared to define a system of patient care guidelines for radiology to address and eliminate inappropriate utilization of imaging services. He indicated that such guidelines could produce savings for the healthcare system without degrading the quality of care. His proposal formed the basis of what became the ACR Appropriateness Criteria (ACR-AC), evidence-based guidelines developed "to assist referring physicians and other providers in making the most appropriate imaging or treatment decision for a specific clinical condition."

Prior to the development of the ACR-AC, the federal Agency for Healthcare Research and Quality (AHRQ, then known as the Agency for Health Care Policy and Research) published attributes for developing acceptable clinical practice guidelines designed by the Institute of Medicine. Major characteristics for acceptable guidelines include *validity* (guidelines should lead to better outcomes), *reproducibility* (another set of experts should be able to produce the same guidelines when using the same methodology and scientific evidence), and *clinical applicability*, among others. The ACR Task Force on Appropriateness Criteria incorporated these attributes into the development of the ACR-AC, and the ACR-AC topics are included in the material posted online by the National Guidelines Clearinghouse (NGC), a publicly available database of evidence-based clinical guidelines compiled by the AHRQ.

The Ambulatory Quality Alliance, a voluntary collaborative of several organizations including the AHRQ, has developed a set of principles to provide guidance for organizations developing appropriateness criteria. The ACR has embraced their definition of appropriateness: "The concept of appropriateness, as applied to healthcare, balances risk and benefit of a treatment, test, or procedure in the context of available resources for an individual patient with specific characteristics. Appropriateness criteria provide guidance to supplement the clinician's judgment as to whether a patient is a reasonable candidate for the given treatment, test or procedure."

Although scientific evidence is intended to be the basis for guidelines like the ACR-AC, the AHRQ acknowledges that judgment and group consensus are a necessary part of the development process. Because of this, development of the ACR-AC takes place under the guidance of expert panels, which for diagnostic imaging are organized along body systems. A large number of physicians volunteer their time for this effort, including nonradiologists representing over 20 medical specialty organizations. Funding and staff support to the panels are provided entirely by the ACR.

Panels are typically composed of more than 10 members, each of whom has expertise in the clinical condition for which the criteria are being developed. The chairs of these panels serve on the Committee on Diagnostic Imaging/Interventional Radiology Appropriateness Criteria, which oversees the activities of all the subspecialty panels.

A separate body, the Committee on Radiation Oncology Appropriateness Criteria, performs the same function for radiation oncology topics.

In addition to the expert panels, other committees also assist in the development and maintenance of the ACR-AC. The Subcommittee on Radiation Exposure assigns relative radiation levels for the procedures included in the AC topics and provides information about radiation dose assessment. The Subcommittee on Appropriateness Criteria Methodology monitors and reviews the methods used in developing and revising the AC topics; it is composed of members from the various expert panels, as well as others with special expertise in relevant fields such as research methodology.

The development of AC topics by the panels is a rigorous process based on a systematic review of available scientific evidence. Topic selection may be based on disease prevalence and morbidity, variability of current practice, cost considerations, and potential for improved care. Topics are intended to be clinically salient and commonly encountered in daily practice. Examples include such entities as "acute chest pain," "headache," and "blunt abdominal trauma." Once a topic is chosen, the clinical conditions to be addressed are defined as specifically as possible, sometimes resulting in a number of variants within each topic. Variants usually reflect a clinical scenario encountered within the topic. For example, the "headache" topic includes such variants as "chronic headache" and "sudden onset of severe headache." With guidance from the panels, ACR staff then perform a search of the peer-reviewed medical literature and compile articles relevant to the condition being studied. The principal topic author then drafts a *narrative*, complete with citations, which summarizes the available evidence in the literature. ACR staff further assist by creating an *evidence table*, which rates the study quality for each article cited in the narrative. Both the narrative and evidence table are reviewed by members of the expert panel, and the author uses their feedback to modify these documents.

After the narrative and evidence table for a topic have been modified and final versions sent to the expert panel, panel members rate the appropriateness of each diagnostic procedure or treatment for each variant. Each member assigns a rating to each procedure based on his or her interpretation of the evidence and personal assessment of the risks and benefits of performing the procedure. Note that when scientific evidence for a specific topic or variant is uncertain or lacking, expert opinion may serve as the primary basis for determinations of appropriateness by panel members.

The process of assigning appropriateness ratings is based on the RAND/UCLA Appropriateness Method (developed by the RAND Corporation and the University of California, Los Angeles) and uses a structured communication technique known as a modified Delphi method. This method allows rater anonymity during the process and is believed to improve the chances of achieving consensus. Appropriateness ratings are assigned on an ordinal scale using integers from 1 to 9, grouped into three categories. Ratings of 1 to 3 are categorized as "usually not appropriate," categories 4 to 6 are designated as "may be appropriate," and categories 7 to 9 are termed "usually appropriate." The "may be appropriate" category results when the evidence is contradictory or unclear, risks and benefits are equivocal or uncertain, there is significant inter-rater disagreement, or special circumstances may influence the risks or benefits of the procedure in question.

An example of the published appropriateness ratings for the clinical condition Suspected Spine Trauma is provided in Table 29.1. In the first variant, a clinical situation in which a patient meets the low-risk criteria for cervical spine imaging by the commonly used National Emergency X-Radiography Utilization Study (NEXUS) criteria or Canadian C-Spine Rule, all of the listed procedures are assigned the lowest possible rating of 1, indicating that ordering imaging studies is usually not appropriate. In the second variant, in which a patient meets clinical criteria for imaging, cervical spine computed tomography (CT) without contrast is assigned the highest possible rating of 9. These ratings make clear that CT, and not radiographs, is the preferred imaging modality in high-risk cases of cervical spine trauma. Note that the Relative Radiation Level for each procedure is provided in the last column.

As of March 2016, the ACR-AC include numerous topics in diagnostic radiology, interventional radiology, and radiation oncology, covering a total of 211 clinical conditions with more than 1000 variants. Diagnostic imaging topics are sorted into 10 subspecialty areas: Breast, Cardiac, Gastrointestinal, Musculoskeletal, Neurologic, Pediatric, Thoracic, Urologic, Vascular, and Women's. Because new scientific evidence about the efficacy and value of imaging modalities for different conditions is continually being introduced, the ACR-AC are frequently reviewed and updated by the expert panels. Topic revisions ideally occur approximately every 3 years.

No matter how expansive or comprehensive they become, of course, the ACR-AC cannot assist in patient care unless referring physicians and other clinicians are aware of their existence and use them to make clinical decisions. Low awareness of the ACR-AC is a problem with roots in the medical education and training process: one study showed that an overwhelming majority (96%) of third- and fourth-year medical students were unaware of the AC as an available resource. Knowledge about the AC also lags among residents in nonradiology specialties, with multiple studies demonstrating poor resident performance when asked to answer multiple-choice questions based on AC topics.

Scarce medical literature has addressed the extent of incorporation of the ACR-AC into clinical practice. A 2009 study revealed exceptionally low utilization of the AC among both residents and attending physicians responding to an online survey, with only 2.4% of 126 respondents reporting using the AC when ordering studies (it should be noted, however, that the study excluded emergency physicians). When respondents were asked which resource served as their first choice when choosing the most appropriate imaging study for patients, the ACR-AC ranked last behind several other options, including Google searches and a panoply of other online resources.

Concerns about poor awareness and knowledge of the ACR-AC have led to several educational efforts targeted at medical students and residents based on the premise that improved awareness of the AC among trainees will lead to improved utilization. Educational interventions taking place as early as during the preclinical curriculum of

TABLE 29.1 ACR Appropriateness Criteria for Suspected Spine Trauma, Acute Cervical Trauma Variants

Radiologic Procedure	Rating	Comments	RRL
VARIANT 1: CERVICAL SPINE IMAGING NOT INDICATED BY NEXUS OR CCR CRITERIA: PATIENT MEETS LOW-RISK CRITERIA			
X-ray cervical spine	1	—	☢☢
CT cervical spine without contrast	1	With sagittal and coronal reformat	☢☢☢
CT cervical spine with contrast	1	—	☢☢☢
CT cervical spine without and with contrast	1	—	☢☢☢
Myelography and postmyelography CT cervical spine	1	—	☢☢☢☢
CTA head and neck with contrast	1	—	☢☢☢
MRI cervical spine without contrast	1	—	O
MRI cervical spine without and with contrast	1	—	O
MRA neck without and with contrast	1	—	O
MRA neck without contrast	1	—	O
Arteriography cervicocerebral	1	—	☢☢☢
VARIANT 2: SUSPECTED ACUTE CERVICAL SPINE TRAUMA: IMAGING INDICATED BY CLINICAL CRITERIA (NEXUS OR CCR); NOT OTHERWISE SPECIFIED			
CT cervical spine without contrast	9	With sagittal and coronal reformat	☢☢☢
X-ray cervical spine	6	Lateral view only; useful if CT reconstructions are not optimal	☢☢
CT cervical spine with contrast	1	—	☢☢☢
CT cervical spine without and with contrast	1	—	☢☢☢
Myelography and postmyelography CT cervical spine	1	—	☢☢☢☢
CTA head and neck with contrast	1	—	☢☢☢
MRI cervical spine without contrast	1	—	O
MRI cervical spine without and with contrast	1	—	O
MRA neck without and with contrast	1	—	O
MRA neck without contrast	1	—	O
Arteriography cervicocerebral	1	—	☢☢☢

ACR, American College of Radiology; *CCR*, Canadian C-Spine Rule; *CT*, computed tomography; *CTA*, computed tomography angiography; *MRA*, magnetic resonance angiography; *MRI*, magnetic resonance imaging; *NEXUS*, National Emergency X-Radiography Utilization Study; *RRL*, relative radiation level.
Rating scale: *1, 2, 3,* Usually not appropriate; *4, 5, 6,* may be appropriate; *7, 8, 9,* usually appropriate.
See the source below for a full definition of the relative radiation level designations in the last column.
From Daffner RH, Hackney DB. ACR appropriateness criteria on suspected spine trauma. *J Am Coll Radiol.* 2007;4(11):762–775.

medical school have shown promise. In a 2013 study, second-year medical students participated in a 3-day radiology elective focused on the ACR-AC, comparative effectiveness in imaging, and the risks of radiation from medical imaging. At the conclusion of this radiology elective, the students demonstrated improvement in their knowledge of appropriate utilization of medical imaging and perceived awareness of the indications, contraindications, and effects of radiation exposure from medical imaging when compared to peers who had participated in a different elective. Participants in the radiology course also reported feeling more confident in their ability to order appropriate imaging studies when investigating common emergency complaints. Without long-term data, however, it remains uncertain if this kind of curricular change can have a meaningful effect on the ordering behavior of budding physicians once they are practicing independently.

Most of the studies addressing the use of the ACR-AC in resident education have examined educational programs within radiology residencies. Some of these studies have

been able to show improved awareness and/or knowledge regarding the AC among radiology residents after exposure to material on imaging appropriateness. Unfortunately, little data exist demonstrating a link between this increased awareness and outcomes for patients and the healthcare system. The only study assessing the broader impact of resident education in this area showed that after participating in lectures about cost-consciousness and hospital charges for abdominal imaging, internal medicine residents ordered fewer abdominal CT and radiographic examinations per patient. This resulted in a cost reduction of $129 per patient. If these results can be replicated on a larger scale and prove to be durable over time, the ACR-AC may be able to fulfill their promise of reducing imaging overutilization and delivering cost savings to the healthcare system.

The ACR-AC also have some limitations. First of all, the appropriateness of imaging in a given scenario basically addresses the initial imaging encounter with the patient and does not discuss further testing as the evaluation progresses, as might be experienced with a diagnostic algorithm or decision-tree approach. Second, although many topics and variants are discussed, the ACR-AC cannot be considered exhaustive in the larger context of all of the possible clinical dilemmas encountered in a busy clinical practice. Third, because the topics are periodically revised and never retired, the committee has limited capacity for introducing new topics. Finally, given the lengthy process of revising topics, rapidly moving developments in a given field may not be reflected in the ACR-AC in a timely fashion.

The ACR is not the only prominent medical specialty organization working to promote evidence-based utilization of imaging services. The American College of Cardiology Appropriate Use Criteria Task Force, in conjunction with several other specialty societies, has published several reports providing AUC for cardiovascular imaging. Topics addressed include cardiac radionuclide imaging, echocardiography, and peripheral vascular ultrasound. Additionally, in 2015 this American College of Cardiology Task Force and the ACR jointly published a major guidelines document in the *Journal of the American College of Cardiology* addressing 20 common clinical scenarios in which patients present to an emergency department with chest pain.

Finally, the efforts of medical organizations in other countries to promote imaging appropriateness bear mentioning. The Cochrane Library, maintained by a global network of collaborators based in the United Kingdom, is a collection of databases that are widely used as high-quality sources of scientific evidence to inform healthcare decision making. The Royal College of Radiology, the British counterpart to the ACR, produces evidence-based radiology referral guidelines similar to the ACR-AC. These guidelines, known as iRefer, are freely available online and as a smartphone application for practitioners in the UK's National Health Service. The Canadian Association of Radiologists also publishes referral guidelines for diagnostic imaging, last updated in 2012.

CLINICAL DECISION SUPPORT

AUC such as the ACR-AC were developed to assist clinicians in making rational, evidence-based choices when ordering diagnostic imaging studies. As noted above, however, bringing about their utilization by clinicians has been challenging. One hurdle has been the lack of accessibility of the ACR-AC at the point of care. A busy physician may not have the time to consult appropriateness criteria before ordering an imaging study or may simply not remember to do so.

Health information technology has provided a possible solution. Interest in systems to aid clinicians in making appropriate clinical decisions has existed since at least the 1950s, but the rapid development of computer and information technology over the past few decades has provided new opportunities to integrate clinical decision algorithms into electronic medical record (EMR) and computerized physician order entry (CPOE) systems. Systems that incorporate these algorithms into the process of order entry are known as CPOE with CDS software, or simply clinical decision support.

CDS systems have drawn attention as a promising mechanism to reduce inappropriate use of medical imaging. When evidence-based guidelines such as the ACR-AC are incorporated into decision algorithms, physicians and other providers have the opportunity to access and use these resources at the point of care. By making appropriateness guidelines a readily available part of routine clinical workflow, computerized CDS has the potential to promote compliance with these guidelines and thereby reduce the volume of unnecessary imaging studies. In addition, CDS systems may provide a time-saving alternative to burdensome preauthorization requirements imposed by third-party payers.

Recently published results describing attempts to implement CDS products have been encouraging. Multiple studies have shown reductions in low-utility imaging after a computerized CDS system was employed. Additionally, one study found that CDS was associated with a 56% relative increase in documented adherence to evidence-based guidelines for imaging in mild traumatic brain injury. This suggests that the decrease in low-utility imaging examinations observed after CDS implementation reflects a shift toward more guideline-concordant ordering patterns.

A major challenge associated with bringing CDS systems into daily clinical work is gaining acceptance from users, namely the referring physicians and other healthcare providers ordering imaging studies. In 2014, one group of authors at the University of Colorado described their difficulties after implementing a third-party CDS in their institution's CPOE system. After receiving negative feedback from clinicians about the unsuitability of the user interface, the authors worked with their IT colleagues to find a solution that would prove more practical to ordering clinicians. They were unsuccessful, however, and eventually discontinued their trial of the CDS product after 12 months of use.

Other centers have shown more success in achieving clinician acceptance of CDS. A 2006 study demonstrated a steady rise in the use of a computerized radiology order entry system for outpatient studies implemented at Massachusetts General Hospital; this increase in usage continued after decision support was added to the system. Decision support was provided for over 70,000 advanced imaging requests, including CT, magnetic resonance imaging, and nuclear cardiology studies. As use of the CDS system rose, the aggregate rate of low-utility imaging examinations ordered declined continuously from 6% during the 1st month of CDS use to 2% by the end of the 12th month. Another group of authors at the University of Virginia described similarly positive results in gaining clinician acceptance of their CDS product, receiving fewer than 10 complaints over a 6-month period during which over 55,000 studies were ordered using the system. These authors credited this to their efforts to educate clinician leaders and encourage physician participation, as well as the user-friendliness of their CDS system.

Efforts to promote and support effective CDS usage are becoming increasingly important for radiologists and physicians in clinical specialties. As part of a national emphasis on value-based care, third-party payers such as the federal Centers for Medicare and Medicaid Services (CMS) are insisting on the use of CDS systems to ensure appropriate, quality-oriented ordering of medical imaging services. The Protecting Access to Medicare Act of 2014 mandates that beginning in 2017, physicians must consult evidence-based AUC through a CDS system before ordering advanced imaging examinations (including CT,

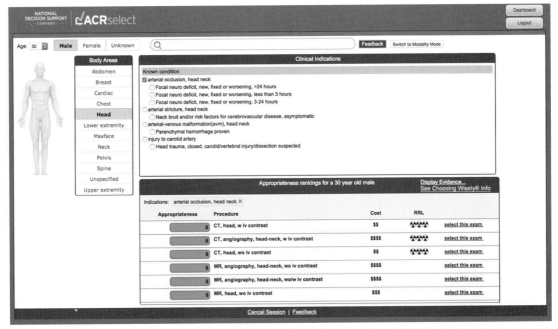

FIG. 29.1 American College of Radiology select user interface demonstrating clinical indications for imaging in the setting of suspected cerebrovascular abnormality. For each indication, a list of possible imaging studies is provided with corresponding appropriateness ratings. Information about relative cost and radiation dose for each exam is also presented to the user. (Courtesy National Decision Support Company.)

magnetic resonance imaging, and nuclear medicine studies). Without confirmation that a CDS system was used, CMS will withhold reimbursement for these studies. The law originally established the start date for this mandate as January 1, 2017; at the time of this writing, that deadline has been postponed.

Multiple CDS software platforms are now commercially available in the United States, all of which incorporate information from the ACR-AC to assist providers when ordering imaging examinations. One of these products, ACR Select, is marketed by the National Decision Support Company, a company that maintains an exclusive relationship with the ACR. ACR Select can be integrated into most major EMR systems, allowing decision support for imaging studies at the point of order. The product uses a series of structured clinical indications to determine the appropriateness score of each imaging study ordered (Fig. 29.1) and can operate in three different modes; the strictest mode prevents clinicians from ordering a study if the appropriateness score from the relevant AC is too low. Additionally, for orders that may be of lower utility, a radiologist can review the decision support session and provide guidance to the clinician on the correct procedure (if any) to be ordered. Other CDS products are offered by Health-Fortis and Medicalis.

SUGGESTED READINGS

American College of Radiology. ACR Appropriateness Criteria. <http://www.acr.org/quality-safety/appropriateness-criteria>.

Bautista AB, Burgos A, Nickel BJ, et al. Do clinicians use the American College of Radiology Appropriateness criteria in the management of their patients? *AJR Am J Roentgenol.* 2009;192(6):1581–1585.

Cascade PN. Setting appropriateness guidelines for radiology. *Radiology.* 1994;192(1):50A–54A.

Covington MF, Agan DL, Liu Y, Johnson JO, Shaw DJ. Teaching cost-conscious medicine: impact of a simple educational intervention on appropriate abdominal imaging at a community-based teaching hospital. *J Grad Med Educ.* 2013;5(2):284–288.

Dillon JE, Slanetz PJ. Teaching evidence-based imaging in the radiology clerkship using the ACR appropriateness criteria. *Acad Radiol.* 2010;17(7):912–916.

Dym RJ, Burns J, Taragin BH. Appropriateness of imaging studies ordered by emergency medicine residents: results of an online survey. *AJR Am J Roentgenol.* 2013;201(4):W619–W625.

Goldzweig CL, Orshansky G, Paige NM, Ewing BA. Electronic health record-based interventions for improving appropriate diagnostic imaging: a systematic review and meta-analysis. *Ann Intern Med.* 2015;162(8):557–565.

Hendee WR, Becker GJ, Borgstede JP, et al. Addressing overutilization in medical imaging. *Radiology.* 2010;257(1):240–245.

Huber T, Gaskin CM, Krishnaraj A. Early experience with implementation of a commercial decision-support product for imaging order entry. *Curr Probl Diagn Radiol.* 2016;45(2):133–136.

Ip IK, Raja AS, Gupta A, Andruchow J, Sodickson A, Khorasani R. Impact of clinical decision support on head computed tomography use in patients with mild traumatic brain injury in the ED. *Am J Emerg Med.* 2015;33(3):320–325.

Leschied JR, Knoepp US, Hoff CN, et al. Emergency radiology elective improves second-year medical students' perceived confidence and knowledge of appropriate imaging utilization. *Acad Radiol.* 2013;20(9):1168–1176.

Rosenthal DI, Weilburg JB, Schultz T, et al. Radiology order entry with decision support: initial clinical experience. *J Am Coll Radiol.* 2006;3(10):799–806.

Rybicki FJ, Udelson JE, Peacock WF, et al. 2015 ACR/ACC/AHA/AATS/ACEP/ASNC/NASCI/SAEM/SCCT/SCMR/SCPC/SNMMI/STR/STS. Appropriate utilization of cardiovascular imaging in emergency department patients with chest pain: a joint document of the American College of Radiology Appropriateness Criteria Committee and the American College of Cardiology Appropriate Use Criteria Task Force. *J Am Coll Cardiol.* 2016;67(7):853–879.

Sheng AY, Castro A, Lewiss RE. Awareness, utilization, and education of the ACR appropriateness criteria: a review and future directions. *J Am Coll Radiol.* 2016;13(2):131–136.

Sistrom CL, Dang PA, Weilburg JB, Dreyer KJ, Rosenthal DI, Thrall JH. Effect of computerized order entry with integrated decision support on the growth of outpatient procedure volumes: seven-year time series analysis. *Radiology.* 2009;251(1):147–155.

Williams A, Sachs PB, Cain M, Pell J, Borgstede J. Adopting a commercial clinical decision support for imaging product: our experience. *J Am Coll Radiol.* 2014;11(2):202–204.

Chapter 30

Internet, Social Media, and Applications

Joseph Fotos

INTRODUCTION

The Digital Revolution began in the latter half of the 20th century with the first uses of digital computers and data storage. The 1970s saw the development of the first microprocessor, Intel's 4004, which marked the advent of the rapidly doubling processor speeds predicted by Moore's Law. These exponential increases in computing power have since drastically changed how businesses and individuals interact by leading to an almost instant sharing of information.

The healthcare industry has been no exception, and the specialty of Diagnostic Radiology has been particularly well suited to take advantage of the many improvements brought about in the continuing Information Age. This is most readily seen in the improvement of industry technologies involving image display and transfer through the use of the Digital Imaging and Communication in Medicine (DICOM) standard and has facilitated digital image processing, instant image manipulation, and the widespread use of picture archiving and communication systems.

Given their penchant for eagerly adopting these new technologies, it is no surprise that radiologists, both in practice and in training, find a wide variety of uses for consumer technologies as well. They are skilled in advanced uses of the Internet, developing social media technologies, and mobile and desktop applications. This chapter specifically discusses uses of these technologies throughout the specialty in the following ways:

Communication and connection: Interpersonal communication technologies and the dissemination of news and information

Community: Technology use involving groups, such as subspecialty societies and meetings

Collaboration: Working with others to complete educational and research projects

Continuing education: Online opportunities for earning continuing medical education (CME) credit

Consultation: Using online encyclopedic resources for self-directed learning and real-time diagnostic assistance

COMMUNICATION, CONNECTIONS, AND COMMUNITY

Electronic Messaging

Perhaps the most ubiquitous communication technology in use today is email. It is used as the primary mode of nonurgent communication for many individuals in the developed world. However, with increasing security concerns regarding the transmission of protected health information, physician use of email for the purposes of discussing specific patients has been discouraged. Various solutions have been implemented, including bolstering security of existing email systems. An important recent solution to this problem has been the implementation of messaging systems housed within the electronic medical record (EMR) itself. Not only has this provided additional robust security for confidential interphysician case discussions but it also has the benefit of adding those messages directly to the patient's chart so that they may be viewed by all healthcare personnel involved in that patient's care. This is of particular importance to the radiologist, who is often faced with the task of combing through the EMR in search of an adequate context for an order with inadequate history. These cataloged conversations often provide insight into the thought processes of the patient's primary physicians, physician extenders, and nursing staff.

There has also been recent development of Health Insurance Portability and Accountability Act (HIPAA) secure text and electronic message systems and applications for use in the hospital setting (Fig. 30.1). These services directly connect ordering clinicians with the entire clinical team, including radiologists, allowing for real-time messaging within a secure environment. These messages can obviate the need for pagers in many cases, which can often result in delayed communication and interaction between members of the healthcare team. Companies include Vocera, TigerText, and Everbridge, which provide mobile applications for popular smartphone operating systems. These applications maintain the security of the messaging information often by routing it through their HIPAA-compliant secure communications servers. Often, these services also offer integration with EMR systems of a hospital or health system as well.

Social Media

Twitter: Website, Mobile and Desktop Apps

Launched in 2006, Twitter is a unique social networking service that consists of short messages of 140 characters or less. These comments submitted by users are termed "tweets." Tweets are readily accessible to the user's "followers," who are other registered users that subscribe to receive them on their user page, termed a "feed." Tweets submitted by users can also be viewed on the submitting user's home page as well. One of the

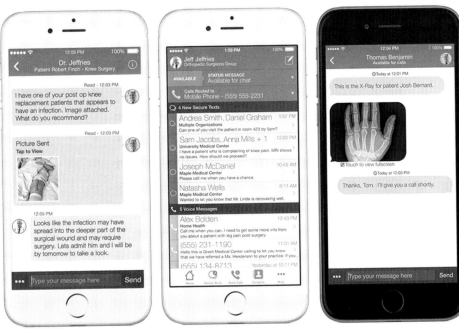

FIG. 30.1 Example of a Health Insurance Portability and Accountability Act–compliant secure text messaging application. This particular product is made by Vocera. (From http://www.vocera.com/products/secure-texting-collaboration.)

AuntMinnie.com
@AuntMinnie

Thank a radiologist? Cancer mortality continues to drop in U.S. bit.ly/1REw3NG #radiology

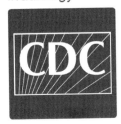

FIG. 30.2 Example of Twitter as a news service. (From https://twitter.com/AuntMinnie/status/708397446070669312.)

defining aspects of this service, though, is the "hashtag," denoted by the pound (#) symbol. Words immediately following the # symbol complete the hashtag (i.e., "#radiology") and become part of a pool of messages that contain that same tag. This is commonly employed by users to add their comments or questions to a given topic that is popular at the time, a phenomenon known as a "trending" topic. Tweets can also be replied to by "tagging" the author within a tweet to bring a message to his or her attention by prefacing his or her username with the "@" symbol (i.e., "@RSNA").

All of the aforementioned mechanics can be combined in multiple ways for many different purposes by many different types of radiology groups and users. For example, it is most commonly used as a simple news delivery service, as seen with the AuntMinnie.com twitter account, which notifies radiologists of important news relevant to their practice (Fig. 30.2).

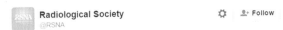

Radiological Society
@RSNA

Residents & Fellows: Don't miss our interactive Career 101 session at 10:30 am, E4351B! bit.ly/1fE8FDZ #RSNA15 #RadRes

FIG. 30.3 Example of Twitter as an active meeting organizer and information service. (From https://twitter.com/RSNA/status/671706388490543104.)

The radiology community might leverage its power most effectively, though, during societal and subspecialty meetings. For example, during the annual meeting of the Radiologic Society of North America (RSNA) in 2015, the meeting organizers, attendees, and industry professionals used the hashtag "#RSNA15" to keep all tweets relevant to the meeting under one easy-to-find trending topic (Fig. 30.3).

Facebook: Website, Mobile Apps

Facebook (launched in 2004) is an incredibly popular social networking service widely used by individuals and businesses for communication. In contrast to Twitter, this service is focused more on interactive discussion, with each user or business establishing a page on which posts are made. Users are then able to add their own comments and questions to any post to which they have access, encouraging an ongoing dialogue. Users are also able to "like" a post, signifying their interest in or support of a post without adding any text. Recent updates have brought the hashtag to Facebook as well, though it is not nearly as ubiquitous as it is on Twitter.

Its use is similar to Twitter in that a large portion of its radiology user base uses the service for news and announcements (Fig. 30.4). Many companies from the radiology industry have also created Facebook pages

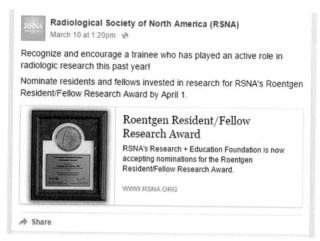

FIG. 30.4 Example of an RSNA Facebook post, announcing an awards opportunity for residents and fellows. (From https://www.facebook.com/RSNAfans/posts/10153884477664892.)

to provide announcements about new products and events. Users can join a group or "like" an organization's page to subscribe to posted updates. They can also expand their own social network by mutually agreeing to be "friends" with other users. The user will then see a series of posts on their home page as a "feed," consisting of updates from "friends" and pages that they have "liked."

LinkedIn: Website, Mobile Apps

Founded in 2002, LinkedIn is a social networking service specifically designed for business professionals and has a structure similar to Facebook. Each user or company has a page on which they post, and comments are then added to that post. This service provides additional details about those with whom you are connected as a user and indicates the number of connections between you and people you might want to contact. The service can also provide information on people who have similar skills and previous work locations to suggest new potential contacts to grow your network (Fig. 30.5). Users can subscribe to news and information in ways similar to Facebook as well. LinkedIn is also useful because it connects businesses that have job openings with those people who may be qualified for them.

Doximity: Website, Mobile Apps

The youngest of the social networks discussed here, Doximity is a service that was launched in 2011 specifically for physicians. It is similar to other networks mentioned previously in that it allows one to connect with colleagues to form a network of contacts. Job postings and news-related posts from reputable sources (including radiology journals and respected public news outlets) are also a feature of the service, similar to LinkedIn. CME credit can be earned through Doximity as well, with customizable subscriptions to articles on selectable topics. The most interesting unique feature, though, is that Doximity also provides users with a HIPAA-secure personal fax number that can be used to send and receive fax messages. These messages can be viewed in the Doximity

mobile app for tablet and phone devices, where they can be signed digitally and sent securely (Fig. 30.6).

ResearchGate: Website, Mobile and Desktop Apps

The largest academic social network (Fig. 30.7), according to a study by *Nature* in 2014, this service emphasizes the sharing of knowledge through published papers and unpublished work (both completed and in progress). Users who join this service upload their research information and are given a "ResearchGate score" that is "calculated based on the publications in [their] profile and how other researchers interact with [their] content." Each paper is also given an "h-index," which measures the "impact of [the user's] work … by looking at the number of highly impactful publications a researcher has published." This is largely based on the number of citations of the paper and the number of highly cited publications in which citations appear.

The service also devotes a large portion of its website to a place where researchers can pose questions to the community. Upon clicking the Questions tab, the user is presented with a list of questions that the algorithm has determined the user may be able to answer based on the information in the user's profile and the content of the user's published work. Questions are also organized by recent questions in the user's field, questions that the user wanted to "follow" for updates, and questions that the user has asked. Finally, all questions within the system are searchable so that any user to can locate information on any topic within the system.

The service also offers a place for job postings, which can be personalized based on the information in the user's profile. Administrators can also post a job to the site. Users can apply for jobs directly within the site, and jobs can be shared so that colleagues can easily recommend job openings to their connections.

CONTINUING EDUCATION

There are many opportunities to obtain CME credits online throughout the medical specialties, including radiology. Perhaps the most accessible of these options is the CME offered by online journals as part of published articles. The RSNA offers hundreds of opportunities to earn CME credit by taking a short posttest after reading through an article (most of which come from its *RadioGraphics* journal). Passing the posttest awards the participant with 1.00 Category 1 CME in most cases. Although residents do not require CME as part of their education, the articles and accompanying posttests provide a useful exercise.

Although not specific to radiology, there are many online CME services that offer courses that can be purchased and taken through any web browser. Examples include NetCE.com and myCME.com. These courses also contain a posttest to be completed to obtain the CME credits, which can be as many as 15 or more credits in some cases.

As bandwidth technology and speeds continue to improve, streaming video services have become much more accessible over the past decade. Following this trend, many societal and education meetings now offer online video streams of lectures that can be used to earn CME credits. The RSNA runs a simultaneous virtual meeting that allows

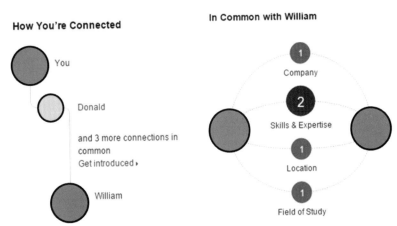

FIG. 30.5 Example of LinkedIn's map of similarities and connections between two individals. (From https://www.linkedin.com/.)

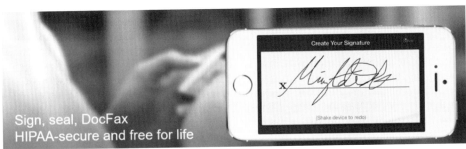

FIG. 30.6 Example of access to a secure fax message that can be signed on a mobile device and sent securely. (From https://www.doximity.com/physicians/docfax.)

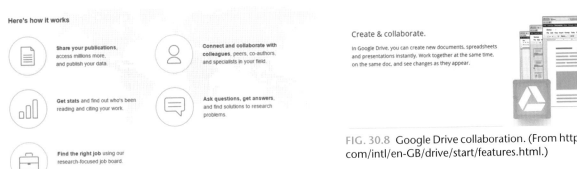

FIG. 30.7 ResearchGate description of service. (From https://www.researchgate.net/about.)

FIG. 30.8 Google Drive collaboration. (From https://www.google.com/intl/en-GB/drive/start/features.html.)

participants to stream lectures live, watch recorded sessions, and even view digital versions of many of the posters presented at the meeting.

COLLABORATION

With the growing popularity of cloud computing, there has been widespread adoption of collaborative services that allow users the ability to simultaneously access resources and work on the same document. These services often offer features such as versioning and trackable changes that create a trail of changes that can be reverted to avoid data loss. They also often provide a comment or chat system to allow a persistent discussion free of the complications of a conference call or the convoluted and often cluttered conversations that develop over email.

Cloud storage and document services, such as Box, Dropbox, Google Drive (Fig. 30.8), and OneDrive/Office 365, also function as collaboration services. For example, when one user shares a document via Google Docs (the document portion of Google Drive), all users who receive the invitation link can be given full permission to view and edit the document. Users can see the document updates as they are editing in the cloud, see which users are currently viewing the document, and even where the text cursor of another user is currently located (indicating the section on which they are focusing). Comments regarding any portion of the document reside along the left side of the screen, allowing users to conduct an ongoing discussion about a specific point or section within the document. Edits are continually tracked, showing the portions that were deleted, portions that were added, and which user performed which action. All of these features combine to form an invaluable service to collaborators positioned across the globe (or even in the same room).

Evernote is used by many as an information-organizing service. Users organize documents and their own notes and pictures into "notebooks" and refine their collection by assigning completely customizable "tags" to any piece of uploaded information for easy sorting at a later time. Evernote also provides a Team Collaboration service by allowing users to share and edit a notebook with others. Although its ability to track and the user's ability to collaborate on a single document are limited (admittedly not the service's goal), its strength is in its convenience in collecting ideas within a team atmosphere and turning them into actionable "to do's" that can be assigned to team members. This service also has a robust optical character recognition feature that makes scanned documents, and even scanned or tablet-based handwritten notes, easily searchable across the system. Evernote also has the advantage of providing integration with other applications and services such as LinkedIn.

Increasing bandwidth and Internet speeds have also led to many new video conferencing technologies. Popular products include GoToMeeting, Adobe Connect, Google Hangouts, Join.Me, and TeamViewer, to name but a few. These services generally share a set of core features. They allow users to participate by phone or through a computer microphone as any ordinary conference call would but add video feeds (often of high quality) from connected webcams for each user. They also offer "screen sharing," which gives users the opportunity to show a video feed of their computer desktop to the other meeting members. This can be used to give a presentation to others through a series of slides but also to illustrate an idea in real time using any available drawing or diagramming program. A chat feature is provided by these services, allowing users to message each other without disturbing the meeting—the modern equivalent of passing notes in class.

All services discussed here are accessible via the company website or through mobile or desktop applications.

CONSULTATION

The number of high-quality online encyclopedic, case-based, and question-based radiology information sources is growing. In many cases the information is complete enough to provide a study source for residents and attending physicians preparing for exams but often succinct enough to provide an efficient real-time source for consultation in the reading room. These sources are well referenced, providing links to the referenced articles if the user wishes to go to the source.

StatDx: Website

StatDx (www.statdx.com), a service provided by Elsevier, is presented in an easily referenced bullet-point format. The information is written by physicians who are often experts in their respective subspecialty fields. The "Key Facts" regarding a diagnosis are presented to the user at the top of the page, which distills the detailed information from the remainder of the page into the most important high-yield features for quick reference. This includes the classic imaging features of an entity, the top differential diagnoses, characteristics on pathology, and the clinical issues relevant to the patient presentation. It closes

with a "Diagnostic Checklist" of items that are felt to be most important to the diagnosis. All of these subheadings are discussed in greater detail within the remainder of the page.

High-quality illustrations are provided, as well as images from all relevant modalities that show the key characteristics of the diagnosis that is discussed in the text. Links to multiple illustrative patient cases are also provided. All images can be downloaded easily into a Microsoft Power-Point slide format for easy incorporation into a poster or presentation.

For an additional charge, the user can also earn Point of Care CME credits for using the service.

RADPrimer: Website

Also created by Elsevier, RADPrimer (www.radprimer.com) offers one of the few available collections of constantly maintained high-quality radiology multiple-choice questions. These questions are organized around the goal of creating a "comprehensive radiology curriculum" by providing a bullet-point formatted page of important points about a broader topic, complete with a pre- and posttest. Questions can also be accessed independently and organized in a self-test in a customizable format including the number of questions, subject area, difficulty, and timed versus tutor formats.

Radiopaedia.org: Website, Mobile Apps

Radiopaedia.org (www.radiopaedia.org) is an "open-edit" service, similar in design to Wikipedia, but specifically designed as a resource for both practicing radiologists and radiology residents. Recognizing the importance of the accuracy of its information (a concern of many regarding the Wiki model), the service employs many volunteer expert section editors who provide oversight of the entire site. They continually review content additions and edits to ensure that information housed within the site is accurate and appropriate for use by medical professionals who may make important patient care decisions based on the information.

The website is organized into two main sections. The first is the "Encyclopedia," which houses all of the articles created for and edited by its contributors. These articles are written by individuals wishing to contribute to this free and open-source project and must be referenced appropriately to be accepted. Images can also be uploaded to an article to provide examples and diagrams. The articles can be found through the search function or through designated categories by type of information (i.e., Anatomy, Physics, Staging, etc.) or by organ system.

Second, the website features a vast collection of "Patient Cases" that can be accessed individually, found linked to a relevant article, or explored through a "Quiz Mode" where cases are presented to a user as unknowns. These cases can be found via the search function or by organ system.

More recently, live and online streamed courses on a wide variety of topics have been provided by this service as well.

Radiology Assistant: Website

Radiology Assistant (www.radiologyassistant.nl) is the "Educational site of the Radiological Society of the Netherlands," initially developed by Dr. Robin Smithuis. This service is divided into organ systems with a comparatively small but very high-yield collection of articles on specific topics that are particularly useful for residents in training as a study source and by practicing radiologists as a quick real-time reference. Examples include the Fleischner Guidelines for pulmonary nodules, updated lung cancer tumor, node, and metastasis staging, and the key imaging features of child abuse (nonaccidental trauma).

IMAIOS: Website, Mobile Apps

The French company IMAIOS (www.imaios.com/en/) provides multiple useful online radiology resources, including e-Anatomy and QEVLAR.

e-Anatomy is an interactive service that provides accurately labeled anatomy on diagrams and real human radiology images. Imaging includes not only radiographs but also high-resolution cross-sectional 3D images in computed tomography, magnetic resonance imaging (often in multiple sequences), and positron emission tomography and computed tomography. Cross-sectional images can be scrolled through because the labels follow their structures. Labels can be searched for, regions or subtypes of structural labels can be displayed, or all labels within a certain proximity of the user's mouse can be displayed.

QEVLAR is a web and mobile application designed specifically for residents to assist with the American Board of Radiology Core Examination preparation. It consists of multiple-choice questions and clinical cases designed by experts in the field to align with those topics tested on the exam.

Yottalook: Website

Yottalook (yottalook.com) is one of the most unique resources discussed here (alongside American Roentgen Ray Society [ARRS] Goldminer described below). This service does not house information, but rather serves as a search engine with specialized algorithms to provide users with information from trusted resources. It consists of four separate search engines: Web, Images, Journals, and Books.

Yottalook Web is designed to search through online radiology resources only, rather than the entire Internet. Yottalook Images had access to approximately 800,000 images at the time of this writing, which are available by searching through peer-reviewed online resources. Yottalook Journals searches through PubMed and online radiology journals. Yottalook Books search results return links to radiology or imaging books.

American Roentgen Ray Society Goldminer: Website

ARRS Goldminer (goldminer.arrs.org) is a robust image search engine specific to radiology resources. Specialized algorithms are used to parse terms in free-text searches, which are matched to standardized language within article figure legends and captions, including the Medical Subject Heading terms. Unlike Yottalook, though, Goldminer only searches peer-reviewed journal articles (including 789 journals at the time of this writing). As such, it does not return image results from radiology encyclopedic websites such as Radiopaedia.

A significant strength of this service lies in its support from the ARRS, which provides CME credit for its use.

Other Mobile Applications

In addition to the services described earlier, which are primarily delivered in a website format with additional mobile application options, there are a large number of resources that have been created as standalone mobile applications. There are myriad such apps, which are widely disparate in their quality. They range from simple calculators (i.e., estimated glomerular filtration rate calculations) to robust anatomic references. Examples of some of these applications are *Diagnostic Radiology: Dynamic Approach to Abdominal Imaging* (an entire imaging textbook), and DexNote, a simple text-based radiology reference tool (both for iOS). Many of these applications suffer from usability issues, though, as noted in a recent review published in the *Journal of the American College of Radiology (JACR)* in March of 2016 (see the Suggested Readings section).

Note that care must be taken with any of these applications to ensure that the information is trustworthy, because they are only subject to a basic application review process (which differs between operating system vendors). Applications in this setting are not subject to a rigorous peer-review process in contrast to the aforementioned web-based services. As with any newly discovered resource, approaching these apps with a healthy measure of caution is always advised.

CONCLUSION

Radiologists and radiology residents have been particularly keen to adopt new online technologies, social media services, and applications. This includes services widely used by the general public but also specialized services created by companies that recognize not only a need but also the desire for new innovative technologies by the radiology community.

SUGGESTED READINGS

Auffermann WF, Chetlen AL, Colucci AT, et al. Online social networking for radiology. *Acad Radiol.* 2015;22:3–13.

Cross T. After Moore's Law. *The Economist.* Available at <http://www.economist.com/technology-quarterly/2016-03-12/after-moores-law>.

Hawkings CM, Duszak R, Rawson JV. Social media in radiology: early trends in twitter microblogging at radiology's largest international meeting. *J Am Coll Radiol.* 2014;11:387–390.

Kahn CE, Thao C. GoldMiner: a radiology image search engine. *AJR Am J Roentgenol.* 2007;188:1475–1478.

Kim MS, Aro MR, Lage KJ, Ingalls KL, Sindhwani V, Markey MK. Exploring the usability of mobile apps supporting radiologists' training in diagnostic decision making. *J Am Coll Radiol.* 2016;13:335–343.

Kind T, Patel PD, Lie D, Chretien KC. Twelve tips for using social media as a medical educator. *Med Teach.* 2014;36(4):284–290.

Lugo-Fagundo C, Johnson MB, Thomas RB, Johnson PT, Fishman EK. New frontiers in education: Facebook as a vehicle for medical information delivery. *J Am Coll Radiol.* 2016;13:316–319.

Prasanna PM, Seagull FJ, Nagy P. Online social networking: a primer for radiology. *J Digit Imaging.* 2011;24(5):908–912.

Radmanesh A. What is a TweetUp?—The ASNR 2015 TweetUp. Available at <http://www.ajnrblog.org/2015/04/21/tweetup-asnr-2015-tweetup/> April 21, 2015.

Ranschaert ER, van Ooijen PMA, McGinty GB, Parizel PM. Radiologists usage of social media: results of the RANSOM survey. *J Digit Imaging.* 2016:1–7.

Van Noorden R. Online collaboration: scientists and the social network. *Nature.* 2014;512:126–129.

Ventola CL. Social media and health care professionals: benefits, risks, and best practices. *Pharm Ther.* 2014;39(7):491–520.

Index

Note: Pages followed by "*b*", "*t*", and "*f*" refer to boxes, tables, and figures respectively.